GERIATRIC PHARMACOLOGY

NOTICE

GERIATRIC PHARMACOLOGY

EDITORS

Rubin Bressler, M.D.

Professor and Head
Department of Internal Medicine
Professor of Pharmacology
University of Arizona Health Sciences Center
Tucson, Arizona

Michael D. Katz, Pharm.D.

Clinical Associate Professor
Department of Pharmacy Practice
College of Pharmacy
University of Arizona
Tucson, Arizona

McGRAW-HILL, INC.
Health Professions Division

New York St. Louis San Francisco Auckland Bogotá Caracas
Lisbon London Madrid Mexico Milan Montreal New Delhi
Paris San Juan Singapore Sydney Tokyo Toronto

To our families and mentors

GERIATRIC PHARMACOLOGY

1234567890 DOCDOC 98765432

ISBN 0-07-007660-X

This book was set in Times Roman by Northeastern Graphic Services, Inc.
The editors were J. Dereck Jeffers and Muza Navrozov;
the production supervisor was Richard Ruzycka;
the cover was designed by Marsha Cohen/Parallelogram; the index was prepared by Tony Greenberg.
R. R. Donnelley & Sons Company was printer and binder.

Library of Congress Cataloging-in-Publication Data

Geriatric pharmacology / edited by Rubin Bressler, Michael D. Katz.
p. cm.
Includes bibliographical references and index.
ISBN 0-07-007660-X:
1. Geriatric pharmacology—Handbooks, manuals, etc. I. Bressler, Rubin, date- . II. Katz, Michael D.
[DNLM: 1. Drug Therapy—in old age. 2. Geriatrics.
3. Pharmacology. WT 100 G366376]
RC953.7.G468 1993
61525'8'0846—dc20
DNLM/DLC
for Library of Congress 92-19631
CIP

Contents

Contributors*

Neil M. Ampel, M.D. [24]
Associate Professor of Medicine
Infectious Disease Section
Department of Internal Medicine
University of Arizona Health Sciences Center
Tucson, Arizona

Edward P. Armstrong, Pharm.D. [13]
Associate Professor
Department of Pharmacy Practice
College of Pharmacy
University of Arizona
Tucson, Arizona

Alan D. Barreuther, Pharm.D. [21]
Clinical Associate Professor
Department of Pharmacy Practice
College of Pharmacy
University of Arizona
Tucson, Arizona

John W. Bloom, M.D. [21]
Associate Professor of Medicine
Respiratory Sciences Center
Department of Internal Medicine
University of Arizona Health Sciences Center
Tucson, Arizona

Robert W. Boyce, R.P.H. [4]
Chief, Pharmacy Services
Indian Health Center
Salem, Oregon

John T. Boyer, M.D. [11]
Professor of Medicine
Chief, Section of Geriatrics
Director, Arizona Center
on Aging—Geriatrics
Department of Internal Medicine
University of Arizona Health Sciences Center
Tucson, Arizona

Rubin Bressler, M.D. [3, 15]
Professor and Head
Department of Internal Medicine
Professor of Pharmacology
University of Arizona Health Sciences Center
Tucson, Arizona

Suzanne Campbell, Pharm.D. [17, 18]
Clinical Assistant Professor
Department of Pharmacy Practice
College of Pharmacy
University of Arizona
Tucson, Arizona

William S. Dalton, M.D., Ph.D. [22]
Associate Professor of Medicine
Director, Bone Marrow Transplant Program
Arizona Cancer Center
University of Arizona
Tucson, Arizona

Robert T. Dorr, Ph.D., R.P.H. [22]
Associate Professor of Pharmacology
Director, Pharmacology Program
Arizona Cancer Center
University of Arizona
Tucson, Arizona

JoLaine R. Draugalis, Ph.D. [1]
Assistant Professor
Department of Pharmacy Practice
College of Pharmacy
University of Arizona
Tucson, Arizona

Timothy C. Fagan, M.D., F.A.C.P. [5]
Associate Professor of Medicine
and Pharmacology
Section of General Medicine
Director, Hypertension Clinic
Department of Internal Medicine
University of Arizona Health Sciences Center
Tucson, Arizona

---

*The numbers in brackets following the contributor name refer to chapter(s) authored or co-authored by the contributor.

Martha P. Fankhauser, M.S. [8]
Clinical Associate Professor
Department of Pharmacy Practice
College of Pharmacy
University of Arizona
Tucson, Arizona

Brian M. Fennerty, M.D. [23]
Assistant Professor of Medicine
Director, GI Endoscopy Laboratory
Department of Internal Medicine
University of Arizona Health Sciences Center
Tucson, Arizona

Paul E. Fenster, M.D. [6]
Associate Professor of Medicine
Section of Cardiology
Department of Internal Medicine
University of Arizona Health Sciences Center
Tucson, Arizona

Walter B. Forman, M.D. [9]
Associate Professor of Medicine—Oncology
Director of Clinical Programs
Cancer Center
University of New Mexico
Albuquerque, New Mexico

George E. Francisco, Pharm.D. [12]
Associate Dean
College of Pharmacy
University of Georgia
Athens, Georgia

Eric P. Gall, M.D. [20]
Professor of Medicine
Chief, Section of Rheumatology/Immunology
Department of Internal Medicine
Director, Arizona Arthritis Center
University of Arizona Health Sciences Center
Tucson, Arizona

Alan J. Gelenberg, M.D. [16]
Professor and Head
Department of Psychiatry
University of Arizona Health Sciences Center
Tucson, Arizona

Richard N. Herrier, Pharm.D. [4]
Chief, Area Pharmacy Branch
Indian Health Service
Phoenix, Arizona

Martin Higbee, Pharm.D. [20, 23]
Associate Professor of Pharmacology
Department of Pharmacy Practice
College of Pharmacy
University of Arizona
Tucson, Arizona

Angela Y. Hirai, Pharm.D. [24]
Clinical Pharmacy Specialist
Department of Pharmacy
Cedars-Sinai Medical Center
Los Angeles, California

Mark Holdsworth, Pharm.D. [9]
Assistant Professor
Department of Pharmacy Practice
College of Pharmacy
University of New Mexico
Albuquerque, New Mexico

David G. Johnson, M.D. [18]
Professor of Medicine and Pharmacology
Chief, Section of Endocrinology
Department of Internal Medicine
University of Arizona Health Sciences Center
Tucson, Arizona

William N. Jones, M.S. [5]
Adjunct Assistant Professor
Clinical Pharmacy Supervisor
Veterans Affairs Medical Center
Department of Pharmacy Practice
College of Pharmacy
University of Arizona
Tucson, Arizona

Amy J. Jones-Grizzle, Pharm.D. [1]
Pharmacoeconomics Fellow
Department of Pharmacy Practice
College of Pharmacy
University of Arizona
Tucson, Arizona

Michael D. Katz, Pharm.D. [10, 11, 16]
Clinical Associate Professor
Department of Pharmacy Practice
College of Pharmacy
University of Arizona
Tucson, Arizona

Robert J. Lipsy, Pharm.D. [14]
Adjunct Assistant Professor
Department of Pharmacy Practice
College of Pharmacy
University of Arizona
Tucson, Arizona

Michael J. Maricic, M.D. [19]
Clinical Assistant Professor of Medicine
Section of Rheumatology
Department of Internal Medicine
University of Arizona Health Sciences Center
Tucson, Arizona

Erwin B. Montgomery, M.D. [14]
Associate Professor
Department of Neurology
University of Arizona Health Sciences Center
Tucson, Arizona

Arshag D. Mooradian, M.D. [7, 17]
Professor of Medicine
Director, Department of Endocrinology
St. Louis University Medical Center
St. Louis, Missouri

Paul E. Nolan, Jr., Pharm.D. [6, 7]
Clinical Associate Professor
Department of Pharmacy Practice
College of Pharmacy
University of Arizona
Tucson, Arizona

Carol J. Rollins, M.S., R.D., Pharm.D. [2]
Adjunct Assistant Professor
Coordinator, Nutrition Support Service
Department of Pharmacy Practice
College of Pharmacy
University of Arizona
Tucson, Arizona

Thomas H. Stanisic, M.D. [12]
Professor of Surgery
Section of Urology
Department of Surgery
University of Arizona Health Sciences Center
Tucson, Arizona

Cynthia Thomson, M.S., R.D. [2]
Clinical Nutrition Research Specialist
Department of Family and Community Medicine
University of Arizona Health Sciences Center
Tucson, Arizona

Kathleen Yochum, R.N., M.P.H., G.N.P. [11]
Director, Continence Clinic
Arizona Center on Aging
University of Arizona Health Sciences Center
Tucson, Arizona

Preface

The elderly constitute an increasing segment of the population of the United States. Because they experience a higher rate of chronic diseases than does the population at large, older individuals utilize a greater proportion of health care services. Although the elderly represent only 12 percent of the total population, they account for 31 percent of all hospital discharges and 42 percent of all acute care hospital days. Physician visits for those over 65 years of age average eight per year, compared to five per year for those under 65. Physician visits, hospitalizations, and the need for nursing home care and home care are expected to increase rapidly into the twenty-first century.

Because of the frequency of chronic illness in the elderly, drug therapy is usually prescribed. The elderly consume 30 percent of all prescription drugs and 40 percent of all nonprescription drugs dispensed and use twice as many prescription drugs as does the general population. In the care of the elderly, 40 percent of physician office visits result in at least two prescriptions being written.

In addition to the frequency of drug use, this patient population presents a variety of unique pharmacotherapeutic problems to the clinician. The pharmacokinetics and the pharmacodynamics of drugs often differ in the elderly. The risk of adverse drug reactions and "therapeutic misadventures" is much more common in the elderly due to the multiplicity of drugs used, potential drug interactions, and pathophysiologic changes.

As our society ages and the availability of efficacious, potent, toxic medications increases, it has become necessary for clinicians to become familiar with the general principles as well as the intricacies of drug therapy in the elderly. Proper use of drugs in the elderly population reduces the chance of an adverse outcome and is likely to maximize therapeutic outcomes and quality of life.

Geriatric Pharmacology provides timely and accurate information concerning the principles of drug use in the elderly and the use of specific drugs and drug classes in this patient population. It is useful to practicing physicians, pharmacists, nurses, and others involved in the care of elderly patients as well as students in the health professions.

This book is unique in several ways. Rather than primarily reviewing internal medicine in the elderly, we have chosen to emphasize the effects of aging on each drug and drug class and the impact of aging on the appropriate choice and monitoring of drug therapy. Our book contains material often not found in other similar texts, including discussions on patient compliance, impotence, osteoporosis, oncology, and nutrition. Also unique is the dual authorship of most chapters in the book, utilizing physician specialists and clinical pharmacists to provide their perspectives. As we have seen in our practices, the joint efforts of physicians and pharmacists have been complementary, resulting in a better therapeutic outcome and better writing.

We would like to express our gratitude to the many individuals who have assisted in this effort. The time and efforts of the chapter authors must be acknowledged. We are indebted to the staff of McGraw-Hill, especially our editor Muza Navrozov, whose patience, understanding, persistence, and good humor are truly appreciated. Finally, we would like to express our thanks to Marie-Anne Robillard and Liz Rosas for their tireless word-processing and secretarial skills.

CHAPTER

1

DEMOGRAPHICS

Amy J. Jones-Grizzle
JoLaine R. Draugalis

The aging process introduces new phases of life accompanied by changes in bodies, minds, and needs. Differences in the elderly's appearance may be obvious, as hair grays, wrinkles appear, or stature shortens. However, many more changes are occurring in the older population, such as a decrease in physical functioning. The elderly lose muscle mass and dexterity as they age as well as hearing and visual capabilities. Another critical difference in the elderly is the decrease in organ capabilities. Because of diminished liver and kidney function, the elderly metabolize medications differently than younger people. Body composition of fat and water is also altered in older persons. These are just a few of the changes that mandate special medical considerations when drug treatment is required. These medical differences become even more important when we are aware of the growth of the elderly population and the extent to which they utilize the health care system.

DEMOGRAPHICS AND PREDICTED GROWTH

Society has come to define the elderly as those aged 65 years or older. However, with the 85-plus age group being one of the fastest growing populations in America, it is oftentimes difficult to think of 65-year-olds as being included in the elderly definition.[1] The elderly population as a whole is increasing at a far more rapid rate than all other age groups. At the beginning of this century, fewer than 1 in 10 Americans reached age 55, with only 1 in 25 surviving to age 65. By 1987, 1 in 5 Americans was 55 or older, and 1 in 8 was at least 65.[1] There are many reasons for this boost in the ranks of the elderly population. Today's large numbers of elderly are attributed to the increased number of births prior to 1920 and after World War II.[2] The current aging of the pre-1920s group, along with a sharp decrease in births after the mid-1960s, has caused a 5-year rise in median age from 27.9 in 1970 to 32.8 in only 17 years—the largest increase in history.[1] Because of decreased numbers of births during the Depression era, the rise in the elderly population will slow over the next 20 years. For several decades thereafter (2010 to 2030), however, the "baby boom" generation (resulting from increased birth rate post-World War II) will dominate the population with one in five Americans over the age of 65.[2] Shortly after this period of rapid growth, we will see a dramatic decline in the elderly as those born during the mid-1960s and 1970s age. However, as the children of the baby boom generation enter the ranks of the elderly (beginning about 2045), another era of rapid growth will emerge. These trends in aging project an increase in median age from 32.8 in 1987 to age 36 by the year 2000, to 42 by the year 2030, and to 46 years of age by the year 2050. The proportion of elderly is also expected to rise from 13 percent in the year 2000, to 21.8 percent by 2030, with a slow increase to 24.5 by the year 2080.[1]

Another factor contributing to the increased numbers of older persons is decreased mortality. With the development of antibiotics and vaccines, dramatic declines in deaths from infectious diseases have resulted. This, along with improvements in sanitation and tremendous advancements in medical technology, has boosted the average life expectancy from 47.3 years in 1900 to 74.7 years in 1987.[1]

Decreases in the average family size today also help explain the increased proportions of the elderly. Today, the average family has less than two children, whereas in 1900, the average family consisted of four children.[1]

HEALTH CARE UTILIZATION

Because the elderly experience a higher rate of chronic conditions than the population at large, older individuals are more likely to utilize health care services than are younger people.[3] This is reflected in the fact that although the elderly represent only 12 percent of the total population, they account for 31 percent of all hospital discharges and 42 percent of all acute care hospital days.[1] The elderly consume 30 percent of all prescription drugs dispensed, are responsible for nearly one-third of the overall $425 billion health care expenditure, and utilize over 50 percent of the $124 billion federal health budget.[3] Physician visits for the 65-plus age group average eight per year compared to five visits per year for those under 65. The projected numbers of elderly will create increased demand for physician care. Physician contacts are estimated to increase 22 percent per year. By the year 2030, a 129 percent increase is predicted with over 570 million physician visits.[1] When comparing hospitalizations of the elderly with the general population, older individuals are admitted more than three times as often, are hospitalized 50 percent longer, and use twice as many prescription drugs as the general population.[1]

Although only about 5 percent of the elderly population reside in nursing homes, approximately 20 percent spend some time in nursing homes during their lifetime.[3] An estimated 1.3 million older persons were cared for in nursing homes during the year 1985. The nursing home population is expected to increase from 1.3 to 2 million by the year 2000 and is then predicted to more than double to 4.6 million by 2040.[1] The rate of use for nursing home facilities has nearly doubled (from 2.5 to 5 percent) since the introduction of Medicare and Medicaid in 1966.[1]

Most people prefer being cared for in their own homes, which is becoming more prevalent as home health care is rapidly expanding. Over 4.5 million visits were funded in 1985 by Medicare alone. Medicare is the largest third-party payer of home health benefits, which currently accounts for greater than $9 billion of the nation's health care expenditures. The projected growth rate is 15 to 20 percent per year.[3]

Informal care provided by friends, spouses, and other relatives is a major source of assistance to the elderly. According to a survey conducted by the Health Care Financing Administration, approximately 2.2 million caregivers provided unpaid assistance to 1.6 million noninstitutionalized elderly persons in 1982.[1]

ECONOMIC FACTORS

As a group, older Americans have lower economic status than their younger counterparts. Loss of income during retirement may contribute to this decreased status, forcing elderly to rely on Social Security benefits, pensions, and assets they have accumulated over their lifetimes. Older persons may become vulnerable to situations out of their control, such as the death of a spouse, disability, or illness. With the high cost of long-term care (often exceeding $23,000 per year), it does not take long to deplete the life savings of older individuals.[3]

In 1987, the median cash income of families with heads aged 65 or older was $20,808 versus a median income of $34,275 for families with heads under age 65. Similar results were demonstrated for individuals not living in families; those 65 and over maintained a median income of $8149, while a median income of $17,117 was observed for individuals under 65.[1]

One of the factors playing a key role in the economic security of the elderly is the high out-of-pocket cost of health care, which consumes a large portion of the elderly's budget. The elderly spend a greater amount, as well as a greater percentage of total expenditures, on health care than the nonelderly.[1] Those aged 65 to 74 spent an average of $1537 (9 percent of their total budget) and persons 75 and over paid an average of $1761 (15 percent of their total budget) in out-of-pocket health care costs in 1986. This compares to an average of $914 (4 percent of their total budget) paid by younger persons.[1]

The major health expense of older Americans is health insurance; they pay more than three times as much as those under 65.[2] In 1987, the elderly paid an average of $728 to receive Medicare coverage.[1] Older persons also spend twice as much on prescription drugs and medical supplies ($326 versus $154) and more for medical services ($669 versus $459) than younger persons.[2]

Medicare paid for 44 percent of the elderly's health care expenses in 1987. Funds were concentrated in acute care; Medicare covered two-thirds of all hospital care (totaling $45 billion) and 60 percent of physician services (totaling $20 billion).[1] Medicaid, a federal-state program, finances approximately 12 percent of the elderly's health care costs, with the majority of money (nearly two-thirds) going toward nursing home care. While Medicare finances less than 2 percent of nursing home care, Medicaid pays for more than 35 percent of long-term care expenditures, which exceeded $11.6 billion in 1987.[1] Despite the sizable contributions of public funds, the elderly remain burdened with paying 29 percent of their total health care costs: "The costs of health care for the elderly not met by Medicare, Medicaid, and out-of-pocket expenditures are funded by private insurance, foundations, and other government sources such as the Veterans Administration, Department of Defense, Indian Health Service, states, and counties."[1]

The inflated cost of health care comes not only from people living longer and requiring more care but also from the rising cost of health care itself. With the elderly population growing at such an accelerated pace, it becomes increasingly important to closely scrutinize spending. Wise choices must be made for optimal utilization of funds. When evaluating services, pharmaceuticals, programs, or procedures, it is crucial to consider all relevant costs and benefits. One way to assess value is by using pharmacoeconomic research. Pharmacoeconomics attempts to balance costs and consequences to determine the most cost-effective alternative. Unlike simple cost analyses, pharmacoeconomic inquiry does not merely isolate costs to arrive at the least expensive choice. In the hospital setting, for example, although drug A may be less costly to purchase than drug B, drug A may require more pharmacy preparation time, more nursing administration time, and more monitoring time or may produce more adverse effects requiring additional treatment or prolonged hospitalization. Examining pharmaceuticals or other health care services in this manner will aid health care professionals and policymakers in the allocation of limited health care resources.

HEALTH STATUS

The chronic conditions responsible for the elderly's disproportionate use of the health care system are the same conditions causing much of the disability seen in older persons. More than four out of five persons 65 and older have at least one chronic condition, with many having multiple conditions. Arthritis, heart disease, hearing impairment, and hypertension are the four most common conditions, which occur in the elderly about five times more often than in the younger population. The above conditions account for almost 60 percent of all chronic diseases experienced by the elderly population.[2] Prevalence of many diseases differs among race and sex; this may be reflected in the fact that 6 out of every 10 elderly are women.[1] These differences will be noted in chapters addressing each specific disease state.

Most hospitalizations of older persons are for acute episodes of chronic diseases rather than for acute conditions. The leading causes of hospitalizations are for circulatory problems (31 percent), including heart disease (21 percent), diseases of the respiratory system (11 percent) and digestive systems (12 percent), and cancer (10 percent).[1] Most physician visits by older persons are also for chronic conditions such as arthritis, diabetes, circulatory problems, and eye problems.[1] Nearly three-quarters of all deaths among the elderly are caused by three chronic diseases: heart disease, cancer, and strokes. Heart disease accounts for nearly half of the deaths in those 65 and older. The risk of dying from the major chronic diseases, however, has been declining (except for cancer) since 1968: "The severity of certain chronic diseases may be reduced in the near future by new technologies."[1] Clinical innovations such as insulin pumps, biotechnology medications [e.g., alteplase (TPA) and erythropoietin (EPO)], and advances in laser therapy may provide beneficial medical technology for older patients.

DRUG USE

The elderly are the largest consumers of pharmaceuticals, accounting for approximately 30 percent of prescription and 40 percent of nonprescription drug use.[3] Older Americans receive more prescriptions, with 40 percent of physician visits involving therapy with at least two drugs, compared with 27 percent of office visits by all individuals. The most commonly prescribed classes of drugs used in the elderly are shown in the table below:[3]

Rank	Therapeutic class
1.	Cardiovascular agents
2.	Diuretics
3.	Analgesics
4.	Gastrointestinal agents
5.	Antidiabetics
6.	Potassium supplements

Some of the factors which influence the use of medications in the elderly include how often the medication must be taken, how expensive therapy is, satisfaction with the physician-patient relationship, how tolerable the medication is, and how seriously the patient views his or her condition.[4] The patient must feel there is the need to take medication; in disease states such as hypertension, where symptoms may be absent, health care professionals must educate the patient in the benefits of drug therapy. Studies have shown that the elderly comply better than young patients when education programs have been implemented.[5] Patient education programs allow the patient to feel more involved in a therapy and provide a better opportunity for communication. Not only can health care providers discover more about patient needs, but patients are able to ask more questions and reveal existing or potential drug-related problems. Ease of administration is important to ensure proper drug use as well. Drug regimens that are complicated or confusing to an elderly patient are likely to be taken incorrectly or not at all. Physicians should always attempt to tailor therapy to the individual's needs. Medications with uncomfortable side effects make it difficult for the elderly to be compliant. Many adverse effects may be deemed worse than the disease itself. The presence of side effects should be taken into account when choosing medication for the elderly, as quality of life is an important consideration. Quality-of-life studies are being conducted more frequently now and are beginning to play a role in the management of care in the elderly. A quality-of-life study performed by Croog et al.[6] examined antihypertensive medications with equal efficacy. Although each drug lowered blood pressure equally well, significant differences were demonstrated in their effects on quality-of-life measures. Results such as these can help physicians achieve the highest level of care for their patients. All the above factors are important to consider because compliance is crucial to effective therapy, as will be discussed in Chap. 4.

Many problems may be associated with drug use in the elderly. Compliance, as already mentioned, is a potential problem in the older population. Noncompliance indicates deviation from the physician's regimen or plan of action. This would include both undermedicating and overmedicating. Reasons for undermedicating could include financial considerations where the patient tries to "stretch" a month's worth of medication into 2 or 3 months. The patient may think a scheduled medication can be taken just when needed or may feel the medication is not working, and therefore why take it? A more subtle reason may exist; the patient may not understand the directions but feels he or she is taking the medication as prescribed. Overmedicating can result from the patient feeling the prescribed dose is not effective or from the "if a little medicine is good, a lot of medicine must be better" theory. Again, confusion may be the reason for noncompliance in this situation. Problems of compliance can be overcome by monitoring the patient's drug use. This should be the joint responsibility of the physician and pharmacist. Talking to patients is the best way to discover noncompliance and the best way to remedy it. Once the reasons for noncompliance are discovered, steps can be taken to either change patient behavior or alter the medication or regimen to better serve the needs of the patient. Another problem more prevalent in the elderly is the incidence of adverse drug reactions (ADRs). Because of greater drug use, older persons experience not only more side effects, but possibly more severe effects. Some of the risk factors for ADRs include age, gender, race (occurring most frequently in older white women), number of medications taken, dosage, treatment duration, and underlying conditions such as renal or hepatic insufficiency. Medication side effects may be manifested in the elderly quite differently from the younger population. Often, the unusual or unexpected reaction may be the rule rather than the exception. Drug-drug interactions are also more probable in the elderly due to increased usage.[3] The greater the number of medications a person is prescribed, the greater the chance of an incompatibility between drugs. Some factors that increase the chance of interaction are multiple medications, multiple physicians, multiple pharmacies, and noncompliance. This increased use of pharmaceuticals, also known as polypharmacy, is associated with noncompliance, adverse drug reactions, drug-drug interactions, and increased cost. It is important to closely monitor drug use in the elderly and even more important that evaluation by health care professionals trained to detect population differences be utilized.

Polypharmacy has traditionally been a problem in nursing home or long-term care patients because they usually have multiple disease states and are further advanced in their illnesses than the noninstitutionalized. Federal regulations designed to decrease polypharmacy and its possible complications were enacted in 1974 requiring skilled nursing facilities to obtain consultant pharmacy services. Monthly drug audits are conducted for each patient. The consultant pharmacist submits findings and recommendations to the administrator, director of nursing, and the primary care physician. In this manner, pharmacists can help physicians best utilize health care resources and give nursing home patients the best possible care: "These reviews have helped decrease polypharmacy, minimized duplication of drugs, prevented significant drug interactions, and reduced inappropriate use of drugs. A review of the literature published between 1975 and 1987 shows an estimated total savings to Medicare during this period of greater than $220 million."[3]

SUMMARY

With the elderly population increasing at such a rapid rate, health care professionals need to prepare for providing care to this special age group. Older persons have unique medical needs and utilize the health care system a great deal more than the younger population. Economic issues will continue to be important in the future, especially with the rising cost of medical technology. Pharmacoeconomic evaluation should continue to be a critical tool in allocating limited health care resources. All socioeconomic and physiologic factors need to be considered when prescribing and monitoring medication for the elderly. When these factors are incorporated into health care, many of the problems associated with drug therapy in the elderly can be avoided.

REFERENCES

1. Aging America Trends and Projections. Serial No. 101-E. U.S. Government Printing Office, Washington, District of Columbia, 1989.
2. Soldo BJ, Agree EM: *Population Bulletin America's Elderly 1988,* vol 43, no 3, Population Reference Bureau, Inc., Washington, District of Columbia, 1988.
3. *The Merck Manual of Geriatrics.* MSD Research Laboratories, Rathway, New Jersey, 1990, pp 193–203.

4. Caldwell JR, Cobb S, Dowling MD, Dejongh D: The dropout problem in antihypertensive treatment: a pilot study of social and emotional factors influencing a patient's ability to follow antihypertensive treatment. *J Chron Dis* 22:579–592, 1970.
5. Morisky DE, Levine DM, Green LW, Smith CR: Health education program effects on the management of hypertension in the elderly. *Arch Intern Med* 142:1835–1838, 1982.
6. Croog SH, Levine S, Testa MA, et al: The effects of antihypertensive therapy on the quality of life. *N Engl J Med* 314:1657–1664, 1986.

CHAPTER

2

NUTRITION

Carol J. Rollins
Cynthia Thomson

As the population over 65 years of age continues to increase, greater attention is focused on the health care requirements of this population. Methods of reducing morbidity and mortality through medical treatment and manipulation of risk factors are sought. In this quest, nutrition is becoming an increasingly recognized factor. The publication of dietary guidelines by various health-related organizations over the past few years attests to this growing interest in the role of nutritional factors in disease, especially the chronic diseases found with increased frequency in the geriatric population. Suboptimal nutrition may, in fact, be one of the major risk factors for morbidity and mortality in all elderly individuals regardless of their overall medical condition. Unfortunately, nutritional assessment is frequently overlooked when evaluating the health status of elderly patients.

The purpose of this chapter is to provide a brief overview of nutrition in the elderly. The emphasis is on nutritional status with the term *malnutrition* used to specify inadequate nutriture. Topics addressed include the incidence of malnutrition, nutritional status assessment, use of the recommended dietary allowances (RDAs)[1] to identify malnourished elderly, factors contributing to malnutrition, nutritional requirements, use of nutritional supplements, nutritional interventions, and food and/or nutrient interactions with medications.

INCIDENCE OF MALNUTRITION

The elderly have repeatedly been identified as a population at risk for nutritional imbalances.[2-6] Various reports indicate that the incidence of malnutrition may be as high as one-third of ambulatory elderly,[6] 35 to 65 percent of hospitalized elderly,[7,8] and 50 to 85 percent of nursing home residents.[9-13] The actual incidence of malnutrition is, however, difficult to determine, since no universally accepted criteria exist for determining nutritional status or for defining malnutrition in the elderly.

Numerous investigators have used anthropometric or biochemical indicators of nutritional status, including vitamin and enzyme activity levels, to identify malnutrition within a study population. Others have used nutrient intake below the RDAs[1] to determine the incidence of malnutrition. In general, malnutrition is reported as more prevalent when nutrient intake below the RDAs is used to define malnutrition. Table 2-1 compares the reported incidences of malnutrition for individual nutrients in healthy, free-living elderly using nutrient intake below the RDAs versus biochemical indicators of nutritional status. Table 2-2 provides the same information for institutionalized elderly.

Nutritional status assessment plays an integral role in identifying malnourished individuals within a population. Thus, to accurately determine the incidence of malnutrition and identify "low-intake" nutrients, it is essential that current nutritional assessment techniques and their limitations be understood. It is also critical to recognize the limitations of using standards, such as the RDAs, to assess adequacy of nutritional intake.

Table 2-1 Incidence of malnutrition in free-living elderly [a]

Nutrient	Intake < RDA,[b] %	Subnormal biochemical indicators,[c] %
Vitamin A	8-65	<0.3
Vitamin D	50-74	2-40
Vitamin E	44	4
Vitamin C	0-42	2-25
Thiamin	3-36	2-25
Riboflavin	2-36	0-28
Niacin	0-4	13
Vitamin B_6	66-85	18
Folacin	55-77	3-60
Vitamin B_{12}	17-39	0-31
Calcium	19-37	No data
Iron	0-4	4
Zinc	43-76	No data

[a]Reported as a percentage of the survey or study respondents. Adapted from Refs. 9-11.

[b]Surveys differed in the fraction or percentage of the RDAs considered indicative of malnutrition and different years of the RDAs were used by different surveys. The most frequently used reference was less than two-thirds of the 1980 RDAs.

[c]Biochemical indicators included serum concentrations, red-cell concentrations, or enzyme activation coefficients, as appropriate for the given nutrient.

Table 2-2 Incidence of malnutrition in institutionalized elderly[a]

Nutrient	Intake < RDA,[b] %	Subnormal biochemical indicators,[c] %
Vitamin A	5-13	0-20
Vitamin D	17-77	48
Vitamin E	No data	3-40
Vitamin C	0-40	0-83
Thiamin	2-30	2-23
Riboflavin	0-34	1-34
Niacin	0-14	33
Vitamin B_6	57-100	1-70
Folacin	37-65	1-57
Vitamin B_{12}	2-9	0-20
Calcium	0-54	2
Iron	0-35	10-31
Zinc	21-58	13

[a]Reported as a percentage of the survey or study respondents. Adapted from Refs. 9, 12, 13.

[b]Surveys differed in the fraction or percentage of the RDAs considered indicative of malnutrition and different years of the RDAs were used by different surveys. The most frequently used reference was less than two-thirds of the 1980 RDAs.

[c]Biochemical indicators included serum concentrations, red-cell concentrations, or enzyme activation coefficients, as appropriate for the given nutrient.

NUTRITIONAL STATUS ASSESSMENT

Assessing the nutritional status of the geriatric population is challenging. Limited data, difficulty obtaining accurate measurements and diet histories, plus the lack of identifiable "norms" for standard nutritional assessment parameters in the elderly limit the accuracy of assessment in this population.[14] Nutritional status assessment may be further obscured by normal changes in body composition associated with aging. These changes make it difficult to differentiate between the normal aging process and the effects of malnutrition. Various components of nutritional status assessment, including diet history, anthropometrics, biochemical evaluation, hematologic evaluation, and physical examination, are reviewed in this section of the chapter. Difficulties associated with application of the parameters to the geriatric population are also presented.

Diet History

A thorough and complete diet history is the backbone of what clinicians assess to be *nutritional risk*. The diet history should include a history of recent food intake, plus detailed information on food frequency, location and sharing of meals, meal preparation, weight history, and use of nutritional supplements.[15] The most commonly employed method of obtaining a history of food intake is the 24-h recall. This method is convenient for both the patient and the clinician, since it requires no record-keeping by the patient and no follow-up visits. A 3-day written food record may replace the 24-h recall when follow-up between the patient and clinician is assured.

Obtaining the diet history for geriatric patients frequently requires a complete patient interview, with inclusion of significant others involved in the individual's care. In fact, the patient's caretaker becomes the primary source for the nutritional history in patients with limited cognitive abilities. Caution is advised, however, when interpreting a 24-h recall of food intake obtained from any elderly individual, either a caregiver or a competent patient, since impairment of short-term memory is known to occur with aging. The 3-day written food record is less subject to error from short-term memory deficit. This method should, therefore, be utilized for collecting dietary intake information from elderly individuals whenever possible. A complete and accurate diet history is especially critical when the RDAs are used as the basis for defining malnutrition. In this case, the diet history is the foundation from which the percentage of the RDAs consumed is determined.

Anthropometrics

Body weight, percentage of ideal body weight, and percentage of usual body weight provide the clinician with essential nutritional status data for formulation of an appropriate nutritional care plan and nutritional goal(s). Nutritional anthropometric measurements (triceps skinfold thickness, midarm circumference, and calculated midarm muscle circumference) also provide important information concerning body fat and somatic protein stores. Decreased lean body mass and increased subcutaneous fat, however, are thought to be a normal consequence of aging. It is estimated that females lose 5 kg of lean body weight between 25 and 70 years of age, while males lose an average of 12 kg during the same time.[16] This decreased body mass primarily represents decreased protein reserves, which translates into reduced ability to respond to a physiologic insult and lower caloric requirements secondary to reduced metabolic activity.[14] Concurrent with the decrease in lean body mass, the elderly experience a decrease in total body water, especially extracellular water.[16,17]

Since both obesity and cachexia are seen in the elderly, the ability to accurately assess body composition in this population is imperative. Accurate assessment, however, has been hindered by difficulty in obtaining measurements in those elderly with limited physical capabilities. Lack of anthropometric standards for the geriatric population has also been an obstacle to accurate assessment. Recent developments make nutritional anthropometry more available and reliable as a nutritional assessment tool for the elderly. For example, a knee height caliper which allows estimation of body stature in nonambulatory patients and those unable to stand erect is now available.[18] Once stature has been estimated, ideal body weight can be determined, a highly inaccurate determination previously. Either a nomogram method or equation method is used to estimate stature after knee height (KH) in centimeters has been measured. The following gender-specific equations are used for the equation method:

$$\text{Stature in men (cm)} = (2.03 \times \text{KH}) - (0.04 \times \text{age in years}) + 64.19$$
$$\text{Stature in women (cm)} = (1.83 \times \text{KH}) - (0.24 \times \text{age in years}) + 84.88$$

Knee height is also useful in determining weight within ± 5 kg in 90 percent of elderly patients.[19] Measurements of calf circumference (CC) and midarm circumference (MAC) in centimeters and subscapular skinfold thickness (SSF) in millimeters are required for this determination. The gender-specific equations for estimating weight are as follows:

$$\text{Weight for men (kg)} = (0.98 \times \text{CC}) + (1.16 \times \text{KH}) + (1.73 \times \text{MAC}) + (0.37 \times \text{SSF}) - 81.69$$

$$\text{Weight for women (kg)} = (1.27 \times \text{CC}) + (0.87 \times \text{KH}) + (0.98 \times \text{MAC}) + (0.4 \times \text{SSF}) - 62.35$$

Standard procedures for measuring triceps skinfold thickness and midarm muscle circumference in recumbent individuals and reference standards for individuals between 62 and 90 years of age are also established.[19,20] These standards include norms for weight, calf circumference, midarm circumference, triceps skinfold thickness, subscapular skinfold thickness, and midarm muscle area. When appropriate reference standards are used along with serial anthropometric measurements over several months, trends in nutritional status can be identified. Monitoring of such trends is critical for prescribing and evaluating nutritional interventions.

Bioelectrical impedance is a relatively new, noninvasive technique for assessment of body composition which has been suggested as an alternative to anthropometric measures. Unfortunately, the data base from which the impedance regression equation was developed included primarily healthy young persons. This makes interpretation of impedance data from the elderly more subject to error.[16]

Biochemical Evaluation

Limited data are currently available on reference standards for biochemical parameters used to assess the nutritional status of elderly patients. The data available are primarily from the Second National Health and Nutrition Examination Survey (NHANES II).[3] This survey collected data on healthy, independent-living elderly men and women between 65 and 74 years of age but excluded those over 74 years. Thus, there are virtually no data on the oldest segment of the geriatric population.

In the elderly it is often difficult to determine if deviations from reference standards are related to the aging process itself, to decreased organ function secondary to chronic diseases, or to changes in nutritional status. Serum albumin, a widely used marker of visceral protein status which is reported to gradually decrease with aging, illustrates this situation.[4] Some clinicians believe the decrease is a normal outcome of either decreased lean body mass or reduced albumin synthesis secondary to decreased liver mass. Others believe the decrease in serum albumin concentration is reflective of dietary protein deficiency and cannot be attributed to the normal aging process. The association of decreased serum albumin concentrations (<3.5 mg/dL) with increased mortality in elderly patients of long-term care facilities[21] and the reported mortality rate of 75 percent for hospitalized elderly with serum albumin concentrations below 2.2 mg/dL[22] suggest a pathologic basis for the decreased albumin concentrations, at least in some cases. Regardless, serial measurements over time with supporting diet history evaluations appear to provide the most relevant nutritional status information to the clinician.

Transferrin and prealbumin (transthyretin) are short-half-life visceral proteins synthesized by the liver and used clinically to detect short-term changes in nutritional status. Both are depressed by inflammatory states and acute stresses, thus limiting their usefulness under these circumstances. No age stratification currently exists for either transferrin or prealbumin reference standards.[4]

The use of transferrin as a short-term indicator of nutritional status in the elderly is controversial. The basis of the controversy is the general state of iron stores in the elderly and the effect of aging per se upon iron status.[4] In general, iron stores are thought to increase with age unless iron deficiency anemia is present.[16,23] Since serum transferrin concentrations are inversely related to iron status, transferrin concentrations generally decrease with age regardless of nutritional status. Conversely, the depressed iron stores associated with iron deficiency anemia raise transferrin concentrations without necessarily reflecting nutritional status. Therefore, a patient with iron deficiency anemia may have a normal serum transferrin concentration despite being undernourished. The presence of iron deficiency anemia in up to half of hospitalized elderly limits the usefulness of transferrin as a nutritional marker in this population.[4] For independent-living elderly, the interpretation of transferrin concentration may be confounded by the presence of iron deficiency anemia in 5 to 15 percent of the population.[2,3] Given the opposing effects of the aging process and iron deficiency on serum transferrin concentrations in the elderly, irrespective of nutritional status, interpretation of serum transferrin as an indicator of nutritional status in the elderly is, at best, difficult.

Lack of age stratification for prealbumin reference standards appears to be appropriate, despite the questionable effect of renal function on prealbumin concentrations.[4,24] In addition, prealbumin appears to be a more discriminating marker of nutritional status in the elderly than either albumin or transferrin.[25] A good correlation between serum prealbumin concentrations and response to specialized nutritional support, irrespective of age, has also been reported.[24] Thus, prealbumin appears to be a better choice than transferrin for routine monitoring of short-term visceral protein status in the elderly.

Nitrogen balance provides a quantitative assessment of nitrogen losses versus nitrogen intake. Nitrogen intake is calculated as grams of protein per day divided by 6.25. Nitrogen losses are generally determined from 24-h urine urea nitrogen excretion in grams plus 4 g of insensible nitrogen losses per day. Insensible losses include unmeasured nitrogen in the urine, such as creatinine and uric acid, plus losses in sweat, skin, and feces. Due to decreased ability to concentrate urine and excrete acid with aging, however, insensible losses of 4 g/day may be an overestimate in the elderly. Insensible losses of 2 to 3 g/day are thought to more accurately reflect nitrogen output in this population.[16] For those elderly exhibiting renal insufficiency, urine urea nitrogen losses may underestimate protein catabolism due to accumulation of urea in the blood as blood urea nitrogen. Use of urea appearance calculations in determining nitrogen balance should provide a more accurate assessment of protein catabolism in such individuals.[26]

Creatinine height index is used to evaluate somatic protein stores. The index is a comparison between measured 24-h urinary creatinine excretion and predicted urinary creatinine for persons of the same height. Standard creatinine coefficients of 23 mg/kg of ideal body weight per 24 h for men and 18 mg/kg of ideal body weight per 24 h for women are based on urinary creatinine elimination in healthy young adults of average musculature.[16] Thus, the "norms" assume both renal function and muscle mass consistent with young adult averages, neither of which is applicable to elderly subjects. Based on creatinine clearance and creatinine excretion data for 548 men ranging in age from 17 to 84 years of age, however, the expected creatinine excretion per kilogram over a period of 24 h is seen to decline by approximately 10 percent per decade over 54 years of age.[27,28] No similar age-adjusted creatinine excretion information is published for women.

Biochemical assessment of specific vitamin status is accomplished by measuring serum, tissue, or urine vitamin concentrations and/or vitamin-dependent enzyme activity. Since biochemical changes precede both physiologic and clinical manifestations of vitamin deficiencies and toxicities, early diagnosis and nutritional intervention are possible using biochemical assessment. There are, however, several problems associated with using vitamin concentrations and vitamin-dependent enzyme activities for nutritional assessment. These problems, discussed below, should be considered when interpreting the "subnormal biochemical indicators" columns of Tables 2-1 and 2-2.

One of the limiting factors for biochemical assessment of specific vitamin status is difficulty obtaining metabolically active tissue for assay. Serum and urine are therefore the most frequently assayed specimens due to their relative ease of collection. Unfortunately, serum vitamin concentrations and urinary excretion often correlate poorly with actual tissue content of the vitamins and with estimated dietary intake. Poor correlation between urinary excretion and tissue content may be accentuated in the geriatric population since the decline in renal function with advancing age makes urinary excretion measurements more prone to error. Difficulty obtaining accurate diet histories from the elderly may also worsen the correlation between biochemical measurements and estimated dietary intake.

Further complications with interpretation of vitamin concentrations and vitamin-dependent enzyme activities in the geriatric population arise from the increased prevalence of medication use and disease states in the elderly. Certain medications and diseases are known to affect specific measurements of vitamin status. For example, tricyclic antidepressants alter riboflavin metabolism and, thus, interfere with measurement of erythrocyte glutathione reductase activity as an indicator of riboflavin nutriture.[29] However, it is not clear that use of tricyclics results in riboflavin deficiency. Similarly, tuberculosis is associated with low serum ascorbate concentrations.[29] It is difficult, however, to know whether the low serum ascorbate reflects impending vitamin C deficiency or simply a lowering of serum concentrations, perhaps as a protective mechanism to reduce availability of ascorbate to the tubercular organisms.

The lack of information regarding age-related changes in vitamin concentrations and enzyme activity also complicate the interpretation of biochemical measurements in the elderly. For instance, it is unclear if a decreased erythrocyte glutathione reductase activation coefficient in the elderly reflects riboflavin malnutrition, since activity decreases with age independent of riboflavin intake.[30] It is reasonable to expect changes as lean body mass is lost with advancing age, but without longitudinal studies to assess the type and magnitude of such changes, it is difficult to determine when deviations from reference standards are related to the aging process and when they represent pathologic changes. In addition, many of the measurements for vitamin concentrations and enzyme activities are expensive, technically difficult, and not readily available. This hinders their application to routine nutritional status assessment.

Hematologic Evaluation

The complete blood count (CBC) is a readily available, easily performed, relatively inexpensive test which provides useful information for evaluating nutritional status. The hematologic parameters of hemoglobin, hematocrit, and mean corpuscular volume (MCV) reflect alterations in hematopoiesis which may occur secondary to protein, iron, folate, or vitamin B_{12} deficiency. Since specific biochemical tests for nutrient status are not included in routine biochemical test profiles, hematologic values consistent with microcytic or macrocytic anemia are often the first evidence of deficiency of these nutrients. Nonnutritional causes of the abnormalities must, of course, be ruled out before the hematologic changes are attributed to poor nutrient intake. When poor diet is the most likely cause of hematologic changes, a complete nutritional status evaluation is appropriate. Multiple nutrient deficiencies are the general rule with poor dietary intake. One or two isolated nutrient deficiencies are more frequently associated with pathologic processes such as vitamin B_{12} deficiency with achlorhydria or iron deficiency with blood loss.

Low values of hemoglobin and hematocrit are commonly reported in the elderly. Iron, folate, and vitamin B_{12} concentrations plus MCV, however, are often inconsistent with anemia.[31] This suggests that hemoglobin and hematocrit concentrations diagnostic of anemia in the elderly may be lower than the current low reference standards. Lower hemoglobin "norms" of 12 g/dL for elderly men and 10 g/dL for women have been suggested to more accurately reflect the true presence of anemia in the elderly.[32] Data from the NHANES II, however, suggest that downward adjustment is required only for elderly men.[3] A hemoglobin concentration of 11.7 g/dL was found to be diagnostic of anemia for women between 45 and 74 years of age. The diagnostic hemoglobin concentration for men was 13.1 g/dL for those 45 to 64 years of age and 12.6 g/dL for those 65 to 74 years of age. Hematocrit and red blood cell reference standards were also lower for elderly men but not for women. No data are currently available to determine if this trend in hematologic parameters continues past the age of 74 years.

By multiplying the total white blood cell count by the percentage of lymphocytes on the differential count, an absolute or total lymphocyte count (TLC) is obtained. The TLC is included among the nutritional assessment parameters employed by some clinicians. A TLC less than 1500 is generally considered indicative of malnutrition. The reliability of the TLC in detecting undernutrition has, however, been questioned.[33] Thus, if the TLC is employed as a nutritional assessment parameter, it should be considered only in relation to other assessment methods.

Nutrition Physical Examination

The final component of nutritional status assessment discussed in this chapter is the nutrition physical examination. In reality, this is often one of the first components of assessment to be completed. The nutrition physical exam is easy to do, inexpensive, relatively reliable, and readily available to the clinician, making it a valuable tool for evaluation of nutritional status in both institutionalized and independently living elderly.

Table 2-3 reports commonly identified nutrition-based lesions and the possible nutrient deficit/excess involved.[34] As with other components of nutritional assessment in the elderly, it is important to consider the effects of medications and disease states on physical findings. Frequently, nonspecific findings consistent with nutrient deficits or excesses are also typical of medication effects or disease states. For example, pitting edema may be associated with a protein-energy deficit, steroid therapy, or congestive heart failure.

DEFINING MALNUTRITION USING THE RDA

Accurate diet histories are essential when using the RDAs to define malnutrition. With appropriate interviewing skills and data collection techniques, it should be possible to obtain acceptable diet histories from most elderly individuals or their caregiver(s). Several problems with this method of determining malnutrition, however, still exist.

Table 2-3 Diagnostic possibilities of selected nutritionally related signs[a]

Body area	Signs	Possibilities
Tongue	Filiform papillary atrophy	Deficit: iron, folic acid, vitamin B_{12}, niacin, other B-complex factors
	Fissuring, edema	Deficit: niacin
	Lobulated with atrophy	Deficit: folic acid
	Scarlet, raw and painful with atrophy	Deficit: niacin, folic acid; possibly vitamin B_{12}, other B-complex factors
	Surface bald, smooth, and beefy red	Deficit: niacin
Gums	Bleeding or red, swollen; interdental gingival hypertrophy	Deficit: ascorbic acid
	Inflammation with generalized stomatitis and ulceration	Deficit: ascorbic acid, folic acid, vitamin B_{12}
Lips and mucous membranes	Inflammation, angular scars, cheilosis/vertical fissuring, ulceration	Deficit: riboflavin
	Pallor	Deficit: iron
Eyes	Corneal vascularization	Deficit: riboflavin, other B-complex factors
	Dull, dry conjunctiva, Bitot's spots	Deficit: vitamin A
	Pallor of everted lower eyelid	Deficit: iron, folic acid
Skin	Decubitus ulcers, delayed wound healing	Deficit: ascorbic acid, zinc, protein; possibly linoleic acid
	Dry, rough, scaling; possibly with headache, diplopia, dizziness	Excess: vitamin A
	Follicular hyperkeratosis (also, see hair)	Deficit: vitamin A, ascorbic acid, linoleic acid
	Hyperpigmentation	Deficit: protein-energy, folic acid, vitamin B_{12}
	Perifollicular petechiae	Deficit: ascorbic acid; possibly vitamin A, linoleic acid
	Petechiae (not perifollicular)	Deficit: vitamin K
	Pitting edema	Deficit: protein-energy
	Reduced turgor, inelastic, "tenting"	Deficit: water, fluids
	Seborrheic inflammation with erythema, thickening, dry, flaky	Deficit: linoleic acid, riboflavin
	Subcutaneous ecchymoses with minor trauma	Deficit: vitamin K, ascorbic acid, protein-energy
Hair	Broken, coiled, swan neck hairs, perifollicular hemorrhages, follicular hyperkeratosis	Deficit: ascorbic acid, vitamin A
	Easily, painlessly pluckable; dry, brittle, lusterless	Deficit: protein-energy, zinc
Nails	Pale, spoon shaped (koilonychia), ridging, brittle, thin, lusterless	Deficit: iron
	Splinter hemorrhages under nails in semicircle lattice in nail bed	Deficit: ascorbic acid
	White spotting	Deficit: zinc

[a]Adapted from Ref. 34, with permission.

One of the most obvious and difficult problems with using the RDAs to define malnutrition in the elderly is that the RDAs do not specifically address requirements of the elderly. By convention, the age demarkation for "elderly" is 65 years and above; yet the oldest age category for the RDAs begins at 51 years.[1] No subgroupings exist within this age category for the usual "elderly" age group or for recognized subcategories of elderly. Thus, when the RDAs are used to define malnutrition in the elderly, the reported incidence of malnutrition may be inaccurate.

A second problem with studies using the RDAs to define malnutrition in the elderly is that the percentage of the RDAs considered indicative of malnutrition varies between investigators. For example, malnutrition has been defined as nutrient intake falling below 100 percent,[9,10] three-quarters,[10] two-thirds,[11] or 50 percent[30] of the RDAs. As the percentage of the RDAs considered indicative of malnutrition decreases, so does the reported incidence of malnutrition. This can be illustrated using pyridoxine intake. When intake below 100 percent of the RDA for pyridoxine is used to indicate malnutrition, 85 to 97 percent of independent community-living elderly can be considered malnourished.[9,10] As the percentage of the RDA decreases to 75 percent, the reported incidence of malnutrition drops to between 80 and 86 percent. At 67 percent of the RDA, the incidence of malnutrition is 54 to 61 percent.[10,11] Finally, at an intake less than 50 percent of the RDA for pyridoxine, approximately half of the elderly are classified as malnourished.[30] Since arguments can be presented to support the use of each reported percentage of the RDAs as the basis for defining malnutrition, the actual incidence of malnutrition remains elusive. This problem could be easily overcome in future studies if investigators agreed to a predetermined percentage of the RDAs as indicating malnutrition.

Pyridoxine also serves to illustrate a problem with inaccurate or incomplete nutrient data. To determine nutrient intake, food consumption data are correlated with nutrient content data. The problem of inaccurate consumption data has been discussed previously. Accurate nutrient content data for the foods consumed are no less important. Unfortunately, nutrient content data for many surveys/studies are based on incomplete nutrient profiles or on data determined by older, less accurate analytical methods. Pyridoxine content, for example, is not available for many entrees, preprepared meals, lamb, veal, or numerous other foods included in a popular "food values" manual.[35] Calculation of nutrient intake using the food values from this manual, thus, underestimates pyridoxine intake for subjects consuming such foods. More accurate and complete nutrient content data are included in recent computer programs based on the revised U.S. Department of Agriculture Handbook 8.[36] Availability of such programs should allow future surveys to determine nutrient intake more accurately.

Another problem with using the RDAs to define malnutrition in the elderly is that the RDAs are designed specifically for meeting the nutritional requirements of normal healthy populations.[1] The RDAs are not intended to, nor do they, address the nutrient requirements of individuals or subpopulations with either acute or chronic illnesses. Considering that approximately 75 percent of the elderly take at least one medication regularly, it is questionable whether the elderly population as a whole meets the criteria of a "healthy population."[37,38] On the other hand, it is questionable whether the small percentage of the elderly population not taking medication regularly can be considered "normal" for this age group. Thus, the applicability of the RDAs in defining malnutrition in the elderly is questionable. Despite this, investigators use the RDAs as a basis for reporting low nutrient intake in elderly patients.

FACTORS CONTRIBUTING TO MALNUTRITION

Malnutrition in the elderly is a multifactorial problem involving physiologic, psychosocial, and financial variables. These variables often intertwine and profoundly affect one another.

Physiologic Variables

Changes in body function which occur due to aging itself or secondary to pathologic processes associated with aging are categorized as physiologic variables. Numerous physiologic variables affect the nutritional status of the elderly. Prominent among these are decreased resting metabolic rate (RMR) and reduced lean muscle mass.[14,16] These two factors appear to be closely linked. Several studies have reported that whole-body RMR, as assessed by oxygen consumption or indirect calorimetry, declines approximately 2 to 4 percent per decade over 40 years of age.[30,39-44] When the RMR is adjusted to fat-free weight, however, much less age-related change is noted. Whether loss of lean muscle mass with aging accounts for the entire age-related decline in RMR is controversial. Tzankoff and Norris[39,40] reported that age-related decreases in creatinine-producing tissue, primarily skeletal muscle, account for the entire decline in RMR. Figure 2-1 illustrates the contribution of muscle versus nonmuscle to whole-body oxygen consumption, a measure of RMR. Since the nonmuscle component is relatively stable, declining oxygen consumption by muscle appears to be primarily responsible for the decline in whole-body oxygen consumption with increasing age. Other studies have found that the lower RMR in older subjects is significantly, but not fully, corrected by adjusting to fat-free weight.[41,42] The age-related decrease in RMR appears, however, to be attenuated by regular participation in aerobic exercise. Physically active older men approximately 50 to 80 years of age are reported to have a RMR about 5 percent below that of active young men, compared to a RMR 17 percent lower for sedentary older men.[41]

The decline in RMR based on age and level of physical activity has important nutritional and medical consequences for the elderly since decreased RMR translates into decreased energy requirements. As energy intake is reduced to match lower requirements, a concomitant decrease in overall nutrient intake occurs and the risk of malnutrition increases. Alternatively, obesity occurs if energy intake

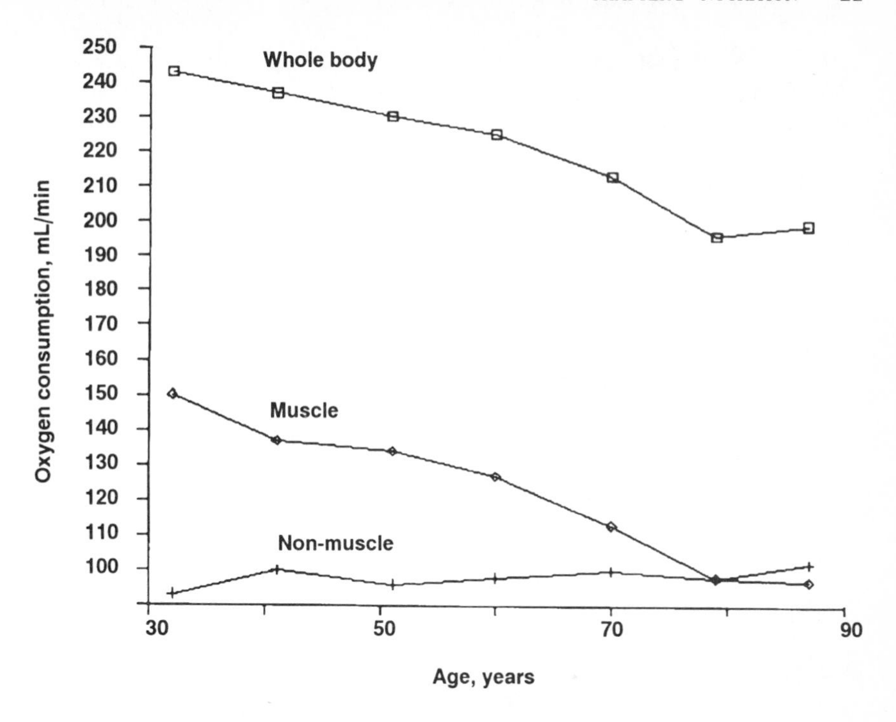

Figure 2-1 Mean changes with age in whole-body, muscle, and nonmuscle oxygen consumption in basal state. Age is the mean (in years) per 10-year age group: 25–34 years (n = 10), 35–44 years (n = 54), 45–54 years (n = 107), 55–64 years (n = 77), 65–74 years (n = 63), 75–84 years (n = 39), and 85–95 years (n = 5). (Adapted from Ref. 39.)

exceeds energy expenditure, thus exposing the person to the numerous medical risks associated with obesity.

Physiologic changes which result in anorexia can also affect nutritional status in the elderly. Factors contributing to anorexia are illustrated in Fig. 2-2.[38] Other physiologic changes with nutritional consequences in the elderly include achlorhydria with associated malabsorption of vitamin B_{12}, folic acid, and ferric iron; altered esophageal motility, dysphagia, or delayed gastric emptying leading to restricted nutrient intake; and decreased intestinal motility with chronic constipation and possible malabsorption secondary to overuse of laxatives.[23,38,45] Failing eyesight may affect nutritional status by interfering with food shopping, cooking, and self-feeding. Xerostoma, which is relatively prevalent in the elderly, increases the risk of malnutrition due to ineffective mastication and swallowing.[5] Likewise, loss of natural teeth, even when replaced by dentures, is associated with mastication problems and reduced nutrient intake. Protein intake appears to be most affected by dentition.[11,46]

Chronic diseases may also be associated with physiologic changes which alter nutritional status. While such changes are not due to aging per se, the incidence of

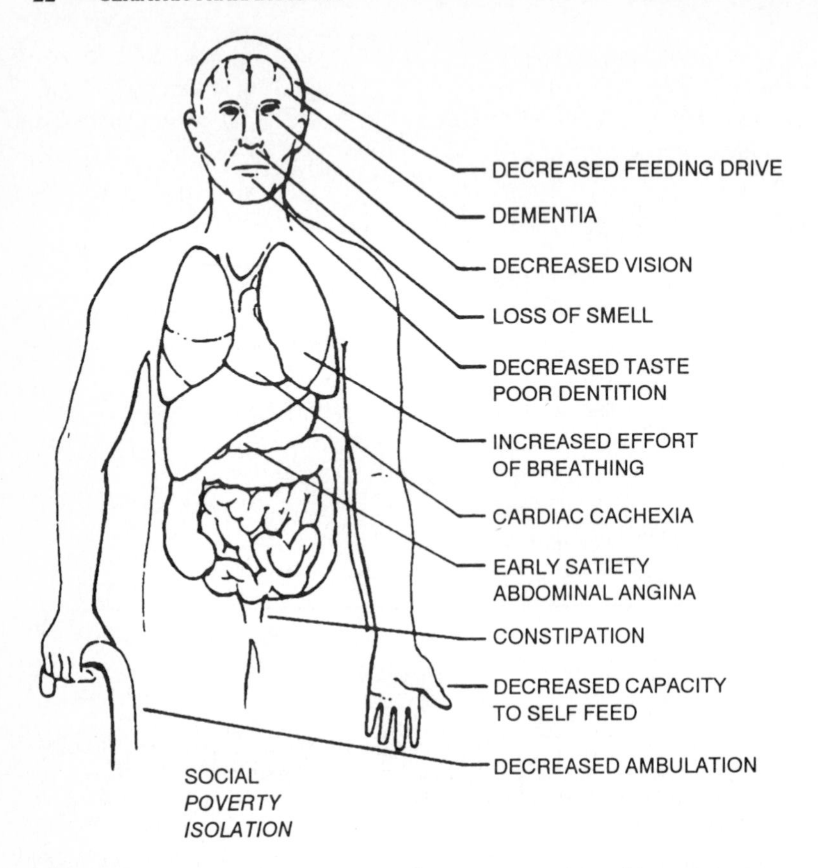

Figure 2-2 Factors contributing to anorexia of aging. (From Ref. 38, with permission.)

these changes increases in the elderly due to the increased incidence of chronic diseases in this age group. Examples illustrating the association between physiologic changes in chronic diseases and nutritional deterioration are presented below.

Shortness of breath secondary to congestive heart failure or chronic obstructive pulmonary disease may be severe enough to interfere with eating. A cycle of weight loss, muscle weakness, increased dyspnea, and further reduction in nutrient intake then occurs. Without nutritional intervention, the result of this cycle is cachexia with eventual heart or respiratory failure. Chronic renal failure is characterized by reduced elimination of metabolic waste products, including those associated with anorexia. Over time, poor nutrient intake secondary to anorexia leads to muscle wasting and multiple nutritional imbalances. Anorexia may also contribute to the poor nutritional status associated with hepatic cirrhosis. The primary cause of malnutrition in cirrhosis, however, is more likely reduced ability of the liver to utilize nutritional substrates for protein synthesis and gluconeogenesis. Depression, dementia, or other cognitive impairments, which occur with increased frequency in the elderly, may also significantly alter nutrient intake.[47] The resulting malnutrition is generally characterized by wasting of body mass, but excessive weight gain may also occur. Weight gain is particularly likely when certain antidepressant medications are prescribed.

Psychosocial Variables

The second group of variables associated with malnutrition in the elderly are psychosocial variables. These variables are characterized by intertwined psychologic and social issues. The most important psychosocial variables include living arrangements, ethnicity, and educational level.

The effect of living arrangements on nutritional status has been addressed by several studies. The NHANES reported lower quality diets for elderly living alone versus those living with a spouse.[2,3] A smaller study, however, found that older adults living alone consumed fewer calories and certain other nutrients than those living with others, but food choices were of equivalent quality.[48] In other words, those living alone simply ate less. This may reflect the tendency of individuals living alone to skip meals more frequently.[49] Dietary intake of men appears to be more influenced by living arrangements than that of women, as evidenced by results of Davis et al.[48] In this study, elderly men living alone were at higher risk of inadequate intake compared to women living alone. Men living with someone, however, had better quality diets than women. Overall, when the dietary adequacy of men was compared to that of women, without regard to living arrangements, men were less likely than women to have poor quality diets.

The connection between living arrangements and dietary intake may be the amount of social interaction which occurs. Improved dietary adequacy of elderly groups has been reported with increased social interaction and social enhancement at mealtime.[50,51] Likewise, dietary problems have been reported to decrease when the elderly perceive visits by friends and relatives as adequate.[47] Other studies have also linked social interaction with dietary adequacy and serve as a premise for congregate meal programs for the elderly.[11,47]

Ethnicity is a psychosocial variable which plays a major role in nutrient intake through its effect on food selection and preparation. Although ethnic foods per se are not nutritionally undesirable, the cumulative effects of certain ethnic dietary habits may place the elderly at increased risk of diet-associated diseases. For example, elderly Mexican-Americans may be at increased risk of cardiovascular disease from the consumption of large quantities of saturated fats and cholesterol-containing foods in their traditional diet. Epidemiologic evidence suggests that this same group may be at increased risk of certain cancers secondary to low intake of vitamin A- and vitamin C-rich foods.[52] Other ethnic influences on nutrient intake include lower iron intake among elderly black females versus white females and lower intakes of thiamine, niacin, and riboflavin in elderly black Americans compared to the elderly in general.[2,3] In some instances, however, low economic status may be as important as ethnicity in affecting nutrient intake.

Educational level may interact with other psychosocial and financial variables to affect nutrient intake in the geriatric population. Intake of vitamin C–rich citrus fruits appears to be the most affected by educational level, independent of ethnic and financial variables.[52] As educational level increases, so does the frequency of citrus fruit intake, and supposedly the vitamin C status.

Financial Variables

Financial variables are intertwined with physiologic and psychosocial variables in affecting nutrient intake of the elderly. Financial status directly affects the quantity and quality of foods which can be purchased. Several studies have shown income to be positively correlated with nutritional status, independent of other variables.[2,3,11,47,52] Physiologic factors can compound the effects of income. For instance, elderly people with chronic diseases requiring medications may be forced to choose between expensive medications and adequate nutrition. Those particularly at risk are the elderly at or near the poverty line but ineligible for assistance programs. Also, limited mobility may force some elderly people to shop at easily accessible convenience stores where the selection of foods is poor and prices are high. The interaction between financial status and psychosocial variables indirectly affects nutrient intake of the elderly through effects on living arrangements, availability of cooking and food storage facilities, and availability of transportation to buy food. Thus, it is obvious that dietary intake of the elderly involves a complex interaction among a multitude of factors. Correcting or improving one of these factors may have little effect on nutritional status unless other factors are also addressed.

NUTRITIONAL REQUIREMENTS

Aging appears to have variable effects on nutritional requirements, increasing the requirement for certain nutrients while decreasing the need for other nutrients. Based on very limited data, however, the requirements for most nutrients are thought to change little due to the aging process itself. This section of the chapter reviews available information regarding changes in nutrient requirements due to aging. Table 2-4 summarizes this information.

Energy Requirements

Energy requirements decrease with advancing age by an estimated 10 percent for each decade past 50 years of age. The downward adjustment for resting energy expenditure is approximately 2 to 4 percent for each decade past 40 years of age, or about one-fifth to one-third of the total decrease in energy requirements.[30,39,44] As discussed previously, loss of metabolically active tissue, reflected in reduced lean body mass, is primarily responsible for the decrease in resting energy expen-

Table 2-4 Changes in nutrient requirements with age[a]

Requirement status	Nutrient	
Increased	Protein (?)	Vitamin B_6
	Vitamin D	Chromium (?)
	Vitamin B_{12}	
Decreased	Energy	
	Vitamin A	
	Folic acid	
No evidence for change	Riboflavin	Biotin
	Thiamin	Pantothenic acid
	Vitamin C	Vitamin E
	Niacin	Vitamin K
No evidence for change in the absence of disease	Sodium	
	Potassium	
	Magnesium	
	Calcium	
	Zinc	

[a]From Ref. 34, with permission.

diture. An age-related decrease in physical activity accounts for most of the remaining fall in energy requirements.[23]

The most frequently used and referenced method for estimating energy requirements continues to be the Harris-Benedict formulas. These gender-specific equations, first published in 1919, were developed using multivariant regression analysis on data from large-scale indirect calorimetry studies.[53] Regression coefficients for weight (W) in kilograms, height (H) in centimeters, and age (A) in years are included in the calculation of basal energy expenditure (BEE):

$$\text{BEE for males: } 66.47 + 13.75W + 5.00H - 6.76A$$
$$\text{BEE for females: } 655.10 + 9.65W + 1.85H - 4.68A$$

Once BEE is calculated, adjustment factors for stress and activity are used to convert resting energy expenditure to estimated daily energy requirements. The clinician must remember that the values obtained from the Harris-Benedict equations are only estimated requirements based on fit to a regression equation. The confidence intervals for these equations are large, with individual requirements varying by more than twofold from calculated values.[54] The only method of accounting for individual variations in energy requirements currently available is indirect calorimetry.

Although the Harris-Benedict equations are widely used and generally considered useful for adults of all ages, their accuracy has been questioned. Newer studies criticize the Harris-Benedict equations for overestimating requirements in the young and underestimating the resting energy requirements of elderly individuals.[54] Also, it is interesting to speculate whether data analyzed by Harris and Benedict in the early 1900s can be considered representative of today's population given the changes which have occurred in demographics over this time span.

Protein

The effect of aging on protein requirements continues to be an area of controversy. Both increased and decreased requirements have been reported.[23,30] Investigators reporting decreased protein needs with advancing age attribute the change to reduced lean body mass. Those reporting increased protein requirements suggest reduced dietary nitrogen retention secondary to lowered caloric intake with aging is responsible. The effects of chronic disease on demand for protein and declining organ function on protein tolerance must also be considered when determining the protein requirements for elderly individuals. In the absence of renal disease, however, the normal age-related decline in renal function should not preclude a high-protein diet (greater than 15 percent of calories from protein) when it is otherwise appropriate. Based on current knowledge, it appears that the RDA of 0.8 g/kg body weight per day for protein[1] is the minimum protein intake that should be recommended for healthy elderly individuals, and 0.9 to 1.0 g/kg/day may be more appropriate for much of the elderly population. Protein intake should, of course, be adjusted according to protein demands and tolerances. For example, protein intake is generally reduced in response to a creatinine clearance below 20 mL/min and increased during periods of metabolic stress. Protein of high biologic value is recommended for the elderly in general but is especially important during periods of metabolic stress.

Fiber

Although fiber is not a nutrient per se, it is a component of the diet which can affect digestion and absorption of nutrients. Fiber may also have a beneficial effect on several diseases which occur frequently in the elderly, including constipation, diverticular disease, hypercholesterolemia, and hyperglycemia. The potential for control of constipation with adequate fiber intake is especially encouraging considering the high usage of pharmaceutical agents, both prescribed and over the counter, for regulation of bowel function in the geriatric population.[30,35]

Intake of 20 to 30 g of dietary fiber per day is recommended for all adults by the American Cancer Society, the American Heart Association, and the U.S. Department of Health and Human Services.[55] For many elderly people, however, this recommendation can be difficult to achieve due to the smaller quantities of food needed to meet their lower caloric requirements. The clinician should also remember that rapid increases in dietary fiber intake can temporarily result in significant gastrointestinal discomfort with reduced overall food consumption. Thus, fiber intake should be gradually increased over several weeks. Fluid intake should also be increased as dietary fiber increases. Inadequate fluid intake combined with increased fiber consumption can lead to fecal impaction, especially when physical activity is limited.

Fluids

Adequate fluid intake is an essential and sometimes overlooked nutritional concern in the elderly. Adequate hydration is necessary for normal functioning of the kidneys, gastrointestinal tract, cardiovascular system, and brain. Fluids are necessary for absorption and metabolism of water-soluble vitamins and for maintenance of normal body temperature.

Fluid requirements normally are 30 to 35 mL/kg body weight per day.[23] Changes do not appear to occur due to aging itself. Fluid requirements in many elderly individuals, however, may be altered by diseases affecting fluid balance. For example, congestive heart failure, renal failure, and ascites are associated with fluid retention which frequently mandates reduced fluid intake. Other individuals may require increased fluid intake secondary to excessive gastrointestinal losses, fever, elevated environmental temperatures, or open wounds, including decubitus ulcers. Altered fluid regulation due to disturbances in thirst and osmoregulatory mechanisms also contributes to fluid imbalances in the elderly.

Vitamins, Minerals, and Trace Elements

Based on available evidence, requirements for most vitamins, minerals, and trace elements do not appear to change with age. The RDAs published in 1989 recognize lower requirements for five nutrients in the "51 or older" age group versus the 25- to 50-year-old group, as shown in Table 2-5.[1] As mentioned previously, energy requirements decrease with age. Since thiamin, riboflavin, and niacin requirements are based on caloric intake, the need for these nutrients also decreases in the older age group. Finally, the requirement for iron in postmenopausal women is recognized as lower than that of the younger age group of women. The requirements for calcium in women was not changed despite possible benefits of increased calcium intake, beginning before 30 years of age, on postmenopausal osteoporosis.[23] Also, data suggesting an increased need for vitamins D, B_6, and B_{12} with aging and decreased requirements for vitamin A and folic acid were not considered adequate to warrant age-related changes in the RDAs for these nutrients at that time.[14,23]

USE OF NUTRITIONAL SUPPLEMENTS

Vitamin and mineral supplement use by the elderly appears to be common but highly variable. Surveys done during the 1980s report that 20 to 98 percent of various segments of the geriatric population used supplements at least intermittently.[10,30,56,57] This is in contrast to less than 1 percent of the elderly using supple-

Table 2-5 Recommended dietary allowances[a]

	Males		Females	
Nutrient	25 to 50 years	≥51 years	25 to 50 years	≥51 years
Vitamin A, μg RE	1000	1000	800	800
Vitamin D, μg	5	5	5	5
Vitamin E, μg a-TE	10	10	8	8
Vitamin C, mg	60	60	60	60
Thiamin, mg	1.5	1.2	1.1	1.0
Riboflavin, mg	1.7	1.4	1.3	1.2
Niacin, mg NE	19	15	15	13
Vitamin B_6, mg	2.0	2.0	1.6	1.6
Folacin, μg	200	200	200	200
Vitamin B_{12}, μg	2.0	2.0	2.0	2.0
Calcium, mg	800	800	800	800
Iron, mg	10	10	15	10
Zinc, mg	15	15	12	12

[a]Selected nutrients. Adapted from Ref. 1.
RE = retinol equivalents, a-TE = alpha-tocopherol.

ments in a 1975 survey.[58] Individuals with higher incomes are generally more prone to supplement use, although 66 percent of a low-income group of elderly in Nevada was noted to use supplements.[59] Attainment of a higher educational level has also been associated with a greater prevalence of supplement use.[57] Other studies in the elderly, however, have found no such correlation.[10,59] Women are more likely to use supplements than men at all ages, and those elderly experiencing difficulty with mastication more commonly use supplements than those without such difficulty.[56] Geographic location also appears to influence supplement use. Individuals in the west, especially California, are most likely to use supplements, while those in the southern United States are least likely to do so.[57,61]

Up to 80 percent of those elderly who use supplements ingest some type of supplement daily.[10,56,61] More than one supplement is consumed on a regular basis by 13 to 45 percent of supplement users.[10,57,60] The types of supplements selected vary considerably from survey to survey, but a few general trends are evident. Overall, approximately half of elderly supplement users take multivitamin/multimineral preparations either daily or intermittently.[62] Vitamin C is the most popular individual vitamin supplement among the elderly, followed by vitamin E. Individual mineral supplements are used less frequently than vitamin supplements, but when used, iron is most frequently consumed, followed by zinc and calcium. Table 2-6 summarizes data on the most popular nutritional supplements used by six survey populations. Caution is advised when comparing the values from different surveys, as done in Table 2-6, since surveys may define "use" differently. Defini-

Table 2-6 Use of popular nutritional supplements by the elderly[a]

Survey location	New Mexico	Boston	Nevada	Ohio	Florida	National
Number in survey	270	691	170	309	3,192	884
Percentage of supplement users	59	50	66	49	41	42
Supplement type[b]						
Combination or multivitamin/multimineral	31/52.5	37/73.5	21/27	37.5/77	31.5/76.5	26/61
Vitamin C	57.5/97.5	40/80	27/41	13.5/28	10.5/25.5	38.5/90.5
Vitamin E	49.5/84	35.5/71	24/36	9.4/19	13.5/32.5	32/75.5
Iron	32.5/55	20.5/41	Not reported	4/8	2/4.5	18/43
Zinc	27.5/47	16/32	8/12	2.5/5	<1/1.5	14/33
Calcium	26/44	13.5/27	16.5/25	6/13	24.5/59	13/31.5

[a]From Ref. 10, 56-60.

[b]Reported as percentage of respondents to survey per percentage of supplement users; values reported to the nearest 0.5%.

tions range from any consumption within the past 2 years to regular ingestion of supplements four or more times within the past week. The method of determining level of supplementation may also differ between surveys. Some surveys use individual supplement ingestion, while others include the content of multivitamin/multimineral preparations with that of individual supplements.

Considering the prevalence of supplement use by the elderly, it is important to assess the possible benefits and risks associated with supplement use. On the benefit side, supplement users tend to have higher intakes of the nutrients supplemented compared to intakes of nonusers.[10,11,56] Depending on the definition of adequate intake, however, supplement use may have only a modest effect on the percentage of the population with adequate intake. For instance, McGrandy et al[11] found that the percentage of elderly receiving less than two-thirds of the RDA for vitamin C changed from 6.2 percent without supplementation to 4.2 percent with supplement use, and calcium changed from 26.5 percent without supplementation to 24 percent with supplement use. Mann et al[62] evaluated the possible benefit of supplement use by doing a randomized, double-blind, placebo-controlled trial that assessed vitamin status by biochemical parameters before and after supplementation with a multivitamin preparation. After 4 months of supplementation, plasma ascorbate and vitamin B_{12} levels and plasma plus erythrocyte folate levels indicated improved status from baseline for these vitamins. The biochemical parameters for these vitamins were also significantly improved in the supplemented group compared to the placebo group. These results suggest that an increased vitamin intake can improve nutritional status on a biochemical basis, at least for the water-soluble vitamins. Table 2-7 summarizes the results of studies using enzyme activation coefficients, which are relatively specific and sensitive biochemical indicators of

Table 2-7 Incidence of vitamin deficiency with and without supplementation in hospitalized and free-living elderly[a]

Nutrient	Hospitalized elderly		Free-living elderly	
Thiamin				
Without supplement	22.9%	23.2%	13.5%	
Supplemented with:				
<5 × RDA (<6 mg)	—	1.9%	6.3%	
5–10 × RDA (6–12 mg)	—	—	—	
>10 × RDA (>12 mg)	None	—	—	
Riboflavin				
Without supplement	11.7%	2.3%	16.2%	2.0-7.2%
Supplemented with:				
<5 × RDA (<7 mg)	—	None	None	None
5–10 × RDA (7–14 mg)	None	—	—	None
>10 × RDA (>14 mg)	—	—	—	—
Vitamin B_6				
Without supplement	19.0%	21.6%		
Supplemented with:				
<5 × RDA (<10 mg)	—	12.5%		
5–10 × RDA (10–20 mg)	1.9%	—		
>10 × RDA (>20 mg)	—	—		

[a]Reported as the percentage of study subjects with enzyme activation coefficients consistent with vitamin deficiency. Adapted from Refs. 63–67.

vitamin status, for assessment before and after supplementation with water-soluble vitamins. Like the study by Mann et al,[62] these results indicate that supplementation improves water-soluble vitamin status at the biochemical level for most patients. It is not clear, however, that improvement in these parameters translates into improved outcomes or direct health benefits from supplementation.

On the risk side of supplement use are concerns of toxicity and diversion of funds from food and medication. The elderly do not appear to be at risk of toxicity from multivitamin/multimineral supplements formulated near RDAs. Individuals ingesting megadoses (10 or more times the RDAs) of one or more vitamins, however, may be at risk of toxicity.[30,56] At least one-quarter of the supplement users in the survey by Garry et al[10] had supplemental intakes 40 times the RDA for vitamin E and 10 to 20 times the RDAs for thiamin, riboflavin, vitamin C, and niacin. Five percent of the supplement users took between 30 and 100 times the RDAs for these nutrients plus vitamins B_6 and B_{12}. A national telephone survey[57] found a similar trend among the respondents 65 years of age or older, except the multiples of the RDAs taken were somewhat lower. For instance, the 95th percentile for vitamin E was 63 times the RDA in the telephone survey[57] versus 100 times in the survey by Garry et al.[10] For vitamin C, the values were 22 times the RDA versus 30 times. In a Boston survey,[56] nearly 40 percent of supplement users exceeded the megadose threshold for vitamin E, over 20 percent took megadoses of thiamin and vitamin C, and more than 10 percent of female supplement users exceeded 10 times the RDAs for riboflavin and vitamins B_6 and B_{12}. Thus, it is obvious that a fairly large number of elderly individuals may be at risk of vitamin toxicity from supplement use.

Despite concern over possible diversion of funds from food and medication purchases to supplement purchases, few surveys have gathered data on the amount of money spent for supplements. In a 1978 Nevada survey,[59] 33 percent of supplement users spent less than $5 per month on supplements, 27 percent spent between $6 and $10, 31 percent spent $11 to $20, and 9 percent spent over $20 per month on supplements. The median income of this group was $200 to $299 per month. Another survey using 1981 data from Ohio[58] found that 73 percent of supplement users spent $5 or less per month on supplements, 6 percent spent $6 to $10, 7 percent spent $11 to $20, and 4 percent spent over $20 per month on supplements. The median income of supplement users in this group was $440 per month. The median percentage of income spent on supplements was 3 percent and the range was from 1 to 8 percent of income. Based on these two surveys, most supplement users were probably not spending a large enough portion of their income on supplements to result in a diversion of funds from food and medication purchases. It is, however, difficult to extrapolate data gathered over 10 years ago to what might be occurring in today's climate of increased health consciousness and advertising for nutritional supplements. Individuals who purchase numerous single-nutrient products or high-potency supplements do, without doubt, spend considerably more than those who purchase a store brand multivitamin/multimineral supplement providing at or near the RDAs.

As a general rule, the elderly should be discouraged from spending large sums of money on vitamin/mineral preparations, especially multiple single-nutrient preparations and high-potency supplements. Many of the elderly believe that supplements give an added health benefit, even when a balanced diet with adequate calories is consumed.[58] In this case, a multivitamin/multimineral product formulated at or near the RDAs should limit the risk of toxicity. Single-nutrient supplements may be appropriate for individuals unable or unwilling to eat products from one of the basic food groups. For instance, calcium supplementation may be appropriate for individuals who eliminate or restrict intake of dairy products. Individuals with documented nutritional deficiencies may also require single-nutrient or high-dose vitamin/mineral therapy.

NUTRITIONAL INTERVENTIONS

Dietary Restrictions

Dietary restrictions for the elderly should be instituted with discretion since undesirable effects may outweigh the benefits for this population. Many elderly patients have difficulty discriminating among food choices and thus either ignore diet instructions or eliminate entire food groups from their diet. Undesirable weight loss or nutrient deficits may result if elimination of entire food groups occurs. Table 2-8 lists some of the more common medical diagnoses of the elderly as well as associated nutritional therapies. The clinician must employ nutritional restrictions based on the individual situation while continuing to monitor the impact of the nutritional therapy, both positive and negative.

Nutrition Support

When elderly patients are unable to obtain adequate nutrition by oral feedings, decisions on the institution of enteral and/or parenteral nutrition must be made. The purpose of this chapter is not to discuss the ethical issues related to artificial feeding but to briefly discuss treatment options. It is important, however, to reinforce the need to discuss potential feeding options with aging patients in advance of when artificial support may be needed. Documentation of the patient's wishes is also critical. Figure 2-3 describes, in an algorithm format, the indications and options for specialized nutritional support.

FOOD/NUTRIENT AND MEDICATION INTERACTIONS

More medications are used by the elderly than by younger persons and multiple medications are frequently used. The elderly are thus at increased risk of adverse medication reactions, including food or nutrient interactions with medications. Such interactions potentially affect medication efficacy, nutritional status, or both. Table 2-9 provides a brief listing of medications commonly used by the elderly and food or nutrient interactions which may be clinically significant. This table contains only a few of the many reported food/nutrient-medication interactions. Many of the effects are nonspecific (i.e., anorexia, nausea, weight change) and develop over time rather than being immediate reactions. The clinician must therefore maintain a high index of suspicion for food/nutrient-medication interactions.

CONCLUSION

Nutritional status is a critical component of overall health status. The elderly are particularly vulnerable to malnutrition due to physiologic changes which occur with aging. Changes in psychosocial and financial positions also increase the risk of altered nutritional status in the geriatric population. Due to relatively nonspecific signs and symptoms, however, malnutrition in the elderly is often overlooked. Such signs and symptoms are simply attributed to the aging process unless the health

Table 2-8 Medical diagnoses and related nutritional therapies

Disease or condition	Standard nutritional therapy	Nutrition-related concerns of therapies
Achlorhydria	No special diet	Can contribute to decreased tolerance to food, B_{12} deficiency, and decreased iron absorption
Cancer	Adequate calories to maintain weight during therapies; reduce fat to 30% of total calories	Nausea, vomiting, mucositis, and diarrhea from therapies may limit intake, leading to inadequate nutrition; altered taste from some therapies; anorexia common
Chronic obstructive pulmonary disease (COPD)	Increase ratio of fats to carbohydrates	May result in delayed gastric emptying, reflux, and nausea; increased risk of CAD (see below)
Chronic renal insufficiency	Protein restriction; decreased sodium, potassium, and fluid may be required	May result in overall decreased intake, resulting in poor nutritional status or dehydration
Congestive heart failure (CHF)	Low-sodium diet	May significantly decrease intake due to reduced taste; supplement potassium as needed if diuretic used is not potassium sparing
Coronary artery disease (CAD)	Reduced cholesterol and fat; increased intake of fish with omega-3 fatty acids	Restrictions could lead to inadequate or unbalanced intake
Decubitus ulcers	Increased calories and protein; zinc, ascorbic acid, and vitamin A supplements may be indicated	Anemia is common; physical therapy is important in conjunction with nutrition
Diabetes mellitus	ADA diet versus liberal diabetic diet	Control of hyperglycemia to allow tissue synthesis versus inadequate intake due to restrictive diet
Hepatitis (active)	Increased calories and protein	Difficult to achieve due to anorexia
Hepatitis (chronic) with cirrhosis	Protein and fluid restriction; decreased sodium	Anorexia may result in deteriorating nutritional status. Limited ability to metabolize nutrients
Osteopenia/ osteoporosis	Increased calcium and vitamin D may be recommended	Increased calcium probably needs to be started at a young age to be effective; adjust diet to meet needs if weight-bearing exercise increased
Peptic ulcer disease (PUD)	No effective diet therapy; avoidance of caffeine, alcohol, and peppermint advised	

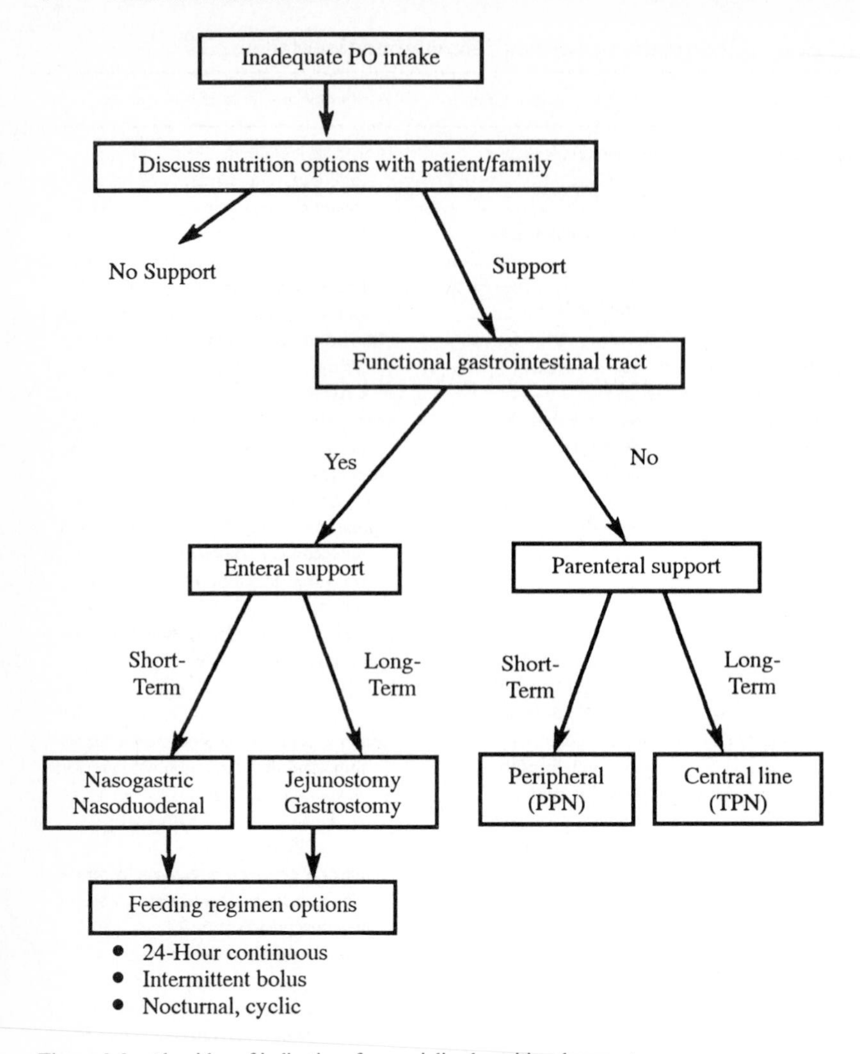

Figure 2-3 Algorithm of indications for specialized nutritional support.

care professional maintains a high index of suspicion for malnutrition. Thus, it is crucial for clinicians to include nutritional status evaluation as part of the overall health status assessment for elderly individuals. To accomplish this, nutritional items should be integrated into the medical history, physical examination, and patient counseling. Specific questions should be asked to obtain information on use of nutritional supplements and medication records should be reviewed for possible food/nutrient interactions. Restrictive diets should be advised only when the benefits clearly outweigh the risks of dietary imbalances, and use of specialized nutritional support should be discussed in advance of its need.

Table 2-9 Food/nutrient and medication interactions[a]

Medication	Dietary implications or effect
Analgesic/anti-inflammatory medications	
Glucocorticoids	Increased appetite; hyperglycemia
Nonsteroidal anti-inflammatory agents	Constipation; nausea; stomatitis
Anticoagulants	
Warfarin	Vitamin E supplements may increase anticoagulant effect; dietary vitamin K may decrease effect
Antihypertensive medications	
Angiotensin I converting enzyme inhibitors	Nausea; anorexia; altered taste or loss of taste with captopril
Beta-adrenergic blockers	Dry mouth; diarrhea; blocks symptoms of hypoglycemia
Clonidine	Dry mouth; blocks symptoms of hypoglycemia
Hydralazine	Anorexia; B_6 supplement may reduce peripheral neuropathy
Methyldopa	Dry mouth; edema; diarrhea; high-protein meal decreases absorption; folate and B_{12} deficiency may occur
Cardiovascular medications	
Calcium channel blockers	Nausea; calcium supplements may decrease effectiveness; low-fat meal prevents flushing with nifedipine
Digoxin	Anorexia; calcium and vitamin D supplements may cause hypercalcemia, which potentiates digoxin effect
Quinidine	Diarrhea; high intake of fruit juice may cause toxicity
Procainamide	Anorexia; bitter taste; sore mouth
Cholesterol-lowering agents	
Cholestyramine or colestipol	Folate deficiency and depletion of fat-soluble vitamins with high dosage and prolonged use
Gemfibrozil	Dry mouth; anorexia; abdominal pain
Diuretics	
Furosemide and other loop diuretics	Increased urinary loss of calcium, potassium, and magnesium
Thiazide diuretics	Decreased urinary loss of calcium; Increased urinary loss of potassium and magnesium; nausea; anorexia
Endocrine medications	
Conjugated estrogens	Edema; Increased risk of folate and B_6 deficiency

(*Continues*)

Table 2-9 (*continued*) Food/nutrient and medication interactions[a]

Medication	Dietary implications or effect
Oral hypoglycemics	Must be used in conjunction with appropriate diabetic diet; high risk of hypoglycemia with long-acting agents
Levothyroxin	Possible decreased glucose tolerance in diabetic
Gastrointestinal medications	
Aluminum hydroxide antacids	Constipation; hypophosphatemia; calcium and vitamin A deficiency
H-2 blockers	Increased risk of vitamin B_{12} deficiency
Metoclopramide	Diarrhea; altered glucose absorption
Laxatives	
Mineral oil	Deficiency of fat-soluble vitamins
Phenolphthalein	Electrolyte changes and malabsorption with abuse of laxatives
Psyllium	Decreased appetite; decreased rate of glucose absorption
Neuropsychiatric medications	
Benzodiazepines	Dry mouth; increased appetite
Fluoxetine	Anorexia; nausea; diarrhea
Tricyclic antidepressants	Dry mouth; increased appetite, especially for carbohydrates
Respiratory medications	
Theophylline	Anorexia; nausea; low-protein and high-carbohydrate diet slows metabolism; charcoal broiled meats increase metabolism
Albuterol; terbutaline	Hyperglycemia may occur in diabetics

[a]Adapted from Refs. 68, 69.

REFERENCES

1. Food and Nutrition Board: *Recommended Dietaty Allowances* 10th ed. Washington, D.C. National Academy of Science, 1989.
2. Abraham S, Carroll MD, Dresser CM, Johnson CL: Dietary intake source data, United States, 1971-1974, Publ. no. PHS 79-1221. Hyattsville, Maryland, Public Health Service, 1979.
3. Carroll MD, Abraham S, Dresser CM: Dietary intake source data, United States, 1976-1980, Vital and health statistics, series 11 no. 231, DHHS Publ. no. PHS 83-1681. Washington, D.C., U.S. Government Printing Office, Washington, D.C., 1983.
4. Morrow FD: Assessment of nutritional status in the elderly: application and interpretation of nutritional biochemistries. *Clin Nutr* 5:112-120, 1986.
5. Rhodus NL, Brown JB: The association of xerostomia and inadequate intake in older adults. *J Am Diet Assoc* 90: 1688-1692, 1990.

6. Linn BS, Jensen J: Malnutrition and immunocompetence in older and younger outpatients. *South Med J* 77: 1098–1102, 1984.
7. Willard M, Gilsdorf RB, Price RA: Protein-calorie malnutrition in a community hospital. *JAMA* 243: 1720, 1980.
8. Bienia R, Ratcliff S, Barbour GL, Kummer M: Malnutrition in the hospitalized geriatric patient. *J Am Geriatr Soc* 30: 433–436, 1982.
9. Rudman D, Arora VD, Feller AG, et al: Epidemiology of malnutrition in nursing homes, in Morley JE, Glick Z, Rubenstein LZ (eds): *Geriatric Nutrition: A Comprehensive Review*. New York, Raven Press, 1990, pp. 325–332.
10. Garry PJ, Goodwin JS, Hunt WC, et al: Nutritional status in a healthy elderly population: dietary and supplemental intakes. *Am J Clin Nutr* 36: 319-331, 1982.
11. McGrandy RB, Russell RM, Hartz SC, et al: Nutritional status survey of healthy noninstitutionalized elderly: nutrient intakes from three-day diet records and nutrient supplements. *Nutr Res* 6: 785–798, 1986.
12. Shaver HJ, Loper JA, Lutes RA: Nutritional status of nursing home patients. *JPEN* 4: 367-370, 1980.
13. Sahyoun NR, Otradovec CL, Hartz SC, et al: Dietary intakes and biochemical indicators of nutritional status in an elderly, institutionalized population. *Am J Clin Nutr* 47: 524–533, 1988.
14. Chernoff R: Physiologic aging and nutritional status. *Nutr Clin Pract* 5: 8–12, 1990.
15. Davis MA, Murphy SP, Neuhaus JM, Lein D: Living arrangements and dietary quality of older U.S. adults. *J Am Diet Assoc* 90: 1667–1672, 1990.
16. Lewis EJ, Bell SJ: Nutritional assessment of the elderly, in Morley JE, Glick Z, Rubenstein LZ (eds): *Geriatric Nutrition: A Comprehensive Review*. New York, Raven Press, 1990, pp. 73–87.
17. Chernoff R, Mitchell CO, Lipschitz DA: Assessment of the nutritional status of the geriatric patient. *Geriatr Med Today* 3: 129–141, 1984.
18. Chumlea WC, Roche AF, Steinbaugh ML: Estimating stature from knee height for persons 60 to 90 years of age. *J Am Geriatr Soc* 33: 116–120, 1985.
19. Chumlea WC, Guo S, Roche AF, Steinbaugh ML: Prediction of body weight for the nonambulatory elderly from anthropometry. *J Am Diet Assoc* 88: 564-568, 1988.
20. Falciglia G, O'Connor J, Gedling E: Upper arm anthropometric norms in elderly white subjects. *J Am Diet Assoc* 88: 569–574, 1988.
21. Rudman D, Feller AG, Nagari HS, et al: Relation of serum albumin concentration to death rate in nursing home men. *JPEN* 11: 360–363, 1987.
22. Harvey DB, Maldawer LL, Bistrian BR, Blackburn GL: Biological measures for the formulation of a hospital prognostic index. *Am J Clin Nutr* 34: 2013-2022, 1981.
23. Chernoff R, Lipschitz DA: Nutrition and aging, in Shils ME, Young VR (eds): *Modern Nutrition in Health and Disease*, 7th ed. Philadelphia, Lea and Febiger, 1988, pp. 982–1000.
24. Sachs E, Bernstein LH: Protein markers of nutritional status as related to sex and age. *Clin Chem* 32: 339–341, 1986.
25. Kergoat MJ, Leclerc BS, PetitClerc C, Imbach A: Discriminant biochemical markers for evaluating the nutritional status of elderly patients in long-term care. *Am J Clin Nutr* 46: 849–861, 1987.
26. Mirtallo JM, Fabri PJ: Effect of nitrogen intake on urea appearance in patients receiving total parenteral nutrition and hemodialysis. *Drug Intell Clin Pharm* 18: 612–616, 1984.
27. Driver AG, McAlevy R: Creatinine height index as a function of age. *Am J Clin Nutr* 33: 2057, 1980 (letter).
28. Rowe JW, Andres R, Tobin FD, et al: The effects of age on creatinine clearance in men: A cross-sectional and longitudinal study. *J Gerontol* 31: 155–163, 1976.
29. Russell RM, Jacob RA, Greenberg LB: Clinical assessment of the nutritional status of adults, in Linder MC (ed): *Nutritional Biochemistry and Metabolism: With Clinical Applications*. New York, Elsevier, 1985, pp. 285–308.
30. Bidlack WR: Nutritional requirements of the elderly, in Morley JE, Glick Z, Rubenstein LZ (eds): *Geriatric Nutrition: A Comprehensive Review*. New York, Raven Press, 1990, pp. 41–72.

31. Guyatt GH, Patterson C, Ali M, et al: Diagnosis of iron-deficiency anemia in the elderly. *JAMA* 88: 205–209, 1990.
32. Lipschitz DA, Mitchell CO, Thompson C: The anemias of senescence. *Am J Hematol* 11: 47–54, 1981.
33. Forse RA, Rompre C, Crosilla P, et al: Reliability of the total lymphocyte count as a parameter of nutrition. *Can J Surg* 28: 216–219, 1985.
34. Kight MA: The nutrition physical examination. *CRN Quart* 2(3): 1–3, 1987.
35. Pennington JAT: *Bowes and Church's Food Values of Portions Commonly Used*, 15th ed. Philadelphia, J.B. Lippincott, 1987.
36. Agriculture Handbook No. 8, Revised. Composition of Foods, Raw, Processed, Prepared. U.S. Department of Agriculture, Washington, D.C.
37. Stewart RB: Drug use in the elderly, in Delafuente JC, Stewart RB (eds): *Therapeutics in the Elderly*. Baltimore, Williams & Wilkins, 1988, pp. 50–63.
38. Silver AJ: Anorexia of aging and protein-energy malnutrition, in Morley JE, Glick Z, Rubenstein LZ (eds): *Geriatric Nutrition: A Comprehensive Review*. New York, Raven Press, 1990, pp. 105–115.
39. Tzankoff SP, Norris AH: Longitudinal changes in basal metabolism in man. *J Appl Physiol* 45: 536–539, 1978.
40. Tzankoff SP, Norris AH: Effect of muscle mass decrease on age-related BMR changes. *J Appl Physiol* 43: 1001–1006, 1977.
41. Poehlman ET, Melby CL, Badylak SF: Relation of age and physical exercise status on metabolic rate in younger and older healthy men. *J Gerontol* 46: B54–58, 1991.
42. Keys A, Taylor HL, Grande F: Basal metabolism and age of adult man. *Metabolism* 22: 579–587, 1973.
43. Poehlman ET, Horton ES: Regulation of energy expenditure in aging humans. *Ann Rev Nutr* 10: 255–275, 1990.
44. Stein TP, Lazarus DD, Chatzidakis C: Human macronutrient requirements, in Rombeau JL, Caldwell MD (eds): *Clinical Nutrition: Enteral and Tube Feeding*, 2nd ed. Philadelphia, W.B. Saunders, 1990, pp. 54–72.
45. Boss GR, Seegmiller JE: Age-related physiological changes and their clinical significance. *West J Med* 135: 434–440, 1981.
46. Gordon SR, Kelley SL, Sybyl JR, et al: Relationship in very elderly veterans of nutritional status, self-perceived chewing ability, dental status, and social isolation. *J Am Geriatr Soc* 33: 334–339, 1985.
47. Fischer J, Johnson MA: Low body weight and weight loss in the aged. *J Am Diet Assoc* 90: 1697–1706, 1990.
48. Davis MA, Murphy SP, Neuhaus JM, Lein D: Living arrangements and dietary quality of older U.S. adults. *J Am Diet Assoc* 90: 1667–1672, 1990.
49. Davis MA, Murphy SP, Neuhaus JM: Living arrangements and eating behaviors of older adults in the United States. *J Gerontol* 43: S96–S98, 1988.
50. Hanson RG: Considering "social nutrition" in assessing geriatric nutrition. *Geriatrics* 33: 49–51, 1978.
51. Ryan VC, Bower ME: Relationship of socioeconomic status and living arrangements to nutritional intake of the older person. *J Am Diet Assoc* 89: 1805–1807, 1989.
52. Bartholomew AM, Young EA, Martin HW, Hazuda HP: Food frequency intakes and sociodemographic factors of elderly Mexican Americans and non-Hispanic whites. *J Am Diet Assoc* 90: 1693–1696, 1990.
53. Harris JA, Benedict FG: *A Biometric Study of Basal Metabolism in Man*. Washington, D.C. Carnegie Institute of Washington, 1919.
54. Owen OE: Resting metabolic requirements of men and women. *Mayo Clin Proc* 63: 503–510, 1988.
55. Cronin FJ, Shaw AM: Summary of dietary recommendations for healthy Americans. *Nutr Today* Nov.-Dec.: 26–34, 1988.

56. Hartz SC, Blumberg J: Use of vitamin and mineral supplements by the elderly. *Clin Nutr* 5: 130-136, 1986.
57. Stewart ML, McDonald JT, Levy AS, et al: Vitamin/mineral supplement use: A telephone survey of adults in the United States. *J Am Diet Assoc* 85: 1585-1590, 1985.
58. Schneider CL, Nordlund DJ: Prevalence of vitamin and mineral supplement use in the elderly. *J Fam Pract* 17: 243-247, 1983.
59. Read MH, Graney AS: Food supplement usage by the elderly. *J Am Diet Assoc* 80: 250-253, 1982.
60. Hale WE, Stewart RB, Cerda JJ, et al: Use of nutritional supplements in an ambulatory elderly population. *J Am Geriatr Soc* 30: 401-403, 1982.
61. McDonald JT: Vitamin and mineral supplement use in the United States. *Clin Nutr* 5: 27-33, 1986.
62. Mann BA, Garry PJ, Hunt WC, et al: Daily multivitamin supplementation and vitamin blood levels in the elderly: a randomized, double-blind, placebo-controlled trial. *J Am Geriatr Soc* 35: 302-306, 1987.
63. Hoorn RKJ, Flikweert JP, Westerink D: Vitamin B-1, B-2 and B-6 deficiencies in geriatric patients, measured by coenzyme stimulation of enzyme activities. *Clin Chim Acta* 61: 151-162, 1975.
64. Vir SC, Love AHG: Thiamine status of institutionalised and non-institutionalised aged. *Int J Vit Nutr Res* 47: 325-335, 1977.
65. Vir SC, Love AHG: Riboflavin status of institutionalised and non-institutionalised aged. *Int J Vit Nutr Res* 47: 336-344, 1977.
66. Vir SC, Love AHG: Vitamin B-6 status of institutionalised and non-institutionalised aged. *Int J Vit Nutr Res* 47: 336-344, 1977.
67. Garry PJ, Goodwin JS, Hunt WC: Nutritional status in a healthy elderly population: riboflavin. *Am J Clin Nutr* 36: 902-909, 1982.
68. Roe DA: *Handbook on Drug and Nutrient Interactions: A Problem-Oriented Reference Guide*, 4th ed. Chicago, The American Dietetic Association, 1989.
69. Allen AM: *Powers and Moore's Food-Medication Interactions*, 7th ed, Smith CH, West J (eds) Pottstown, Pennsylvania, Zaneta M. Pronsky and Associates, 1991.

CHAPTER

3

ADVERSE DRUG REACTIONS

Rubin Bressler

The elderly population has increased over the past 75 years and is projected to further increase to 25 percent of the population by the early part of the twenty-first century. Although a number of factors have favored more prolonged life, elderly people experience more chronic disease and multiple chronic diseases and are treated with multiple drugs. The elderly have a higher incidence of arthritis, asthma, chronic lung disease, diabetes mellitus, hypertension, cardiovascular diseases, and cancers. Treatment of these diseases with drugs holds the potential for adverse drug reactions in an age group with a propensity for such reactions.[1,2]

An adverse drug reaction may be viewed as a response to a drug that is noxious and unwanted and that occurs at doses that are usually therapeutic. The definition includes *idiosyncrasy* (an inordinate response to a usual dose) and *hypersensitivity* (signs and symptoms resulting from an immune response to a standard dose). Drug interactions are modifications of the effect of a drug when used in association with another drug. These interactions can result in augmentation or diminution of drug activity and account for a proportion of adverse drug reactions.

In recent years, considerable attention has been paid to factors influencing drug therapy in elderly patients. Elderly patients have an increased frequency of adverse drug reactions. These reactions have been attributed to both *pharmacokinetic* (the time course of drug absorption, distribution, metabolism, and excretion) and *pharmacodynamic* (the clinical aspects of physiologic responses to drug actions, i.e., compensatory homeostatic responses) deficiencies in the elderly patient.[3,4]

Most adverse drug reactions in the elderly are not idiosyncratic. They are extensions of the expected effects of the drug. In order to understand the pathogenesis of the problem, the effects of aging on pharmacokinetics and pharmacodynamics are discussed and the effects of aging on drug absorption, distribution, metabolism, excretion, and sensitivity reviewed.

Adverse drug reactions may be responsible for over 10 percent of elderly patient hospital admissions and for lengthening hospital stays. A number of these adverse drug effects might be obviated by the physician anticipating the specific toxic effect of prescribed drugs and by considering the possible effect of the patient's age and illness on the pharmacokinetics of the drug used.[5-7]

Drug absorption is basically unimpaired in the elderly in spite of decreased gastrointestinal blood flow, increased gastric pH, and diminished intestinal motility.[2,8,9] Obviously disease of the gastrointestinal tract will influence drug absorption. Drugs which influence the absorption of other drugs, such as cholestyramine, and anticholinergic drugs may delay the absorption of other drugs.[5,8,9]

Drug distribution is influenced by a number of age-related changes. These include a decrease in lean body mass and water content and an increase in adipose tissue.[10]

The increase in adipose tissue favors deposition of lipophilic drugs, such as diazepam and other long-acting benzodiazepines, as well as of digitoxin and synthetic steroids. Water-soluble drugs reach higher plasma levels in elderly patients because of the lesser quantity of body water and muscle into which the compound can distribute. A number of the commonly used drugs are water-soluble, including procainamide, quinidine, propranolol, theophylline, warfarin, and a number of sedatives and hypnotics.[11-14]

Hydrophilic drugs like acetaminophen, digoxin, and cimetidine are distributed less in the elderly because of decreased body muscle mass, decreased body water, and in subjects with heart disease, hypertension, or diabetes mellitus, decreased blood flow to body organs.[15,16] This situation occurs in the elderly because drug distribution is determined by body composition (muscle-lipid-water), plasma protein binding of drugs, and perfusion of organs by blood.

The pharmacokinetics of drugs used in patients with congestive heart failure has been found to be altered. Drug actions were potentiated by both decreased hepatic perfusion and the reduced liver size of elderly patients, which is often congested in heart failure states. These factors decrease clearance of drugs whose elimination is dependent on hepatic inactivation. Drugs whose elimination depends on renal excretion reach higher steady-state plasma levels because of the intrinsic decrement in renal function accompanying aging and the decreased renal perfusion in heart failure. Drug efficacy can be delayed by a longer distribution time. Excessive drug action may be experienced because of the decreased rate of drug inactivation or elimination.[17-19]

PROTEIN BINDING OF DRUGS

A number of drugs are highly bound to plasma proteins (85 to 99 percent), primarily albumin. However, the free drug determines pharmacologic action, since bound drug cannot reach target tissues. Bound drug serves as an inactive drug reservoir.

Albumin is the major protein which binds acidic drugs and is reduced by 12.5 percent in the elderly.[20,21] Alpha-1-acid glycoproteins, which bind basic drugs, are not depressed in elderly people. Significant augmentation of pharmacologic effects is expected from drug displacement from albumin or low serum albumin when the drug is highly protein bound and has a small volume of distribution. Albumin may be further depleted by a number of diseases common in elderly people. These include congestive heart failure, chronic renal disease, rheumatoid arthritis, hepatic cirrhosis, malnutrition, and some cancers.[21] Decreased binding of drugs to plasma proteins has been found to underlie some adverse effects in the elderly. It is now recognized that reduced narcotic doses are required in the elderly because of increased sensitivity to the drugs' respiratory depressant action and the decreased protein binding of the narcotic. In a time study of meperidine plasma concentration following intravenous injection in surgical patients and normal subjects, the older patients had higher unbound (free) drug fractions.[22] It was found that the diminished warfarin binding capacity in the elderly was proportional to lower plasma albumin levels.[23] Some drugs that are highly protein bound include warfarin, phenytoin, tolbutamide, indomethacin, and furosemide.

In the elderly patient, a decrease in serum albumin may result in higher concentrations of unbound active drug. A number of drugs are extensively bound to plasma proteins (80 percent or more), and although decreased levels of serum albumin may result in depressed total plasma levels of drugs like warfarin, propranolol, quinidine, phenytoin, and tolbutamide, their unbound concentrations may be in the therapeutically active range.[24] Although drug binding decreases with aging, the free fraction is increased by 50 percent in only a few drugs (diflunisal, naproxen, salicylate, and valproic acid). Because most laboratories report total plasma drug levels, one can be misled by a slightly depressed but therapeutically effective plasma drug concentration. Renal disease, with its decreased serum albumin, its frequent acidosis, and the effect of uremia itself on drug binding, is a clinical state where drug binding is characteristically decreased (see Table 3-1).

DECREASED HOMEOSTATIC MECHANISMS

Age decrements are more marked in physiologic adjustments that require the integrated activity of several organ systems than in those that involve a single system. The impairments of renal, hepatic, cardiac, respiratory, neuromuscular, and endocrine vitality with aging result in a slower rate of recovery following a variety of physiologic displacements. Aging is characterized by a diminution of the adaptive capacity to a variety of inputs. The reduced homeostatic responses of the elderly result in adverse drug reactions that may be compensated for in the younger patient. Decreased cardiac outputs, lowered plasma volumes, diminished vasomotor controls, and decreased glucose tolerance all give rise to a greater frequency of

Table 3-1 Factors affecting drug disposition in elderly patients

Age-related physiologic change	Pathologic condition	Therapeutic and environmental factor
Absorption		
Increased gastric pH	Achlorhydria	Antacids
Decreased absorptive surface	Diarrhea	Anticholinergics
Decreased splanchnic blood flow	Postgastrectomy	Cholestryramine
Decreased gastrointestinal motility	Malabsorption syndromes	Drug interactions
	Pancreatitis	Food or meals
Distribution		
Decreased cardiac output	Congestive heart failure	Drug interactions
Decreased total body water	Dehydration	Protein-binding displacement
Decreased lean body mass	Edema or ascites	
Decreased serum albumin	Hepatic failure	
Increased α_1-acid glycoprotein	Malnutrition	
Increased body fat	Renal failure	
Metabolism		
Decreased hepatic mass	Cancer	Dietary composition
Decreased hepatic blood flow	Congestive heart failure	Drug interactions
	Fever	Insecticides
	Hepatic insufficiency	Tobacco (smoking)
	Malnutrition	
	Thyroid disease	
	Viral infection or immunization	
Excretion		
Decreased renal blood flow	Hypovolemia	Drug interactions
Decreased glomerular filtration rate	Renal insufficiency	
Decreased tubular secretion		

Source: Adapted from Vestal and Dawson, *Handbook of the Biology of Aging*, 2nd ed. Van Nostrand Reinhold, New York, 1985, p 749. By permission.

adverse reactions in response to a variety of drugs. Moreover, the elderly are frequently afflicted with several chronic diseases that may necessitate multiple-drug therapy.

The impaired homeostatic capacity, multiple chronic illnesses, and multiple-drug therapy afford greater opportunity for adverse drug reactions. Because of decreased capacity for cardiovascular homeostasis, elderly patients are more prone to postural hypotension secondary to the use of diuretics, sympatholytics, nitrates, phenothiazines, tricyclic antidepressants, quinidine, procainamide, and antihypertensive drugs. Adverse drug reactions are also more common in the elderly because of the multiplicity of drugs required, their long-term use, and the occurrence of drug-drug interactions.

The inability to respond normally to postural changes, changes in blood pressure, blood glucose, temperature, or augmentation of cardiac output with exercise may create difficulty in compensating for drug effects.[25] Recently, it was shown that both the sympathetic response and the parasympathetic response of the iris are reduced with age. These findings, coupled with observations of diet-associated hypotension, suggest that baroreceptor function is reduced in the elderly.[26,27]

Elderly patients experience adverse drug reactions even with the most careful medical care. Sedative-hypnotic agents depress mentation and cerebral circulation, resulting in manifold mental and physical changes. The combination of alcohol, barbiturates, and tranquilizers is poorly tolerated by elderly subjects.[28-30]

Hallucinations and other forms of disturbed cerebral function, as well as glaucoma or urinary retention, may follow the administration of antiparkinsonian, sympathomimetic, or anticholinergic drugs.[31-33] An apparent suicide may be, in fact, an accidental death when sedatives have been prescribed injudiciously or if they are taken repeatedly by an increasingly confused aged person.

A general rule of therapeutics is that the correct dose for every patient should be empirically determined. In the elderly, it is especially important to individualize therapy. When one deals with such patients, unusual responses, including tolerance, hypersensitivity, and toxicity, should all be suspected and carefully evaluated.

HEPATIC DRUG ELIMINATION

Drug metabolism in the liver is often a two-phase process. Phase I consists of oxidations, reductions, and hydrolytic reactions, and phase II consists of conjugative reactions. Hepatic drug metabolism generally serves to inactivate drugs, but in some instances it may activate them. Drug metabolism usually produces more water-soluble compounds which are capable of excretion in the urine or bile. Phase I drug metabolism involves the hepatic cytochrome P-450 family of enzymes.[34,35] There may be as much as a sixfold difference in rates of cytochrome P-450 drug metabolism among individuals.[34]

Categories of drug metabolism are based on hepatic extraction ratios and hepatic capacity for phase I drug metabolism. The degree of hepatic drug extraction from blood perfusing the liver relates to the degree of dependence of drug elimination on hepatic blood flow. Drugs with high extraction ratios are very dependent on hepatic blood flow and undergo extensive first-pass metabolism.[3-5,36]

The elimination of drugs with low hepatic extraction ratios is a function of the drug's plasma protein binding and the liver's capacity to metabolize the drug.

When the extraction ratio is high (0.7 or more), most of the drug is removed from perfusing blood by the liver regardless of the degree of protein binding, and clearance approaches hepatic blood flow. This occurs in the case of narcotics, analgesics, propranolol, verapamil, tricyclic antidepressants, theophylline, and a number of glucuronide conjugates. Drugs with low extraction ratios (0.3 or less) such as warfarin, phenytoin, and nonsteroidal anti-inflammatory drugs have clearances based on free-drug concentrations and therefore plasma protein binding.[5,37,38]

Considerable amounts of drug can be extracted and metabolized by the liver. However, the process is capable of being saturated. Saturation of first-pass (flow-limited) drug uptake results in large increases in systemic drug concentrations with small increases in drug dose (dose-dependent kinetics). Increased systemic bioavailability has been shown for a number of highly extracted drugs in elderly subjects. These include propranolol, labetalol, verapamil, and chlormethiazole.[5,39-42] This is not unexpected since drugs with high rates of metabolism are both saturable and are dependent on hepatic blood flow, which is reduced in the elderly.[34,43,44] The decrease in hepatic blood flow ranges from 12 to 40 percent (see Table 3-2).

Evidence derived from human studies suggest that the combination of decreased hepatic blood flow and reduced size of the liver may be responsible for decreased drug clearance in the elderly.[36,38,45,46]

When highly extracted drugs are used at therapeutic doses which are saturable or near saturable, decreases in drug absorption from the gastrointestinal tract can reduce systemic bioavailability.

Drugs which have low extraction ratios are considered to have low intrinsic clearance by the liver. They have a capacity-limited metabolism, which is a function of liver size and plasma protein binding.[38,47,48] Although plasma protein is decreased in the elderly and protein binding of drugs is decreased by some disease states, the liver size is decreased.[21,45-51]

The study of drugs with capacity-limited metabolism in the elderly has been complicated by the large variation of interindividual responses and the confounding influences of gender, smoking, diet, environment, chronic diseases, and use of other drugs. However, a decreased metabolism of some drugs has been demonstrated in the elderly.[52-54]

Some studies have found that phase I metabolism of imipramine, amitriptyline, and thioridazine is decreased in elderly subjects.[55,56] A majority of studies have shown that drug metabolism decreases with aging but that the decrement is selective and does not apply to all drugs.[5,36,38,57-59]

Whereas the phase I pathways of drug metabolism may be reduced or unchanged in the elderly, the phase II (conjugation) pathway is unaltered in the elderly.[37,58] Drugs like chlordiazepoxide, diazepam, clorazepate, and prazepam have been shown to have a prolonged elimination in the elderly. They are subject to both phase I (oxidative) and phase II (conjugative) metabolism. The elimination of oxazepam, lorazepam, and temazepam, drugs subject to only phase II metabolism, is unaltered in the elderly.

The evidence that phase I drug metabolism is decreased in the elderly is based in large part on studies in rats. A number of studies of age-related changes in hepatic drug metabolizing enzymes have been carried out in human liver biopsy specimens. These studies have failed to demonstrate any correlation between gender, age, and liver drug metabolizing enzyme activity (P-450 reductase)[58,59] (see Table 3-3).

An effect of age on the stereoselective disposition of a chiral drug has been

Table 3-2 Comparison of pharmacokinetic parameters of several flow-dependent (high extracted) drugs in young and old subjects

	Old subjects			Young subjects		
Drug	Vd, L/kg	$t_{1/2}$, h	Cl	Vd, L/kg	$t_{1/2}$, h	Cl
Indocyanine green	41.1 ± 5.3	4.7 ± 0.57 (min)	6.1 ± 0.6 (mL/min/kg)	41.6 ± 6.4	3.1 ± 0.3 (min)	7.1 ± 1.2 (mL/min/kg)
Lidocaine	0.85 ± 0.17	2.1 ± 0.14	5.0 ± 1.2 (mL/min/kg)	0.7 ± 0.2	1.5 ± 0.18	5.3 ± 1.5 (mL/min/kg)
Nortriptyline	—	45 (23.5–79)	18.8 (L/h) (8.3–38.4)	—	26.8	54 + 24 (L/h)
Propranolol	4.2 ± 0.5	5.6 ± 0.6	9.0 ± 0.9 (mL/min/kg)	3.8 ± 0.3	4.5 ± 0.4	10.6 ± 1.3 (mL/min/kg)
Morphine	4.7 ± 0.2	4.4 ± 0.25	12.4 ± 1.23 (mL/min/kg)	3.2 ± 0.3	2.95 ± 0.5	14.7 ± 0.9 (mL/min/kg)

Source: Wilkinson and Shand: A physiological approach to hepatic drug clearance. *Clin Pharmacol Ther* 18:377–390, 1975. Used by permission.

Table 3-3 Relation of age to clearance of drugs cleared by hepatic biotransformation

Drug or metabolite	Initial pathway of biotransformation[a]
Evidence suggesting age-related reduction in clearance	
Antipyrine[b]	Oxidation (OH, DA)
Diazepam[b]	Oxidation (DA)
Chlordiazepoxide	Oxidation (DA)
Desmethyldiazepam[b]	Oxidation (OH)
Desalkylflurazepam[b]	Oxidation (OH)
Clobazam[b]	Oxidation (DA)
Alprazolam[b]	Oxidation (OH)
Quinidine	Oxidation (OH)
Theophylline	Oxidation
Propranolol	Oxidation (OH)
Nortriptyline	Oxidation (OH)
Small or negligible age-related change in clearance	
Oxazepam	Glucuronidation
Lorazepam	Glucuronidation
Tempazepam	Glucuronidation
Warfarin	Oxidation (OH)
Lidocaine	Oxidation (DA)
Nitrazepam	Nitroreduction
Flunitrazepam	Oxidation (DA), nitroreduction
Isoniazid	Acetylation
Ethanol	Oxidation (alcohol dehydrogenase)
Metoprolol	Oxidation
Digitoxin	Oxidation
Prazosin	Oxidation

[a]OH denotes hydroxylation and DA dealkylation.

[b]Evidence suggests that the age-related reduction in clearance is greater in men than in women.

Source: Adapted from Greenblatt, Seller, and Shader: Studies of the relation of age to the clearance of drugs cleared by hepatic biotransformation. *N Engl J Med* 306:1083, 1982. By permission of the *New England Journal of Medicine.*

shown.[60] The enantiomers of hexobartibal were studied in young and elderly subjects. The clearance of the (-) enantiomer was twice as rapid in the young subjects, whereas the clearance of the (+) enantiomer was not influenced by age. It has also been shown that age and gender may be determinants of the stereoselective elimination of mephobarbital. The study showed that the elimination of the (-) enantiomer was more rapid in young males than young females and that the same gender difference was evident in the elderly. However, the elderly subjects eliminated the (-) enantiomer less rapidly than the young subjects.[61]

INDUCTION OF DRUG METABOLISM IN THE ELDERLY

Enzyme induction is associated with an increased synthesis of hepatic enzymes. The augmentation or regression of these enzymes occurs over a period of days to weeks. It has been ascertained that drug-induced enzyme induction capacity may be reduced in the elderly.[62-65] However, enzyme induction by smoking is unaltered.[66,67] Lower doses of a drug must be used if an inducing drug is being simultaneously used. Moreover, a reduction in drug dose is important when an inducing drug is withdrawn, since the therapeutic dose used may become an overdose.

RENAL EXCRETION OF DRUGS IN THE ELDERLY

Many drugs both active and inactive are excreted by the kidney. Decreased renal function affects pharmacokinetics of a drug if it is more than 60 percent excreted by the kidney. Renal blood flow decreases by around 1 percent a year after age 50, and renal clearances in the elderly without renal disease are around 60 to 70 mL/min.[68-70] When the glomerular filtration rate falls below 30 mL/min, drugs whose elimination is primarily renal accumulate producing higher blood levels of drug for longer periods of time. Such drugs include digoxin, procainamide, lithium, atenolol, amphotericin, pentamidine, cimetidine, allopurinol, primidone, chlorpropamide, and many commonly used antibiotics.[68]

Renal function in the elderly may not be accurately assessed by serum creatinine (Table 3-4). The decrease in muscle mass and turnover results in a lower serum creatinine.[70] Creatinine clearance is a more accurate measure of renal

Table 3-4 Cross-sectional age differences in creatinine clearance, serum creatinine, and 24-hour creatinine excretion

Age, years	Subjects, *n*	Creatinine clearance, $mL/min/1.73\ m^2$	Serum creatinine concentration, mg/100 mL	Creatinine excretion, mg/24 h
17-24	10	140.2[a] ± 3.7	0.808 ± 0.026	1790 ± 52
25-34	73	140.1 ± 2.5	0.808 ± 0.010	1862 ± 31
35-44	122	132.6 ± 1.8	0.813 ± 0.009	1746 ± 24
45-54	152	126.8 ± 1.4	0.829 ± 0.008	1689 ± 18
55-64	94	119.9 ± 1.7	0.837 ± 0.012	1580 ± 22
65-74	68	109.5 ± 2.0	0.825 ± 0.012	1409 ± 25
75-84	29	96.9 ± 2.9	0.843 ± 0.019	1259 ± 45

[a]Values indicate mean ± 1 SEM.

Source: Adapted from Rowe JW, Andrew R, Tobin JD, et al.: Cross-sectional age differences in creatinine clearance, serum creatinine, and 24-hour creatinine excretion. *J Gerontol* 31:155-163, 1976. By permisssion from the Gerontological Society of America.

function in the elderly.[70,71] Several methods of estimates of creatinine clearance from serum creatinine have been validated.[72] Examples of impairment of renally excreted drugs in the elderly are shown in Tables 3-5 and 3-6.

Phase II drug metabolism reactions such as conjugation usually inactivate drugs. Recent studies have shown that a conjugated metabolite of morphine, morphine-6-glucuronide, is 40 times as potent as morphine.[73] It has been found that around 80 percent of the opiate's analgesic action derives from morphine-6-glucuronide after a single dose of morphine and possibly even more at steady state.[5,73] The use of morphine in patients with impaired renal function resulted in prolonged effects and toxicity due to the accumulation of morphine-6-glucuronide.[74,75] The central nervous system depressant effects of opiates including respiratory depression are especially dangerous in the elderly, who are more sensitive to the drugs. Meperidine is oxidatively demethylated in the liver to the still active and more toxic normeperidine, which is renally eliminated. Both renal disease and/or decreased renal function in the elderly can produce excess drug effects with meperidine.

PHARMACODYNAMIC CHANGES IN THE ELDERLY

A number of studies in elderly subjects have shown alterations in some aspects of neural function and responses to certain stimuli and drugs.

Changes in autonomic nervous system function have been found in elderly

Table 3-5 Excretion of digoxin in young and elderly subjects

Group	Number	Age, years	Digoxin clearance, mL/min/1.73 m^2	Blood half-life, h
Young	9	27 ± 4	83 ± 17	51
Old	5	77 ± 4	53 ± 9	73

Source: Adapted from Ewy G, Kapadia GG, Yao L, et al: Digoxin metabolism in the elderly. *Circulation* 39:449–453, 1960. By permission from American Heart Association.

Table 3-6 Renal excretion of penicillin in the elderly according to sex and age groups

	Men, age 50–70		Women, age 30–65	
Number of patients	9	18	7	8
Creatinine clearance, mL/min	93.2	40.3	112.0	61.4
Penicillin half-life, min	23.7	55.5	20.7	39.1

Source: Adapted from Mølholm Hansen J, Kampmann J, Laursen H: Average values (±SD) in different age groups. *Lancet* i:1170, 1970. By permission.

people. The respiratory variation of heart rate during β-adrenergic blockade is an index of cardiac parasympathetic activity. Parasympathetic activity has been found to be reduced in the elderly, whereas plasma norepinephrine and blood pressure are increased, indicating increased cardiovascular sympathetic activity.[76,77] Baroreceptor sensitivity has been shown to be decreased with aging.[77,78]

Sensitivity of elderly subjects to both adrenergic agonist isoproterenol stimulation and β-adrenergic blockade by propranolol has been shown to be reduced.[79] Stimuli such as exercise, which causes increases in plasma catecholamines, do not reliably increase heart rate in elderly subjects.[80,81] This is consonant with the studies showing decreased β-adrenergic responsiveness in the elderly.[82,83] Cardiac output during exercise in healthy elderly subjects is normal by virtue of a greater stroke volume and increased end-systolic and end-diastolic volumes. There is a lesser use in heart rate compared to young exercising subjects probably as a consequence of a decrease in adrenergically mediated cardiovascular reflexes with aging.[80,83,84]

Studies on the arterial system of elderly subjects have shown attenuated responses to β-adrenergic stimulation.[85,86] Elderly subjects have responses to both alpha-adrenergic stimulation and blockade, which are comparable to younger subjects.[87-89]

DRUG SENSITIVITY

Clinical observations have indicated that elderly patients have lower dose requirements for warfarin anticoagulation.[90] Elderly patients had a greater degree of anticoagulation even with lower doses of warfarin (Fig. 3-1).

The increased sensitivity to warfarin anticoagulation was ascertained to be due to a greater decrease in clotting factor synthesis in the elderly compared to younger subjects at the same warfarin concentrations.[91]

Elderly subjects appear to be more sensitive to sedative drugs.[92,93] A number of clinical pharmacologic studies on the pharmacokinetics of the commonly used benzodiazepines in the elderly have been done. These are discussed in Chap. 8. These studies have established a greater sensitivity of elderly subjects to benzodiazepines.[94-96]

Studies on drugs used as analgesics in elderly patients have shown a decrease in narcotic requirements. These studies, like other studies on sensitivity to drugs, have not separated pharmacodynamic from pharmacokinetic contributions to the analgesic response (see Chap. 9). The degree of postoperative pain relief afforded by fixed doses of intramuscular narcotics correlated positively with age. The elderly required decreased doses compared to younger patients.[97] However, pharmacokinetic studies of narcotic use in the elderly have shown a reduced clearance.[98,99] The study of sensitivity to narcotics in the elderly subject entails simultaneous measurements of pharmacokinetic and pharmacodynamic parameters. This is a difficult assessment, but it has been done.[100] It has been shown that electroencephalographic quantification of narcotic effects on the brain allowed the simultaneous measurement of serum

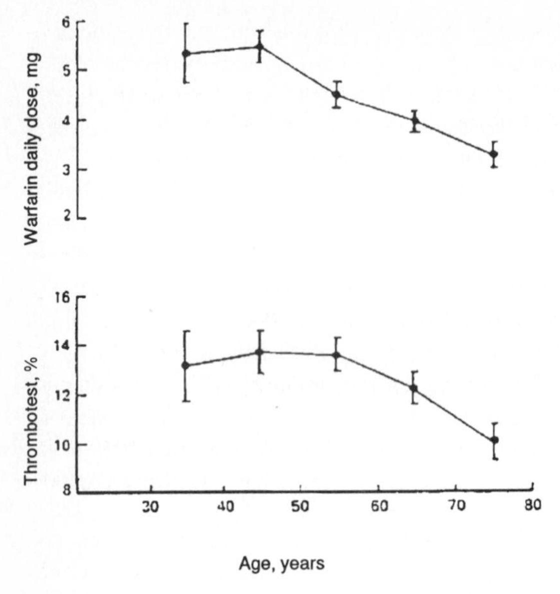

Figure 3-1 Mean ± SD of mean daily dose of warfarin given and thrombotest values for patients in the age ranges shown. *(From O'Malley K, Stevenson IM, Ward CA, Wood AJJ, Crooks J: Determination of anticoagulant control in patients receiving warfarin.* Br J Clin Pharmacol *4:309–314, 1977. Used with permission.)*

narcotic concentrations and brain effects over time. These studies demonstrated increased brain sensitivity to narcotics in elderly subjects.[100,101]

DRUG INTERACTIONS

The incidence of a number of diseases increase as people age. The prevalence of diabetes mellitus, osteoporosis, cancers, hypertension, and cardiovascular diseases all increase with age. Moreover, it is not unusual for elderly people to be afflicted with more than one disease. Chronic diseases are usually treated with drugs, and it is not unusual to have patients being treated with multiple drugs for several diseases by several physicians. In addition to the number of drugs prescribed by physicians for the elderly patient, patients also use over-the-counter drugs for headaches, joint pains, coryza, constipation, allergies, dyspepsia, etc. This health care scene of drug utilization is a fertile one for adverse drug reactions deriving from drug-drug interactions. Drug interactions are in part a function of the number of drugs used.[6,7,33,102]

Although compliance and confusion may contribute to the adverse effects of multiple-drug therapy, there are often pharmacokinetic bases and sometimes pharmacodynamic bases for these unwanted effects.[103,104] These adverse drug effects could be decreased by a better awareness of drug handling by elderly subjects.

Mechanisms by which drug-drug interactions can occur include (1) inhibition of drug absorption; (2) decreased hepatic blood flow; (3) inhibition of renal excretion; (4) inhibition or stimulation of drug metabolism; (5) displacement from albumin binding; and (6) pharmacodynamic effects of drugs on tissue responses. A listing of some drug interactions is shown in Table 3-7.[105]

Some commonly used drugs act as inhibitors of drug metabolism by competing for binding sites. Drugs like erythromycin, cimetidine, valproic acid, dextropropoxyphene, propranolol, phenothiazines, and sulfonamides are inhibitors with maximal effects at around their steady-state concentrations. Warfarin is a widely used drug in the elderly whose metabolism is inhibited by allopurinol, metronidazole, and trimethoprim-sulfamethoxazole. Phenytoin hydroxylation is inhibited by isoniazid, benzodiazepines, and phenothiazines. The inhibitory effects are more pronounced at higher doses of phenytoin because of saturation of the hydroxylating enzymes (dose-dependent kinetics).[106,107]

Drugs which decrease hepatic blood flow such as vasodilators and β-adrenergic blocking agents decrease elimination of drugs with high hepatic extraction ratios. Hydralazine increases the bioavailability of propranolol and metoprolol but not β blockers with low extraction ratios like atenolol, nadolol, and acebutolol.[108]

Drug interactions occur when several renally excreted drugs are used simultaneously. There is competition for the renal tubular carrier systems. The clearance of digoxin by renal and nonrenal systems is decreased by quinidine, verapamil, and amiodarone.[109-111] Nonsteroidal anti-inflammatory drugs and thiazide diuretics decrease lithium clearance.[112,113] These interactions may be more significant in the elderly where renal function is decreased by the aging process.

Cimetidine, which is cleared in part in the unmetabolized state by the kidney, is partially cleared and metabolized by the liver. Cimetidine binds to hepatic cytochrome oxidase in a dose-dependent manner and inhibits the metabolism of a number of drugs including warfarin, phenytoin, and theophylline.[114]

DECREASED HOMEOSTATIC MECHANISM

Age decrements are more marked in physiologic adjustments that require the integrated activity of several organ systems than in those involving a single system. The impairment of renal, hepatic, cardiac, respiratory, neuromuscular, and endocrine vitality with aging results in a slower rate of recovery following a variety of physiologic displacements. Aging is characterized by a diminution of the adaptive capacity to a variety of stimuli. The reduced homeostatic responses of the elderly result in adverse drug reactions that might be compensated for in the younger patient. Decreased cardiac output, lowered plasma volume, diminished vasomotor control, and decreased glucose tolerance all prepare the way for a greater frequency of adverse drug reactions in response to a variety of drugs. Moreover, the elderly

Table 3-7 Clinically important drug interactions

Primary drugs	Interacting drug(s)	Mechanism	Effect
Augmented drug effects			
Warfarin	Phenylbutazone	IM, DA	Hemorrhage
	Metronidazole	IM	
	Aspirin	OM	
Antidiabetic sulfonylureas, (tolbutamide, chlorpropamide)	Sulfaphenazole	IM	Hypoglycemia
	Chloramphenicol	IM	
	Phenylbutazone	IM, DA, IE	
	Warfarin	IM	
Phenytoin	Phenylbutazone	IM	Nystagmus
	Chloramphenicol	IM	Cerebellar ataxia
	INH	IM	Sedation
Azathioprine	Allopurinol	IM	Bone marrow suppression
Methotrexate	Sulfisoxazole	DA	Bone marrow suppression
	Aspirin	IE	
Digoxin	Diuretics	OM	Digitalis intoxication
	Quinidine	OM	
Propranolol	Cimetidine	HBF	Bradycardia
Sedative-hypnotics	Ethanol	OM	Excessive sedation
Decreased drug effects			
Warfarin	Barbiturates	SM	Loss of anticoagulant control
	Rifampin	SM	
	Glutethimide	SM	
	Disopyramide	SM	
Prednisone	Barbiturates	SM	Decreased steroid effects
Steroidal orally administered contraceptives	Rifampin	SM	Loss of contraceptive effects
Quinidine	Barbiturates Rifampin	SM	Decreased antiarrhythmic effect
Lincomycin	Kaolin-pectin	IA	Decreased drug bioavailability
Tetracycline	Antacids-iron	IA	
Tolbutamide	Thiazide diuretics	OM	Decreased hypoglycemic effects
Chlorpropamide	Corticosteriods	OM	

DA = displacement from albumin binding; HBF = decreased hepatic blood flow; IA = inhibition of drug absorption; IE = inhibition of renal excretion; IM = inhibition of drug metabolism; OM = other mechanisms (pharmacodynamic effects of drugs on tissue responses); SM = stimulation of drug metabolism.

are not infrequently afflicted with several chronic diseases, which may necessitate use of multiple-drug therapy.

The impaired homeostatic capacity, multiple chronic illnesses, and multiple-drug therapy afford greater opportunity for adverse drug reactions. Because of decreased capacity for cardiovascular homeostasis, elderly patients are more prone to develop postural hypotension secondary to the use of diuretics, sympatholytics, nitrates, phenothiazines, tricyclic antidepressants, quinidine, procainamide, and antihypertensive drugs. Adverse drug reactions are also more common in the elderly because of the multiplicity of drugs required, their long-term use, and the occurrence of drug-drug interactions.

Elderly patients experience adverse drug reactions even with the most careful medical care. Sedative hypnotics depress mentation and cerebral circulation, resulting in manifold mental and physical changes. The combination of alcohol, barbiturates, and tranquilizers is poorly tolerated by elderly subjects and is therefore contraindicated.

Hallucinations and other forms of disturbed cerebral function may follow the administration of antiparkinsonian, sympathomimetic, or anticholinergic drugs in addition to the risk of glaucoma and urinary retention. The supposed suicide may in fact be an accidental death when sedatives are prescribed injudiciously or taken repeatedly by an increasingly confused old person.

In summary, adverse drug responses in the elderly are the result of a composite of pathophysiologic characteristics of the aging process. Anoxic, anemic, and hypothyroid states increase sensitivity to morphine, barbiturates, and sedative drugs.

A general rule of therapeutics is that the correct dose for every patient must be empirically determined. In the elderly it is especially important to individualize therapy. When one deals with these patients, unusual responses, including tolerance, hypersensitivity, and toxicity, should be suspected and carefully evaluated.

AVOIDANCE OF ADVERSE DRUG REACTIONS IN THE ELDERLY

The avoidance of adverse drug reactions is a rational goal but is difficult in the elderly patient. Age-related impairment of renal excretion and hepatic metabolism and less adaptive homeostatic mechanisms of the cardiovascular, renal, respiratory, neurologic, and endocrine systems make the older patient more sensitive to usual drug doses and to drug-drug interactions. Some guidelines to drug therapy in the elderly patient follow:

1. Establish a diagnosis before treating. Drug therapy ideally should be considered for a definite period of time or a definite symptomatic or biochemical end point. Treatment should be aimed at altering the natural history of a disease

(hypertension, depression, psychosis, arteriosclerotic disease) and not merely be a symptomatic intervention. The gain-risk aspect of drug therapy in the elderly must be considered because of the higher frequency and severity of adverse drug reactions.

2. Review the elderly patient's drug regimen frequently and be alert to the possibility that other physicians are prescribing drugs for the patient. The elderly patient with multiple diseases usually is treated with multiple drugs. These include drugs directed against specific diseases as well as nonprescription drugs, such as aspirin, sympathomimetics, antihistamines, caffeine, and anticholingerics. Periodic drug review and compliance evaluation are worthwhile.
3. Minimize the number of drugs being used. Review the pharmacologic actions of the drug(s) being used and their mode of inactivation or elimination from the body (e.g., renal excretion, hepatic metabolism). Monitor the patient for both therapeutic and adverse effects until steady-state levels have been reached (five half-lives); this may be up to twice the time period for the younger patient. Use the lowest dose that is effective in the individual patient with careful attention to and monitoring of the patient during the drug induction period. Adjust the maintenance dose downward if advancing age is associated with impairment of the major mode of drug elimination.
4. When one encounters symptoms that mimic stereotypes associated with old age (forgetfulness, weakness, confusion, anorexia, anxiety), suspect a drug reaction as a contributing factor, especially if the patient is receiving a psychotropic drug, sedative-hypnotic, or drugs affecting cardiac output or the renal system.

REFERENCES

1. Bender AD: Pharmacologic aspects of aging: a survey of the effect of increasing age on drug activity in adults. *J Am Geriatr Soc* 12:114-134, 1964.
2. Vestal RE: Clinical pharmacology, in Hazzard WR, Andres R, Bierman EL, Blass JP (eds): *Principles of Geriatric Medicine*. New York, McGraw-Hill, 1990, pp 201-211.
3. Tsujimoto G, Hashimoto K, Hoffman BB: Pharmacokinetic and pharmacodynamic principles of drug therapy in old age. Part I. *Int J Clin Pharmacol Ther Toxicol* 27:13-26, 1989.
4. Tsujimoto G, Hashimoto K, Hoffman BB: Pharmacokinetic and pharmacodynamic principles of drug therapy in old age. Part II. *Int J Clin Pharmacol Ther Toxicol* 27:102-116, 1989.
5. Dawling S, Crome P: Clinical pharmacokinetic considerations in the elderly: an update. *Clin Pharmacokinet* 17:236-263, 1989.
6. Adams KRH, Al-Hamouz S, Edmund E, et al: Inappropriate prescribing in the elderly. *J Roy Coll Phys Lond* 21:39-41, 1987.
7. Gosney M, Tallis R: Prescription of contraindicated and interacting drugs in elderly patients admitted to hosptial. *Lancet* 2:564-567, 1984.
8. Nielson CP, Cusack BJ, Vestal RE: Geriatric clinical pharmacology and therapeutics, in Speight TM (ed): *Avery's Drug Treatment*, 3d ed. Baltimore, Williams and Wilkins, 1987, pp 162-193.

9. Plein JB, Plein EM: Aging and drug therapy. *Ann Rev Gerontol Geriatr* 2:211-254, 1981.
10. Bender A: The effect of increasing age on the distribution of peripheral blood flow in man. *J Am Geriatr Soc* 13:192-198, 1965.
11. Forbes GB, Reina JC: Adult lean body mass declines with age: some longitudinal observations. *Metabolism* 19:653-663, 1970.
12. Schulz P, Turner-Tamiyasu K, Smith G, et al: Amitriptyline disposition in young and elderly normal men. *Clin Pharmacol Ther* 33:360-366, 1983.
13. Christensen JH, Andreasen F, Jansen JA: Pharmacokinetics and pharmacodynamics of thiopentone. *Anaesthesia* 37:398-404, 1982.
14. Klotz U, Avant GR, Hoyumpa A, et al: The effects of age and liver disease on the disposition and elimination of diazepam in adult man. *J Clin Invest* 55:347-359, 1975.
15. Divoli M, Abernethy DR, Amels B, Greenblatt DJ: Acetaminophen kinetics in the elderly. *Clin Pharmacol Ther* 31:151-156, 1982.
16. Cusack B, Horgan J, Kelly JG, et al: Digoxin in the elderly: pharmacokinetic consequences of old age. *Clin Pharmacol Ther* 25:772-776, 1979.
17. Shammas FV, Dickstein K: Clinical pharmacokinetics in heart failure. *Clin Pharmacokinet* 15:94-113, 1988.
18. Thomson PD: Alterations in pharmacologic response induced by cardiovascular disease, in Melmon KL (ed): *Cardiovascular Drug Therapy.* Philadelphia, F. A. Davis, 1974, pp 55-61.
19. Thomson PD, Melmon KL, Richardson JA, et al: Lidocaine pharmacokinetics in advanced heart failure, liver disease and renal failure in humans. *Ann Intern Med* 78:499-508, 1973.
20. Greenblatt DJ: Reduced serum albumin concentration in the elderly: a report from the Boston Collaborative Drug Surveillance Program. *J Am Geriatr Soc* 27:564-567, 1979.
21. Wallace SM, Verbeeck RG: Plasma protein binding of drugs in the elderly. *Clin Pharmacokinet* 12:41-72, 1987.
22. Mather LE, Tucker GT, Pflug AE, et al: Meperidine kinetics in man: intravenous injection in surgical patients and volunteers. *Clin Pharmacol Ther* 17:21-30, 1975.
23. Hayes MJ, Langman MJS, Short AH: Changes in drug metabolism with increasing age. I. Warfarin binding and plasma proteins. *Br J Clin Pharmacol* 2:69-72, 1975.
24. Levy RH, Moreland TA: Rationale for monitoring free drug levels. *Clin Pharmacokinet* 9(suppl):1-9, 1984.
25. Rodehefferf RJ, Gerstenblith GMD, Becker LG, et al: Exercise cardiac output is maintained with advancing age in healthy human subjects: cardiac dilatation and increased stroke volume compensation for a diminished heart rate. *Circulation* 69:203-213, 1984.
26. Pfeifer MA, Weinberg CR, Cook D, et al: Differential changes of autonomic nervous system function with age in man. *Am J Med* 75:249-258, 1983.
27. Gerstenblith G, Lakatta EG, Weisfeldt ML: Age changes in myocardial function and exercise response. *Prog Cardiovasc Dis* 19:1-21, 1976.
28. Learoyd BM: Psychotropic drugs and the elderly patient. *Med J Australia* 1:1131-1133, 1972.
29. Vestal RE, McGuire EA, Tobin JD, et al: Aging and ethanol metabolism. *Clin Pharmacol Ther* 21:343-354, 1977.
30. Sellers EM, Frecher RC, Romach MK: Drug metabolism in the elderly: Confounding of age, smoking and ethanol effects. *Drug Metab Rev* 14:225-250, 1983.
31. Thomspon TL, Moran MG, Nies AS: Psychotropic drug use in the elderly. *N Engl J Med* 308:134-138, 194-199, 1938.
32. Vestal RE, Cusack BJ: Pharmacology of aging, in Schneider EL, Rowe JW (eds): *Handbook of the Biology of Aging*, 3d ed. San Diego, California, Academic Press, 1990, pp 349-383.
33. Abrass IB: Drug therapy, in Kane RL, Ouslander JG, Abrass IB (eds): *Essentials of Clinical Geriatrics,* 2d ed. New York, McGraw-Hill, 1989, pp 341-361.
34. Vestal RE, Dawson GW: Pharmacology and aging, in Finch CE, Schneider EL (eds): *Handbook of the Biology of Aging*, 2d ed. New York, Van Nostrand, 1985, pp 744-819.
35. Nebert DW, Gonzalez FJ: Cytochrome P450 gene expression and regulations. *Tips* 165:160-164, 1985.

36. Vestal RE: Aging and determinants of hepatic drug clearance. *Hepatology* 9:331-334, 1989.
37. Montamat SC, Cusack BJ, Vestal RE: Management of drug therapy in the elderly. *N Engl J Med* 321: 303-309, 1989.
38. Durnas C, Loi CM, Cusak BJ: Hepatic drug metabolism and aging. *Clin Pharmacokinet* 19:359-389, 1990.
39. Castleden CM, George CF: The effect of aging on the hepatic clearance of propranolol. *Br J Clin Pharmacol* 7:49-54, 1979.
40. Kelly JG, McGarry K, O'Malley K, O'Brien ET: Bioavailability of labetalol increases with age. *Br J Clin Pharmacol* 14:304-305, 1982.
41. Nation RL, Vine J, Triggs EJ, Learoyd B: Plasma level of chlormethiazole and two metabolites after oral administration to young and aged human subjects. *Eur J Clin Pharmacol* 12:137-145, 1977.
42. Storstein L, Larsen A, Midtbo K, Saevareid L. Pharmacokinetics of calcium channel blockers in patients with renal insufficiency and in geriatric patients. *Acta Med Scand* 681(suppl 1):25-30, 1984.
43. Geokas MC, Haverback BJ: The aging gastrointestinal tract. *Am J Surg* 117:881-892, 1969.
44. Wilkinson GR, Shand DG: A physiological approach to hepatic drug clearance. *Clin Pharmacol Ther* 18:377-390, 1975.
45. Wynne HA, Cope LH, Mutch E, et al: The effect of age upon liver volume and apparent liver blood flow in healthy man. *Hepatology* 9:297-301, 1989.
46. Woodhouse KW, Wynne HA: Age-related changes in liver size and hepatic blood flow: the influence on drug metabolism in the elderly. *Clin Pharmacokinet* 15:287-296, 1988.
47. Pirtiaho HI, Sotaniemi EA, Alquist J, et al: Liver size and indices of drug metabolism in alcoholics. *Eur J Clin Pharmacol* 13:61-67, 1978.
48. Homeida M, Robert CJC, Halliwell M, et al: Antipyrine clearance per unit volume liver: an assessment of hepatic function in chronic liver disease. *Gut* 20:596-601, 1979.
49. Gersovitz M, Munro HN, Udall J, Young VR: Albumin synthesis in young and elderly subjects using a new stable isotope methodology: response to level protein intake. *Metabolism* 29:1075-1086, 1980.
50. McLachlan MSF: The aging kidney. *Lancet* 2:143-145, 1978.
51. Williams FM, Wynne H, Woodhouse KW, Rawlins MD: Plasma aspirin esterase: the influence of old age and frailty. *Age Aging* 18:39-42, 1989.
52. O'Malley K, Crooks J, Duke E, Stevenson JH: Effects of age and sex on human drug metabolism. *Br Med J* 3:607-609, 1971.
53. Vestal RE: Drug use in the elderly: a review of problems and special considerations. *Drugs* 16:358-382, 1978.
54. Greenblatt DJ, Seller EM, Shader RI: Drug disposition in old age. *N Engl J Med* 306:1081-1088, 1982.
55. Abernethy DR, Greenblatt DJ, Shader RI: Imipramine and desipramine disposition in the elderly. *J Pharmacol Exp Ther* 232:133-138, 1985.
56. Cohen BM, Sommer BR: Metabolism of thioridazine in the elderly. *J Clin Pharmacol* 8:336-339, 1988.
57. Ouslander JG: Drug therapy in the elderly. *Ann Intern Med* 95: 711-722, 1981.
58. Swift CG, Triggs EJ: Clinical pharmacokinetics in the elderly, in Swift CG (ed): *Clinical Pharmacology in the Elderly*. New York, Marcel Dekker, 1987, pp 31-82.
59. Wynne HA, Mutch E, James OFW, et al: The effect of age upon the affinity of microsomal monooxygenase enzymes for substrate in human liver. *Age Aging* 17:401-405, 1988.
60. Drayer DE: Pharmacokinetic differences between drug enantiomers in man, in Wainer IW, Drayer DE (eds): *Drug Stereochemistry: Analytical Methods and Pharmacology*. New York, Marcel Dekker, 1988, pp 209-225.
61. Hooper WD, Qing MS: The influence of age and gender on the stereoselective metabolism and pharmacokinetic of mephobarbital in humans. *Clin Pharmacol Ther* 48:633-640, 1990.
62. Salem SAM, Rajgayaben P, Shepard AMM, Stevenson IH: Reduced induction of drug metabolism in the elderly. *Age Aging* 7:68-73, 1978.

63. Vestal RE, Wood AJJ, Branch RA, et al: Effects of age and cigarette smoking on propranolol disposition. *Clin Pharmacol Ther* 26:8-15, 1979.
64. Jusko WJ, Gardiner MJ, Mangione A, et al: Factors affecting theophylline clearances: age, tobacco, marijuana, congestive heart failure, obesity, oral contraceptives, benzodiazepines, barbiturates and ethanol. *J Pharmaceut Sci* 68:1358-1366, 1979.
65. Branch RA, Herman RJ: Enzyme induction and β-adrenergic receptor blocking drugs. *Br J Clin Pharmacol* 21:371-376, 1984.
66. Bonde J, Pedersen LE, Bodtker S, et al: The influence of age and smoking on the elimination of disopyramide. *Br J Clin Pharmacol* 20:453-458, 1985.
67. Crowley JJ, Cusack BJ, Jue SG, et al: Aging and drug interactions: II. Effect of phenytoin and smoking on the oxidation of theophylline and cortisol in healthy men. *J Pharmacol Exper Ther* 245:513-523, 1988.
68. Rowe JW: Aging, renal function and response to drugs. *Aging* 16:115-130, 1981.
69. Davies DE, Shock NW: Age changes in glomerular filtration rate, effective renal plasma flow and tubular excretory capacity in adult males. *J Clin Invest* 29:496-507, 1950.
70. Rowe JW, Andres R, Tobin JD, et al: The effect of age on creatinine clearance in men: a cross-sectional and longitudinal study. *J Gerontol* 31:155-163, 1976.
71. Shock NW: Age changes in renal function, in Cowdreys L (ed): *Problems of Aging*. Baltimore, Williams and Wilkins, 1952, pp 614-630.
72. Luke DR, Halstenson CE, Opsahl JA, Matzke GR: Validity of creatinine clearance estimates in the assessment of renal function. *Clin Pharmacol Ther* 48:503-508, 1990.
73. Shimomura K, Kamata O, Veki S, et al: Analgesic effect of morphine glucuronides. *Tohoku J Exper Med* 105:45-52, 1971.
74. Osborne RJ, Joel SP, Selvin ML: Morphine intoxication in renal failure: the role of morphine-6-glucuronide. *Br Med J* 292:1548-1549, 1986.
75. Sawe J, Suensson JO, Odar-Cederlof I: Kinetics of morphine in patients with renal failure. *Lancet* 2:211, 1985.
76. Halter J: Alterations of autonomic nervous system function, in Andres R, Bierman EL, Hazzard WR (eds): *Principles of Geriatric Medicine*. New York, McGraw-Hill, 1985, pp 218-230.
77. Rowe JW, Troen BR: Sympathetic nervous system and aging in man. *Endocrinol Rev* 1:167-178, 1980.
78. Gribbin B, Pickering TG, Sleight P, Peto R: Effect of age and high blood pressure on baroreceptor sensitivity in man. *Circulat Res* 29:424-431, 1971.
79. Vestal RE, Wood AJJ, Shand DG: Reduced beta-adrenoreceptor sensitivity in the elderly. *Clin Pharmacol Ther* 26:181-186, 1979.
80. Lakatta EG: Age-related alterations in the cardiovascular response to adrenergic mediated stress. *Fed Proc* 39:3173-3177, 1980.
81. Fleg JL, Lakatta EG: Cardiovascular disease in old age, in Rossman I (ed): *Clinical Geriatrics*, 3d ed. Philadelphia, Lippincott, 1986, pp 169-196.
82. Roth GS, Hess GD: Changes in the mechanism of hormone and neurotransmitter action during aging: Current status of the role of receptor and postreceptor alterations. *Mech Aging Dev* 20:175-194, 1982.
83. Lakatta EG, Yin FCP: Myocardial aging: functional alterations and related cellular mechanisms. *Am J Physiol* 242(Heart Circ Physiol): H927-H941, 1982.
84. Lakatta EG, Gernstenblith G, Angell CS, et al: Diminished inotropic response of aged myocardium to catecholamines. *Circ Res* 36:262-269, 1975.
85. Strozzi C, Cocco G, Destro A, et al: Disorders in peripheral arterial system in asymptomatic elderly. Plethysmographic semiology at rest, during postural efforts and pharmacological tests. *Gerontology* 25:24-34, 1979.
86. Van Brummelen P, Buhler FR, Kiowski W, Amann FW: Age related decrease in cardiac and peripheral vascular responsiveness to isoprenaline: studies in normal subjects. *Clin Sc (OXF)* 60:571-577, 1981.

87. Elliott HL, Summer DJ, McLean K, Rein JL: Effect of age on the responsiveness of vascular alpha-adrenoreceptors in man. *J Cardiovasc Pharmacol* 4:388–392, 1982.
88. Stevens MJ, Lipe S, Moulds RFW: The effect of age on the responses of human isolated arteries and veins to noradrenaline. *Br J Clin Pharmacol* 14:750–752, 1982.
89. Scott PJW, Reid JL: The effect of age on the responses of human isolated arteries to noradrenaline. *Br J Clin Pharmacol* 13:237–239, 1982.
90. O'Malley K, Stevenson IM, Ward CA, et al: Determination of anticoagulant control in patients receiving warfarin. *Br J Clin Pharmacol* 4:309–314, 1977.
91. Shepherd AMM, Hewick OS, Moreland TA, Stevenson IH: Age as a determinant of sensitivity to warfarin. *Br J Clin Pharmacol* 4:315–320, 1977.
92. Greenblatt DJ, Allen MD: Toxicity of nitrazepam in the elderly: A report from the Boston Collaborative Drug Surveillance Program. *Br J Clin Pharmacol* 5:407–413, 1978.
93. Reidenberg MM, Levy M, Warner H, et al: Relationship between diazepam dose, plasma level, age and central nervous system depression. *Clin Pharmacol Ther* 23:371–374, 1978.
94. Greenblatt DJ, Allen MD, Shader RI: Toxicity of high dose flurazepam in the elderly. *Clin Pharmacol Ther* 21:355–361, 1977.
95. Castleden CM, George CF, Marcer D, Hallett C: Increased sensitivity to nitrazepam in old age. *Br Med J* 1:10–12, 1977.
96. Swift CG, Haythorne JM, Clarke P, Stevenson IH: The effect of aging on measured responses to single doses of oral temazepam. *Br J Clin Pharmacol* 11:413–414, 1981.
97. Kaiko RF: Age and morphine analgesia in cancer patients with postoperative pain. *Clin Pharmacol Ther* 28:823–826, 1980.
98. Helmer H, van Peer A, Woestenborgh R, et al: Alfentanil kinetics in the elderly. *Clin Pharmacol Ther* 36:239–243, 1984.
99. Owens JA, Sitar DS, Berger L, et al: Age-related morphine kinetics. *Clin Pharmacol Ther* 34:364–368, 1983.
100. Scott JC, Stanski DR: Decreased fentanyl and alfentanil dose requirement with age. A simultaneous pharmacokinetic and pharmacodynamic evaluation. *J Pharmacol Exp Ther* 240:159–166, 1987.
101. Scott JC, Ponganis KV, Stanski DR: EEG quantification of narcotic effect: the comparative pharmacodynamics of fentanyl and alfentanil. *Anesthesiology* 62:234–241, 1985.
102. McInnes GT, Brodie MJ: Drug interactions that matter: a critical reappraisal. *Drugs* 36:83–110, 1988.
103. Blaschke T, Cohen S, Tatro D: Drug-drug interactions and aging, in Jarvic L (ed): *Clinical Pharmacology and the Aged Patient*. New York, Raven, 1981, pp 11–26.
104. Nolan L, O'Malley K: Prescribing for the elderly. Part II. Prescribing patterns: differences due to age. *J Am Geriatr Soc* 36:1245–1254, 1988.
105. Nolan L, O'Malley K: Prescribing for the elderly. Part I: Sensitivity of the elderly to adverse drug reactions. *J Am Geriatr Soc* 36:142–149, 1988.
106. Perucca E, Rickens A: Drug interactions involving drugs used in the treatment of epilepsy, in Petrie JC (ed): *Clinically Important Adverse Drug Interactions*, vol 2. Amsterdam, Elsevier, 1984, pp 99–146.
107. Miller RR, Porter J, Greenblatt DJ: Clinical importance of the interaction of phenytoin and isoniazid. *Chest* 75:356–358, 1979.
108. McLean AJ, Wilhelm D, Heinzow BG: Stable oral availability of atenolol coadministered with hydralazine. *Drugs* 25(suppl 2):131–135, 1983.
109. Doering W: Quinidine-digoxin interaction. *N Engl J Med* 301:400–404, 1979.
110. Moysey JO, Jaggarao NSV, Grundy EN, Chamberlain DA: Amiodarone increases plasma digoxin concentrations. *Br Med J* 282:272, 1981.
111. Petersen KE, Thayssen P, Klitgaard NA, et al: Influence of verapamil on the inotropism and pharmacogenetics of digoxin. *Eur J Clin Pharmacol* 25:199–206, 1983.
112. Hurtig HI, Dyson WL: Lithium toxicity enhanced by diuresis. *N Engl J Med* 290:748–749, 1974.

113. Jefferson JW, Greisi JH, Carroll J, Baudhuin M: Drug-drug and drug-disease interactions with nonsteroidal antiinflammatory drugs. *Am J Med* 81:948, 1986.
114. Smith SR, Kendall MJ: Randitidine versus cimetidine: a comparison of their potential to cause clinically important drug interactions. *Clin Pharmacokinet* 15:44–56, 1988.

CHAPTER

4

COMPLIANCE WITH PRESCRIBED DRUG REGIMENS

Richard N. Herrier
Robert W. Boyce

Over the last 20 years, patient noncompliance with prescribed drug therapy has become increasingly recognized as a major contributor to poor therapeutic outcomes.[1-9] Inadequate long-term nonadherence to treatment regimens has been cited as the major problem in controlling hypertension.[2] Research estimates that noncompliance is responsible for over 10 percent of all hospital admissions as well as 300,000 hospital admissions and 125,000 deaths annually among patients with cardiovascular diseases.[8,9] Estimates of the cost of noncompliance due to additional outpatient visits, hospitalizations, nursing home admissions, and emergency room visits range from 13 to 22 billion dollars each year.[9]

Pharmacists, nurses, and physicians, through their professional organizations and state licensing boards, have implemented standards of practice and regulations that include compliance enhancement and patient education activities as major professional responsibilities. In response, educational institutions have increased their efforts at improving health professional skills in these areas. The Omnibus Budget Reconciliation Act (OBRA), passed in 1990, and recent white papers by the Inspector General of the Department of Health and Human Services[8] and the Commissioner of the Food and Drug Administration[10] have given notice of a more active role of the federal government in this significant problem.

The opinions expressed in this document are those of the authors and do not necessarily reflect the views of the Indian Health Service, U.S. Public Health Service, or the Department of Health and Human Services.

NONCOMPLIANCE IN THE ELDERLY

Most health care professionals assume that, among elderly patients, compliance with prescribed treatment regimens is far below published averages of 40 to 50 percent for all age groups. However, the compliance literature fails to support this assumption, and some studies indicate better compliance among certain groups of elderly patients than is seen in the general population.[11] While rates of compliance with prescribed medications have not been shown to be related to age, the elderly are at greater risk of encountering compliance problems because of their higher rate of medication use, including more complex multidrug regimens, resulting from a higher incidence of chronic disease.[8] Adults aged 65 and over represent over 12 percent of the current population and consume 30 percent of all prescription medication prescribed. This population percentage is expected to double over the next four decades.[8]

In addition to risks associated with higher frequency and complexity of drug use, traditional compliance-enhancing strategies appear to be more prone to failure in this age group due to unique problems seen in the elderly.[7, 8, 12, 13] Vision and hearing impairment occurs more frequently among the elderly. Ninety percent of patients over 60 require correction of vision. In older patients nearly one-eighth are considered legally blind and over one-third may have cataracts. Color vision is also negatively impacted by age. Almost a third have hearing impairment severe enough to interfere with normal speech and communication. Lack of dexterity, decreased mobility, decreased ability to recall information, social isolation, limited income, and impaired mental status have also been cited as important factors in reducing the effectiveness of compliance-enhancing strategies in the elderly.[7]

ASSESSING COMPLIANCE

Patient adherence with prescribed drug therapy is a dynamic process. It is well established that compliance rates with drug therapy for chronic diseases such as diabetes and hypertension decrease over time.[3, 5] In addition, the fluctuations that occur in daily life (e.g., schedule changes, intercurrent acute illness, special life events) make "perfect adherence" a difficult goal for even the most motivated patients to attain.

Similarly, accurate assessment of the degree of compliance is a difficult goal to attain for providers. Almost all methods currently used tend to overestimate compliance, can be easily defeated by patients, or are difficult to interpret due to interpatient variability.[7, 9]

Achievement of treatment goals (e.g., normal blood pressure or glucose level) can be a good indicator of compliance. However, by adhering to the therapy only for a short period of time prior to the provider visit, patients can present with disease parameters that make them appear compliant and under good control. Pill counts and self-reporting can be effective, but pill dumping and adjustments of the treatment record may mask noncompliant behavior. Computerized recording devices and drug blood levels, while appearing to be the most accurate, have similar limitations that allow patients to mask less than optimal compliance.

One of the most frequently used assessment methods is patient interviewing. Because many studies have shown the severe limitations of this approach, it has been incorrectly labeled as unreliable and stimulated searches for better assessment methods.[9, 14] However, most of these studies used interview techniques (closed-ended questions) and approaches (questions that imply negative feedback if improperly answered) which facilitated the patient's ability to mask noncompliance and avoid negative provider feedback. This use of less than optimal interview technique probably accounts for much of the discrepancy between interview results and actual compliance noted in the research literature.

The exact wording of the questions is important.[15, 16] Open-ended questions such as "How are you taking your medicine?"; "What kind of problem are you having with your medication"; "How do you feel about your medication?"; or "What was the hardest part about taking your medication?" are appropriate to begin questioning. Preceding open-ended questions with a statement also encourages factual responses, e.g., "Most patients find it difficult to remember to take all their pills. What kind of problems have you been having?" (or "How did it go for you?"). If compliance problems are acknowledged, then specific open-ended questions can be used to further delineate problems. Once you have a good idea as to the specifics of the patient's compliance problems, a supportive open-ended question such as "What can we do to make it easier for you to remember?" will open a supportive dialogue aimed at helping patients find ways to improve their compliance.

Even if all techniques used to assess compliance have limitations, there are some practical actions that providers can take to maximize the accuracy of their compliance assessment.

1. *Have realistic expections.* Providers need to recognize the difficulties involved for anyone to perfectly adhere to long-term drug therapy. During initial education efforts, acknowledge your awareness of the difficulties involved, note that it will take a while to get into the new routine of taking medicines, alert patients to your plan to monitor compliance regularly, and reassure them that you will be supportive in helping them work out any problems.

2. *Use nonthreatening open-ended questions.* Use appropriate open-ended questions to ascertain the level of the patient's compliance and specific problems associated with medicine taking.

3. *Be supportive not punitive.* As a provider, avoid internalizing patient's noncompliance, e.g., assuming it is your failure or a rejection of you and your efforts. Similarly, avoid viewing patient failures as character defects or a lack of effort or concern. These traps lead to negative feedback to the patient, unwanted critical parental behavior by the provider, and ultimately patient's hiding true compliance problems from the provider. If the approach to the patient is realistic, recognizes inherent difficulties, and attempts to create a partnership to work out

compliance problems, the patient can be truthful about actual compliance without fear of reprisal.

4. *Use several methods.* In addition to creating a proper environment and using open-ended questions during the interview, the provider should periodically or routinely use one or more additional compliance assessment methods simultaneously, e.g., attainment of desired outcomes, pill counts, medication refill record check, and drug blood levels.[9]

PRACTICAL STRATEGIES FOR IMPROVING COMPLIANCE

Patient-focused Approaches

Assess noncompliance risk factors Patients should be evaluated for problems that may either interfere with the patient's ability to comply or reduce the effectiveness of compliance-enhancing strategies. Some of the evaluation can be done by record review, e.g., looking for a past history of compliance behavior, drugs used in other diseases, and the presence of diagnoses that interfere with compliance (e.g., mental retardation, alcoholism, dementia). Careful patient interview can reveal potential problems, e.g., inability to communicate in English, impaired mental status, low levels of social and family support, inability to pay for therapy, hearing difficulties, patient preference for level of involvement with treatment decisions, health beliefs or cultural values that may interfere with desired behavior, and patient attitudes about their disease and medicine taking. Patient health beliefs play a major role in determining patient compliance.[3,5-7,17] In some cultures, illness is regarded as punishment for inappropriate behavior and must be endured for true healing to take place. In that situation, taking medication to cure or control the illness would be contrary to patient values. Patients who attempt to deny their illness may see treatment as a constant reminder and negative symbol of their vulnerability. Others fear medication and may feel that they or society are overmedicated. Physical assessment may be required to assess patient mobility, manual dexterity, vision, and hearing.

Maintain flexible, individualized approach to patients Patient satisfaction, derived primarily from the quality of the patient-provider relationship, is an important factor in enhancing compliance.[11,18,19] How well the provider creates a relationship that matches the patient's perceived needs has a major impact on determining patient satisfaction. This requires the provider to develop an individualized approach for each patient.

In recent years, there has been increasing advocacy in the literature for active involvement of the patient as a partner in health care decisions as an effective tool to improve patient satisfaction, compliance, and patient outcomes.[20] In particular, patients born after 1940 generally place higher values on knowledge and assertiveness and prefer significant levels of knowledge about their illness and a more active involvement in the decisions regarding treatment. In contrast, the current generation of geriatric patients, with their greater awe and admiration for providers plus a greater respect for authority and rules, exhibit a lower desire to be actively involved.[21] Race, culture, sex, and the disease also have impact on the level of involvement the patient desires. Unfortunately, patient attitudes and beliefs about the severity of disease and the value of treatment as well as their preferences regarding the level of involvement in care decisions are not static but fluctuate or permanently shift based on levels of acceptance of their chronic illness, life experiences, and new knowledge. Patients who normally prefer a more passive role may at times want to be very involved in decisions, and patients who usually insist on active involvement may periodically choose to play a more passive role.

To aid in determining individual levels of desire for active involvement, some authors have classified patients according to a *locus of control* theory.[6,20] *Externals* tend to be fatalistic and see life events as a result of powers beyond their personal control and understanding, e.g., luck, chance, fate, deities. Externals tend to prefer the traditional directive role of the provider and passive role as a patient. *Internals* perceive that life events are a function of his or her behavior or actions and prefer a more active role in the patient-provider relationship.

There are three significant implications of these findings for providers. First, as the current nongeriatric population ages, there will be a continually growing patient demand for a more active role in treatment decisions. To maximize opportunities for compliant behavior, providers dealing with geriatric patients will need to shift from a directive style to that of a partnership as their primary role. Second, using patient preferences for levels of involvement, attitudes, and beliefs, providers will need to select a relationship style appropriate to each patient. Finally, the provider must remain sensitive to changes in those preferences, continually assessing them and adjusting the patient-provider relationship according to patient preferences in order to maintain a strong patient-provider relationship.

Use stepwise approach to implement patient education and therapeutic regimens Because of the demands of a busy workload and need to perform at high professional levels, providers may, at the time of initial diagnosis, overload the patient with a comprehensive educational program and a long list of major behavioral changes to implement. Considering modern social learning theory, it is not suprising that patients view the treatment as a more serious problem than the disease, which may result in significant compliance problems and poor control of their illness.[22,23] In the end, the provider's zealous efforts may lead to the outcomes he or she was trying to prevent—disease complications secondary to inadequate treatment.

Applied to patient compliance, one aspect of social learning therapy, the self-efficacy concept, proposes that patients' perception of their capability to carry out provider recommendations strongly influences what they will attempt and how much effort they will expend to overcome barriers to compliance.[20,23] Patients tend to avoid activities they believe exceed their capabilities but will try those they feel capable of performing. Combining self-efficacy with traditional learning principles and the health belief model strongly suggests that an incremental approach to patient education and the implementation of therapeutic regimens is the most efficient and likely to achieve long-term success.[23] This is particularly true with chronic diseases such as mild to moderate hypertension or non-insulin-dependent diabetes mellitus, where small delays in implementing therapy will not adversely effect long-term outcomes or complications.

Drug Regimen–focused Approaches

Minimize cost of therapy Forty percent of the population over 65 have incomes near or below the poverty level and may not be able to afford newer and generally more expensive drugs.[8] Inability to pay for medication and the high cost of prescriptions is the second most common reason for noncompliance.[24,25] When considering the cost of therapy, one needs to include costs of ancillary items.[8] In a diabetic patient, those items such as blood glucose testing machines, testing strips, and syringes may exceed the cost of therapy or are not covered by third-party payors.

In addition to minimizing economic costs associated with a particular treatment regimen, the provider must limit the personal costs, i.e., side effects of medication and personal inconvenience. Side effects of medication may be a significant factor in up to 25 percent of patients discontinuing or altering their medication regimen.[8] Negative effects perceived by the patient as being caused by the drug therapy may have an even greater impact.[19] In general, drug regimens with higher degrees of patient inconvenience or those requiring significant behavior changes have higher incidences of noncompliance by patients.[5,6,7,19] Patients whose regimen consists of several types of intervention, i.e., diet, blood testing, and pill taking, will have different rates of compliance for each intervention, the relative rates determined by the relative degree of behavior change or inconvenience as perceived by the patient. In one study among type II diabetics medication adherence rates were considerably higher (87 percent) than rates of adherence to other aspects of the regimen—diet, exercise (50 percent), and blood glucose testing (60 percent).[26]

Simplify the treatment regimen The more complex the drug regimen, the more likely patients will have problems adhering to it. Decreasing the number of pills per dose, the number of drugs in the treatment regimen, or the number of doses per day have all been associated with improved compliance.[3,5-9] However, when selecting a drug regimen or changing a current regimen, the provider must be aware of the differences between the pharmacokinetic (half-life) and pharmacodynamic (duration of desired response) properties of each drug used to treat a particular disease. For example, methyldopa and propranolol have kinetic half-lifes that indicate the need to administer the drug three to four times a day to maintain adequate blood levels. However, clinical trials show that the antihypertensive effects for a single dose last long enough to allow once or twice daily dosing in many patients. Similarly, data showing improved compliance rates by decreasing the frequency of doses may be misleading. Interpreting studies measuring compliance relative to dosage frequency is made difficult by three factors—differing definitions of compliance, questionable research methods, and a built-in sample bias—because the vast majority of patients who participate are either highly motivated or already compliant. A careful review of the literature[3,7,27-29] shows an improvement in compliance rates for drugs that are taken once a day when compared to those taken three or four times daily. However, there appears to be little difference in compliance rates between drugs taken once vs. twice daily. Advantages in compliance rates and outcomes of twice daily regimens over thrice daily regimens and twice daily over four times per day regimens are minimal or unclear.

Other effective strategies Shortening the duration of treatment whenever possible has been shown to enhance compliance.[19] Similarly, "tailoring" the regimen—linking medication taking to daily activities and, for multidrug regimens, matching pill-taking frequencies (e.g., one pill from each bottle is taken upon awakening and at bedtime)—also improves compliance rates.[30,31]

The selection and modification of a drug regimen that optimizes compliance is a complicated process that is best accomplished by combining objective data about the various choices with patient variables, e.g., disease and individual psychosocial parameters. Objective evaluation is becoming increasingly difficult. Highly sophisticated and subtle marketing techniques used by pharmaceutical manufacturers, including advertising and promotional literature, have significant impact on prescriber decisions and are very difficult for an individual provider to detect. In addition, much of the current medical literature contains built-in bias due to the influence of pharmaceutical manufacturers funding many of the studies. Unfortunately, it is uncommon to find appropriate and fair comparisons of newer agents against equally effective and inexpensive alternatives or large studies comparing the relative efficacy of all the alternatives used in treating a particular disease.

One resource for objective comparative analysis of drug literature is the pharmacist. In particular, clinical pharmacists, found in hospitals, managed-care facilities, nursing homes, and outpatient clinics, are an excellent source of objective patient-oriented information and advice regarding optimal drug regimens. Similar assistance can be obtained from pharmacy-based drug information centers and literature reviews done as part of a facility's pharmacy and therapeutics process.

Provider-focused Approaches

Be pragmatic Compliance with prescribed drug therapy is a difficult process, and adherence to the treatment regimen will almost always be imperfect even in the most motivated patients. Therefore, the provider must realize that adherence will be imperfect and, in managing the care of the patient, will assume that the patient is exhibiting some degree of noncompliance. If a patient's degree of disease control changes or a side effect occurs, providers should first look for compliance problems as a cause for the change in patient status.[19] For example, in diabetic patients on insulin who experience more frequent episodes of hypoglycemia or whose blood glucose control deteriorates, many providers will alter the dosage of insulin. Instead, the provider should first check for compliance problems by having the patient draw up his or her insulin dose. This enables easy detection of dosing problems due to poor vision, poor techniques, or inadequate understanding. A careful history may reveal other problems such as changes in diet or exercise, temporary unavailability of insulin, or lack of clean syringes.

The initial postdiagnosis education and compliance support efforts are generally the most intense. However, a large number of initially compliant patients will demonstrate noncompliant behavior later in the course of therapy. It has been estimated that over 50 percent of initially compliant hypertensive patients had discontinued treatment one year after initial diagnosis.[5] Therefore, the provider must remain vigilant for adherence problems, regularly evaluating compliance even in patients who have been "doing well" for many years.

Finally, a commonsense approach to changing drug therapy should be utilized. At a time when providers are continuously bombarded with new drugs and new *state-of-the-art* therapy, the old saying "If it ain't broke, don't fix it" should be the provider's guiding principle. Current marketing strategies use subtle techniques to imply that the patient may not be getting the "best state of the art therapy." Many of the purported disadvantages of older, less expensive products in the treatment of chronic diseases are duration of risk and dose related. These disadvantages, established by comparing older studies which used higher doses over long periods of time, may not be valid in geriatric populations. Given the shorter life expectancy of geriatric population, the effectiveness of newer low-dose, low-side-effect regimens using older products, and the much higher cost of newer drugs, the provider must carefully weigh whether there are any real advantages in switching a 75-year-old hypertensive controlled on a once daily 12.5-mg dose of hydrochlorothiazide to a newer state-of-the-art drug at 10 to 25 times the cost of the current regimen.

Treat the patient not the disease As providers, we tend to perceive our role as the diagnosis and treatment of diseases. Guided by that perception, providers may treat patients and their diseases primarily on a technical level and get frustrated and angry if patients do not follow instructions or, despite providers' best efforts, achieve only partially satisfactory treatment results.

Given this situation, it is not surprising to find poor patient-provider communication, poor patient-provider relationships, and low patient satisfaction levels with provider communication or attitudes listed as major contributors to noncompliance.[18-20,22,24] One author strongly suggests that noncompliance in diabetes is due in large part to the failure of providers to recognize that their goal is not treating disease, but helping patients treat their disease.[22] The precept "help patients treat their disease" is applicable to all chronic diseases. Recent trends toward replacing the more negative term *compliance* with the less blame-placing term *adherence* is another attempt to alter providers' perceptions and facilitate a more cooperative approach to facilitating patient adherence.3,7

Use effective patient education techniques The literature describing the efficacy of patient education in improving patient compliance and outcomes is confusing and at times contradictory.[1-9,23,24,30,31] Depending on reader bias, the literature can be used to support positions regarding the impact of patient education on compliance ranging from none to significant. However, there are several important issues and actions that can be used as guidelines to effective patient education.

Understand the scope of impact of patient education activities To effectively adhere to prescribed drug regimens, the patient must (1) have an understanding of his or her disease and its treatment, e.g., how to take the medication, the importance of medication in producing outcomes, and the skills needed to administer the treatment; (2) be self-motivated to comply; and (3) make changes in behavior, e.g., take pills, change the diet, or exercise.

Regardless of whether the disease is acute or chronic, patient understanding of how to use the medicine is the foundation for compliance; i.e., if patients do not understand how to properly take their medication, they will not be able to comply effectively.[11] Patient education activities primarily have positive impacts on patient understanding. In addition, patient education can positively impact patient health beliefs, enhancing self-motivation by reducing barriers to motivation and compliance.[5,6,23] Therefore, educational activities that lead to better understanding and influence health beliefs are the essential building blocks in achieving adherence with prescribed drug regimens.

However, the relative impact of patient education varies with the nature of the illness and its treatment. In patients with acute disorders, patient understanding is a major determinant to eventual compliance. Self-motivation of patients to adherence of prescribed treatment is relatively easy to achieve, since compliance is easily linked to getting rid of the symptoms (e.g., pain, fever, nausea) associated with the illness. Similarly, patients do not have to make prolonged or major changes in behavior. The compliance literature confirms the significant positive impact of education on patient compliance with the brief periods of treatment required in acute disorders and the relatively minor roles motivation and behavior change play in these situations.[1-9,32]

In contrast, patient education, while still required as a foundation, has less impact on compliance in patients on prolonged drug therapy required with chronic disease than does self-motivation or levels of behavior changes required. Self-motivation is more difficult because many chronic diseases are asymptomatic and the treatment, aimed at preventing complications, may produce unwanted symptoms. Similarly, patients with chronic diseases are asked to make major, permanent lifestyle changes which may include alterations in diet and exercise as well as using prescribed medication on a daily basis for the remainder of their life. A review of the compliance literature confirms that in patients with chronic disorders, patient education ranks third in importance when compared to self-motivation and the behavior change required.[1-9,33,34] While much of the literature shows little or no impact of patient education on compliance with prolonged therapy, it is misleading. Most studies utilize relatively ineffective styles of education or ignore the essential nature of patient understanding of eventual compliance. Several studies show patient education activities do improve compliance over short periods of time through enhancing patient understanding or modifying patient health beliefs that were barriers to adherence.[6,35,36]

Actively involve patients in educational process The traditional approach to patient education, in which the provider gives the information and the patient passively receives it, is not consistent with effective learning methods. The traditional approach fosters lower retention levels of key information and provides no method of reliable verification of patient understanding.[37,38]

Since adults prefer to be more actively involved in the learning process, current trends in adult patient education favor an interactive approach as the most effective teaching technique. When compared to traditional educational approaches, actively involving the patient significantly improves patient understanding, patient satisfaction, compliance, and outcome.[4,11,16,38-41] Effective techniques to actively involve the patient in the learning process include the use of open-ended questions, patient demonstration, skill practice, and discussion. In addition to better educational results, this interactive approach also facilitates easy identification of language and cultural barriers or impairments in vision, hearing, and mental status. The interactive approach also provides multiple opportunities to verify patient understanding of key elements of information needed to comply.

Verify patient understanding Providers spend considerable time educating patients through either traditional or interactive educational approaches. However, on most occasions they leave out the most important step, i.e., having the patient verify to the provider either verbally or through patient demonstration of techniques that he or she has an adequate understanding to allow compliance.[42] Pharmacists in the Indian Health Service (IHS) are taught to close each patient consultation session with a nonthreatening open-ended question to verify patient understanding, e.g., "Just to make sure I didn't leave anything out, please tell me (or show me) how you are going to use your medication?"[11,16] For consultation of patients on chronic medication they utilize the *show-and-tell* technique, in which pharmacists *show* the medication to the patient and ask the patient to *tell* them key elements of understanding needed to comply. Two open-ended questions—What is the medication for? How do you take medication?— allow the pharmacist or provider to verify understanding or to correct misunderstandings. A third question—What kind of problems are you having?—incorporates Sbarbaro's approach to detect any negative effects the patient perceives are caused by the drug therapy.[16,19]

Presentation of educational material Meta-analysis of the compliance literature has shown that the most effective education technique is *one-to-one* verbal counseling between a provider and patient.[43] Written material, such as patient package inserts (PPI's), has been advocated as a preferred educational method. However, written material used alone has little or no effect in improving patient understanding.[5,6,44-46] While not effective by itself, written material does have a place in patient education as an adjunct to one-to-one verbal counseling to enhance patient understanding. The design of the written material is a critical factor in determining its usefulness. Morrow and colleagues have studied and outlined the pertinent design factors needed to develop the most effective forms of written educational materials for geriatric patients.[47] Similarly, several authors have identified key factors in organizing and designing effective individual or group verbal instructional methods.[3,16,38,48] The use of technical or medical jargon should be avoided in both written and verbal instruction efforts. Many authors cite its use as a significant barrier to improving patient understanding.[1-9]

Use behavior-oriented approaches Since compliance with long-term drug therapy is so dependent on making significant behavioral changes, behavior modification techniques are very effective in enhancing adherence to chronic drug therapy.[31,34] While there are many effective techniques listed, most share the same psychosocial foundation as current persuasion techniques used in marketing and sales.[49]

Regular visits to same provider The simple act of developing a good patient-provider relationship, spending time with the patient, and demonstrating genuine concern evoke a powerful stimulus (i.e., principle of reciprocity) to comply with the provider's wishes.[49]

Self-monitoring/self-reporting Having patients monitor their blood pressure or blood glucose has been shown to enhance compliance. Similarly, just having patients write down results of self-monitoring or medication-taking activity results in better adherence. These types of activity strengthen patient commitment to the treatment regimen.[3,5,6,30,31]

Increase frequency of follow-up visits For patients with compliance problems, simply increasing the frequency of follow-up visits or other forms of increased attention (phone calls, postcard reminders) will increase adherence through a health-related version of the *hawthorne effect*.[3,5,6,30,31]

Use support groups While the compliance literature is less clear about support groups, they are effective in facilitating patient adjustments, changing health beliefs, increasing commitment to treatment plans, and, through a sharing of concerns and problems, enhancing levels of self-efficacy.

Use contingency contracting Contingency contracting has been shown to be an effective tool in enhancing compliance. It takes advantage of two behavioral principles—commitment-consistency and reinforcement-reward—for positive outcomes. A contract is negotiated between the provider and the patient regarding the desired behavior. To be effective, the contract must be written and include rewards for specific positive behaviors. In general, the more public the contract (e.g., declaration before a support group), the greater the eventual compliance.[3,5,6,30,35,49,50]

Enlist the aid of family In geriatric patients with compliance problems, utilizing spouses, children, relatives, or caretakers to provide support, supervise medication taking, or administer medication is a particularly effective method to enhance compliance.[6,51]

Use compliance aids if indicated For motivated patients with compliance problems that have not responded to repeated attempts to enhance compliance or who have special problems, e.g., poor vision, there are a variety of compliance aids available. Aids ranging from mechanical devices to enable vision-impaired diabetics to draw up the proper insulin dose to prescription bottles that "beep" when the next dose is due are readily available. Bond and Hussar[9] have recently published an excellent discussion of available compliance aids.

Utilize non-physician providers The compliance literature strongly supports a multidisciplinary approach to compliance enhancement. In particular, pharmacists and nurses have been used to enhance compliance through activities ranging from patient education and monitoring compliance to managing the care of patients under physician-approved guidelines or protocols.[6,52,53,54]

Within the IHS, a comprehensive health maintenance organization, pharmacists play a major role in enhancing patient adherence to prescribed drug regimens.[16,55,56] Pharmacists fill all prescriptions from the patient's permanent medical record. Using this data base, which includes laboratory tests and complete physician and pharmacy records, IHS pharmacists review all drug orders for compliance, appropriateness, and potential adverse effects. If problems are detected, they are resolved with the prescriber prior to dispensing. In addition to their responsibility for assuring the appropriateness of therapy, IHS pharmacists are responsible for verifying that each patient understands how to properly utilize his or her medication. Pharmacist-patient consultation takes place in a private environment, usually in a private consultation room, which is part of the outpatient pharmacy. IHS pharmacists utilize an innovative and effective interactive counseling technique that maximizes patient involvement and minimizes professional time expended.[16] All IHS pharmacists are taught these innovative counseling techniques as well as other compliance monitoring and enhancement methods in a week-long course, IHS Clinical Pharmacy Training Seminar. At many sites, certified IHS pharmacists, using guidelines approved by the medical staff, manage the care of patients requiring continuous drug therapy, between annual physician visits. Pharmacists have the latitude to adjust doses and change medication within the limits of the protocols. Problems which arise that cannot be handled by the pharmacist are referred to the physician for appropriate action.

In summary, the optimal approach to enhancing compliance in geriatric patients is in the individualized use of a combination of strategies listed. Assessing compliance, a good patient-provider relationship, actively involving the patient in treatment decisions, simplifying the drug regimen, effective use of interactive patient education technique, and the use of behavior modification techniques combined with the use of a multidisciplinary team approach to compliance enhancement will yield positive results with most patients.

REFERENCES

1. Sackett DL, Haynes RB (eds): *Compliance with Therapeutic Regimens.* Baltimore, Johns Hopkins University Press, 1976.
2. Haynes RB, Taylor DW, Sackett DL (eds): *Compliance in Health Care.* Baltimore, Johns Hopkins University Press, 1979.
3. Meichenbaum D, Turk, DC: *Facilitating Treatment Adherence.* New York, Plenum Press, 1987.
4. Ley P: *Communicating with Patients: Improving Communication Satisfaction and Compliance.* London, Croom Helm, 1988.
5. Eraker SA, Kirscht JP, Becker MH: Understanding and improving patient compliance. *Ann Intern Med* 100: 258–268, 1984.
6. Becker MH: Patient adherence to prescribed therapies. *Medical Care* 23: 539–555, 1985.
7. Pesznecker BL, Patsdaughter C, Moody KA, Albert M: Medication regimens and the home health care client: A challenge for health care providers. *Home Health Care Serv Quart* 11: 9–68, 1990.
8. Kusserow RP: Medication regimens causes of non-compliance. Office of Inspector General, Department of Health and Human Services (Report OEI-0489-89121), March 1990.
9. Bond WS, Hussar DA: Detection methods and strategies for improving medication compliance. *Am J Hosp Pharm* 48: 1978–1988, 1991.
10. Bressler, DA: Communicating with patients about their medication. *N Engl J Med* 325: 1650–1651, 1991.
11. Weingarten MA, Cannon BS: Age as a major factor affecting adherence to medication for hypertension in a general practice population. *Fam Pract* 5: 294–296, 1988.
12. King K: Strategies for enhancing compliance in the dialysis elderly. *Am J Kidney Dis* 16: 351–353, 1990.
13. Portnoy E: Enhancing communication with elderly patients. *Am Pharm* NS25: 506, 1985.
14. Kass MA, et al: Compliance with topical pilocarpine. *Am J Ophthalmol* 101: 515, 1986.
15. Bartlett EE: The stepped approach to patient education. *Diabetes Educ* 14: 130, 1987.
16. Gardner M, Boyce RW, Herrier RN: *Pharmacist-Patient Consultation Program: An Interactive Approach to Verify Patient Understanding.* New York, Pfizer, 1991.
17. Haurtin-Roberts S: Health beliefs, compliance and hypertension. *JAMA* 264: 2864, 1990.
18. Coleman VR: Physician behavior and compliance. *J Hypertens* 3: 69, 1985.
19. Sbarbaro JA: The patient-physician relationship: Compliance revisited. *Ann Allergy* 64: 325, 1990.

20. Steele DJ, et al: Beyond advocacy; a review of the active patient concept. *Patient Educ Counsel* 10: 3, 1987.
21. Massey M: *The People Puzzle: Understanding Yourself and Others.* Reston, Virginia, Reston Publishing, 1979.
22. Anderson RM: Is the problem of noncompliance all in our heads? *Diabetes Educ* 11: 31-34, 1985.
23. Rosenstock IM: Understanding and enhancing patient compliance with diabetic regimens. *Diabetes Care* 8: 611, 1985.
24. Clark LT: Improving compliance and increasing control of hypertension: needs of special hypertensive populations. *Am Heart J* 121: 664, 1991.
25. Col N, Fanale JE, Kronholm P: The role of medication non compliance and adverse drug reactions in hospitalization of the elderly. *Arch Intern Med* 150: 841, 1990.
26. Ary DV, Toobert D, Wilson W, Glasgow RE: Patient perspective on factors contributing to non adherence to diabetes regimen. *Diabetes Care* 9: 168-172, 1986.
27. Eisen SA, Miller DK, Woodward RS, et al: The effect of prescribed daily dose frequency on patient medication compliance. *Arch Intern Med* 150: 1881-1884, 1990.
28. Kubacka RT, Juhl RF: Attitudes of patients with hypertension or arthritis towards the frequency of medication administration. *Am J Hosp Pharm* 432: 2499-2501, 1985.
29. Kass MA, Gordon M, Morley RE, et al: Compliance with topical timolol treatment. *Am J Ophthalmol* 103: 188-193, 1987.
30. Haynes RB, Sackett DL, Taylor DW: Practical management of low compliance with antihypertensive therapy: A guide for the busy practitioner. *Clin Invest Med* 1: 175-180, 1979.
31. Haynes RB, Wang E, De Mota Goems M: A critical review of interventions to improve compliance with prescribed medications. *Patient Educ Counsel* 10: 155-166, 1987.
32. Williams RL, Maiman LA, Broadbent DN, et al: Educational strategies to improve compliance with an antibiotic regimen. *Am J Dis Child* 140: 216-220, 1986.
33. Bloomgarden ZT, Karmally W, Metzger J, et al: Randomized, controlled trial of diabetic patient education: improved knowledge without improved metabolic status. *Diabetes Care* 10: 263-272, 1987.
34. Cameron R, Best JA: Promoting adherence to health behavior change interventions: recent findings from behavioral research. *Patient Educ Counsel* 10: 139-154, 1987.
35. DeBlaquiere P, Christensen DB, Carter WB, Martin TR: Use and misuse of metered dose inhalers by patients with chronic lung disease *Am Rev Respir Dis* 140: 910-916, 1989.
36. Gonzalez-Fernandez RA, Rivera M, Torres D, Quiles J, et al: Usefulness of a systemic hypertension in-hospital educational program. *Am J Cardiol* 65: 1384-1386, 1990.
37. Tarnow KG: Working with adult learners. *Nursing Educator* 4: 34-40, 1979.
38. Hanson SL, Pichert JW: Patient education: the importance of instructional time and active patient involvement. *Medical Teacher* 7: 313-322, 1985.
39. Self TH, Brooks JB, Lieberman P, Ryan MR: The value of demonstration and the role of the pharmacist in teaching the correct use of pressurized bronchodilators. *Can Med Assoc J* 128: 129-131, 1983.
40. Orth JE, Stiles WB, Scherwitz L, Vallbona C: Patient exposition and provider explanation in routine interviews and hypertensive patients' blood pressure control. *Health Psychology* 6: 29-42, 1987.
41. Etzwiler DD: Diabetes management: the importance of patient education and participation. *Post Grad Med* 80: 67-72, 1986.
42. Robinson ML: Improving patients prescription compliance. *Internist* 25: 31-32, 1984.
43. Mullen PD, Green LW: Meta-analysis points way towards more effective medication teaching. *Promoting Health* 6: 6-8, 1985.
44. Green LW, Mullen PO, Stainbrook GL: Programs to reduce drug errors in the elderly: direct and indirect evidence form patient education. *J Geriatr Drug Ther* 1: 3-18, 1986.
45. De Tullio PL, Eraker SA, Jepson C, et al: Patient medication instruction and provider interactions: effects on knowledge and attitude. *Health Ed Quart* 13: 51-60, 1986.

46. Johnson MW, Mitch WE, Sherwood J, et al: The impact of a drug information sheet on the understanding and attitude of patients about drugs. *JAMA* 256: 2722-2724, 1986.
47. Morrow D, Leiver V, Sheikh J: Adherence and medication instructions: review and recommendations. *J Am Geriatr Soc* 36: 1147-1160, 1988.
48. Worcester MI, O'Connor K: Tailoring teaching and the elderly in home care. *Home Health Care Serv Quart* 11: 69-120, 1990.
49. Cialdini RB: *Influence, the New Psychology of Modern Persuasion.* New York, Quill Press, 1984.
50. Janz NK, Becker MH, Hartman PE: Contingency contracting to enhance patient compliance: A review. *Patient Educ Counsel* 5: 165-178, 1982.
51. Doherty WJ, Schrott HG, Metcalf L, Iasiello-Vailas L: Effects of spouse support and health beliefs on medication adherence. *J Fam Pract* 17: 837-841, 1983.
52. Gryfe CI, Gryfe BM: Drug therapy of the aged: the problem of compliance and the roles of physicians and pharmacists. *J Am Geriatr Soc* 32: 301-307, 1984.
53. Kazis LE, Friedman RH: Improving medication compliance in the elderly, strategies for the health care provider. *J Am Geriatr Soc* 36: 1161-1162, 1988.
54. Church RM: Pharmacy practice in the Indian Health Service. *Am J Hosp Pharm* 44: 771-775, 1987.
55. Church RM: The expanded role of pharmacists in the public health service: An overview of a pharmacy practice model. *Hosp Form* 24: 256-532, 1989.
56. Herrier RN, Boyce RW: Pharmacist-managed patient care services and prescriptive authority in the U.S. public health service. *Hosp Form* 25: 67-80, 1990.

CHAPTER

5

HYPERTENSION

William N. Jones
Timothy C. Fagan

Hypertension is one of the most common medical disorders in the United States. The risks of uncontrolled hypertension have been well documented.[1] The Framingham Study has shown that systolic blood pressure (SBP) and diastolic blood pressure (DBP) correlate with the development of stroke, coronary heart disease (CHD), and congestive heart failure (CHF).[2] In fact, SBP is a slightly better predictor of morbidity than DBP. Eight other observational studies involving over 400,000 people (96 percent male) have demonstrated a risk for untreated hypertension.[3] Whelton and Klag[4] have reviewed the effects of hypertension and the development of renal dysfunction. Their analysis shows that development of renal failure in patients is related to uncontrolled hypertension.

The prevalence of systolic-diastolic and isolated systolic hypertension (ISH) increases with age; approximately 45 to 60 percent of people 65 to 74 years old have hypertension. Women and Caucasians have lower prevalence than males and blacks.[5] ISH has been found in 5 to 7 percent of white and black men and women in various studies.[6]

At least 15 clinical trials have been reported which clearly demonstrate the benefits of treating hypertension.[7-10] The treatment of malignant hypertension was shown to be effective in reducing morbidity and mortality. With the high frequency of morbid and mortal events associated with malignant hypertension, controlled clinical trials were not needed. In 1967 the Veterans Administration (VA) Cooperative Study Group on Antihypertensive Agents demonstrated the markedly reduced cardiovascular morbidity and mortality associated with treating men with severe hypertension. Other major clinical trials have shown that antihypertensive therapy alters the natural history of hypertension, even in patients with mild hypertension and in patients over 60 years old. Most of the studies were no longer than 5 years in duration; only the U.S. Public Health Service (USPHS) trial followed patients blindly for over 6 years. Blinding to both investigators and patients occurred only in the European Working Party on Hypertension in the Elderly (EWPHE) study, VA cooperative studies, and USPHS studies. The drug therapy most commonly used in the studies was a step-care regimen with a thiazide or thiazide-like diuretic and additional nondiuretic therapy as needed, although the Medical Research Council (MRC) study was a single-blind, parallel comparison of placebo, bendroflumethiazide, and propranolol in 17,354 patients. End-organ disease was allowed for enrollment in VA, EWPHE, MRC, and Hypertension Detection and Follow-up Program (HDFP) studies. In spite of these limitations, both "soft" and "hard" endpoints were found to be altered by antihypertensive therapy. Progression to more severe hypertension, cardiomegaly, left ventricular hypertrophy (LVH), proteinuria, and retinopathy (i.e., soft endpoints) have been demonstrated repeatedly as nonmorbid or nonmortal endpoints. The hard endpoints of death or morbid events, such as stroke, have clearly been reduced by the use of antihypertensive agents. The mortality in the HDFP was 3.5 times higher when prior end-organ dysfunction was present upon entry. Both fatal and nonfatal strokes have been consistently reduced in the HDFP, VA, EWPHE, MRC, and Australian National Blood Pressure Trial (ANBP) studies. The effects of antihypertensive therapy on cardiovascular endpoints have been mixed and somewhat disappointing. A 38 percent reduction in fatal cardiovascular events was found in the EWPHE study. Deaths from myocardial infarction were reduced by 26 percent in the entire group and by 46 percent in patients with mild hypertension in the HDFP study. A non-statistically significant 55 percent reduction in ischemic heart disease was found in the ANBP study. The results of the MRC trial were a 2 percent increase in CHD in the diuretic group and a 13 percent fall in CHD in the propranolol group. The Multiple Risk Factor Intervention Trial (MRFIT) also reported a 2 percent increase in myocardial infarction-related deaths in the stepped-care treated patients (diuretic initially).

One of the controversial areas of hypertension is the generally disappointing result in reductions in the rate of myocardial infarction compared to reductions in the rate of cerebrovascular accident (CVA). The most important reason is frequently overlooked. The relationship between blood pressure and stroke is much steeper than the relationship between blood pressure and myocardial infarction.[1] Thus, for any given reduction in blood pressure, a much larger reduction in CVA than myocardial infarction is to be expected. Various authors debate the effect of thiazide diuretics as a contributing factor to the CHD outcomes. It is possible that the current trials are too small, the patients had CHD prior to enrollment, other factors contribute to CHD, no true change occurs, or some drugs increase CHD. It is also possible that most trials have been too short. Interestingly, mortality rates in the MRFIT were 10.6 percent lower overall, and 7.7 percent lower for CHD in the special intervention group, in a 10.5-year follow-up.[11] The greatest difference between the early reports and the longer term MRFIT follow-up is a 24 percent reduction in myocardial infarction-associated deaths in the later reports. As in the early reports, a difference remained between men with and without any electrocardiogram (ECG) abnormality at baseline with regard to myocardial infarction; patients with abnormal ECGs had a higher death rate. This report supports the suggestion that hypertension trials need longer durations to assess the CHD effects.

Is it possible to lower the DBP too far and thereby increase mortality? This has been a subject of debate for several years. A variety of problems are possible in making this analysis. However, several studies show that deaths from myocardial infarction appear to have a *J-curve* appearance (i.e., mortality rises with the lowest SBP or DBP) when the SBP is less than 150 mmHG and/or DBP is less than 85 mmHg. It is conceivable that patients without critical coronary stenosis could develop ischemia if perfusion pressure is too low at a normal blood pressure.[12] Further research will be needed before the optimal DBP range can be adequately defined.

Specific findings in elderly patients in clinical trials are limited. In a VA study, 81 men 60 to 75 years old with a mean blood pressure of 178/102 mmHg were examined in a double-blind, placebo-controlled trial. Morbid cardiovascular events occurred in 62.8 percent of the control group versus 28.9 percent of the drug-treated patients. In the ANBP 582 patients, 60 to 69 years old were randomized to placebo or drug therapy (thiazide, methyldopa, or beta blocker). Death, stroke, myocardial infarction, or CHF were reduced by 39 percent in the treated group. Mortality after 5 years in the HDFP, in patients 60 to 69 years old, was 17.2 percent lower in the stepped-care group versus referred-care patients, primarily due to lower cardiovascular mortality. The EWPHE trial included 840 patients who were older than 60 years. Patients were treated with placebo or thiazide plus triamterene. Methyldopa was added if blood pressure was not controlled. After nearly 4.5 years cardiovascular mortality was significantly reduced by 38 percent in the treated patients; although overall mortality was reduced, it was statistically unchanged.[13] In the group of patients continuing in the double-blind study, a reduction in death from myocardial infarction of 60 percent, a 52 percent reduction in stroke, and a 90 percent reduction in progressive hypertension were found. Patients over 79 years old appeared to have no benefit from treatment. The relatively small size of the groups may have contributed to the failure to find statistically significant differences.

The Systolic Hypertension in the Elderly Program (SHEP) is a major placebo-controlled, randomized, double-blind clinical trial assessing the effect of antihypertensive therapy in patients with ISH. Patients with SBP 160 to 219 mmHg and DBP below 90 mmHg were eligible for the study. The blood pressure goals were lowering of SBP by 20 mmHg if the SBP initially was 160 to 179 or SBP less than 160 if originally over 180 mmHg. This study has presented early results supporting the view that elderly patients with ISH will comply with medications and can be safely treated.[14,15] Patients were treated with chlorthalidone, 12.5 to 25 mg daily; atenolol 25 to 50 mg or reserpine 0.05 to 0.1 mg daily were added if SBP was not at goal. In the final results, 2365 patients were in the active treatment group and 2371 in the placebo group. These patients were followed for up to 5 years (mean 4.5 years). Diuretic therapy alone was given to 46 percent of the active group, and 69 percent were treated with first- or first- and second-step agents. Other active medications, not described, were given to 21 percent, and 9 percent did not receive therapy. In the placebo group, active antihypertensive therapy was prescribed in 13 percent after 1 year, 33 percent at 3 years, and 44 percent after 5 years. Most of these patients developed sustained DBP exceeding 90 mmHg during the follow-up. After 5 years of follow-up the mean decreases in SBP and DBP in the active treatment group were 26 and 9 mmHg, respectively. The overall reduction in SBP in the placebo patients was approximately 15 mmHg. SBP 11 to 14 mmHg lower was found in the active treatment group throughout the 5 years of the study. Goal SBP was reached in 65 to 72 percent of the active treated patients and in 32 to 40 percent of the placebo group over the 5-year follow-up. Stroke incidence was 5.2 per 100 participants in the active group and 8.2 per 100 participants in the placebo group with a relative risk of 0.64 in the active treatment group. The incidence of stroke was lower in the active treatment group in each age group: 60 to 69, 70–79, and 80 years and older. Nonfatal cardiovascular events were lower in the active treatment group, relative risk ranging from 0.46 for left ventricular failure to 0.86 for angioplasty. Total mortality, mortality associated with myocardial infarction, sudden cardiac death, and other cardiovascular mortality were lower in the active treatment group. Combined nonfatal and fatal endpoints of the SHEP were lower in the active treatment group (289 versus 424, 32 percent reduction with active treatment).[10] These results clearly support treating elderly patients with ISH. They are particularly impressive since more than one-third of the placebo patients were treated with active drugs during the study. Potential criticism of this study includes selection of elderly participants free of other illnesses, which makes extrapolation to less healthy patients more difficult, and choice of diuretics as baseline therapy.

ETIOLOGY AND PATHOPHYSIOLOGY OF HYPERTENSION

The basis for the increased prevalence of hypertension in the elderly is only partially understood and is clearly multifactorial. The decrease in aortic compliance and increase in aortic volume with age, as well as decreased compliance in large arteries and increased resistance in small arteries and arterioles, are the major pathophysiologic changes associated with hypertension in the elderly.[16] However, the etiologic factors producing the vascular changes, which underlie the increase in blood pressure, are unclear. In industrialized societies DBP and, to an even greater extent, SBP increase with age, but in some primitive cultures this does not occur.[16] This suggests that some aspects of life in highly technologic societies may be critical factors in increasing hypertension with increasing age. Possible sociocultural etiologic factors include diet, obesity, low level of physical activity, stress, high alcohol consumption, and high rates of smoking.

Daily intake in excess of 1 oz of pure ethanol is clearly associated with elevated blood pressure. Obesity has been shown to have a weak, but positive, association with increased blood pressure in the elderly.[16] Promotion of large-vessel atherosclerosis by smoking, with resultant decreased arterial compliance, is also a factor. Well-conditioned individuals tend to have lower blood pressure than less well conditioned individuals.[16] Older individuals are often less active than younger individuals. Therefore, a sedentary lifestyle and consequent deconditioning may also contribute to increased blood pressure in elderly patients.

Several other potential etiologic factors are involved in hypertension in the elderly. Baroreceptor sensitivity decreases so that adjustments in blood pressure, after acute rises, occur less quickly and completely. Less rapid and complete responses to changes in position, meals, stress, and drugs contribute to wider swings in blood pressure in older hypertensive patients. Decreased dilation of blood vessels in response to $beta_2$-adrenergic stimulation and cholinergic stimulation may contribute to increased peripheral resistance and increased blood pressure in the elderly. Decreases in activity of the renin-angiotensin system may contribute to an increased prevalence of postural hypotension. A blunted heart rate increase in response to $beta_1$-adrenergic stimulation may also contribute to an increased prevalence of postural hypotension.

Decreased glomerular filtration and tubular excretion with advanced age may decrease clearance and increase plasma concentrations of drugs which are primarily eliminated by the kidney. In some instances, this decrease may lead to increased antihypertensive response and/or toxicity in older patients. Decreased renal blood flow and glomerular filtration may lead to decreased ability to excrete sodium and increased blood pressure on that basis. Thus, in older patients, the role of dietary sodium may become more important. Much remains to be elucidated regarding the factors leading to increased blood pressure in highly technologic societies.

DIAGNOSIS

The World Health Organization (WHO) criteria for hypertension are SBP > 160 mmHg and/or DBP > 95 mmHg. A DBP greater than 90 mmHg is considered as hypertensive by the Fourth Joint National Committee on Detection, Evaluation, and Treatment of High Blood Pressure (JNC). The JNC classifies hypertension as mild, moderate, and severe if the DBP is 90 to 104 mmHg, 105 to 114 mmHg, and greater than 115 mmHg, respectively. All patients should have hypertension confirmed before any treatment regimen is begun. The JNC recommends confirmation within 2 months if mild or within 2 weeks if moderate hypertension. Patients with severe hypertension should have immediate evaluation.[17]

The exact value of blood pressure at which to initiate treatment is unknown. Kaplan suggests that patients with consistent DBP over 95 mmHg should receive therapy.[3] Patients at greater risk of stroke (e.g., blacks in the United States, diabetics, and those with CHD) should have treatment started at over 90 mmHg. It should be remembered that women have fewer complications of hypertension than men at equal DBP, which suggests the level necessitating treatment of blood pressure could be higher in women.[3] The JNC recommendations are to use nonpharmacologic therapy when DBP is 90 to 94 mmHg and periodically monitor for progression of hypertension.[17]

Establishing the correct diagnosis is particularly important in the elderly. Pseudohypertension may occur in elderly patients. If the artery is not distensible due to calcification, overestimation of the blood pressure can occur. Osler's maneuver may be helpful in evaluating the elderly patient's blood pressure. This bedside technique requires monitoring the radial or brachial pulse when inflating the blood pressure cuff. If the artery is palpable when the systolic pressure is exceeded, the patient is *Osler positive*; if the artery is no longer palpable, the patient is *Osler negative.*[18] In the elderly, supine and standing blood pressures should be measured, since orthostatic hypotension may occur in as many as 24 percent of individuals.[19] Elevated blood pressure only at the physician's office, or "white coat" hypertension, may result in unnecessary and expensive treatment. Similarly, failing to confirm the diagnosis, especially of mild hypertension, over several months may result in prescribing treatment inappropriately. Having patients measure blood pressures at home with reliable equipment may increase the accuracy of diagnosis.[20] It is also important to use correct technique and to use an appropriately sized cuff and bladder in order to make an accurate diagnosis. Muscular and/or obese patients need larger cuffs to ensure a more accurate measurement.

THERAPEUTICS OF HYPERTENSION

Mostly short-term studies have shown that some nonpharmacologic therapies of hypertension are effective in lowering DBP by 5 to 10 mmHg. Patients with DBP in the range of 90 to 94 mmHg are the best candidates for nonpharmacologic therapy alone. Restriction of salt, reduction in weight, moderation of alcohol ingestion, and aerobic and/or rhythmic exercise can be successful in treating mild hypertension and/or lowering other cardiovascular risk factors. Increased ingestion of potassium and/or calcium as means to lower blood pressure are not clearly established at the present time.[17] Lowering saturated fat intake and cessation of smoking are behaviors which can reduce independent risk factors for myocardial infarction.

If after using nonpharmacologic therapy for several months the blood pressure is not fully controlled, drug therapy is indicated for elderly patients. The JNC has presented an individualized approach to the management of hypertension.[17] Several options are available for initial therapy.

General Considerations

A wide variety of agents is commercially available to control hypertension. Despite many claims, very small, if any, differences in controlling blood pressure can be identified with various agents. However, in black and elderly patients some differences appear to exist.[21] On average, these patients may respond less well to beta blockers and angiotensin converting enzyme inhibitors (ACEIs). Selection of drug therapy should be individualized and based on the goals of therapy of hypertension. Patients with DBP exceeding 95 mmHg without end-organ damage or those with other risks (e.g., smokers, diabetics, CHD patients) or end-organ damage (e.g., renal dysfunction, CHF, or LVH) and DBP above 90 mmHg should be candidates for drug therapy. Initially blood pressure should be lowered to below 140/90 mmHg. The long-term goal should be prescribing therapy which controls the blood pressure, is tolerated by the patient, and is affordable. Shulman et al[22] have reported that 22 percent of controlled or mild hypertensives and 36 percent of moderate or severe hypertensives had difficulty purchasing medication. They also found that 16 percent of patients could not afford prescription refills at least one time. Positive long-term outcome requires flexibility in order to achieve normal blood pressure without adverse effects. The overall endpoint should be reduction in the risk of renal, cardiovascular, and/or cerebrovascular complications of untreated hypertension.

As a general rule, therapy should be started at low doses with gradual titration until the blood pressure reaches acceptable values. Metabolic capacity and renal excretion of drugs are decreased in the elderly. Consideration of the changes in pharmacokinetics and pharmacodynamics may prevent adverse events, such as orthostatic hypotension, from occurring. The other major consideration is the concomitant diseases which each patient may have. Accomplishing treatment of two disorders with a single drug individualizes therapy and should result in overall lower costs and fewer adverse events (e.g., use of a beta blocker for a patient with both hypertension and angina).

Diuretics Thiazide diuretics have been used for more than 30 years. Each major clinical trial assessing treatment of hypertension has included a diuretic as first-line therapy. These drugs differ in potency (the dose required to produce the same pharmacologic response) and half-life, but the intrinsic activities of the drugs are equal.

Hydrochlorothiazide is the most frequently prescribed agent in this class. The exact mechanism of action of thiazide diuretics as antihypertensive drugs is not known. Initially the drugs cause saluresis, volume depletion, and reduced cardiac output. Over weeks to months plasma volume returns toward normal and total peripheral resistance falls along with the blood pressure. The cardiac output tends to return to pretreatment levels. Alterations in intracellular sodium and/or calcium occur and may be related to the lowering of peripheral resistance.[23]

The advantages of thiazide diuretics are once daily dosing, limited titration (most patients respond well to the lowest dose), documented efficacy, additive effects with nearly all other antihypertensive agents, and low cost. Some studies have suggested that thiazide diuretics may protect against osteoporosis and hip fractures,[24] which may be a secondary advantage in the elderly. However, results of other studies do not support this advantage.[25] About 50 percent of hypertensive patients have mild hypertension which can be controlled with thiazide diuretics alone. A higher percentage of blacks and older patients appear to respond to thiazides compared to beta blockers.[26-28] Doses of thiazides should be 12.5 to 50 mg/day of hydrochlorothiazide or its equivalent. Both 12.5 and 25 mg of hydrochlorothiazide daily are effective.[29-31] Higher doses also produce hypokalemia, hypercalcemia, and hyperuricemia more commonly.

Hypokalemia, hyperlipidemia, hyperuricemia, and hyperglycemia are commonly discussed disadvantages of thiazides. In clinical studies kaliuresis is clearly dose related. Using moderate to large doses (about 100 mg hydrochlorothiazide or equivalent), the mean decrease in serum potassium is 0.6 to 0.7 meq/L. Reducing sodium intake reduces kaliuresis in diuretic-treated patients. Adding a potassium-sparing diuretic (e.g., triamterene, spironolactone, or amiloride) also reduces the frequency of hypokalemia. The effect of thiazides on potassium should be of greater concern in the elderly patient concurrently treated with digitalis glycosides or in whom hypokalemia is a preexisting condition. Data are conflicting regarding the risk of ventricular arrhythmias in diuretic-treated patients.[32] With the conflicting data that hypokalemia is safe, hypokalemia (i.e., K < 3.5 meq/L) should be avoided.

Very clearly, a small increase in total and low-density lipoprotein (LDL) serum cholesterol (6 to 10 percent) occurs during thiazide diuretic therapy. The effect on high-density lipoprotein (HDL) cholesterol is either no change or a small decrease (0 to 2 percent). Fortunately, the effect appears to be transient; in a VA cooperative study the total serum cholesterol values rose for about 12 weeks but were at pretreatment values after 12 months of therapy. Data regarding HDL and LDL cholesterol are not presented.[26,27] In the MRFIT study total, LDL, and HDL cholesterol were lower than baseline after 6 years of follow-up in the group prescribed diet and diuretics.[33] Whether the changes in cholesterol seen with diuretics affect patient outcome is unknown and should not preclude use of these agents, but it may be considered as an additional factor in selecting antihypertensive therapy.

Hyperuricemia occurs commonly with thiazide diuretics. Patients should not receive therapy for drug-induced, asymptomatic hyperuricemia. A nondiuretic treatment strategy should be considered if the pretreatment uric acid is above the normal range, but mild diuretic-induced hyperuricemia (uric acid less 9 mg/dL) does not contraindicate thiazide or loop diuretic therapy. The frequency of gout in thiazide-treated patients is less than 5 percent per year. If gout occurs, consideration should be given to an alternative drug in order to avoid adding another agent to control this adverse effect of the thiazide.

Hyperglycemia may be a problem for some patients receiving thiazide diuretics. The VA Cooperative Study Group assessed the effect of hydrochlorothiazide in doses of 50, 100, or 200 mg daily on serum glucose and on 2 h glucose tolerance in a subgroup. A total of three hydrochlorothiazide patients received oral hypoglycemic agents after the short- and long-term phases of the study. The average rise in fasting plasma glucose (FPG) was 4.7 to 6.4 mg/dL in the short- and long-term phases. Fewer than 5 percent of the patients had an increase in FPG to over 139 mg/dL. Eleven percent of the hydrochlorothiazide patients developed an abnormal 2-h glucose tolerance test. The patients taking 100 or 200 mg hydrochlorothiazide had markedly higher FPG and more frequent abnormal glucose tolerance tests compared to the patients taking 50 mg.[34] Berglund et al[35] found 1 of 53 men (1.9 percent) treated with bendroflumethiazide 2.5 to 5 mg daily developed overt diabetes in 10 years of follow-up. The precise reason for hyperglycemia developing with diuretic-treated patients is unknown. Recently, higher plasma insulin levels in conjunction with higher plasma glucose levels have been described in hypertensive patients compared to normals.[36] In elegant metabolic studies this *insulin resistance* appears to be mildly exacerbated by a thiazide and a beta blocker but not by an ACEI or a selective alpha$_1$ antagonist.[37-39] It is possible that hypokalemia contributes to this effect of thiazides. Diabetic patients may require modification of antidiabetic treatment. Correction of hypokalemia may reverse the hyperglycemic effects of diuretics, although this is not a uniform finding.

A less commonly discussed adverse effect of thiazide diuretics is sexual dysfunction. In the MRC trial 22.6 percent of the men reported impotence while taking bendroflumethiazide compared to 10.1 percent with placebo and 13.2 percent with propranolol. Impotence resolved with discontinuation of thiazide therapy.[28] Impotence due to drugs may be a particular problem in elderly male patients who have less "potency reserve."

Chlorthalidone is a "thiazide-like" diuretic which is significantly longer acting than hydrochlorothiazide. Chlorthalidone was used as initial therapy in the SHEP study.[10] It has similar efficacy and adverse effects when compared to hydrochlorothiazide. Chlorthalidone has been associated with significant volume depletion and electrolyte disturbances, particularly in the elderly. This is due in part to its long duration of action, but primarily it is due to use of excessive doses. In the SHEP trial, the maximum dose was 25 mg/day.[10] Despite potassium supplements for patients with serum potassium below 3.5 meq/L, 4 percent of patients had serum potassium below 3.2 meq/L at some time during the study, and 4 percent of patients also had serum sodium below 130 meq/L at some time during the study. Chlorthalidone is highly effective in elderly patients at doses of 12.5 to 25 mg/day, and this dose range should not be exceeded in elderly patients.

The loop diuretics, furosemide, bumetanide, and ethacrynic acid, have been reported to be less or equally effective antihypertensive agents compared to thiazides. These agents are best used to manage hypertension when the patient has renal failure (i.e., serum creatinine above 2 to 2.5 mg/dL) or CHF which cannot be controlled with a thiazide.

In summary, thiazide diuretics are effective in controlling hypertension. They may be particularly effective in the elderly patients. Doses of 12.5 to 25 mg daily of hydrochlorothiazide should produce an adequate response in many patients and reduce the frequency of adverse effects.

Beta blockers A total of 11 beta-adrenergic receptor antagonists (beta blockers) are commercially available in the United States. Propranolol, atenolol, and metoprolol are the three most commonly prescribed beta blockers. Differences between beta blockers include potency, routes of metabolism and/or excretion, half-life, relative selectivity for $beta_1$ and $beta_2$ receptors, lipid solubility, and intrinsic sympathomimetic activity (ISA). A summary of these differences is listed in Table 5-1. Whether greater lipophilicity is associated with more frequent central nervous system effects is debatable. It is also important to note that some studies support once daily dosing of beta blockers with short half-lives.[40] Therefore, longer half-lives or sustainedrelease products may have little advantage over other beta blockers. Having positive ISA has limited advantages in terms of controlling hypertension, although some patients, who develop significant bradycardia or bronchospasm with a beta blocker without ISA, may have fewer problems with pindolol or acebutolol. The antihypertensive efficacy of beta blockers in hypertension is equal among these drugs even though potency differs. Labetalol has some alpha blocking activity in combination with its beta blocking effects. However, in comparative, crossover trials as monotherapy, labetalol has not been more effective than other beta blockers.

The beta blockers competitively inhibit the activity of the sympathetic nervous system. Several mechanisms of action have been proposed for the beta blockers as antihypertensive agents. Initially the heart rate and cardiac output decline and peripheral resistance increases. In responding patients, the peripheral resistance returns toward baseline over time. Beta blockers inhibit renin release, which may be a part of the overall mechanism of action. From animal studies, small doses of

Table 5-1 Pharmacologic and pharmacokinetic properties of oral beta blockers in the United States

Drug	$Beta_1$ selectivity[a]	ISA[a]	Systemic availability, %	Metabolism/ excretion	Protein binding, %	Lipid solubility[a]	Half-life, h
Acebutolol	+	+	40–50	Hepatic/renal	25	+/++	3–4
Atenolol	++	-	50	Renal	10	+	6–7
Betaxolol	+	-	90	Hepatic	50	++	14–22
Carteolol	-	++	85	Renal	20–30	+	6–7
Labetalol[b]	-	-	25	Hepatic/renal	50	+/++	6–8
Metoprolol	++	-	50	Hepatic	12	++/+++	3–7
Nadolol	-	-	30	Renal	30	+	10–24
Penbutolol	-	+	>90	Hepatic	80–98	+++	5
Pindolol	-	+++	>90	Hepatic/renal	50	++	3–4
Propranolol	-	-	30	Hepatic	90	+++	3–5
Timolol	-	-	50–75	Hepatic	10	+/++	3–5

[a] +, low; ++, moderate; +++, high; -, absent.
[b] Also has alpha-blocking activity.

beta blockers injected directly into the cerebral ventricles result in a prompt fall in systemic blood pressure,[23] suggesting a central mechanism of action.

The traditional view is that beta blockers are less effective in the elderly than diuretics.[41] In the VA cooperative study,[27] propranolol in doses of 40 to 320 mg twice daily controlled blood pressure in 52.8 percent of the patients completing 12 months of treatment, while 65.5 percent of the patients treated with hydrochlorothiazide were controlled in this study. Other studies have shown metoprolol and nadolol to be effective in controlling blood pressure in patients 55 to 65 years old.[42,43] Clearly, beta blockers do control blood pressure in older people. However, the rate of control may be somewhat less than with diuretics.

Beta blockers are effective antianginal and antidysrhythmic agents in addition to their antihypertensive actions. Secondary prevention of myocardial infarction is a major indication for some beta blockers (e.g., propranolol, timolol, metoprolol, atenolol). The antianginal and antidysrhythmic properties of beta blockers without ISA should be considered when selecting therapy for patients with angina, after a myocardial infarction, or with dysrhythmias. Other properties shared by some beta blockers without ISA include efficacy in migraine prophylaxis and treatment of senile tremor.[28]

The MRC trial was a 5-year comparison of placebo, bendroflumethiazide, and propranolol in 17,354 patients. As noted previously, strokes were markedly reduced in the treated patients while CHD mortality was not statistically reduced. Interestingly, in the group of men who did not smoke, CHD morbidity and mortality were decreased. Smokers should be encouraged to stop smoking as an independent risk for CHD. However, in patients who do smoke, selection of a beta blocker which does not undergo oxidative metabolism might be considered since metabolism may be stimulated.

Contraindications for beta blockers are CHF, asthma, severe peripheral vascular disease, severe cardiac conduction abnormalities, and possibly diabetes mellitus. In diabetes mellitus, beta blockers may inhibit insulin release from beta cells in the pancreas, partially mask symptoms of hypoglycemia, and impair recovery of blood sugar to normal levels when hypoglycemia occurs. Symptoms of hypoglycemia are partially masked by beta blockers. However, since sweating is a parasympathetically mediated event, this symptom of hypoglycemia is not impaired by beta blockers. Hirsch and coworkers have utilized an elegant euglycemic clamp technique in the presence and absence of propranolol to show that beta blockade does not cause absolute hypoglycemia unawareness but shifts the glycemic thresholds for symptoms to lower plasma glucose concentrations in patients with type I diabetes mellitus.[44] Patients who are treated with insulin should receive special counseling regarding the difference in symptoms of hypoglycemia if a beta blocker is used to treat hypertension. Type I diabetics are at much greater risk of hypoglycemia than are type II diabetics, even when the type II patients are receiving insulin, because of the relative insulin resistance in type II patients. In type II patients impairment of insulin release by beta blockers is a problem which is rarely present in insulinopenic type I patients.

In nondiabetic patients propranolol has been found to cause a small rise in FPG of 4 to 4.7 mg/dL. In the VA cooperative study no patients taking propranolol had a glucose level exceeding 199 mg/dL after an oral glucose tolerance test.[34] The development of diabetes is uncommon in propranolol-treated patients. In a 10-year study, Berglund et al noted that diabetes developed in 5/53 (9.4 percent) of the patients taking propranolol. In this group one patient also received a diuretic and another was receiving glucocorticoid therapy when the diagnosis of diabetes was established.[35]

Beta blockers without ISA may cause an increase in total cholesterol (TC) and LDL cholesterol (LDL-C) and a decrease in HDL cholesterol (HDL-C), although the changes are fairly small. The increases in TC and LDL-C are in the range of 3 to 4 percent. TC/HDL-C ratios increase 10 to 20 percent with atenolol, nadolol, metoprolol, and propranolol. Pindolol and acebutolol cause either a small decrease in TC or no change. The HDL-C rises about 4 percent with ISA positive agents. Labetalol has little or no effect on TC.[33] Although these biochemical changes occur, no data are currently available which assess the outcomes of patients treated with beta blockers to determine if these small changes in lipid metabolism are clinically important. Because trials to provide these data would have to be very large and have confounding variables, it is unlikely that this information will ever be available. The significance of these changes and their implications for therapy must remain a matter of clinical judgment.

Adverse effects associated with beta blockers include fatigue, asthma, CHF, insomnia, nightmares, depression, and cognitive side effects. Impotence was reported in about 13 percent of the men randomized to propranolol in the MRC trial. The frequency of impotence with propranolol was intermediate to that which occurred with hydrochlorothiazide (22.6 percent) and placebo (10.1 percent).[28] A withdrawal syndrome may occur with beta blockers. Withdrawal symptoms are typically sympathetic manifestations (e.g., tachycardia, hypertension, angina, myocardial infarction). This syndrome is particularly important when the beta-blocker doses are large, the patient is concurrently taking a central alpha-agonist agent, and/or the pretreatment blood pressure is very high. A conservative approach would be to taper beta blockers if discontinuation is necessary.

The beta blockers are effective antihypertensive agents in elderly as well as young patients. However, a somewhat lower response rate may be expected in older patients. Therapy should be initiated with lower doses and slowly titrated to control blood pressure.

Angiotensin converting enzyme inhibitors Currently captopril, enalapril, lisinopril, fosinopril, benazepril, and ramipril are the commercially available ACEIs. Other members of this class are in various stages of development and approval (e.g., spirapril, perindopril, quinapril). These drugs inhibit the metabolic conversion of angiotensin I to angiotensin II, the most potent vasoconstrictor known. The converting enzyme also degrades bradykinin. Therefore, enzyme inhibition also increases concentrations of this potent vasodilator. A central mechanism may also be involved in the hypotensive effects of ACEIs, since angiotensin II increases adrenergic outflow from the brain.[45] Differences between these drugs are potency, metabolic/excretory pathways, and half-life. These drugs are very similar when used clinically. A summary of pharmacologic and pharmacokinetic properties appears in Table 5-2.

Captopril is rapidly absorbed with about 70 percent bioavailability. Ingestion with food may reduce captopril's bioavailability, although this change has not been proven to be clinically significant. The half-life is about 2 h. Approximately one-half of a captopril dose is rapidly metabolized to captopril-cysteine disulfide and the disulfide dimer of captopril. About 40 to 50 percent of captopril is excreted unchanged in the urine, but the metabolites are also renally excreted.

Enalapril is a prodrug, which is rapidly deesterified in the liver to enalaprilat. Peak serum concentrations are reached in about 4 h. The lysine analog of enalapril, lisinopril, is more slowly absorbed than the other ACEIs. The half-life of these two ACEIs is 11 to 12 h. Approximately 40 percent of an oral dose of enalapril is absorbed. Bioavailability of lisinopril is about 25 percent, and peak concentrations occur in about 8 h, which corresponds to the peak hypotensive effect. Although different bioavailabilities are reported for these ACEIs, it is unclear if the effective doses of these drugs are different.

Ramipril is also a prodrug of the ACEI ramiprilat. The half-life of ramipril is about 4.5 h, although a very long terminal elimination half-life of 110 h suggests tight binding to angiotensin converting enzyme. Between 50 and 60 percent of administered ramipril is absorbed from the gastrointestinal tract.

Fosinopril sodium is hydrolyzed after absorption to fosinoprilat. Administration as the sodium salt improves absorption, which averaged 36 percent in healthy volunteers. Taken with food, absorption of fosinopril may be slowed while the extent of absorption is not changed. Typically, the peak in blood levels occurs 3 h after a dose, although the lowest blood pressure after doses occurs between 12 and 16 h. In

Table 5-2 Pharmacologic and pharmacokinetic properties of oral angiotensin converting enzyme inhibitors available in the United States

Drug	Sulfhydryl group	Pro-drug	Metabolism/ excretion[a]	Systemic availability, %	t_{max}, h	Half-life, h
Benazepril	No	Yes	Hepatic/renal	40	2	10.5
Captopril	Yes	No	Hepatic/renal	70	1	2
Enalapril	No	Yes	Renal	40	4	11
Fosinopril	No	Yes	Renal/hepatic	36	3	12
Lisinopril	No	No	Renal	25	8	12
Ramipril	No	Yes	Renal	55	3	4.5

[a]Primary route is shown above the slash; only one route is listed if the other route clears a minor or negligible portion.

healthy volunteers, 46 percent of an intravenous dose was recovered in the urine and 44 percent in the feces. As renal function declines, hepatic clearance increases. Therefore, the total body clearance of fosinoprilat remains constant at any degree of renal insufficiency. According to the manufacturer, 12 healthy subjects 65 to 74 years of age had the same absorption, distribution, protein binding, and excretion as 12 healthy subjects aged 20 to 35 years. The half-life is about 12 h.

Benazepril HCl is also a prodrug. Benazeprilat results from hydrolysis in the liver. Peak benazeprilat plasma concentrations occur 1 to 2 h after ingestion when taken fasting and 2 to 4 h after ingestion when taken with food. The half-life is 10 to 11 h. Benazeprilat is extensively metabolized in the liver; only 20 percent of benazeprilat is excreted in the urine, and about 12 percent is excreted unchanged in bile. Pharmacokinetics in a group of younger (21 to 39 years) and older (66 to 74 years) volunteers were very similar with single and multiple doses.

Enalapril, lisinopril, and ramipril are excreted primarily in the urine; elderly patients may have exaggerated responses to these drugs since glomerular filtration rates are less in this group of patients. Fosinoprilat has renal and hepatic excretion while benazeprilat has primarily hepatic excretion. No evidence of an exaggerated response to these drugs in patients with hepatic insufficiency was found. Differences in pharmacokinetics do not result in clinically important therapeutic differences if pharmacokinetic differences are considered at the outset of treatment when the therapeutic plan is developed.

Clinical studies have documented that ACEIs will lower blood pressure significantly.[39] For example, 51 percent of patients over 60 years old responded to captopril monotherapy, with black and white patients responding equally.[46] All ACEIs except captopril are effective in many patients when given once daily. Captopril is effective when given twice daily, while a few studies document once daily efficacy. In elderly patients initial doses of captopril should not exceed 12.5 mg twice daily initially. Maximum doses of captopril should be 150 mg daily, although a flat relationship between dose and maximum response has been noted, because binding to angiotensin converting enzyme is essentially complete at low doses. However, as with any drug, an increase in dose will increase duration of effect. Enalapril and lisinopril should be given in doses of 2.5 to 40 mg daily with lower doses being used initially. Ramipril doses range from 2.5 to 10 mg once daily. Benazepril and fosinopril should be given initially in 10-mg daily doses. Dosage adjustments between 20 and 40 mg daily may be needed to control blood pressure at 24 h; some patients may require 30-mg daily or twice daily dosing. ACEIs and diuretics produce additive hypotensive effects, and combination therapy might be considered, instead of using higher ACEI doses. Patients with diabetes and CHF would be excellent candidates for ACEI therapy. Diabetic proteinuria appears to be reduced and insulin sensitivity is increased by ACEI therapy.[47] Numerous trials have documented the effectiveness of ACEIs in CHF.[23]

Adverse effects of ACEIs are of some concern. Initially very high doses of captopril were used to manage hypertension. Rarely, patients developed proteinuria and agranulocytosis. With the findings that lower ACEI doses are very effective, these severe toxic reactions are very rare. However, patients should be counseled to report any signs of infection (e.g., fever). Patients with bilateral renal artery stenosis or renal artery stenosis in a solitary kidney may develop acute renal failure when ACEIs are prescribed. Severe hyperkalemia and angioedema are also rare adverse effects of any ACEIs. Patients should have follow-up evaluation of renal function and electrolytes to reduce the patient's risk for these serious or life-threatening adverse events. Patients should also be informed to seek immediate medical care if dyspnea or rapid facial, neck, or tongue swelling occur. Nonproductive, chronic coughing may occur in 10 to 15 percent of patients taking ACEIs. This side effect is reversible when the drug is discontinued, although coughing may resolve very slowly. Patients who are volume depleted, due to diuretic treatment, for example, can develop severe hypotension.[17] No apparent adverse effects on glucose or lipid metabolism are known to occur with ACEIs.[33]

Nonsteroidal anti-inflammatory drugs (e.g., indomethacin, aspirin) have been noted to interfere with the hypotensive effects of ACEIs. The former agents are known to inhibit cyclooxygenase and reduce renal vasodilator prostaglandin excretion. Lithium toxicity has rarely been noted in patients treated concurrently with ACEIs.[23]

Calcium channel antagonists Seven voltage-dependent calcium channel antagonists, commonly referred to as *calcium channel blockers* (CCBs), are capable of lowering blood pressure and are commercially available, although nimodipine and bepridil are not indicated for treatment of hypertension. These drugs are chemically very different, but all are effective in lowering blood pressure. Vasoconstriction and myocardial contractility are dependent upon calcium entry into cells, possibly through heterogenous channels. Once calcium enters a vasoactive cell, it binds to calmodulin, resulting in activation of actin-myosin and contraction. The overall mechanism of these agents is reducing the entry of calcium into cells and slowing contractility or automaticity. The pharmacologic effects of CCBs are listed in Table 5-3.[48]

Immediate-release verapamil can be given twice daily. Comparing response and pharmacokinetics in the young, elderly, and very elderly, a longer half-life (3.8, 8, and 7.4 h, respectively) and greater hypotensive response (7.3, 13.5, and 15.9

Table 5-3 Pharmacologic properties of calcium channel blockers

Effect	Nifedipine[a]	Verapamil	Diltiazem
Heart rate	+/+[b]	+/–	+/–
Contractility	+/–	–/–	–
Atrioventricular conduction	+/–	–/–	–
Vasodilation	+/+	+	+

[a]Nifedipine represents dihydropyridine CCBs (e.g., nicardipine, isradipine, felodipine, amlodipine).
[b]+/+, marked increase; +, increase; +/–, no change or decrease; –, decrease; –/–, marked decrease.

mmHg fall in mean blood pressure, respectively) have been reported.[49] Immediate-release nifedipine, nicardipine, and diltiazem need to be given at least three times daily to control blood pressure. Sustained-release products for verapamil, nifedipine, and diltiazem, which allow once or twice daily dosing, are now commercially available. Each of the CCBs should be started at lower doses and titrated to controlled blood pressure. The ranges of daily doses used in hypertension are as follows: verapamil 120 to 480 mg, diltiazem 90 to 360 mg, nifedipine 30 to 120 mg, and nicardipine 60 to 120 mg. Isradipine, the newest commercially available CCB, is effective in doses of 2.5 to 10 mg twice daily. All CCBs are effective in lowering blood pressure and provide additional, but less than additive, hypotensive effects in combination with diuretics.

The CCBs have been suggested to have greater efficacy than other agents in blacks and the elderly.[17] In a recent review, data supporting greater efficacy of CCBs were not found for elderly hypertensives compared to diuretics and beta blockers, although blacks may respond more frequently to CCBs than to ACEIs.[50]

Adverse reactions which occur most commonly with the dihydropyridine CCBs are vasodilator effects (flushing, headaches, ankle edema, reflex tachycardia). Sustained-release nifedipine appears to cause vasodilator adverse reactions less commonly than immediate-release nifedipine. These agents can occasionally cause angina when excessive vasodilation or hypotension occurs. Verapamil and diltiazem are more likely to cause bradycardia and conduction abnormalities. The most common adverse effect of verapamil is constipation, which requires stopping verapamil in less than 10 percent of patients, but it is more of a problem in elderly patients, in whom constipation is a common complaint. All three classes of CCBs have been rarely reported to cause CHF and hepatitis. Although qualitatively similar, diltiazem causes adverse reactions less frequently than verapamil, nifedipine, or nicardipine.[48] No significant adverse metabolic reactions have been reported with CCBs at therapeutic doses.[33] However, in overdose situations severe hyperglycemia may occur.

Sympatholytic agents Various drugs affecting adrenergic tone have sites of action in the central nervous system and peripherally. The peripheral $alpha_1$ antagonists commercially available are prazosin, terazosin, and doxazosin. Each of these drugs reduces peripheral resistance by competitively blocking postsynaptic alpha-adrenergic receptors. This mechanism allows for feedback inhibition to presynaptic $alpha_2$ receptors, resulting in less reflex tachycardia[51] than observed with vasodilators such as hydralazine. Prazosin is rapidly absorbed, has a half-life of about 3 h, and is commonly given 2 or 3 times daily. The newer agents, terazosin and doxazosin, have longer durations of action and can be given once or twice daily. The range of daily doses for each of these agents is as follows: prazosin 2 to 20 mg, terazosin 1 to 40 mg, and doxazosin 1 to 16 mg. The $alpha_1$ antagonists have been used as monotherapy for mild hypertension successfully, although they are not included as first-line therapy by the JNC. Recent information supports use of these drugs in men with benign prostatic hypertrophy, since they relax the bladder sphincter.[52] Although objective and subjective improvement has occurred, placebo controls have generally been lacking. In patients with hypertension and symptomatic prostatic hypertrophy, a trial of an $alpha_1$ antagonist may be considered.

With all three of these drugs about 10 to 15 percent of patients discontinue therapy due to an adverse reaction, primarily due to dizziness, vertigo, and weakness. Other adverse effects include fatigue, tachycardia, nausea, headache, nasal congestion, and impotence. One advantage of $alpha_1$ antagonists may be the small decrease in TC and rise in HDL-C,[33] although no major clinical trials have used any of these agents to determine if the biochemical changes result in positive outcomes related to CHD.

Centrally acting $alpha_2$ agonists include methyldopa, clonidine, guanabenz, and guanfacine.[23] These drugs stimulate inhibitory centers in the brain and reduce sympathetic outflow from the central nervous system. The primary differences among this group of agents are potency. No therapeutic difference is apparent between these four drugs except dose. All of these agents cause drowsiness, dry mouth, depression, decreased cognitive function, postural hypotension, and impotence. Methyldopa can also rarely cause hepatitis, fever, hemolytic anemia, thrombocytopenia, and a systemic lupus erythematosus (SLE)-like syndrome, which the other members of this class do not. A withdrawal syndrome, or *rebound hypertension*, is commonly associated with clonidine but may occur with any of these agents when used in high doses and abruptly discontinued. Withdrawal symptoms may occur more commonly when any of these drugs is combined with a beta blocker, due to continued beta blockade and unopposed vasoconstrictor alpha-adrenergic stimulation. Clonidine transdermal patches cause skin rashes, most of which are not severe, in about 20 percent of patients.

Clonidine, methyldopa, and guanabenz are most often given twice daily. Guanfacine has a longer duration of action and can be given once daily. Typical daily dose ranges for this group of antihypertensives are as follows: Clonidine 0.1 to 0.4 mg, guanabenz 4 to 16 mg, guanfacine 1 to 3 mg, and methyldopa 250 to 1000 mg. Maximum doses of these drugs are 1.2, 32, 3, and 2000 mg, respectively. Clonidine is also available as a transdermal system which slowly releases 0.1 to 0.3 mg/day. When the transdermal patch is used, the onset is slower (2 to 3 days), but each patch is effective for 7 days. With high doses, clonidine and other $alpha_2$ agonists can paradoxically raise blood pressure.

Reserpine inhibits uptake of norepinephrine into adrenergic neurons, which results in reduced peripheral vascular resistance. Catecholamines are also reduced in the central nervous system, which may be the reason for the sedative and depressive effects of reserpine. Advantages of reserpine include once daily dosing, ease of titration, and the fact that it is the least expensive antihypertensive agent available.[23]

Adverse effects of reserpine include nasal congestion, cognitive functional impairment, and depression. Patients with past history of depression should not receive reserpine. However, elderly patients have tolerated low doses of reserpine well in comparison to metoprolol, methyldopa, and hydralazine, each in combination with hydrochlorothiazide.[53,54] Daily doses of reserpine should never exceed 0.25 mg, and in combination with a diuretic, doses as low as 0.05 mg daily are effective.[23]

Guanethidine and guanadrel are actively taken into adrenergic neurons. Initially, norepinephrine release is inhibited, and subsequently storage granules are depleted, resulting in peripheral vasodilation. Based upon the depletion of norepinephrine from storage granules, orthostatic hypotension is a fairly common problem associated with these agents. Fluid retention, diarrhea, and failure of ejaculation occur with guanethidine. Guanadrel is a shorter acting agent and has similar adverse effects but appears to be better tolerated than guanethidine (possibly related to lower doses of guanadrel commonly being used). Since orthostatic hypotension is a concern in the elderly, these drugs should be avoided if possible in this subgroup or in any patients with orthostatic hypotension.

Direct-acting vasodilators Hydralazine and minoxidil are the two commercially available *direct-acting* vasodilators for oral use. The mechanisms of action of these drugs are different. Hydralazine causes relaxation of smooth muscle in peripheral arteriolar walls; at least part of this effect is mediated through endothelial-derived relaxing factor (EDRF) or nitric oxide (NO). Minoxidil appears to be a prodrug. Minoxidil sulfate causes vasodilation, apparently through effects on potassium channels. Both drugs can hyperpolarize vascular smooth muscle, which results in calcium or potassium being unable to enter cells. A lowering of peripheral resistance results in lowering the blood pressure. As peripheral resistance falls, stroke volume, heart rate, and possibly myocardial oxygen consumption rise. Angina may occur when myocardial oxygen consumption increases. Tachyphylaxis to direct vasodilators occurs when they are used alone, due to the reflex tachycardia and fluid retention which occur as peripheral resistance falls. In the elderly, baroreceptor reflexes may be impaired and less tachycardia may be observed.[23]

Headache, fluid retention, reflex tachycardia, and precipitation of angina in patients with CHD are common adverse effects of hydralazine and minoxidil. Hydralazine can cause a reversible systemic lupus erythematosus syndrome which occurs rarely at doses of less than 200 mg daily. Minoxidil commonly produces hypertrichosis which slowly resolves if minoxidil is stopped. Pleural and pericardial effusions as well as nonspecific ST changes on the ECG can occur with minoxidil therapy. Based upon the adverse reactions of these drugs, they are used in combination with other antihypertensive agents when severe, uncontrolled hypertension that is unresponsive to other therapy is present.[23]

The major differences between hydralazine and minoxidil are potency and duration of action. Minoxidil is much more potent and longer acting compared to hydralazine. It also has a greater maximum effect at tolerable doses. Hydralazine is well absorbed and has a half-life of about 2 to 3 h. Although the half-life is short, it can be given twice daily. Hydralazine is typically given in doses of 25 to 100 mg two or three times daily, while minoxidil doses are 2.5 to 80 mg daily given in one or two doses.

Approach to Treating Elderly Hypertensives

Confirming that the patient has hypertension by repeating blood pressure measurements over weeks to months is important for the majority of hypertensive patients with SBP < 180 mmHg and DBP 90–114 mmHg. Using this time to establish a diagnosis also allows for implementation and assessment of the efficacy of nonpharmacologic treatment.

In patients with DBP 90 to 95 mmHg and SBP < 160 mmHg and without end-organ damage or other CHD risk factors, drug therapy should be delayed. After a trial of nonpharmacologic therapy patients with coexisting risk factors and/or persistent DBP > 95 mmHg or SBP > 160 mmHg should have drug therapy. Important differences in efficacy between classes of drugs are fairly small. Diuretics may be more effective in controlling hypertension in black and elderly patients.[21] Demographic and pathologic characteristics of patients are very helpful in designing pharmacotherapeutic regimens. Managing hypertension and a concomitant illness with a single drug helps to keep regimens simple and less costly. Avoiding drugs which may worsen concomitant illness or interact with medications for that illness is also of paramount importance. Individualized treatment can follow the JNC guidelines.[17] It is important to recall that the ideal antihypertensive drug does not exist (Table 5-4).[28] A compilation of various diseases and drugs which should be preferred or avoided to treat hypertension is provided in Table 5-5.

Therapy with one drug in a small dose and in a simple regimen should be undertaken. Most drugs can be given once or twice daily, although a sustained-release preparation may be needed. In a recent study of hypertensive patients, compliance was 96 percent with once, 93 percent with twice, and 84 percent with thrice daily regimens.[55] These results suggest that compliance with medication

Table 5-4 Ideal antihypertensive drug characteristics

Controls SBP and DBP in 100% of patients with mild hypertension
Well tolerated and without serious adverse effects
Long duration of effect (to allow 1-2 daily doses)
For elderly, reduces peripheral resistance, maintains cardiac output
Few drug-drug interactions
Reduces cardiovascular morbidity and mortality in clinical trials
Additive responses with other antihypertensives
Absence of adverse metabolic effects
Absence of pseudotolerance
Few contraindications
Inexpensive

Source: Modified from Ref. 28.

Table 5-5 Choices among antihypertensive agents

Condition	Drugs to consider[a]	Drugs to avoid
Angina	BBs, CCBs	Hydralazine, minoxidil
CHF	Diuretics, ACEIs, hydralazine, $alpha_1$ blockers, nitrates	BBs, CCBs?
Chronic obstructive pulmonary disease/asthma	CCBs, $alpha_1$ blockers, $alpha_2$ agonists, ACEIs	BBs
Depression	ACEIs, CCBs, diuretics, vasodilators	Reserpine, $alpha_2$ agonists, BBs?
Diabetes	ACEIs, CCBs, $alpha_1$ blockers, $alpha_2$ agonists	BBs, diuretics
Migraine headache	BBs, CCBs, clonidine	Vasodilators
Myocardial infarction prophylaxis	Non-ISA BBs	—
Osteoporosis	Thiazide diuretics?	Loop diuretics?
Prostatic hypertrophy	$Alpha_1$ antagonists	—
Renal failure	Loop diuretics, CCBs, ACEIs, vasodilators, BBs	ACEIs[b]
SVT	BB, verapamil, diltiazem	Vasodilators, dihydropyridine CCBs
Ulcer disease	$Alpha_2$ agonists, CCBs, BBs	Reserpine, guanethidine

[a]BB, beta blocker; CCB, calcium channel blocker; ACEI, angiotensin converting enzyme inhibitor; non-ISA BB, beta blocker without intrinsic sympathomimetic activity.

[b]ACEI can cause acute renal failure if bilateral renal artery stenosis is present.

regimens is the same with once or twice daily therapy, and once or twice daily therapy can be individualized to fit each patient's lifestyle. The quality of life is important for a largely asymptomatic disease. A great deal of flexibility should occur in prescribing therapy for elderly patients with hypertension in order to not worsen the quality of life. Although ACEIs are heavily promoted as improving quality of life, some patients will have to discontinue therapy with ACEIs due to fatigue, sexual dysfunction, headache, nightmares, coughing, hyperkalemia, anxiety, neutropenia, and acute renal failure. Croog et al[56] have reported greater improvement in well being with captopril compared to methyldopa and propranolol. However, more patients taking captopril (33 percent) required the addition of hydrochlorothiazide than either methyldopa- (28 percent) or propranolol- (22 percent) treated patients, suggesting that the doses may not have been equivalent. Worsening of general well being, physical symptoms, and sexual dysfunction were reported in 18.8 to 30.9

percent of the captopril-treated subjects. Although captopril was associated with statistically less frequent adverse effects than the methyldopa- or propranolol-treated patients, quality of life may be a clinically important problem with all three drugs in individual patients. The cost of therapy should be considered as a portion of the quality of life. As first-line therapy, costs are least with diuretics, reserpine, some beta blockers, hydralazine, and generic verapamil compared to other beta blockers, ACEIs, central agents, $alpha_1$ antagonists, and other CCBs. In one study, patients reported being unable to afford medications with substantial frequency,[22] which may be exacerbated in the elderly with limited, fixed incomes. Compliance, control of blood pressure, and subsequent hypertensive complications may occur if medications are not affordable. Anticipation of adverse effects as part of the monitoring also helps to reduce the frequency of repeating laboratory tests unnecessarily. For example, after about 1 week the maximum hypokalemic effect of diuretics is usually seen.[57] Measuring serum electrolytes very frequently may be unnecessary unless doses or drugs are changed. After baseline electrolytes, follow-up might be considered in about 6 weeks and, if normal, in another 6 to 12 months.

If patients fail to respond in 1 to 3 months to monotherapy at optimal dose, it is possible to switch to alternative monotherapy or add an agent with a different mechanism of action (e.g., diuretic added to beta blockers, CCBs, or ACEIs). In patients treated with appropriate agents with different mechanisms of action but who fail to attain goal blood pressure, the clinician should consider noncompliance, inadequate dosing, drug-drug interactions, or intercurrent illness. Collaboration between physicians, pharmacists, nurses, and patients can improve compliance. Patient education regarding the long-term sequelae of uncontrolled hypertension and determining the patient's attitude regarding medication taking are responsibilities of the physician, nurse, and pharmacist. Monitoring medication taking by counting tablets or capsules at return visits or assessing prescription refill histories may identify noncompliant patients. Simplification of complex regimens and ritualizing times of taking medications may improve patient compliance. If noncompliance is due to adverse reactions, therapy should be modified to attain control of blood pressure without intolerance. Doses may be increased with the caveat that elderly patients may have exaggerated responses to medications. Common drug-drug interactions for antihypertensive agents are listed in Table 5-6. A very common drug combination observed by the authors in elderly patients is an ACEI and a nonsteroidal anti-inflammatory agent (NSAID). Patients prescribed NSAID therapy can have loss of hypotensive effects when hypertension is treated with ACEIs. A rise in blood pressure may also occur in patients treated with other antihypertensive agents when an NSAID is added to the regimen.

The SHEP results support the conclusion that patients with ISH should receive therapy.[15] Patients with SBP > 160 mmHg should benefit from treatment with low-dose antihypertensive therapy if nonpharmacologic treatment fails. The endpoint of treatment should be to lower the SBP to 140 to 160 mmHg.[17]

A currently unanswered question is whether antihypertensive therapy must be continued for life. The JNC recommendation is that patients with mild hypertension

Table 5-6 Common drug-drug interactions with antihypertensive agents

Antihypertensive	Interacting Drugs
Diuretics	Increase lithium serum concentration; NSAIDs decrease hypotensive effect
Sympatholytics	Tricyclic antidepressants decrease effect of guanethidine (+) and clonidine (+/-); hypertension with sympathomimetics
Beta blockers	Reduced absorption with cholesterol-binding resins; cimetidine may reduce metabolism and increase effect of BBs with extensive metabolism; verapamil + BBs may cause CHF; NSAIDs may reduce antihypertensive effect
ACE inhibitors	NSAIDs may reduce antihypertensive effect; hyperkalemia with potassium sparing diuretics/KCl; occasionally may increase serum lithium concentrations
Calcium channel blockers	Hypotension possible with quinidine; increased digoxin levels with verapamil; cimetidine may increase CCB effect; nicardipine and diltiazem may increase cyclosporine serum concentrations

who have had controlled blood pressure for at least 1 year can have medications gradually reduced and withdrawn as long as blood pressure remains controlled.[17] Maintenance of nonpharmacologic therapy may be important to controlling blood pressure in these patients. In several clinical trials 21 to over 50 percent of the patients on various antihypertensive agents had controlled blood pressure for as long as 12 to 30 months after discontinuing treatment.[58-60] From a pharmacotherapeutic standpoint, using the lowest dose or maintaining control without pharmacologic treatment is most likely to achieve the goal of controlling blood pressure without adverse effects.

REFERENCES

1. Stokes III J, Kannel WB, Wolf PA, et al: Blood pressure as a risk factor for cardiovascular disease. The Framingham Study—30 years of follow-up. *Hypertension* 13(suppl I): I13–I18, 1989.
2. Kannel WB, Gordon T, Schwartz MJ: Systolic versus diastolic blood pressure and the risk of coronary heart disease. The Framingham Study. *Am J Cardiol* 27: 335–346, 1971.
3. Kaplan NM: Hypertension in the population at large, in *Clinical Hypertension*. Williams & Wilkins, Baltimore, MD, 1990, pp 1–25.
4. Whelton PK, Klag MJ: Hypertension as a risk factor of renal disease. Review of clinical and epidemiological evidence. *Hypertension* 13(suppl I): I-19–I-27, 1989.
5. Harlan WR, Hull AL, Schmouder RL, et al: High blood pressure in older Americans. The first National Health and Nutrition Examination survey. *Hypertension* 6: 802–809, 1984.
6. The Working Group on Hypertension in the Elderly: Statement on hypertension in the elderly. *JAMA* 256: 70–74, 1986.

7. Gifford Jr RW: Review of the long-term controlled trials of usefulness of therapy for systemic hypertension. *Am J Cardiol* 63: 8B–16B, 1989.
8. Gifford Jr RW: Long-term trials in hypertension. *J Hyperten* 8(suppl 2): S17–S22, 1990.
9. Collins R, Peto R, MacMahon S, et al: Blood pressure, stroke, and coronary heart disease. Part 2, short-term reduction in blood pressure: overview of randomized drug trials in their epidemiological context. *Lancet* 335: 827–838, 1990.
10. SHEP Cooperative Research Group: Prevention of stroke by antihypertensive drug treatment in older persons with isolated systolic hypertension. *JAMA* 265: 3255–3264, 1991.
11. The Multiple Risk Factor Intervention Trial Research Group: Mortality rates after 10.5 years for participants in the Multiple Risk Factor Intervention Trial. Findings related to a priori hypotheses of the trial. *JAMA* 263: 1795–1801, 1990.
12. Berglund G: Goals of antihypertensive therapy. Is there a point beyond which pressure reduction is dangerous? *Am J Hyperten* 2: 586–593, 1989.
13. Davidson RA, Caranasos GJ: Should the elderly hypertensive be treated? Evidence from clinical trials. *Arch Intern Med* 147: 1933–1937, 1987.
14. Hulley SB, Furberg CD, Gurland B, et al: Systolic Hypertension in the Elderly Program (SHEP): antihypertensive efficacy of chlorthalidone. Am J Cardiol 56: 913–920, 1985.
15. Hulley SB, Feigal D, Ireland C, et al: Systolic Hypertension in the Elderly Program (SHEP). The first three months. *J Am Geriatr Soc* 34: 101–105, 1986.
16. Byyny RL: Hypertension in the elderly, in Laragh JH, Brenner BM (eds): *Hypertension. Pathophysiology, Diagnosis, and Management.* Raven, New York, 1990, pp 1869–1887.
17. The 1988 Report of the Joint National Committee on Detection, Evaluation, and Treatment of High Blood Pressure. *Arch Intern Med* 148: 1023–1038, 1988.
18. Messerli FH: Osler's maneuver, pseudohypertension, and true hypertension in the elderly. *Am J Med* 80: 906–910, 1986.
19. Caird FI, Andrews GR, Kennedy RD: Effect of posture on blood pressure in the elderly. *Br Heart J* 35: 527–530, 1973.
20. Kaplan NM: Misdiagnosis of systemic hypertension and recommendations for improvement. *Am J Cardiol* 60: 1383–1386, 1987.
21. Moser M: Relative efficacy of, and some adverse reactions to, different antihypertensive regimens. *Am J Cardiol* 63: 2B–7B, 1989.
22. Shulman NB, Martinez B, Brogan D, et al: Financial cost as an obstacle to hypertension therapy. *Am J Public Health* 76: 1105–1108, 1986.
23. Kaplan NM: Treatment of hypertension: drug therapy, in *Clinical Hypertension*, 5th ed. Williams & Wilkins, Baltimore, MD, 1990, pp 182–267.
24. Wasnich R, Davis J, Ross P, Vogel J: Effect of thiazides on rates of bone mineral loss: a longitudinal study. *Br Med J* 301: 1303–1305, 1990.
25. Heidrich FE, Stergachis A, Gross KM: Diuretic use and the risk of hip fractures. *Ann Intern Med* 115: 1–6, 1991.
26. Veterans Administration Cooperative Study Group on Antihypertensive Agents: Comparison of propranolol and hydrochlorothiazide for the initial treatment of hypertension. I. Results of short-term titration with emphasis on racial differences in response. *JAMA* 248: 1996-2003, 1982.
27. Veterans Administration Cooperative Study Group on Antihypertensive Agents: Comparison of propranolol and hydrochlorothiazide for the initial treatment of hypertension. II. Results of long-term therapy. *JAMA* 248: 2004–2011, 1982.
28. Gifford Jr RW, Borazanian RA: Traditional first-line therapy. Overview of medical benefits and side effects. *Hypertension* 13(suppl I): I-119–I-124, 1989.
29. Beerman B, Groschinsky-Grid M: Antihypertensive effect of various doses of hydrochlorothiazide and its relation to the plasma level of the drug. *Eur J Clin Pharmacol* 13: 195, 1978.
30. Degnbol B, Dorph S, Marner T: The effect of different diuretics on elevated blood pressure and serum potassium. *Acta Med Scand* 193: 407, 1973.

31. Berglund G, Andersson O: Low doses of hydrochlorothiazide in hypertension: antihypertensive and metabolic effects. *Eur J Clin Pharmacol* 10:177, 1976.
32. Freis ED: The cardiotoxicity of thiazide diuretics: review of the evidence. *J Hypertens* 8(suppl 2): S23–S32, 1990.
33. Houston MC: New insights and new approaches for the treatment of essential hypertension: selection of therapy based on coronary heart disease risk factor analysis, hemodynamic profiles, quality of life, and subset analysis. *Am Heart J* 117: 911–951, 1989.
34. Veterans Administration Cooperative Study Group on Antihypertensive Agents: Propranolol or hydrochlorothiazide alone for the initial treatment of hypertension. IV. Effect on plasma glucose and glucose tolerance. *Hypertension* 7: 1008–1016, 1985.
35. Berglund G, Andersson O, Widgren B: Low-dose antihypertensive treatment with a thiazide diuretic is not diabetogenic. A 10 year controlled trial with bendroflumethiazide. *Acta Med Scand* 220: 419–424, 1986.
36. Ferranini E, Buzzigoli G, Bonadonna R, et al: Insulin resistance in essential hypertension. *N Engl J Med* 317: 350–357, 1987.
37. Pollare T, Lithell H, Berne C: A comparison of effects of hydrochlorothiazide and captopril on glucose and lipid metabolism in patients with hypertension. *N Engl J Med* 321: 868–873, 1989.
38. Pollare T, Lithell H, Mörlin C, et al: Metabolic effects of diltiazem and atenolol: results from a randomized, double-blind study with parallel groups. *J Hyperten* 7: 551–559, 1989.
39. Pollare T, Lithell H, Selinus I, Berne C: Application of prazosin is associated with an increase of insulin sensitivity in obese patients with hypertension. *Diabetologia* 31: 415–420, 1988.
40. Carter BL, Gersema LM, Williams GO, Schabold K: Once-daily propranolol for hypertension: a comparison of regular release, long-acting, and generic formulations. *Pharmacotherapy* 9: 17–22, 1989.
41. Buhler FR, Burkart F, Lutold BE, et al: Antihypertensive beta-blocking action as related to renin and age: a pharmacologic tool to identify pathogenic mechanisms in essential hypertension. *Am J Cardiol* 36: 653–669, 1975.
42. Wikstrand J, Westergren G, Berlund G, et al: Antihypertensive treatment with metoprolol or hydrochlorothiazide in patients aged 60 to 75 years. Report from a double-blind international multicenter study. *JAMA* 255: 1304–1310, 1986.
43. Freis E: Age and antihypertensive drugs (hydrochlorothiazide, bendroflumethiazide, nadolol, and captopril). *Am J Cardiol* 61: 17–21, 1988.
44. Hirsch IB, Boyle PJ, Craft S, Cryer PE: Higher glycemic thresholds for symptoms during β-adrenergic blockade in IDDM. *Diabetes* 40: 1177–1186, 1991.
45. Frohlich ED: Angiotensin converting enzyme inhibitors. Present and future. *Hypertension* 13(suppl I): I125–I130, 1989.
46. Tuck ML, Katz LA, Kirkendall WM, et al: Low-dose captopril in mild to moderate geriatric hypertension. *J Am Geriatr Soc* 34: 693–696, 1986.
47. McAreavey D, Robertson JIS: Angiotensin converting enzyme inhibitors and moderate hypertension. *Drugs* 40: 326–345, 1990.
48. Dustan HP: Calcium channel blockers. Potential medical benefits and side effects. *Hypertension* 13(suppl I): I137–I140, 1989.
49. Abernethy DR, Schwartz JB, Todd EL, et al: Verapamil pharmacodynamics and disposition in young and elderly hypertensive patients. Altered electrocardiographic and hypotensive responses. *Ann Intern Med* 105: 329–336, 1986.
50. Zing W, Ferguson RK, Vlasses PH: Calcium antagonists in elderly and black hypertensives: therapeutic controversies. *Arch Intern Med* 151: 2154-2162, 1991.
51. Grimm Jr RH: Alpha$_1$-antagonists in the treatment of hypertension. *Hypertension* 13(suppl I): I131–I136, 1989.
52. Lepor H: Role of long-acting selective alpha$_1$-blockers in the treatment of benign prostatic hyperplasia. *Urol Clin North Am* 17: 651–659, 1990.

53. Materson BJ, Cushman WC, Goldstein G, et al: Treatment of hypertension in the elderly: I: Blood pressure and clinical changes. Results of a Department of Veterans Affairs Cooperative Study. *Hypertension* 15: 348–360, 1990.
54. Goldstein G, Materson BJ, Cushman WC, et al: Treatment of hypertension in the elderly: II. Cognitive and behavior function. Results of a Department of Veterans Affairs Cooperative Study. *Hypertension* 15: 361–369, 1990.
55. Eisen SA, Miller DK, Woodward RS, et al: The effect of prescribed daily dose frequency on patient medication compliance. *Arch Intern Med* 150: 1881–1884, 1990.
56. Croog SH, Levine S, Testa MA, et al: The effects of antihypertensive therapy on the quality of life. *N Engl J Med* 314: 1657–1664, 1986.
57. Morgan DB, Davidson C: Hypokalemia and diuretics: an analysis of publications. *Br Med J* 280: 905–908, 1980.
58. Levinson PD, Khatri IM, Freis ED: Persistence of normal BP after withdrawal of drug treatment in mild hypertension. *Arch Intern Med* 142: 2265–2268, 1982.
59. Finnerty FA: Step-down treatment of mild systemic hypertension. *Am J Cardiol* 53: 1304–1307, 1984.
60. Freis ED, Thomas JR, Fisher SG, et al: Effects of reduction in drugs or dosage after long-term control of systemic hypertension. *Am J Cardiol* 63: 702–708, 1989.

CHAPTER

6

ANTIARRHYTHMIC DRUGS

Paul E. Fenster
Paul E. Nolan, Jr.

PATHOPHYSIOLOGY AND CLINICAL SIGNIFICANCE OF SUPRAVENTRICULAR AND VENTRICULAR ARRHYTHMIAS

Abnormalities of the cardiac rhythm are quite common in the elderly. Aging is associated with changes in the structure and function of the cardiac conduction system. These changes, especially if associated with alterations due to chronic ischemic heart disease, hypertensive heart disease, cardiomyopathy, or valvular disease, predispose the elderly to a variety of bradyarrhythmias or tachyarrhythmias. Most of these arrhythmias are transient and are asymptomatic or produce only mild symptoms and require neither treatment nor extensive evaluation. However, in some individuals, the arrhythmia episodes are prolonged or recur frequently, producing symptoms that are quite disturbing or that adversely affect cardiac function, so therapy is indicated. In some cases, ventricular arrhythmias indicate an increased risk of sudden cardiac death. There are some clinical conditions in which carefully selected antiarrhythmic drugs may decrease the risk of sudden death.

This chapter reviews the common types of cardiac arrhythmias and their clinical significance and reviews the clinical pharmacology of the major antiarrhythmic agents.

Bradyarrhythmias

Heart rate declines with age. This is probably due to degenerative changes within the sinus node and alterations in autonomic modulation of heart rate. Sinus node dysfunction may produce persistent, inappropriate sinus bradycardia, sinus pauses, or sinus arrest. These may be associated with an increased prevalence of paroxysmal supraventricular tachycardia (brady-tachy syndrome).

Bradycardia may be due to atrioventricular (AV) block. The block may be within the AV nodal region or within the intraventricular His-Purkinje system. Depression of AV nodal conduction is common, usually asymptomatic, and associated with a good prognosis. AV block due to depressed intraventricular conduction is more likely to progress to high-grade AV block and to require implantation of a permanent pacemaker.

Any of these bradycardias may be caused by drugs, especially antiarrhythmic drugs. Any antiarrhythmic agent, but especially digitalis, beta-adrenergic blockers, verapamil, diltiazem, amiodarone, and the IC class of antiarrhythmics may depress sinoatrial (SA) nodal or AV nodal function. The IA agents, IC agents, and amiodarone may depress intraventricular conduction. The use of these drugs should be decreased or discontinued, if possible, prior to considering placement of a permanent pacemaker.

The symptoms produced by bradycardia may be subtle in the elderly. A slight decrease in cardiac output may be manifest as diminished exercise capacity. Decreased cerebral perfusion may produce impaired mentation or fatigue. More frequent or prolonged episodes of bradycardia may produce low-output, congestive heart failure or syncope.

Supraventricular Tachycardias

Almost all supraventricular tachycardias are caused by reentry or by enhanced automaticity. Atrial tachycardias arise above the AV node. Atrial tachycardias caused by enhanced automaticity include sinus tachycardia, ectopic atrial tachycardia, and multifocal atrial tachycardia. Atrial tachycardias due to reentry include atrial fibrillation, atrial flutter, and sinoatrial node reentrant tachycardia.

Atrioventricular nodal tachycardias include atrioventricular nodal reentrant tachycardia (AVNRT) and a rhythm due to enhanced automaticity, accelerated ectopic junctional tachycardia. Supraventricular tachycardia may also occur via a reentry mechanism utilizing an accessory pathway. The most common of these is atrioventricular reciprocating tachycardia (AVRT).

Ventricular Arrhythmias

The presence of ventricular ectopy is a common finding, even in individuals without heart disease. The prevalence of ventricular ectopy is increased in the elderly population. Ventricular ectopy is more common in individuals with any form of heart disease or pulmonary disease or any acute or chronic systemic illness or metabolic disturbance. Ventricular arrhythmias are commonly a result of drug toxicity or overuse of common stimulants.

In the vast majority of cases, ventricular ectopy is asymptomatic. However, in some individuals, these arrhythmias indicate an increased risk of sudden cardiac death. The prognostic significance of ventricular arrhythmias depends on the type and severity of heart disease and the specific arrhythmia. The risk of arrhythmic death is higher in patients with coronary artery disease, especially in the presence of prior myocardial infarction. The risk is increased further if there is associated left ventricular dysfunction. The prognostic significance of ventricular arrhythmias is not as well established in patients with cardiomyopathy or other forms of heart disease. The risk of arrhythmic death also increases with increasing frequency and complexity of the ventricular arrhythmia. The risk is extremely high in patients with recurrent sustained ventricular tachycardia or those resuscitated from an episode of ventricular fibrillation.

THERAPEUTIC STRATEGY OF DRUG USE

Approach to Supraventricular Tachycardia

Most supraventricular tachycardias (SVTs) are associated with a benign prognosis, so treatment depends on the frequency and severity of arrhythmia-related symptoms. There are some notable exceptions to this general rule: (1) Chronic atrial fibrillation, whether paroxysmal or persistent, is associated with a significant risk of systemic emboli in the elderly and in patients with any form of organic heart disease. Chronic anticoagulation reduces the embolic risk.[1-3] (2) Accessory pathways may have a short refractory period, facilitating a rapid ventricular response to atrial fibrillation, with risk of hemodynamic compromise or ventricular fibrillation. (3) Incessant tachycardia may result in myocardial dysfunction with clinical congestive heart failure.

Drug therapy to terminate or prevent SVT, if indicated, should be guided by the mechanism of the arrhythmia. The distinction between reentry and enhanced automaticity is clinically important.

AVNRT and AVRT can often be terminated by carotid sinus pressure, Valsalva maneuver, or facial immersion in cold water. These maneuvers increase vagal tone and thereby alter the critical balance of conduction velocity and refractory period in the AV node, thereby terminating the tachycardia.

The most effective drugs for terminating AVNRT and AVRT are adenosine and verapamil. The extremely short duration of action of adenosine is a significant advantage over verapamil. Verapamil has a negative inotropic effect and may cause prolonged hypotension.

Paroxysms of AVNRT may be prevented with chronic drug therapy that alters conduction velocity or refractory period in the AV node. Verapamil and diltiazem are both highly effective. Other effective agents include digitalis, quinidine, procainamide, disopyramide, beta-adrenergic blockers, flecainide, encainide, propafenone, and amiodarone.

These same medicines are effective in preventing episodes of AVRT. However, drugs that slow conduction in the accessory pathway are preferred for prophylaxis, since drugs lacking this property could be hazardous should atrial fibrillation occur. Drugs that slow accessory pathway conduction and prolong refractoriness include quinidine, procainamide, disopyramide, flecainide, encainide, propafenone, and amiodarone.

Sinus node reentry tachycardia and atrial reentry tachycardia may be difficult to prevent with drugs. Verapamil is often effective.

Atrial fibrillation is probably the most common symptomatic supraventricular arrhythmia. The prevalence of atrial fibrillation increases with age. The hazards of atrial fibrillation in a patient with an accessory pathway have been mentioned above. In other patients, the most serious consequence of chronic atrial fibrillation is systemic embolism. The risk of embolism is increased in the elderly, but it is reduced by chronic warfarin.[1-3] Therefore, chronic anticoagulation with warfarin is indicated, although the benefit must be weighed against the risk of bleeding complications. The role of aspirin in the prevention of emboli in atrial fibrillation in the elderly is uncertain.

Atrial fibrillation can often be terminated, and recurrences prevented, if it is due to an underlying medical problem that can be resolved. Examples of this include atrial fibrillation due to thyrotoxicosis, pulmonary embolism, or acute heart failure.

The treatment of chronic persistent atrial fibrillation is control of the heart rate. The ventricular response to atrial fibrillation can usually be controlled with a beta-adrenergic blocker or verapamil or diltiazem. Other effective agents include flecainide, encainide, propafenone, and amiodarone. However, there are considerable risks associated with the use of these other drugs. Flecainide, encainide, and propafenone slow AV nodal conduction rate, but they do not prolong the refractory period. The refractory period determines the maximum number of impulses per second that may traverse the AV node. In some individuals, the ventricular response to atrial fibrillation may actually increase with flecainide, encainide, or propafenone. Therefore, when using a IC agent to control the ventricular response, the AV node should also be depressed by using digitalis, a beta blocker, or verapamil or diltiazem. Amiodarone may cause any of a large variety of adverse effects during chronic administration.

Digitalis helps control the ventricular rate in stable patients at rest, but it is usually inadequate during exercise or acute illness.

Recurrences of paroxysmal atrial fibrillation may often be prevented by quinidine, procainamide, or disopyramide. For patients in whom these drugs are ineffective, flecainide, encainide, propafenone, or amiodarone may be useful. However, the risks mentioned above again apply. Digitalis, beta-adrenergic blockers, verapamil, and diltiazem are only modestly effective in preventing recurrences of atrial fibrillation.

The atrial tachycardias due to enhanced automaticity are, in general, more difficult to control than those due to reentry. Ectopic atrial tachycardia may be slowed by digoxin, beta blockers, or verapamil. The rhythm is sometimes prevented by flecainide, encainide, or amiodarone.

Multifocal atrial tachycardia is seen predominantly in elderly patients with acute illness or in patients with chronic obstructive pulmonary disease. The best therapeutic approach is to treat the underlying disease. Verapamil often helps control the rate and may restore sinus rhythm.

Approach to Ventricular Arrhythmias

In most individuals, ventricular ectopy requires no treatment. These arrhythmias are usually asymptomatic or produce mild palpitations that are best treated with reassurance as to their benign nature. In patients with coronary artery disease and complex ventricular arrhythmias, the goal of therapy is the reduction in the risk of arrhythmic death. The best means of achieving this goal is uncertain. Beta blockers reduce the risk of death when administered chronically after myocardial infarction. However, the Cardiac Arrhythmia Suppression Trial (CAST)[4] demonstrated that antiarrhythmic drugs (flecainide or encainide) administered in doses that substantially suppress arrhythmias are associated with an *increased* risk of sudden death. This is probably due to the tendency of antiarrhythmic drugs to worsen arrhythmias in some patients. Unfortunately, this tendency cannot be reliably detected by cardiac rhythm monitoring. It is likely that electrophysiologic testing is better for guiding the selection of a specific antiarrhythmic drug for a specific patient. Non-drug therapies, including electrophysiologically guided catheter or surgical ablation of the site of origin of the arrhythmia or implantation of an automatic defibrillator, may be effective in many drug-resistant cases.

CLINICAL PHARMACOLOGY OF ANTIARRHYTHMIC DRUGS

Antiarrhythmic drugs are most often classified by the modified Vaughan Williams scheme, which is based on the electrophysiologic effect of the drugs (Table 6-1). This scheme has significant shortcomings, most notably the difference in effects of a given drug on normal and abnormal cardiac tissue, the alteration in effect due to the action of drug metabolites, and the properties of some drugs that are characteristic of more than one class. Nonetheless, the classification system is widely used and is a convenient shorthand approach for identifying the major electrophysiologic actions of the antiarrhythmic drugs.

The class I drugs block the fast inward sodium channel, decreasing the maximum depolarization rate of the action potential. These agents are subclassified as IA, IB, or IC depending on their effects on intracardiac conduction and refractoriness. The IA agents, quinidine, procainamide, and disopyramide, increase ventricular refractoriness and prolong the QT interval. The IB agents lidocaine, tocainide, and mexiletine shorten action potential duration and re-

Table 6-1 Classification of antiarrhythmic drugs

Class I: Drugs that block the fast inward sodium current

A. Drugs that reduce transmembrane phase 0 upstroke velocity and prolongation of action potential duration:
- Quinidine
- Procainamide
- Disopyramide

B. Drugs that produce less reduction in the transmembrane phase 0 upstroke velocity and shorten repolarization and refractoriness:
- Lidocaine
- Tocainide
- Mexiletine
- Phenytoin

C. Drugs that markedly reduce the upstroke velocity of phase 0 of the transmembrane action potential and thereby slow conduction:
- Flecainide
- Encainide
- Lorcainide
- Propafenone

No subclass:
- Moricizine

Class II: Drugs that block beta adrenoreceptors

- Propranolol
- Timolol
- Atenolol
- Metoprolol
- Others

Class III: Drugs that block potassium channels and prolong repolarization and refractoriness

- Amiodarone
- Bretylium
- *N*-acetylprocainamide
- Sotalol

Class IV: Drugs that block the slow calcium channel of the AV and sinus nodes

- Verapamil
- Diltiazem

fractoriness, producing little change in PR, QRS, or QT intervals. The IC drugs flecainide, encainide, and propafenone slow conduction velocity but do not change repolarization. They prolong the PR and QRS intervals. The class II drugs are the beta-adrenergic blockers. The class III drugs prolong action potential duration and refractoriness. This class includes amiodarone, sotalol, bretylium, and *N*-acetylprocainamide. The class IV drugs are selected calcium channel blockers, such as verapamil and diltiazem.

Monitoring Antiarrhythmic Drug Therapy

In most patients, antiarrhythmic drug therapy is evaluated by the clinical response. If the desired therapeutic response, such as relief of palpitations or suppression of ectopy, is achieved and there are no adverse symptoms or objective evidence of drug toxicity, then measurement of serum drug concentration is not necessary. However, there are several clinical settings in which knowledge of the serum drug concentration may be helpful. The drug level may clarify the situation when the clinical response is unexpected at the administered dose, such as the occurrence of drug toxicity at a low dose. In this instance, the serum drug level may differentiate abnormal metabolism or elimination of the drug from unusual sensitivity to the drug.

Serum drug levels may be helpful when the pharmacokinetics of the drug are altered. This may occur in a patient with hepatic, renal, or cardiac dysfunction or when a drug that interacts with the antiarrhythmic agent is administered concomitantly.

Serum drug levels may be helpful in evaluating compliance with the prescribed dosing regimen. The serum level may also be helpful in determining the appropriate dose when changing dosage forms (conventional versus sustained release) or when changing commercial brands.

Quinidine

Quinidine (Fig. 6-1) and quinine are alkaloids derived from cinchona bark. Quinidine is effective in the treatment of a wide variety of supraventricular and ventricular arrhythmias and is the most widely used antiarrhythmic agent. However, the drug has a narrow therapeutic range and potentially serious cardiac and noncardiac toxicity. Therefore, the dose must be individualized, and patients receiving the drug must be monitored closely.

Clinical pharmacology (Table 6-2) Estimates of the clinical pharmacokinetic and pharmacodynamic parameters of quinidine are highly dependent upon the analytical methods utilized. Specific assays, such as high-pressure liquid chroma-

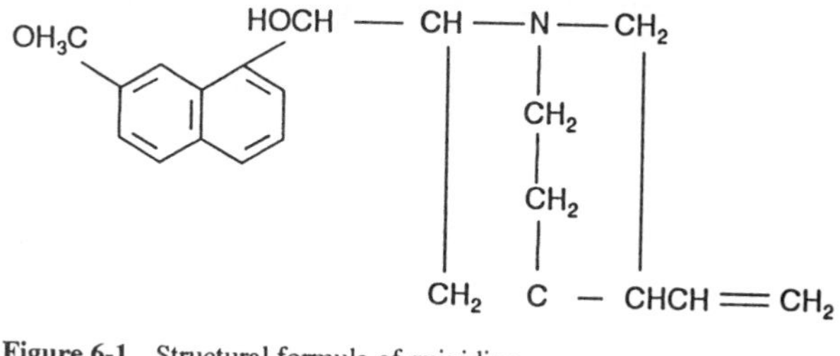

OH_3C — HOCH — CH — N — CH_2

CH_2

CH_2

CH_2 C — CHCH = CH_2

Figure 6-1 Structural formula of quinidine.

Table 6-2 Clinical pharmacology of antiarrhythmic drugs

	Major route of metabolism/ elimination	Elimination half-life	Active metabolites	Usual clinical dose range	Age-related alterations in pharmacokinetics
Quinidine	Hepatic; renal elimination of metabolites	5–6 h	Several	600–1800 mg/day	Prolonged $T_{1/2}$ decreased clearance
Procainamide	Renal 45–60%, hepatic 40-55%	2.6–4.6 h	*N*-acetylprocainamide	2–6 g/day	Prolonged $T_{1/2}$ decreased clearance
Disopyramide	Renal 50%, hepatic 50%	7 h	Mono- *N*-dealkyl disopyramide	400–800 mg/day	Prolonged $T_{1/2}$ decreased clearance
Lidocaine	Hepatic	3 h (during IV infusion)	MEGX	1–4 mg/min IV infusion	Prolonged $T_{1/2}$ decreased clearance
Tocainide	Hepatic 50–70%, renal 30–50%	11–14 h	None	1200–1800 mg/day	Probably prolonged $T_{1/2}$ decreased clearance
Mexiletine	Hepatic 77-98%	12 h	None	600–1200 mg/day	Prolonged $T_{1/2}$

Moricizine	Hepatic	3–4 h	Several	600–900 mg/day	Probably prolonged $T_{1/2}$ decreased clearance
Flecainide	Hepatic 50–90%, renal 10–50%	14 h	2	200–400 mg/day	Prolonged $T_{1/2}$ decreased clearance
Encainide	Hepatic, except in poor metabolizers	1–2 h; 6–11 h in poor metabolizers	ODE and MODE	—	Probably prolonged $T_{1/2}$ of ODE and MODE
Propafenone	Hepatic	2–10 h; 10–32 h in poor metabolizers	2	450–900 mg/day	—
Amiodarone	Hepatic	53 days	Desethylamiodarone	200–600 mg/day	Probably prolonged $T_{1/2}$ decreased clearance
Bretylium	Renal	7–9 h	None	1–2 mg/min IV infusion	Probably prolonged $T_{1/2}$
Adenosine	Erythrocytes, endothelial cells	Seconds	None	6–12 mg IV bolus	—

Note: $T_{1/2}$, elimination half-life; ODE, *O*-demethylencainide; IV, intravenous; MODE, 3-methoxy- *O*-demethylencainide; MEGX, monoethylglycinexylidide.

tography (HPLC), can differentiate quinidine from dihydroquinidine (a contaminant found in all quinidine preparations) and from the various quinidine metabolites.[5] Therefore, relative to the pharmacokinetic parameters obtained from studies using nonspecific assays, the use of specific HPLC assays results in reduced estimates of serum quinidine concentrations, bioavailability, area under the curve, elimination half-life, and amount of quinidine eliminated in the urine and increased estimates of total body clearance.[5] In addition, the therapeutic serum concentration guidelines for quinidine are broader when a nonspecific assay is used than when a specific one is used. Therefore, a knowledge of the assay procedure used in a clinical pharmacologic investigation of quinidine is important in the interpretation of both pharmacokinetic and pharmacodynamic data.

Absorption Quinidine undergoes some first-pass hepatic removal.[6] The mean absolute bioavailability of quinidine sulfate (83% quinidine base) is 70 percent in young healthy individuals.[7] In older patients, the absolute bioavailability is 87 percent.[8] Mean peak plasma concentrations are observed at about 1.5 h following administration.

A sustained-release preparation of quinidine sulfate is bioequivalent to the standard product.[9] Maximal serum concentrations are observed at 3.3 h for the sustained-release preparation. Serum concentrations of the sustained-release product demonstrate much less interdose fluctuation than do concentrations of the standard formulation.

Quinidine gluconate tablets (62% quinidine base) are more slowly absorbed than conventional quinidine sulfate tablets.[10] Peak serum concentrations occur 3.6 h after the dose. The extent of absorption of quinidine gluconate is comparable to that of quinidine sulfate.

The bioavailability of quinidine polygalacturonate (60% quinidine base) is comparable to that of quinidine sulfate.[11]

Distribution The volume of distribution of quinidine averages 2.5 L/kg. Approximately 87 percent is protein bound.[12] The protein binding of quinidine is concentration independent. The volume of distribution and protein binding of quinidine do not vary significantly with age.[13]

The protein binding of quinidine is increased in trauma patients,[12] following acute myocardial infarction, subsequent to cardiac surgery,[14] and in survivors of prehospital cardiac arrest.[15] The protein binding of quinidine decreases in chronic liver disease to approximately 73 percent.[16,17] This reduction may be the result of decreases in serum albumin concentrations. Heparin increases free fatty acids, which displace quinidine from binding sites,[18] decreasing the protein binding.

Elimination and metabolism Quinidine is eliminated primarily by hepatic metabolism.[6] Only 18 percent of an intravenous dose[8] and only 13 percent of an oral dose[6] of quinidine is excreted unchanged in the urine.

The renal elimination of quinidine occurs in part via glomerular filtration and correlates with creatinine clearance.[13] Neither hemodialysis[19] nor peritoneal dialysis[20] has a clinically significant impact upon the systemic removal of quinidine. Quinidine also undergoes active renal tubular secretion.[21] The renal excretion of quinidine varies inversely with urine pH.[22]

In young healthy subjects, the elimination half-life of quinidine averages 5.7 h. In healthy elderly subjects, the average elimination half-life is 9.7 h.[13]

The mean total body clearance of quinidine is 4.04 mL/min/kg in young healthy volunteers and 2.64 mL/min/kg in healthy elderly subjects.[13] The reduction is due to decreases in both renal and hepatic clearances.

The principal metabolites of quinidine are 3-hydroxyquinidine, 2′-oxoquinidinone, quinidine 10,11-dihydrodiol, quinidine *N*-oxide, and *O*-desmethylquinidine.[23-25] Most metabolites of quinidine likely contribute to both the therapeutic and the toxic effects of the parent compound.

Dihydroquinidine, a contaminant of all commercial quinidine preparations, is detected in the plasma of patients who take quinidine chronically.[25] Dihyroquinidine may contribute to both the therapeutic and the toxic effects of quinidine.

Conditions that alter pharmacokinetics ***Hepatic disease*** Patients with biopsy-proven cirrhosis have a significantly prolonged half-life (9 vs. 6 h) and a larger volume of distribution (3.8 versus 2.5 L/kg) than matched controls.[17] However, the total clearance is not altered. The unbound serum concentration of quinidine tends to increase in patients with hepatic disease.[16,17]

Congestive heart failure In congestive heart failure, the volume of distribution and the total body clearance of quinidine are significantly decreased. The renal clearance is also significantly reduced in patients with heart failure. However, the half-life is not significantly changed.[26] Congestive heart failure reduces the rate, but not the extent, of quinidine absorption following the oral administration of quinidine.[27]

Pharmacokinetic and pharmacodynamic drug interactions Quinidine doubles the serum digoxin concentrations.[28,29] The magnitude of the increase may be related to the dose or the serum concentration of quinidine.[28] Quinidine decreases the volume of distribution, total body clearance, renal clearance, and nonrenal clearance of digoxin.[29] The volume of distribution of digoxin is diminished in part because of the reduced binding of digoxin to skeletal muscle.[30] The decreases in the renal and nonrenal clearance of digoxin result from inhibition of the renal and biliary secretion of digoxin by quinidine.[31] Digoxin toxicity may develop after quinidine is added, so reduction in the digoxin dose is advised prior to starting quinidine.

When coadministered with procainamide, quinidine increases both steady-state serum procainamide and *N*-acetylprocainamide concentrations.[32] Quinidine decreases total body clearance and prolongs the half-life of procainamide. The interaction may result from the competitive inhibition of the renal tubular secretion of procainamide (and *N*-acetylprocainamide) by quinidine.

Quinidine selectively inhibits cytochrome P-450, the hepatic enzyme principally responsible for the oxidation of debrisoquine and sparteine along with the oxidation of about 30 clinically prescribed drugs.[33,34] Therefore, quinidine can theoretically inhibit the oxidation of these drugs, especially in those individuals who are extensive metabolizers. For example, quinidine alters the pharmacokinetics of propafenone,[35] encainide,[36] flecainide,[37] and metoprolol.[38] Quinidine increases steady-state plasma propafenone concentrations twofold and decreases both the oral clearance of propafenone and the steady-state plasma concentrations of 5-hydroxypropafenone in extensive metabolizers. Quinidine has no effect on steady-state plasma concentrations of propafenone in poor metabolizers.[35] In extensive metabolizers of encainide, quinidine decreases the total body clearance and nonrenal clearance of encainide and prolongs the half-life.[36] In poor metabolizers neither the pharmacokinetics nor the electrocardiographic effects of encainide are modified by quinidine. Quinidine inhibits the sequential steps in the metabolism of flecainide in extensive metabolizers, resulting in a decrease in the total body clearance of flecainide.[37] The duration of the beta-blocking effects of metoprolol is prolonged by the concurrent administration of quinidine as a result of a reduction in the oxidative metabolism of metoprolol.[38]

Several drugs have been shown to decrease the elimination of quinidine and elevate the plasma concentrations of quinidine. Cimetidine decreases the clearance of quinidine by 36 percent, increases the half-life of quinidine by 55 percent, raises peak quinidine plasma levels, and potentiates the electrocardiographic effects of quinidine.[39] Amiodarone increases the serum concentrations of quinidine an average of 32 percent within 24 h of initiation of amiodarone therapy.[40] Verapamil slightly increases the half-life of quinidine and decreases the oral clearance of quinidine from 17 L/h to approximately 11 L/h by impairing the metabolism of quinidine.[41] The administration of intravenous verapamil to patients on oral quinidine may result in marked hypotension.[42] The probable mechanism is the additive $alpha_1$- and $alpha_2$-adrenergic blockade with the combination of quinidine and verapamil.

Some drugs enhance the elimination of quinidine. Phenytoin and phenobarbital produce a 50 percent decrease in the half-life of quinidine, most likely due to the enhanced metabolism of quinidine.[43] Rifampin decreases the half-life of quinidine almost threefold and increases the oral clearance of quinidine.[44] The coadministration of nifedipine decreases the serum concentration of quinidine in an occasional patient as a consequence of nifedipine-mediated increases in the total body clearance of quinidine.[45]

Adverse reactions Quinidine prolongs the QT interval in a generally dose-related manner. However, marked prolongation of the QT interval may occur in some patients on low doses and at low serum concentrations. Marked prolongation of the

QT interval (over 500 ms) is associated with an increased risk of torsades de pointes. The arrhythmia may be responsible for syncope or sudden death. For this reason, some experts advise hospitalization of all patients in whom quinidine treatment is initiated. The risk of torsades is increased by hypokalemia, hypomagnesemia, or bradycardia. The treatment of torsades requires discontinuation of quinidine and any other agent causing QT prolongation. Pacing or increasing the heart rate with isoproterenol is effective treatment until the quinidine effect diminishes. Intravenous magnesium sulfate is also effective.

Exacerbation of arrhythmias may occur without marked QT prolongation. However, the rate of proarrhythmia is low for the three IA antiarrhythmic agents. Stanton et al[46] evaluated the incidence of serious new ventricular tachyarrhythmias associated with the initiation of antiarrhythmic drug therapy in patients who were being treated for ventricular tachycardia or fibrillation. A serious new arrhythmia was attributed to quinidine in only 1 of 167 patients.

The most common adverse effect from quinidine is diarrhea, which is due to a direct gastric irritant effect. This occurs in up to 30 percent of patients, and it may be more common with quinidine sulfate than with the slower release formulations. Other gastrointestinal effects include nausea, vomiting, abdominal pain, and anorexia. The frequency of occurrence of these adverse effects may be reduced by taking quinidine with meals.

Quinidine has anticholinergic effects and may thereby enhance AV nodal conduction. Quinidine may also slow the rate of atrial flutter and, in conjunction with the anticholinergic effect, permit 1 : 1 conduction through the AV node. This may cause an increase in the ventricular response to atrial fibrillation. Therefore, an AV nodal blocking agent such as digoxin, a beta blocker, or an appropriate calcium channel blocker such as verapamil or diltiazem should be administered prior to quinidine in patients with atrial fibrillation.

Quinidine causes alpha-adrenergic blockade that produces peripheral vasodilation, and hypotension may occur. This is more likely in patients who are also receiving other vasodilators. Quinidine usually is not a myocardial depressant unless large doses are given intravenously at a rapid rate.

At high serum concentrations, quinidine may produce cinchonism, with tinnitus, hearing loss, visual disturbances, confusion, and gastrointestinal symptoms.

Allergic reactions to quinidine include rash, fever, and, rarely, anaphylaxis. An immune-mediated thrombocytopenia is an uncommon event. This is due to antibodies to quinidine-platelet complexes.

Procainamide

Procainamide (Fig. 6-2), like quinidine, suppresses both supraventricular and ventricular arrhythmias. The two agents have similar electrophysiologic effects, but the clinical response to one may differ from the response to the other. Procainamide may be administered orally or intravenously. Chronic oral administration is associated with a high incidence of side effects.

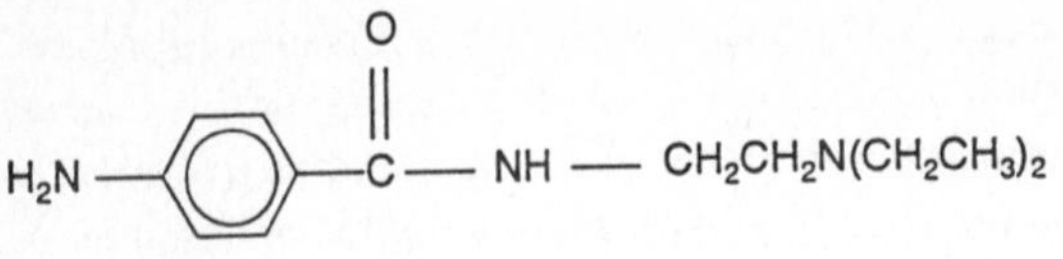

$$H_2N-C_6H_4-\overset{O}{\overset{\|}{C}}-NH-CH_2CH_2N(CH_2CH_3)_2$$

Procainamide

Figure 6-2 Structural formula of procainamide.

Clinical pharmacology (Table 6-2) ***Absorption*** The absolute bioavailability of conventional procainamide capsules ranges from 75 to 95 percent. Peak concentrations occur within 2 h of the dose.[47] The bioavailability of sustained-release procainamide tablets (Procan-SR by Parke-Davis and Pronestyl-SR by E. R. Squibb & Sons) is similar to that of the conventional-release product.[48] However, for clinical purposes the bioequivalence of different procainamide products cannot be assumed. Arrhythmias have recurred after switching from one form of procainamide to another.[49] When changing from conventional to sustained-release formulations or when changing from one sustained-release preparation to another, plasma procainamide levels may need to be measured.

Distribution The volume of distribution of procainamide ranges from 2.0 to 3.8 L/kg (mean 2.7 L/kg).[50] The protein binding of procainamide averages only 16 to 20 percent.[51] This indicates that most of the procainamide in the body is stored in tissues, and changes in the protein binding of procainamide would not be anticipated to alter the pharmacodynamic response.

Elimination and Metabolism The half-life of procainamide averages 3.4 h in healthy subjects (2.6 to 4.6 h).[50] The mean total body clearance is 9.4 mL/min/kg (7.9 to 13.2 mL/min/kg).[50] Both the half-life and the total body clearance are dependent upon the renal function and the acetylator phenotype of the individual.

Procainamide is both renally excreted and hepatically metabolized. Renal clearance averages approximately 5 mL/min/kg in healthy subjects.[50] In general, this is between 45 and 60 percent of the total body clearance of procainamide and is independent of of procainamide acetylator status. The renal clearance of procainamide considerably exceeds creatinine clearance,[51] indicating that procainamide is both filtered and secreted by the kidney.

The principal metabolite of procainamide is *N*-acetylprocainamide (NAPA). The acetylation of procainamide is bimodally distributed; individuals are genetically either fast or slow acetylators.[52] The rate of acetylation has important clinical consequences, as slow acetylators are more likely to develop procainamide-induced lupuslike syndrome.[52] The steady-state concentration ratio of serum NAPA to serum procainamide can be utilized to determine acetylator status in patients with good renal function.[51] A ratio equal to or greater than 1.0 is consistent with a fast acetylator phenotype.

NAPA is an active metabolite with class III antiarrhythmic action.[53] In individuals with normal renal function, approximately 85 percent of the amount of NAPA in the body is eliminated by the kidney both by glomerular filtration and by active tubular secretion.

A decrease in the elimination of both procainamide and NAPA occurs with aging. Both the ratio of procainamide clearance to creatinine clearance and the ratio of NAPA clearance to creatinine clearance decline with increasing age.[54] The total body clearance for procainamide averages 4.3 mL/min/kg for patients over 60 years old, whereas the mean value is 7.7 mL/min/kg for patients under 60 years of age.[55] The total body clearance of NAPA in elderly patients without cardiac failure is also decreased.[56] The decline in the elimination of procainamide and NAPA is predominantly the result of age-related decreases in glomerular filtration and renal tubular secretion.

Conditions that alter pharmacokinetics ***Renal impairment*** Renal dysfunction decreases the elimination of both procainamide and NAPA. In functionally anephric patients, the half-life of procainamide averages 14 h.[57] In patients with less severe renal impairment, the mean half-life is 11 h.[58] The average half-life for NAPA in functionally anephric patients is 42 h.[59]

The clearance of procainamide during hemodialysis averages 67 mL/min.[60] For NAPA, the mean dialysis clearance is 48 mL/min.[61] However, due to the multicompartmental pharmacokinetic nature and extensive tissue distribution of procainamide and NAPA, only small amounts of either would be anticipated to be removed by hemodialysis. Continuous ambulatory peritoneal dialysis is inefficient in removing either procainamide or NAPA. Dosage replacement following either hemodialysis or peritoneal dialysis should be guided by the clinical status of the patient and by the serum concentration.

Hepatic dysfunction In chronic hepatic disease, the amount of procainamide excreted in the urine is reduced by 50 percent.[62] This decrease in the urinary excretion of procainamide is greatest in patients with ascites. Assuming that there is no alteration in bioavailability, these findings suggest that doses of procainamide should be reduced 50 percent in patients with chronic hepatic dysfunction. Clinical assessment plus serum concentration monitoring should be used as guidelines for dosage adjustment.

Obesity A study of obese individuals suggests that loading doses of procainamide should be based upon ideal body weight and that maintenance doses should be based upon total body weight.[63]

Congestive heart failure For patients with moderate congestive heart failure (CHF) the total body clearance of procainamide averaged 3.5 mL/min/kg. The mean total body clearance for a similar group of patients without CHF was 6.9 mL/min/kg.[55]

Pharmacokinetic drug interactions The H_2-receptor blockers cimetidine[64] and ranitidine[65] decrease the elimination and increase the serum concentrations of procainamide. The predominant mechanism is impairment in the renal clearance of procainamide probably via competitive inhibition of renal tubular secretion. However, inhibition of the nonrenal clearance of procainamide may also occur. The magnitude and occurrence of the interaction between ranitidine and procainamide may be dependent upon the dose of ranitidine. Initial procainamide dosage reductions in the range of 20 to 30 percent would appear to be reasonable when cimetidine is concomitantly prescribed. Similar reductions may be necessary during concurrent procainamide and ranitidine treatment, especially when ranitidine doses are greater than 300 mg/day.

Amiodarone increases the serum concentrations of procainamide and NAPA.[40] In patients taking chronic procainamide, a 20 percent reduction in the dose of procainamide is required following initiation of amiodarone to maintain stable serum procainamide levels. The combination of amiodarone and procainamide results in further increases in the QRS duration and the QTc interval. This drug combination should be used only with great caution.

Trimethoprim decreases the renal clearance of procainamide and NAPA and the total body clearance of procainamide.[66] The mean serum levels of procainamide and NAPA are increased 69 and 50 percent, respectively, by trimethoprim. Procainamide doses initially should be reduced approximately 50 percent when trimethoprim is concurrently administered.

Ethanol reduces the half-life and increases the total body clearance of procainamide.[67] These effects are most prominent in slow acetylators. The probable mechanism of the interaction is induction of the *N*-acetylation of procainamide by ethanol.

Adverse effects Procainamide may provoke or worsen ventricular arrhythmias. However, this potential risk of proarrhythmia is low. In the large clinical electrophysiologic study of Stanton et al,[46] procainamide provoked serious ventricular arrhythmias in none of 77 patients under treatment for serious ventricular arrhythmias. Procainamide should not be used in patients with the prolonged QT syndrome, a history of torsades de pointes, or hypokalemia. As with all antiarrhythmic agents, careful monitoring is appropriate, especially when initiating drug treatment of serious ventricular arrhythmias.

The most common adverse reaction to chronic procainamide that requires drug discontinuation is development of a lupuslike syndrome. The syndrome is uncommon in the first 6 months of therapy but occurs in 15 to 25 percent of patients after more than 1 year. The syndrome usually begins as mild arthralgias but eventually progresses to arthritis, malar rash, and pleural and pericardial effusions. Cardiac tamponade may occur. Renal involvement rarely occurs. The syndrome is reversible with discontinuation of procainamide.

Over 70 percent of patients on chronic procainamide treatment develop antinuclear antibodies. The drug should not be discontinued for this laboratory abnormality if symptoms and signs of the lupuslike syndrome are absent.

The lupuslike syndrome does not develop in response to *N*-acetylprocainamide. Slow acetylators of procainamide seem to be more prone to developing the syndrome and develop it sooner than rapid acetylators.[52]

Procainamide may induce neutropenia or agranulocytosis. This rare adverse event may be more common when a sustained-release formulation is used. With any form of procainamide, the white blood count should be checked every 2 weeks for the first 3 months of treatment. Thereafter, the risk of neutropenia is quite low.

Other adverse reactions that are common, but usually not serious, include nonspecific gastrointestinal and central nervous system (CNS) symptoms such as anorexia, nausea, fatigue, lightheadedness, inability to concentrate, and altered sensorium.

Disopyramide

Disopyramide (Fig. 6-3), like quinidine and procainamide, is useful in the treatment of a variety of supraventricular and ventricular arrhythmias. Clinical application of this drug is limited by negative inotropic and anticholinergic effects.

Clinical pharmacology (Table 6-2) Disopyramide is unique among currently available antiarrhythmic drugs in that it demonstrates serum concentration-dependent protein binding.[68] As the serum concentration of total (bound plus unbound) disopyramide increases, the unbound fraction of the total serum concentration of disopyramide also increases. Pharmacokinetic and pharmacodynamic parameters determined from total serum concentrations of disopyramide will differ from those

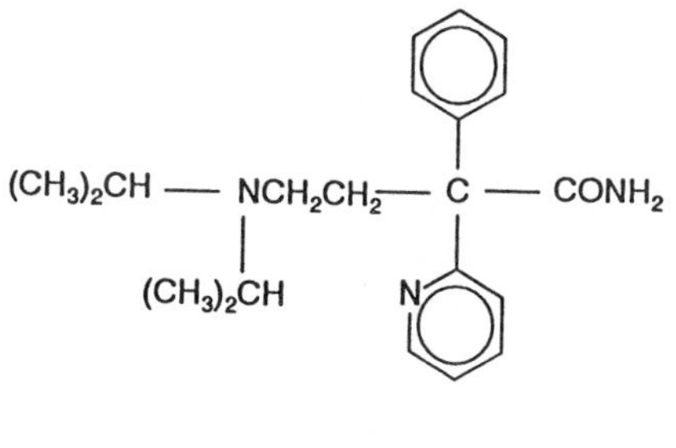

$(CH_3)_2CH$ — NCH_2CH_2 — C — $CONH_2$

$(CH_3)_2CH$ N

Disopyramide

Figure 6-3 Structural formula of disopyramide.

determined from the unbound concentrations. For example, disopyramide is a restrictively cleared drug, and therefore the total body clearance can be estimated as total body clearance of unbound drug times the fraction of unbound drug. From this it can be discerned that the total body clearance of disopyramide is dependent upon the fraction of unbound drug. Consequently, as the fraction unbound decreases with time following dosage administration, the total body clearance will decrease (i.e., total body clearance is time dependent). However, the clearance of unbound drug remains constant. Therefore, for disopyramide it remains important to distinguish between pharmacokinetic parameters determined from concentrations of unbound drug and those calculated from total serum concentrations of disopyramide.

Absorption The absolute bioavailability of unbound disopyramide in normal volunteers averages 85 percent.[69] The absolute bioavailability of total disopyramide can be as low as 52 percent.[70] This discrepancy between the extent of absorption of unbound disopyramide and total disopyramide is consistent with the nonlinear protein binding of disopyramide. With increasing doses, the amount of disopyramide absorbed as determined from concentrations of the drug unbound is directly proportional to the dose.[71] However, the increases in the amount of disopyramide absorbed as determined from total concentrations is less than proportional to the dose. Peak concentrations of both total and unbound disopyramide generally occur after between 0.5 and 2 h, and these observations are dose independent.[71]

The controlled-release product of disopyramide is bioequivalent to the immediate-release preparation at steady state.[72] The controlled-release product demonstrates less intersubject variability in absorption. When switching from the immediate-release to the controlled-release product, it is recommended that therapy be initiated with the controlled-release product 6 h following the last dose of the immediate-release preparation.

Distribution The fraction of disopyramide that is not bound to plasma proteins increases with increasing total serum concentrations.[68] Following a single intravenous bolus dose of disopyramide, the percentage of unbound drug can range from about 10 percent to approximately 60 percent over a total serum concentration range of 1 to 7 μg/mL.[73] There are marked interindividual differences in the percentage of unbound drug, however. In patients who take disopyramide chronically, the percentage of unbound drug at steady state ranges from 4 to 37 percent.[74]

In normal volunteers, the average volume of distribution of unbound disopyramide ranges from 1.4 to 2.8 L/kg,[69,73] and for total disopyramide it ranges from 0.4 to 0.6 L/kg. The volume of distribution of total disopyramide is increased in the elderly.[75]

Elimination and metabolism The mean half-life of unbound disopyramide in normal subjects is 5 to 6 h.[69,73] The half-life of total disopyramide is 7 h. Both are prolonged in the elderly.[75,76] The total body clearance of unbound disopyramide averages 3.2 to 5.4 mL/min/kg.[69,73] For total disopyramide, the mean total body clearance ranges from 0.7 to 1.2 mL/min/kg and is time dependent.[69,73] The total body clearance of total and unbound disopyramide is decreased in the elderly.[75,76]

Approximately 50 percent of the total body clearance of unbound disopyramide is due to renal elimination.[73] Unbound disopyramide undergoes both glomerular filtration and renal tubular secretion.[71] In normal subjects, the renal clearance of total disopyramide averages 0.6 mL/min/kg for 12 h following dosage administration and then significantly decreases over the subsequent 24 h.[73] This time-dependent decrease in renal clearance results from the binding of disopyramide to saturable plasma protein. The renal clearance of unbound disopyramide is not time dependent, and the mean value ranges from 1.8 to 3.4 mL/min/kg in normal volunteers.[69]

Conditions that alter pharmacokinetics ***Renal dysfunction*** For total disopyramide, the volume of distribution, total body clearance, and amount excreted in the urine are significantly reduced and the half-life increased in chronic renal disease.[77] However, dosage reductions of disopyramide appear to be necessary only for creatinine clearances of less than 40 mL/min due to the saturable protein binding of disopyramide. As the concentration of unbound disopyramide increases due to renal dysfunction, the unbound fraction also increases. Because the total body clearance of total disopyramide will increase with the increasing free fraction, the total serum concentration of disopyramide will decrease. Therefore, in patients with renal disease an increase in the plasma concentration of total disopyramide is evident only when renal impairment is considerable. The loading doses of disopyramide should also be reduced in patients with severe renal dysfunction.[77]

The pharmacokinetics of unbound disopyramide have also been investigated in patients with chronic renal failure.[78] Total body clearance and renal clearance are reduced, and half-life is increased.

Based upon total plasma concentrations of disopyramide, hemodialysis does not appreciably remove disopyramide from the body.[79] The dialysis clearance of unbound disopyramide remains to be investigated, however. Postdialysis replacement of disopyramide appears to be unnecessary, but it should be guided by the clinical response of the patient.

Hepatic disease The total body clearance of unbound disopyramide is significantly reduced in patients with hepatic cirrhosis.[80] The free fraction of disopyramide is increased. The dose of disopyramide should be initially reduced approximately 25 percent in patients with hepatic cirrhosis.

Congestive heart failure The total body clearance and renal clearance of both unbound and total disopyramide are decreased in patients with left ventricular dysfunction.[69] The half-life of unbound and total disopyramide is longer in patients with cardiac dysfunction. For patients with heart failure for whom disopyramide is prescribed, dosage reductions in the range of 15 to 25 percent appear to be reasonable initially.

Pharmacokinetic and pharmacodynamic drug interactions The pharmacokinetics of disopyramide are influenced by hepatic enzyme inducers. Phenytoin decreases serum concentrations and shortens the half-life of total disopyramide.[81,82] These pharmacokinetic effects may decrease the antiarrhythmic activity of disopyramide. Rifampin[83] and phenobarbital[84] also enhance the metabolism of disopyramide.

Stereospecific aspects of disopyramide pharmacokinetics Disopyramide exists as a racemic mixture of the R(-) and S(+) enantiomers. These enantiomers exhibit different pharmacologic and pharmacokinetic properties. Clinical data suggest that the S(+) enantiomer is more effective than the R(-) enantiomer in preventing induction of atrial flutter.[85] The S(+) enantiomer also produces greater anticholinergic effects.[86] The enantiomers seem to exert approximately equivalent negative inotropic effects.[87]

Adverse effects As with all antiarrhythmic agents, the most serious adverse effect is arrhythmia aggravation. In the study of Stanton et al,[46] this was a relatively uncommon event for each of the drugs with IA-type electrophysiologic effects. Serious ventricular arrhythmias were provoked in 1 percent of patients being treated with disopyramide for ventricular arrhythmias. However, disopyramide should not be administered to patients with long QT syndrome, hypokalemia, or a history of torsades de pointes.

Disopyramide exerts a clinically significant negative inotropic effect. This effect has been used therapeutically in patients with obstructive cardiomyopathy. The drug should be avoided in all other patients with a history of CHF or with significant impairment of left ventricular function.

The most common adverse effects from disopyramide are due to the drug's dose-related anticholinergic effects. These include urinary retention, constipation, dry mouth, dry eyes, and esophageal reflux. The elderly are especially prone to develop these adverse effects. These side effects may be ameliorated by concomitant administration of a cholinesterase inhibitor such as physostigmine or neostigmine. The drug is contraindicated in patients with glaucoma or obstructive uropathy.

Lidocaine

Lidocaine (Fig. 6-4) is the most widely used intravenous antiarrhythmic drug. Lidocaine is usually the drug of first choice for the acute suppression of ventricular arrhythmias, but it has no role in the therapy of supraventricular arrhythmias.

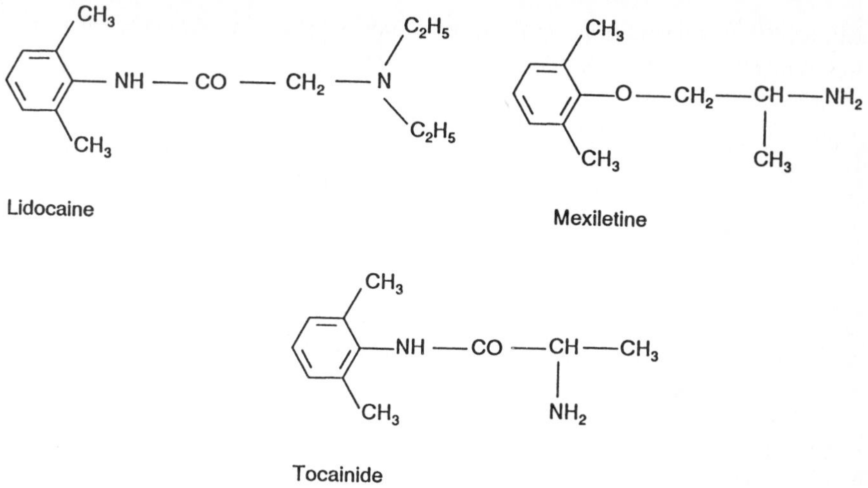

Lidocaine

Mexiletine

Tocainide

Figure 6-4 Structural formulas of lidocaine, mexiletine, and tocainide.

Although the drug has frequently been given prophylactically in the setting of acute myocardial infarction, this practice has recently been questioned. Lidocaine use requires careful monitoring not only to assess the antiarrhythmic response but also to prevent serious toxicity.

Clinical pharmacology (Table 6-2) ***Absorption*** Lidocaine is usually administered intravenously because the drug undergoes significant hepatic first-pass elimination following oral administration.[88] When hepatic metabolism is impaired, bioavailability increases. The bioavailability of lidocaine in cirrhotic patients is 91 percent.[88]

Distribution Following the administration of an intravenous bolus, the disposition of lidocaine occurs in two phases (i.e., according to a two-compartment model). This pattern of disposition has important dosing implications. During the initial phase, lidocaine is distributed rapidly to well-perfused tissues such as those of the heart, brain, kidney, and lung (i.e., the central compartment). This initial disposition phase is generally completed within 30 min in healthy volunteers.[89] The antiarrhythmic effect of lidocaine correlates with the concentration of the drug in the central compartment. During the second phase, lidocaine is distributed more slowly to adipose tissue and skeletal muscle (i.e., the peripheral compartment).[90] The peripheral tissues release lidocaine back into the circulation more slowly, and the drug is eliminated. The mean volumes of distribution for the central and peripheral compartments are 0.48 L/kg [89] and 2.8 L/kg, respectively.[91]

Lidocaine is bound to serum proteins, albumin, and alpha$_1$-acid glycoprotein (AAG), an acute-phase reactant.[92] Approximately 70 percent of the total lidocaine concentration is bound in normal subjects. Approximately 20 percent of the total lidocaine concentration is bound to albumin and 50 percent to AAG.

Metabolism and elimination Lidocaine is extensively metabolized in the liver.[90] Normal individuals eliminate less than 3 percent of a dose unchanged in the urine.[93,94] The hepatic extraction ratio for lidocaine, the amount removed from the circulation during a single pass through the liver, ranges from 61 to 81 percent.[95] The rate of lidocaine metabolism is primarily determined by hepatic blood flow, which is directly related to cardiac index.[90] The clearance of lidocaine is also influenced by hepatic enzyme inducers and inhibitors.[90] Therefore, changes in either hepatic blood flow or the intrinsic metabolic capability of the liver will likely alter the elimination of lidocaine.

Lidocaine undergoes sequential oxidative *N*-deethylation to initially form monoethylglycinexylidide (MEGX) and subsequently glycinexylidide (GX).[90] MEGX and GX are intermediate metabolites. The principal metabolite found in the urine is 4-hydroxy-2,6-xylidine, which accounts for 73 percent of an administered dose.[94] It is unlikely that this metabolite is pharmacologically active.

MEGX and GX possess antiarrhythmic activity.[90] MEGX is 80 percent as potent as lidocaine, and GX is about 20 percent as potent based upon a guinea pig atrial model of oubain-induced arrhythmias.

The elimination half-life and total body clearance of MEGX are similar to those of lidocaine.[96] In cardiac patients without heart failure, the average ratio of MEGX to lidocaine is 0.21.[97] However, in some patients with heart failure [97] and in those with renal failure,[98] concentrations of MEGX have approached or exceeded those of lidocaine. These elevated concentrations of MEGX have been associated with toxic effects.

After an intravenous bolus dose, the elimination half-life of GX is 10 h, and approximately 50 percent of the dose is eliminated in the urine unchanged in healthy subjects.[99] GX accumulates in patients with diminished renal function.[98] The concentration ratio of GX to lidocaine usually does not exceed 0.43 and typically is much lower.

MEGX most likely contributes to both the antiarrhythmic and the toxic effects of lidocaine, and GX probably contributes to the occurrence of adverse effects. Patients with heart failure may be potentially at a greater risk for developing "lidocaine" toxicity secondary to the accumulation of MEGX. Patients with renal failure may be potentially at a greater risk for developing "lidocaine" toxicity secondary to the accumulation of GX.

The terminal elimination half-life of lidocaine is approximately 1.7 h in young healthy individuals.[89,91] The elimination half-life averages 2.3 h in healthy elderly male individuals.[91] After intravenous bolus dosing, the total body clearance averages almost 20 mL/min/kg. However, when lidocaine is administered as an intravenous infusion for 24 h or more, the half-life is prolonged to 3 h and the total body clearance is reduced to about 12 mL/min/kg in young subjects. In elderly females, the total body clearance of lidocaine averages 18 mL/min/kg.[91]

The mechanism of the decline in the rate of lidocaine elimination during continuous infusion appears to be inhibition of lidocaine metabolism.[96,100] Lidocaine and MEGX inhibit the hydroxylation of each other.[100] The increased formation of lidocaine metabolites that occurs during prolonged continuous infusions may reduce the metabolism of lidocaine.

Conditions that alter pharmacokinetics ***Congestive heart failure*** There is an inverse relationship between the cardiac index and steady-state lidocaine concentrations due to changes in hepatic blood flow.[90] The total body clearance of lidocaine may be reduced 40 to 60 percent in patients with heart failure.[93] The volume of distribution in heart failure is also significantly decreased.[93] Therefore, the loading dose and the infusion rate of lidocaine should be reduced in the presence of heart failure; the greatest reduction should be made in patients with the most severe heart failure.

Hepatic disease In subjects with chronic hepatic disease, lidocaine elimination is decreased and protein binding is decreased, resulting in a significant increase in unbound drug.[93] The half-life of lidocaine may be prolonged to almost 7 h and the total body clearance decreased to 6 mL/min/kg.[93]

Renal disease Renal disease minimally influences the pharmacokinetics of lidocaine.[93,94] However, GX may accumulate in patients with severe renal impairment and contribute to drug toxicity.[98]

Obesity Lidocaine is highly lipophilic. Abernethy and Greenblatt[101] found that obese males and females have markedly longer half-lives and increased absolute volumes of distribution when compared to nonobese subjects. However, total body clearance was similar for the obese and nonobese groups. When the volume of distribution was corrected for total body weight, there were no differences between the obese and nonobese subjects. These results suggest that loading doses of lidocaine should be based upon total body weight, and infusion rates need not be adjusted in the presence of obesity.

Pharmacokinetic drug interactions Cimetidine, but not ranitidine, may decrease the clearance and volume of distribution of lidocaine and increase its half-life and plasma concentration.[102] However, the effects of cimetidine on the pharmacokinetics of lidocaine appear to be relatively small. Nonetheless, clinicians should be aware that the potential for lidocaine toxicity may be enhanced when cimetidine is coadministered. The mechanisms of the interaction may be cimetidine-mediated decreases in both hepatic blood flow and hepatic oxidative metabolism.

Several beta-adrenergic receptor antagonists alter the pharmacokinetics of lidocaine. Propranolol decreases the clearance of lidocaine by 40 percent and increases the half-life from 1.1 to 1.7 h.[103] The major mechanism by which these effects occur is the direct inhibition of lidocaine metabolism by propranolol.[104] Propranolol-mediated decreases in hepatic blood flow may also play a role. Neither atenolol[105] nor pindolol[106] significantly affects lidocaine clearance.

Adverse reactions Studies have suggested that minor but common adverse effects on the CNS, which include drowsiness, blurred vision, numbness of the tongue and lips, speech disturbances, dizziness, and nausea, have generally occurred at total lidocaine concentrations of 3 to 6 μg/mL. More severe CNS disturbances, including mental confusion, poor respiratory effort, seizure, marked sedation, and coma, usually have been observed at total lidocaine concentrations of greater than 6 μg/mL. Serum concentrations of unbound lidocaine correlate better with the severity of CNS toxicity than do total lidocaine concentrations.[107] Excessive lidocaine dosages can also depress myocardial function and inhibit the sinus node. Block below the bundle of His may occur, although this is uncommon.

Considerable overlap has been observed between therapeutic concentrations of lidocaine (i.e., usually 2 to 6 μg/mL) and toxic concentrations. Some of this overlap may be attributed to failure to quantify lidocaine metabolites MEGX and GX, which in some patients may contribute to the occurrence of adverse effects. Another possible explanation for the overlap may be the variability in the protein binding of lidocaine, which can result in differences in concentrations of unbound lidocaine.

Tocainide

Tocainide (Fig. 6-4) is structurally similar to lidocaine. The replacement of one of the methyl groups results in a compound that has markedly less hepatic first-pass elimination, so tocainide may be administered orally or intravenously. Tocainide produces electrophysiologic effects similar to those of lidocaine. Both drugs have minimal effect on the surface electrocardiogram. Like lidocaine, tocainide suppresses ventricular arrhythmias, but it has little effect on supraventricular arrhythmias.

Clinical pharmacology (Table 6-2) ***Absorption*** Tocainide is rapidly and virtually completely absorbed following oral administration.[108] Tocainide demonstrates dose-independent absorption over a dosage range of 10 to 1000 mg. The ingestion of tocainide with food results in slower absorption and a 40-percent reduction in maximal tocainide concentrations, but the extent of absorption remains unchanged.[108]

Distribution In healthy subjects, the reported volume of distribution of tocainide has ranged from 1.62 L/kg[108] to 2.9 L/kg.[109] In patients administered tocainide within 24 h of onset of acute myocardial infarction, the mean volume of distribution was 3.2 L/kg.[109]

Metabolism and elimination Tocainide undergoes both renal elimination and hepatic biotransformation.[108-110] Thirty to 50 percent of an administered dose is excreted in the urine as unchanged tocainide.[108,109] Alkalinization of the urine markedly reduces the renal clearance and prolongs the elimination half-life of unchanged tocainide.[108] Within the physiologic range of urine pH, this effect is probably minor. None of the metabolites of tocainide is pharmacologically active.

In healthy volunteers, the average elimination half-life of tocainide is 11 to 14 h and total body clearance is 2.1 to 2.6 mL/min/kg.[108,109] In patients who were administered intravenous tocainide within 24 h of acute myocardial infarction, half-life was found to be 14.5 h and the total body clearance was 2.6 mL/min/kg.[109]

Conditions that alter pharmacokinetics Decreases in either renal or hepatic function result in alterations in the pharmacokinetics of tocainide. In patients who are on hemodialysis for renal failure, the mean half-life of tocainide is 22.3 h and the total body clearance averages 1.34 mL/min/kg.[111] Hemodialysis removes approximately 25 percent of the amount of tocainide within the body at the start of dialysis. In patients with creatinine clearance of 10 to 55 mL/min, the average half-life is 19 h and the total body clearance is 1.34 mL/min/kg. Accordingly, tocainide dosage should be decreased in patients with renal failure. However, creatinine clearance per se is a poor estimator of the half-life of tocainide due to the significant nonrenal elimination of tocainide in renal failure.

In patients with decompensated cirrhosis and moderate renal dysfunction, the half-life of tocainide averages 27 h and the mean total body clearance is 1.8 mL/min/kg.[112] These findings are similar to those in individuals with severe renal impairment.

In patients with ventricular arrhythmias and chronic congestive heart failure, there is a decreased mean total body clearance of tocainide (1.36 mL/min/kg) compared to that in patients without CHF (1.85 mL/min/kg).[113] In patients with acute myocardial infarction and secondary mild left ventricular failure, the average half-life is 15.6 h.[114] Therefore, CHF diminishes the elimination of tocainide to a variable degree, probably due to the severity of the cardiac impairment. Tocainide doses should be decreased accordingly.

Pharmacokinetic drug interactions The coadministration of rifampin with tocainide results in significant shortening of half-life, 9.4 vs. 13.2 h, and increases the oral clearance of tocainide, 2.10 vs. 1.56 mL/min/kg.[115] These changes probably occur as a consequence of increases in the nonrenal clearance of tocainide. However, phenobarbital, which induces the activity of glucuronyl transferase, the enzyme responsible for the formation of the principal metabolite of tocainide, does not alter tocainide metabolism or pharmacokinetics.

Neither cimetidine nor ranitidine affects the half-life or renal clearance of tocainide. However, it appears that cimetidine, but not ranitidine, may decrease the absorption of tocainide. Allopurinal may increase the half-life of tocainide. There is no interaction between tocainide and digoxin.

Stereospecific aspects of tocainide pharmacokinetics The chemical structure of tocainide contains an asymmetric carbon atom, and the drug is administered clinically as a 50-percent racemic mixture. The R(-) and S(+) enantiomers of tocainide demonstrate different pharmacologic properties.[116,117]

The R(-) enantiomer of tocainide is more pharmacologically active[116] and more rapidly metabolized than the S(+) enantiomer.[117] The dissimilarities in the pharmacologic and pharmacokinetic properties between the enantiomers may account for some of the reported differences in antiarrhythmic response and adverse effects of tocainide.

Adverse reactions The most common adverse reactions to tocainide are nonspecific CNS and gastrointestinal reactions. These include dizziness, nausea, paresthesia, tremor, headache, vomiting, skin rash, and confusion. These are usually mild, dose related, and reversible with dose reduction. Drug discontinuation is necessary in approximately 20 percent of patients taking tocainide.

Tocainide has minimal hemodynamic effects. The drug may be used in patients with CHF, but smaller doses may be required.

Bone marrow depression with neutropenia, anemia, or agranulocytosis has been reported in 0.18 percent of patients receiving tocainide. This usually occurs within the first 12 weeks of therapy.

Pulmonary fibrosis has been reported in about 0.11 percent of patients on tocainide. This occurred after 3 to 18 weeks of treatment, and most patients reported to have pulmonary fibrosis were seriously ill prior to receiving tocainide.

Mexiletine

Mexiletine (Fig. 6-4) is structurally similar to lidocaine and tocainide and has similar electrophysiologic effects. Mexiletine was originally developed as an anorexiant and anticonvulsant; its antiarrhythmic properties were recognized later.

Clinical pharmacology (Table 6-2) ***Absorption*** The absolute bioavailability of conventional mexiletine capsules averages 80 to 87 percent, indicating a minimal effect of hepatic first-pass metabolism on the absorption of mexiletine.[118] The absorption of mexiletine is independent of dose. Peak plasma concentrations are generally attained within 2 to 4 h.[118]

In the elderly, the rate of absorption is significantly slower, but the extent of absorption is similar to that in younger subjects.[119] The absorption of mexiletine is delayed and slower in patients with a recent myocardial infarction. This effect may occur secondary to the vagolytic properties of coadministered narcotic analgesics, which prolong the gastric emptying time. Nonetheless, the extent of mexiletine absorption appears to be relatively unaffected by recent myocardial infarction. Most patients with chronic ventricular arrhythmias demonstrate absorption pharmacokinetics that are similar to those of healthy elderly subjects.

Distribution Mexiletine is extensively distributed to body tissues with a volume of distribution of 5.5 to 6.6 L/kg.[120] In acute myocardial infarction, the volume of distribution increases to over 8 L/kg,[121] perhaps reflecting a decrease in cardiac output and hepatic blood flow with a subsequent decrease in metabolic elimination. However, 7 to 14 days after infarction the volume of distribution decreases to normal.

Mexiletine is approximately 70 percent protein bound. However, only 1 percent of total body mexiletine is in the blood, so alterations in protein binding would not be anticipated to be clinically significant.

Metabolism and elimination Mexiletine is extensively metabolized in the liver.[122] In addition, mexiletine undergoes conjugation with glucuronic acid. The metabolites are not pharmacologically active.[123] The renal excretion of unchanged mexiletine ranges from 1.4 to 23 percent in young, as well as elderly, healthy volunteers.[119]

The elimination half-life averages 12 h[118] and remains relatively constant following escalating doses of mexiletine. In general, healthy elderly subjects demonstrate a modestly prolonged half-life, 14.4 h, relative to younger individuals.[119]

Within 24 h of an acute myocardial infarction, the half-life of mexiletine is prolonged to 15 h, but it decreases to 11 h 1 to 2 weeks following the infarction.[121] The acute change is possibly due to decreased hepatic blood flow.

Conditions that alter pharmacokinetics Chronic hepatic impairment and clinically severe CHF alter the pharmacokinetics of mexiletine.[124,125] At equivalent doses of mexiletine, patients with ventricular arrhythmias and cirrhosis demonstrate a 3.5-fold increase in steady-state peak plasma concentrations of mexiletine compared to patients with ventricular arrhythmias and normal hepatic function.[124] This finding corresponds to a 70-percent reduction in total body clearance in patients with chronic hepatic disease. The mean half-life of mexiletine is modestly prolonged to about 15 h in patients with CHF.[125] A twice-daily dosing regimen could be utilized in this patient subgroup.

The average half-life in patients with creatinine clearances of less than 10 mL/min (15.7 h) was significantly longer than in patients with creatinine clearances of at least 75 mL/min (10.35 h) and in patients with creatinine clearances of between 10 and 30 mL/min (13.76 h).[126] In patients with creatinine clearances of less than 3 mL/min, the mean half-life was 22.3 h.[127] Hemodialysis does not significantly affect the elimination of mexiletine.[127] Peritoneal dialysis has also been ineffective in the removal of mexiletine. Failure to decrease the dosage of mexiletine in patients with severe renal impairment has resulted in both cardiac and extracardiac adverse effects.

Pharmacokinetic drug interactions Metoclopramide significantly shortens and atropine significantly lengthens the time to maximal mexiletine plasma concentrations.[128] In addition, atropine reduces the observed peak plasma level of mexiletine. However, the amount of mexiletine absorbed is unaltered by either metoclopramide or atropine. Magnesium-aluminum antacids lengthen the time to maximal plasma concentration of mexiletine but do not change either the amount of mexiletine absorbed or the observed maximal level of mexiletine.[129]

Inducers of the hepatic mixed-function oxidase enzyme system increase the total body clearance and decrease the elimination half-life of mexiletine. Rifampin, phenytoin, and cigarette smoking shorten the elimination half-life of mexiletine an average of 41, 51, and 36 percent, respectively.[130-132] The total body clearance of mexiletine is increased by approximately 50 percent by each of these substances as a result of increases in nonrenal clearance. Therefore, both the total daily dose and the frequency of administration of mexiletine should be increased in patients who are also taking rifampin or phenytoin or in those who are chronic cigarette smokers. In contradistinction to these findings, neither cimetidine nor ranitidine, two histamine-2 receptor antagonists with varying inhibitory effects on the hepatic microsomal enzyme system, significantly alter the metabolism of mexiletine. Mexiletine significantly prolongs the half-life and decreases the total body clearance of theophylline via inhibition of cytochrome P-450 isozymes.[133]

Stereospecific aspects of mexiletine pharmacokinetics Mexiletine contains an asymmetric carbon atom. This results in the existence of two enantiomers, R(-) and S(+) mexiletine. The pharmacokinetic data reported above are based on total [R(-) plus S(+)] concentrations of mexiletine since mexiletine is administered clinically as the racemate. However, differences in the pharmacokinetics of the two enantiomers of mexiletine are significant, and these differences may explain some of the interindividual differences in mexiletine pharmacokinetics. The R(-) enantiomer is twice as potent as the S(+) enantiomer in terms of binding to sodium channels on myocytes.[134]

Adverse effects The reported occurrence of intolerable side effects from mexiletine ranges from 5 to 50 percent, with most studies reporting 20 to 30 percent. In 12 clinical trials that included information on the adverse effects of mexiletine, 105 (22 percent) of a total of 487 patients had side effects that limited the use of the drug.[135] Campbell et al [136] reported a significant correlation between the plasma concentration of mexiletine and the severity of side effects, although other investigators do not agree. Gastrointestinal disturbances, usually nausea or vomiting, are the most frequent side effects. They may be reduced by administering the drug with meals.

Central nervous system side effects are somewhat less common and include a fine tremor of the hands, dizziness, blurred vision, dysarthria, ataxia, drowsiness, and confusion.

As with any antiarrhythmic medication, the potential exists for exacerbation or provocation of arrhythmias. For mexiletine, however, this has been reported relatively infrequently in patients undergoing noninvasive or electrophysiologic evaluation[46] for arrhythmias. As with other class IB antiarrhythmic agents, provocation of torsade de pointes is a very rare outcome of mexiletine treatment.

Hemodynamically significant cardiac side effects, such as marked bradycardia or hypotension, are unusual with mexiletine. Mexiletine does not cause significant depression of cardiac function at the usually administered doses.

Thrombocytopenia is a very rare side effect of mexiletine. It may be observed within days of initiating therapy and is rapidly reversible after drug discontinuation. The mechanism is unknown.

Moricizine

Moricizine (Fig. 6-5) is a phenothiazine derivative that was first developed in the Soviet Union. A class I agent with properties that make it difficult to subclassify, moricizine suppresses both atrial and ventricular arrhythmias. Interest in moricizine was heightened when it was chosen as one of the antiarrhythmics for the CAST in post-myocardial infarction patients. The encainide and flecainide treatment groups in the CAST showed an excessive mortality rate when compared to the group that received a placebo.[4] The CAST II trial of moricizine versus placebo also showed a trend toward decreased survival among patients treated with moricizine.

Clinical pharmacology (Table 6-2) Moricizine is well absorbed. However, the bioavailability is 30 to 40 percent due to first-pass metabolism.[137] Peak plasma levels occur 1 to 1.5 h after oral ingestion. The drug is rapidly and virtually completely metabolized in the liver.[138] Multiple metabolites are formed. Some of the metabolites probably contribute to the antiarrhythmic effect. The elimination half-life in normal patients is 3 to 4 h.[137] In cardiac patients, the half-life is 6 to 13 h, probably due to decreased cardiac output, liver blood flow, and rate of drug metabolism.[138]

Moricizine is 92 to 95 percent bound to plasma proteins,[138] especially albumin and alpha-acid glycoprotein. Therefore, small decreases in protein binding, as may

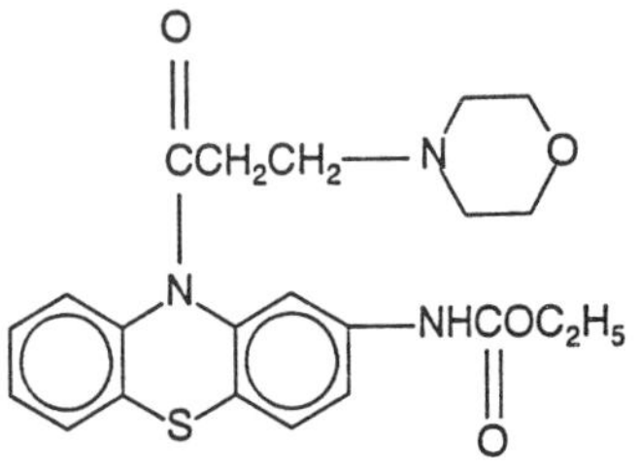

O
||
CCH_2CH_2—N O
N
S —$NHCOC_2H_5$
||
O

Moricizine

Figure 6-5 Structural formula of moricizine.

occur due to displacement of moricizine by other drugs, could markedly increase the concentration of free, active moricizine.

Pharmacokinetic drug interactions Cimetidine decreases the clearance of moricizine, probably by inhibition of hepatic microsomal enzymes. The half-life of moricizine is prolonged approximately 33 percent by cimetidine.[139]

Moricizine probably does not alter the pharmacokinetics of digitalis.

Adverse effects Moricizine is generally well tolerated. The most common adverse effects are nonspecific gastrointestinal symptoms, especially nausea. These are reported by about 10 percent of patients and can often be reduced or eliminated by taking the drug during meals. Nonspecific CNS symptoms, such as dizziness, anxiety, visual disturbances, paresthesias, or depression, are also reported by about 10 percent of patients. Other possible but uncommon noncardiac adverse effects include fever, thrombocytopenia, and abnormal liver enzymes.

Depression of intraventricular conduction with fascicular block may occur, but it is uncommon.

As with all antiarrhythmic agents, there is some proarrhythmic potential. Careful evaluation of the cardiac rhythm is required after initiation of antiarrhythmic drug therapy.

Flecainide

Flecainide (Fig. 6-6) was the first member of the class IC antiarrhythmic agents that was developed. Flecainide produces marked suppression of nonsustained ventricular arrhythmias, although it has a less consistent effect in patients with sustained arrhythmias. Because of its negative inotropic effect, flecainide should be used with caution in patients with depressed ventricular function. Flecainide use is associated with a significant risk of lethal proarrhythmia in patients with histories of myocardial infarction and ventricular arrhythmias. Flecainide may be most useful for treating supraventricular tachycardias in patients who do not have structural heart disease.

Clinical pharmacology (Table 6-2) Flecainide is well absorbed after oral administration and is 95 percent bioavailable.[140,141] Peak plasma concentrations of

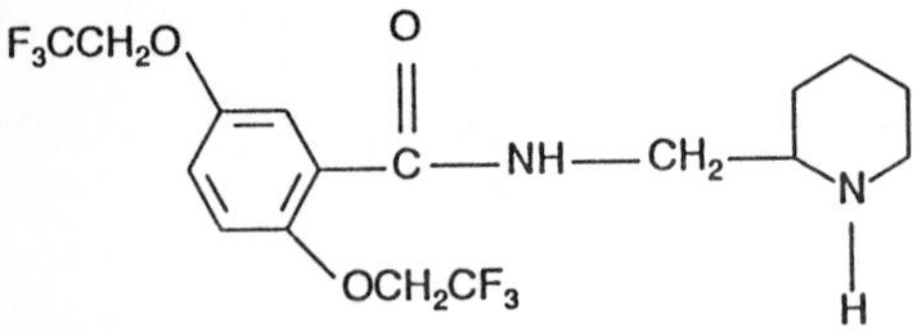

Flecainide

Figure 6-6 Structural formula of flecainide.

flecainide are attained between 1.5 to 3.0 h and are proportional to the dose.[141] The volume of distribution of flecainide is large, averaging nearly 9 L/kg.[141] Flecainide is extensively distributed to several tissues including the heart.[141] A mean of 27 percent (range 10 to 50 percent) of a single dose is excreted unchanged in the urine.[140,141] The remainder of the drug is biotransformed into two major metabolites, *meta-O*-dealkylated flecainide and its lactam, both of which are conjugated in the liver and then undergo renal excretion.[140] Both metabolites are active, but they are less potent than the parent compound.[142] It is unlikely that the metabolites of flecainide contribute significantly to the effect of flecainide in most patients.[143] Flecainide is only 32 to 47 percent bound by plasma proteins.[143]

In normal patients, the elimination half-life of flecainide is about 14 h (with a range of 7 to 23 h).[141] This half-life generally permits administration twice a day. In elderly patients and in patients with heart failure, clearance is reduced and the elimination half-life is prolonged to about 19 h (range 14 to 26 h).[144] In patients with end-stage renal disease, the half-life is prolonged up to 50 h, and the total clearance is decreased by approximately 40 percent.[141]

Drug interactions Flecainide interacts pharmacokinetically with digoxin, cimetidine, and propranolol. In normal volunteers, the digoxin trough serum concentration is higher, and the peak digoxin serum level is 13 percent higher when flecainide is also administered.[145] Flecainide and propranolol appear to raise each other's plasma concentration and to exert additive negative inotropic effects.[146] Cimetidine reduces the total clearance of flecainide by 13 to 27 percent and prolongs the elimination half-life.[147] Plasma concentrations of flecainide have also reportedly been elevated by concomitant amiodarone therapy.[148]

Adverse effects Proarrhythmic events resulting from flecainide were assessed in 1330 patients who were followed for an average of 10 months.[149] Proarrhythmic events occurred in 6.8 percent of patients overall, were serious in 2.3 percent, and were lethal in 1 percent. The incidence of proarrhythmia appeared to be related to the baseline arrhythmias. Serious nonlethal proarrhythmic events occurred in 6.6 percent of patients with sustained ventricular tachycardia, in less than 1 percent of patients with nonsustained ventricular tachycardia, and in only one of the patients with isolated ventricular premature complexes. However, in the CAST there was an excessive number of deaths and nonfatal cardiac arrests in patients taking flecainide or encainide compared to patients taking a placebo.[4] The CAST investigators concluded that neither flecainide nor encainide should be used in the treatment of patients with asymptomatic or minimally symptomatic ventricular arrhythmias after myocardial infarction, even though these drugs are usually effective in suppressing ventricular arrhythmias.

Whether it is used alone or in combination with other drugs, flecainide must be used with caution, even in patients with a history of symptomatic sustained ventricular tachycardia or fibrillation. Fontaine and associates found that when flecainide and amiodarone are used in an effort to control such patients, there is not only an increased incidence of cardiac decompensation but also an increase in the cardiac pacing threshold.[150] This drug combination can also produce torsade de pointes.

Noncardiac side effects include CNS symptoms, such as dizziness and difficulty with visual accommodation,[143] but these occur uncommonly. These adverse effects can usually be eliminated by reducing the dose. Gastrointestinal side effects are rare.

Propafenone

Propafenone (Fig. 6-7) was first synthesized in 1970 and has been available for clinical use in Germany since 1977. Clinical trials have shown that propafenone is effective in suppressing both ventricular and supraventricular arrhythmias, including those in patients with the Wolff-Parkinson-White syndrome. Although propafenone is generally well tolerated, it may prolong AV conduction and aggravate existing AV block. The drug has a negative inotropic effect and should be used cautiously in patients with a history of CHF or depressed ejection fraction.

Clinical pharmacology (Table 6-2) ***Absorption*** Orally administered propafenone is well absorbed. Peak serum levels are obtained approximately 2 h after administration of a 150-mg dose and 3 h after a 300-mg dose.[151] The half-life of propafenone ranges from 2 to 8 h following a single dose of 100 or 300 mg. The relationship between dose and steady-state concentration is nonlinear. When the dose is increased from 300 to 900 mg/day, the serum concentration increases almost 10-fold.[151] This suggests that a saturable first-pass hepatic enzyme process is responsible for the metabolism of propafenone.

Distribution Propafenone is distributed in the body according to a two-compartment model. The volume of distribution of the central compartment at steady state is approximately 3 to 4 L/kg. Propafenone is most widely distributed in the lungs, liver, and heart, with the lowest amount of drug appearing in fat and the brain.

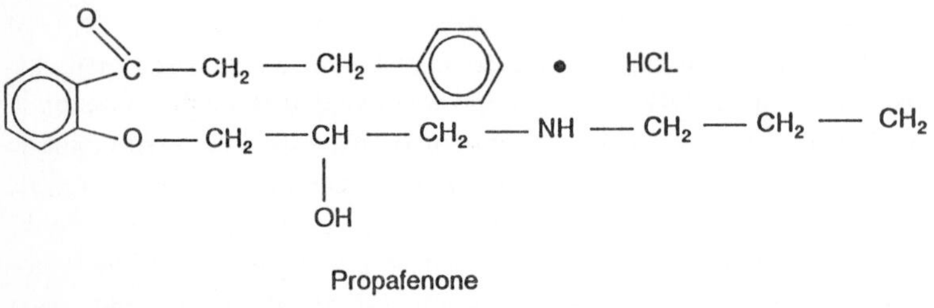

Propafenone

Figure 6-7 Structural formula of propafenone.

The drug is 80 to 90 percent bound to the protein alpha$_1$-acid glycoprotein in human plasma.

Metabolism and elimination Propafenone is extensively metabolized. Eleven metabolites have been identified, two of which are active.[152] The two active metabolites, 5-hydroxypropafenone and *N*-depropylpropafenone, have concentrations in humans of less than 20 percent of propafenone. Less than 1 percent of the drug is eliminated unchanged in the urine.

There are two genetically determined patterns of propafenone metabolism. Ninety percent of patients are extensive metabolizers who show shorter elimination half-lives, lower plasma concentrations, higher oral clearance, and detectable amounts of metabolites of 5-hydroxypropafenone. Poorer metabolizers do not form the 5-hydroxy metabolite and exhibit longer elimination half-lives that range from 10 to 32 h, higher plasma concentrations, a linear dose-response relationship, and nondetectable levels of 5-hydroxypropafenone.

Ten percent of Caucasians are poor metabolizers. Because the difference in the blood concentrations of propafenone between rapid and slow metabolizers decreases at high doses and there is a lack of the active 5-hydroxy metabolites in slow metabolizers, the recommended dosing regimen is the same for all patients.[152,153]

The clearance of propafenone is decreased in patients with hepatic dysfunction.[154] There appears to be no difference in metabolism between patients with normal renal function and those with renal impairment or severe renal failure.[155]

Drug interactions A number of commonly used drugs, including digoxin, warfarin, cimetidine, and beta-adrenergic blockers, have been reported to interact with propafenone. Nolan and associates[156] studied the effects of propafenone on digoxin kinetics in healthy volunteers. The kinetics were evaluated following intravenous administration of digoxin alone, after propafenone 150 mg every 8 h, and after propafenone 300 mg every 8 h. Total body clearance of digoxin was decreased after treatment with the higher dose of propafenone. The area under the curve for digoxin was increased by 23 percent. The renal clearance and the half-life of digoxin were not altered.[156] Therefore, the digoxin dose should be decreased approximately 25 percent and serum levels monitored in patients who receive concomitant propafenone therapy.

Propafenone may inhibit the metabolism of warfarin, and consequently prothrombin times may be increased in patients receiving both propafenone and warfarin. Concomitant administration of propafenone and beta blockers such as propranolol or metoprolol has been shown to increase concentrations of propranolol and metoprolol; therefore, when these drugs are used concomitantly, the metoprolol dose should be decreased.[151] The dose of propafenone should be reduced in patients receiving concomitant cimetidine, as cimetidine coadministration increases propafenone concentration by 20 percent. Small doses of quinidine completely inhibit the hydroxylation pathway, making all patients in effect slow metabolizers.[152]

Adverse effects In general, propafenone is well tolerated. The majority of adverse effects are noncardiac in nature and include unusual taste sensation (a bitter or metallic taste), dizziness, headache, and gastrointestinal complaints. Cardiac side effects include development of first-degree block, intraventricular conduction delay, bundle branch block, or heart failure. Proarrhythmia has been reported in patients who receive propafenone.

Amiodarone

Amiodarone (Fig. 6-8) is a potent drug that suppresses a variety of supraventricular and ventricular arrhythmias. Amiodarone is a class III antiarrhythmic agent, which means that its principal electrophysiologic action is to prolong the cardiac action potential and consequently the duration of the refractory period in several cardiac tissues.[157] These effects are predominantly observed with chronic administration of amiodarone and may be due in part to selective blockade of triiodothyronine (T3) action on the myocardium. Amiodarone also demonstrates class I activity and weak calcium channel blocking effects (i.e., class IV activity).[157] In addition, amiodarone is a noncompetitive alpha- and beta-adrenergic receptor antagonist and may demonstrate anticholinergic effects.[157]

Clinical pharmacology (Table 6-2) The clinical pharmacokinetics of amiodarone have principally been determined in young, healthy volunteers.[158] Following single oral doses of amiodarone, absorption of amiodarone is slow and the absolute bioavailability averages 35 percent.[158] Amiodarone appears to be principally eliminated via hepatic *N*-dealkylation to form *N*-desethylamiodarone.[157] This metabolite is electrophysiologically and pharmacokinetically similar to amiodarone. *N*-desethylamiodarone significantly contributes to the antiarrhythmic and the toxicologic effects of amiodarone.

After single intravenous doses of amiodarone, total body clearance averages 8.6 L/h; steady-state volume of distribution is approximately 4900 L. The terminal elimination half-life averages 25 days.[158] In contrast to these findings, the mean

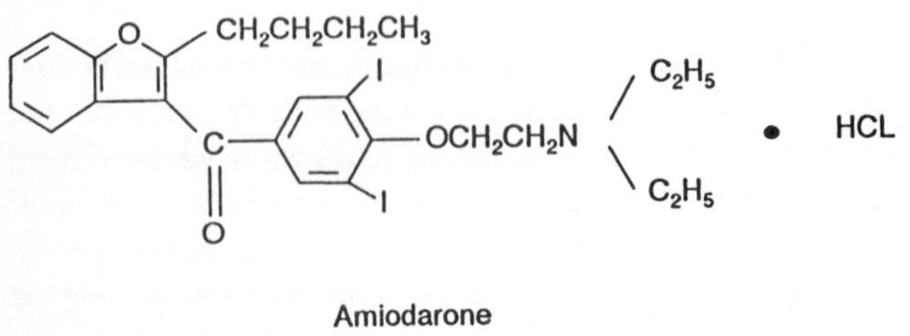

$CH_2CH_2CH_2CH_3$ I I C O OCH_2CH_2N C_2H_5 C_2H_5 • HCL

Amiodarone

Figure 6-8 Structural formula of amiodarone.

terminal elimination half-life of amiodarone was 53 days in patients whose chronic amiodarone therapy was discontinued.[158] These findings suggest that amiodarone demonstrates time-dependent pharmacokinetics so that the clearance of amiodarone decreases with chronic administration.

Information describing the clinical pharmacokinetics of amiodarone in the elderly is lacking. Nonetheless, advanced age (i.e., greater that 60 years of age) may predispose patients to develop amiodarone toxicity.[159] This finding may represent differences in the pharmacokinetics and/or pharmacodynamics of amiodarone in the elderly.

There is also little information regarding the clinical pharmacokinetics of amiodarone in disease states. Renal dysfunction appears to have a negligible impact upon the elimination of either amiodarone or its principal metabolite, *N*-desethylamiodarone.[160]

The use of serum concentration monitoring of amiodarone remains controversial. Rotmensch and co-workers[161] suggested a therapeutic range of 1 to 2.5 μg/mL for amiodarone and believed that serum *N*-desethylamiodarone concentrations did not furnish supplemental therapeutic information. Other investigators have advocated targeting amiodarone dosing to achieve 10 to 15 percent prolongation of the QT interval.[162] Other potentially useful pharmacodynamic endpoints include the development of corneal microdeposits[163] and the rise in serum reverse T3 concentrations.[164]

Pharmacokinetic drug interactions Amiodarone pharmacokinetically and pharmacodynamically interacts with a number of other drugs.[165] The coadministration of amiodarone results in increased serum concentrations of digoxin, quinidine, procainamide, flecainide, aprindine, warfarin, and phenytoin, and patients may be at risk for developing drug-induced toxicity as a result of the increases in serum concentration. For these drugs, dosage reductions in the range of 20 to 50 percent are generally recommended when amiodarone is concomitantly administered. Amiodarone also potentiates the pharmacologic effects of beta-adrenergic antagonists and diltiazem.[165] Phenytoin appears to increase the metabolic conversion of amiodarone to *N*-desethylamiodarone.[166] The clinical consequences of this interaction remain to be determined.

Adverse effects Most patients who chronically ingest amiodarone develop adverse effects.[167] The majority of side effects may be managed by dosage reduction. However, some adverse effects, such as pulmonary fibrosis or hepatitis, are life-threatening and require discontinuation of amiodarone. Certain side effects may be related to either the cumulative dose or serum concentrations of amiodarone and desethylamiodarone. The incidence of adverse effects increases with continued administration, but the occurrence of intolerable side effects necessitating withdrawal of amiodarone decreases with continued use.[159] Patients 60 years of age or older may be at greater risk for developing amiodarone-induced adverse effects.[159]

Amiodarone-induced adverse effects involve a variety of organ systems including the cardiovascular, pulmonary, gastrointestinal, neurologic, ophthalmologic, dermatologic, and thyroid systems.[167] Only a small number of patients will have worsening of CHF or hypotensive episodes during chronic amiodarone treatment. However, rapidly administered intravenous amiodarone, especially at doses greater than 5 mg/kg, may cause acute myocardial depression and hypotension in patients with underlying left ventricular dysfunction. The most common proarrhythmic effects of amiodarone involve the sinus node and include symptomatic sinus bradycardia, sinoatrial block, and sinus arrest. Amiodarone infrequently produces ventricular proarrhythmic effects including torsade de pointes.

Up to 13 percent of amiodarone-treated patients may develop manifestations and symptoms of pulmonary toxicity, and as many as 10 to 20 percent of these may die of cardiopulmonary complications.[167] The mechanism of the pulmonary toxicity may be immune mediated. Although abnormal baseline pulmonary function studies may not identify high-risk patients, some investigators find the studies predictive for development of pulmonary toxicity.

The most common adverse effects of amiodarone involve the gastrointestinal system.[167] Symptoms include anorexia, nausea, constipation, abdominal pain, and diarrhea. These symptoms may be dose related.

Hepatic concentrations of amiodarone greatly exceed those in the plasma. Mild elevations of serum aspartate aminotransferase levels occur in 15 to 20 percent of patients taking amiodarone. The degree of elevation may correlate with serum concentrations of amiodarone and desethylamiodarone. Clinically apparent amiodarone-induced hepatitis is rare. Liver biopsy should be considered for patients with persistent elevations of serum aminotransferase levels.

Neurologic side effects occur in 5 to 74 percent of patients taking amiodarone.[167] The most common symptoms are tremor, ataxia, and neuropathy. These and other neurologic effects may be dose dependent.

Virtually 100 percent of patients on amiodarone develop corneal microdeposits. However, only a small number of patients have visual complications such as blurring of vision, blue-green halo vision, or photophobia, all of which may resolve with a reduction in the dose of amiodarone.

Dermal photosensitivity and blue-grey discoloration of the skin, especially in sun-exposed areas, are the most commonly reported amiodarone dermatologic adverse effects.[167] Both of these adverse effects appear related to dose and duration of amiodarone therapy. Amiodarone and desethylamiodarone are concentrated in the skin. Patients should be cautioned to wear protective clothing and to avoid prolonged sun exposure.

The incidence of thyroid abnormalities typically ranges from 0 to 11 percent in patients taking amiodarone, but up to 49 percent of patients have developed thyroid derangements.[167] Each 200-mg tablet of amiodarone contains 75 mg of iodine. Essentially all patients develop alterations in thyroid function tests. In addition, amiodarone may cause either hyper- or hypothyroidism. Hyperthyroidism may require treatment with standard antithyroid drugs, potassium perchlorate, beta-adrenergic antagonists, and/or corticosteroids. Hypothyroidism can be managed with thyroid replacement with a therapeutic goal of normalization of serum T4 and perhaps thyroid-stimulating hormone (TSH) levels.

Bretylium Tosylate

Bretylium (Fig. 6-9) is an antiarrhythmic agent available for intravenous or intramuscular use. The drug has class III electrophysiologic effects. Bretylium initially releases norepinephrine from postganglionic adrenergic neurons and then inhibits further release as well as reuptake.[168]

Pharmacokinetics (Table 6-2) Bretylium is extensively distributed throughout the body but selectively accumulates in the sympathetic ganglia and adrenergic neurons. Bretylium is eliminated almost exclusively by active tubular secretion in the kidneys.[169] The drug is not metabolized by the liver. The elimination half-life averages 7 to 9 h, but interindividual variation is considerable. The half-life is greatly prolonged in renal failure.[170]

Adverse effects Initial intravenous administration of bretylium is usually associated with a transient rise in blood pressure and tachycardia and often with an increase in frequency of arrhythmias. These events are probably due to the initial release of norepinephrine. Nausea and vomiting are also common.[171] The subsequent inhibition of norepinephrine release is associated with hypotension. Orthostatic hypotension usually occurs. Supine hypotension may occasionally be seen and can be treated with vasopressor catecholamines.[172] Other adverse effects include bradycardia, worsening heart failure, proarrhythmia, drowsiness, and fatigue.

Adenosine

Adenosine is an endogenous purine nucleoside that plays a major role in maintaining the myocardial balance between oxygen supply and oxygen demand. Adenosine is released in the coronary circulation during myocardial ischemia. The

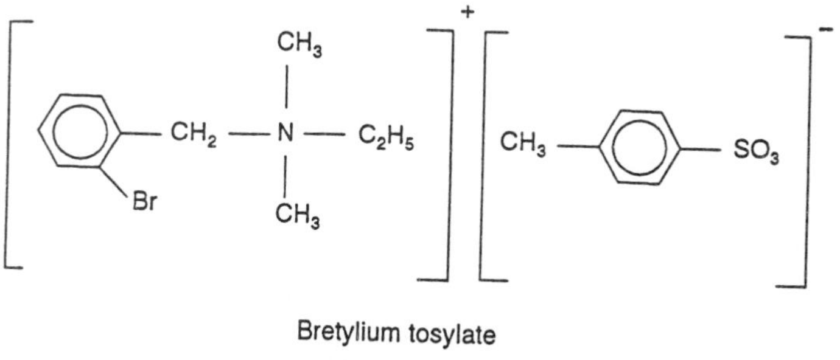

Figure 6-9 Structural formula of bretylium tosylate.

stimulation of cell surface adenosine receptors inhibits adenyl cyclase and, consequently, the synthesis of cyclic adenosine monophosphate (AMP). This results in the following actions that help restore oxygen balance: dilation of coronary resistance vessels, inhibition of the hemodynamic and metabolic effects of beta-adrenergic stimulation, and inhibition of sinus node automaticity and AV node conduction, thereby slowing the heart rate. Adenosine also inhibits platelet aggregation, inhibits superoxide anion generation by neutrophils, and is the probable cause of anginal pain.

Intravenously administered adenosine exerts a potent depressant effect on AV nodal conduction and is exceptionally effective in terminating supraventricular tachycardias that utilize the AV node as part of a reentrant pathway.

Clinical pharmacology (Table 6-2) After intravenous injection, adenosine is rapidly cleared from the circulation by erythrocytes and endothelial cells,[173] which metabolize adenosine to the inactive compound inosine and to adenosine monophosphate. The elimination half-life is several seconds.

Pharmacokinetic drug interactions Dipyridamole inhibits the uptake and subsequent degradation of adenosine. The effects of exogenously administered adenosine are therefore increased in the presence of dipyridamole.[174,175] Patients taking dipyridamole either should not receive adenosine or should be given lower doses.

Methylxanthines competitively block the adenosine receptor. Therefore, in the presence of theophylline or pharmacologic levels of caffeine or other methylxanthines, the usual doses of adenosine may not be effective.[176]

Adverse effects Adenosine commonly produces mild proarrhythmic effects. Sinus bradycardia or AV block, lasting only a few seconds, are a consequence of the physiologic effect of the drug. Atrial and ventricular ectopy are also common. Atrial fibrillation occasionally occurs.[177,178]

Chest discomfort occurs in about one-third of patients. This is a consequence of the stimulation of adenosine receptors. Transient dyspnea, flushing, cold sweats, or headaches are also common. The median duration of these symptoms is less than 1 min.[173,177-180]

REFERENCES

1. Petersen P, Boysen G, Godtfredsen J, et al: Placebo-controlled, randomized trial of warfarin and aspirin for prevention of thromboembolic complications in chronic atrial fibrillation: the Copenhagen AFASAK study. *Lancet* 1: 175, 1989.
2. Stroke Prevention in Atrial Fibrillation Study Group Investigators. Preliminary report of the Stroke Prevention in Atrial Fibrillation Study. *N Engl J Med* 322: 863, 1990.
3. The Boston Area Anticoagulation Trial for Atrial Fibrillation Investigators. The effect of low-dose warfarin on the risk of stroke in patients with non-rheumatic atrial fibrillation. *N Engl J Med* 323: 1505, 1990.

4. The Cardiac Arrhythmia Suppression Trial Investigators. Preliminary report: effect of encainide and flecainide on mortality in a randomized trial of arrhythmia suppression after myocardial infarction. *N Engl J Med* 321: 406, 1989.
5. Guentert TW, Upton RA, Holford NHG, et al: Divergence in pharmacokinetic parameters of quinidine obtained by specific and nonspecific assay methods. *J Pharmacokinet Biopharm* 7: 303, 1979.
6. Ueda CT, Williamson BJ, Dzindzio BS: Absolute quinidine bioavailability. *Clin Pharmacol Ther* 20: 260, 1976.
7. Guentert TW, Upton RA, Holford NHG, et al: Gastrointestinal absorption of quinidine from some solutions and commercial tablets. *J Pharmacokinet Biopharm* 8: 243, 1980.
8. Conrad KA, Molk BL, Chidsey CA: Pharmacokinetic studies of quinidine in patients with arrhythmias. *Circulation* 55: 1, 1977.
9. Gibson DL, Smith GH, Koup JR, et al: Relative bioavailability of a standard and a sustained-release quinidine tablet. *Clin Pharm* 1: 366, 1982.
10. Ochs HR, Greenblatt DJ, Woo E, et al: Single and multiple dose pharmacokinetics of oral quinidine sulfate and gluconate. *Am J Cardiol* 41: 770, 1978.
11. McGilveray IJ, Midha KK, Rowe M, et al: Bioavailability of 11 quinidine formulations and pharmacokinetic variation in humans. *J Pharm Sci* 70: 524, 1981.
12. Edwards DJ, Axelson JE, Slaughter RL, et al: Factors affecting quinidine protein binding in humans. *J Pharm Sci* 73: 1264, 1984.
13. Ochs HR, Greenblatt DJ, Woo E, et al: Reduced quinidine clearance in elderly persons. *Am J Cardiol* 42: 481, 1978.
14. Garfinkel D, Mamelok RD, Blaschke TF: Altered therapeutic range for quinidine after myocardial infarction and cardiac surgery. *Ann Intern Med* 107: 48, 1987.
15. Kessler KM, Lisker B, Conde C, et al: Abnormal quinidine binding in survivors of prehospital cardiac arrest. *Am Heart J* 107: 665, 1984.
16. Perez-Mateo M, Erill S: Protein binding of salicylate and quinidine in plasma from patients with renal failure, chronic liver disease and chronic respiratory insufficiency. *Eur J Clin Pharmacol* 11: 225, 1977.
17. Kessler KM, Humphries WC, Black M, et al: Quinidine pharmacokinetics in patients with cirrhosis or receiving propranolol. *Am Heart J* 96: 627, 1978.
18. Kessler KM, Leech RC, Spann JF: Blood collection techniques, heparin and quinidine protein binding. *Clin Pharmacol Ther* 25: 204, 1979.
19. Woie L, Oyri A: Quinidine intoxication treated with hemodialysis. *Acta Med Scand* 195: 237, 1974.
20. Hall K, Meatherall B, Krahn J, et al: Clearance of quinidine during peritoneal dialysis. *Am Heart J* 104: 646, 1982.
21. Notterman DA, Drayer DE, Metakis L, et al: Stereoselective renal tubular secretion of quinidine and quinine. *Clin Pharmacol Ther* 40: 511, 1986.
22. Gerhardt RE, Knouss RF, Thyrum PT, et al: Quinidine excretion in aciduria and alkaluria. *Ann Intern Med* 71: 927, 1969.
23. Drayer DE, Lowenthal DT, Restivo KM, et al: Steady-state serum levels of quinidine and active metabolites in cardiac patients with varying degrees of renal function. *Clin Pharmacol Ther* 24: 31, 1978.
24. Rakhit A, Holford NHG, Guentert TW, et al: Pharmacokinetics of quinidine and three of its metabolites in man. *J Pharmacokinet Biopharm* 12: 1, 1984.
25. Thompson KA, Murray JJ, Blair IA, et al: Plasma concentrations of quinidine, its major metabolites, and dihydroquinidine in patients with torsades de pointes. *Clin Pharmacol Ther* 43: 636, 1988.
26. Ueda CT, Dzindzio BS: Quinidine kinetics in congestive heart failure. *Clin Pharmacol Ther* 23: 158, 1978.
27. Ueda CT, Dzindzio BS: Bioavailability of quinidine in congestive heart failure. *Br J Clin Pharmacol* 11: 571, 1981.

28. Rodin SM, Johnson BJ: Pharmacokinetic interactions with digoxin. *Clin Pharmacokinet* 15: 227, 1988.
29. Hager WD, Fenster P, Mayersohn M, et al: Digoxin-quinidine interaction. Pharmacokinetic evaluation. *N Engl J Med* 300: 1238, 1979.
30. Schenck-Gustafsson K, Jogestrand T, Nordlander R, et al: Effect of quinidine on digoxin concentration in skeletal muscle and serum in patients with atrial fibrillation. Evidence for reduced binding of digoxin in muscle. *N Engl J Med* 305: 209, 1981.
31. Hedman A, Angelin B, Arvidsson A, et al: Interactions in the renal and biliary elimination of digoxin: stereoselective difference between quinine and quinidine. *Clin Pharmacol Ther* 47: 20, 1990.
32. Hughes B, Dyer JE, Schwartz AB: Increased procainamide plasma concentrations caused by quinidine: a new drug interaction. *Am Heart J* 14: 908, 1987.
33. Speirs CJ, Murray S, Boobis AR, et al: Quinidine and the identification of drugs whose elimination is impaired in subjects classified as poor metabolizers of debrisoquine. *Br J Clin Pharmacol* 22: 739, 1986.
34. Brinn R, Brosen K, Gram LF, et al: Sparteine oxidation is practically abolished in quinidine-treated patients. *Br J Clin Pharmacol* 22: 194, 1986.
35. Funck-Bretano C, Kroemer HK, Pavlou H, et al: Genetically-determined interaction between propafenone and low dose quinidine: role of active metabolites in modulating net drug effect. *Br J Clin Pharmacol* 27: 435, 1989.
36. Funck-Bretano C, Turgeon J, Woosley RL, et al: Effect of low dose quinidine on encainide pharmacokinetics and pharmacodynamics. Influence of genetic polymorphism. *J Pharmacol Exp Ther* 249: 134, 1989.
37. Munafo A, Buclin T, Steinhauslin F, et al: Disposition of flecainide in subjects taking quinidine. *Clin Pharmacol Ther* 47: 156, 1990 (abstr).
38. Schlanz KD, Yingling KW, Verme CN, et al: Metoprolol pharmacodynamics and quinidine-induced inhibition of polymorphic drug metabolism. *Pharmacotherapy* 10: 232, 1990 (abstr).
39. Hardy BG, Zador IT, Golden L, et al: Effect of cimetidine on the pharmacokinetics and pharmacodynamics of quinidine. *Am J Cardiol* 52: 172, 1983.
40. Saal AK, Werner JA, Greene HL, et al: Effect of amiodarone on serum quinidine and procainamide levels. *Am J Cardiol* 53: 1264, 1984.
41. Edwards DJ, Lavoie R, Bechman H, et al: The effect of coadministration of verapamil on the pharmacokinetics and metabolism of quinidine. *Clin Pharmacol Ther* 41: 68, 1987.
42. Maisel AS, Motulsky HJ, Insel PA: Hypotension after quinidine plus verapamil. Possible additive competition at alpha-adrenergic receptors. *N Engl J Med* 312: 167, 1985.
43. Data JL, Wilkinson GR, Nies AS: Interaction of quinidine with anticonvulsant drugs. *N Engl J Med* 294: 699, 1976.
44. Twum-Barima Y, Carruthers SG: Quinidine-rifampin interaction. *N Engl J Med* 304: 1466, 1981.
45. Munger MA, Jarvis RC, Nair R, et al: Elucidation of the nifedipine-quinidine interaction. *Clin Pharmacol Ther* 45: 411, 1989.
46. Stanton MS, Prystowsky EN, Fineberg NS, et al: Arrhythmogenic effects of antiarrhythmic drugs: a study of 506 patients treated for ventricular tachycardia. *J Am Coll Cardiol* 14: 209, 1989.
47. Koch Weser J: Pharmacokinetics of procainamide in man. *Ann NY Acad Sci* 179: 370, 1971.
48. Baker BA, Reynolds JR, Gleckel L, et al: Comparative bioavailability between two oral sustained-release procainamide products. *Clin Pharm* 7: 135, 1988.
49. Grubb BP: Recurrence of ventricular tachycardia following conversion from proprietary to generic procainamide. *Am J Cardiol* 63: 1532, 1989.
50. Manion CV, Lalka D, Baer DT, et al: Absorption kinetics of procainamide in humans. *J Pharm Sci* 66: 981, 1977.
51. Reidenberg MM, Drayer DE, Levy M, et al: Polymorphic acetylation of procainamide in man. *Clin Pharmacol Ther* 17: 723, 1975.
52. Weber WW, Hein DW: *N*-acetylation pharmacogenetics. *Pharmacol Rev* 37: 25, 1985.
53. Singh BN, Feld G, Nadamanee K: Arrhythmia control by selective lengthening of cardiac

repolarization: role of N-acetylprocainamide, active metabolite of procainamide. *Angiology* 37: 930, 1986.

54. Reidenberg MM, Camacho M, Kluger J, et al: Aging and renal clearance of procainamide and acetylprocainamide. *Clin Pharmacol Ther* 28: 732, 1980.
55. Bauer LA, Black D, Gensler A, et al: Influence of age, renal function and heart failure on procainamide clearance and N-acetylprocainamide serum concentrations. *Int J Clin Pharmacol Ther Toxicol* 27: 213, 1989.
56. Galeazzi RL, Omar-Amberg C, Karlaganis G: N-acetylprocainamide kinetics in the elderly. *Clin Pharmacol Ther* 29: 440, 1981.
57. Gibson TP, Atkinson AJ, Matusik E, et al: Kinetics of procainamide and N-acetylprocainamide in renal failure. *Kidney Int* 12: 422, 1977.
58. Lima JJ, Conti DR, Goldfarb AL, et al: Clinical pharmacokinetics of procainamide infusions in relation to acetylator phenotype. *J Pharmacokinet Biopharm* 7: 69, 1979.
59. Stec GP, Atkinson AJ, Nevin MJ, et al: N-acetylprocainamide pharmacokinetics in functionally anephric patients before and after perturbation by hemodialysis. *Clin Pharmacol Ther* 26: 618, 1979.
60. Gibson TP, Lowenthal DT, Nelson HA, et al: Elimination of procainamide in end stage renal failure. *Clin Pharmacol Ther* 17: 321, 1975.
61. Gibson TP, Matusik EJ, Briggs WA: N-acetylprocainamide levels in patients with end-stage renal failure. *Clin Pharmacol Ther* 19: 206, 1976.
62. Du Souich P, Erill S: Metabolism of procainamide and p-aminobenzoic acid in patients with chronic liver disease. *Clin Pharmacol Ther* 22: 588, 1977.
63. Christoff PB, Conti DR, Naylor C, et al: Procainamide disposition in obesity. *Drug Intell Clin Pharm* 17: 516, 1983.
64. Christian CD, Meredith CG, Speeg KV: Cimetidine inhibits renal procainamide clearance. *Clin Pharmacol Ther* 36: 221, 1984.
65. Somogyi A, Bochner F: Dose and concentration dependent effect of ranitidine on procainamide disposition and renal clearance in man. *Br J Clin Pharmacol* 18: 175, 1984.
66. Kosoglou T, Rocci ML, Vlasses PH: Trimethoprim alters the disposition of procainamide and N-acetylprocainamide. *Clin Pharmacol Ther* 44: 467, 1988.
67. Olsen H, Morland J: Ethanol-induced increase in procainamide acetylation in man. *Br J Clin Pharmacol* 13: 203, 1982.
68. Hinderling PH, Bries J, Garrett ER: Protein binding and erythrocyte partitioning of disopyramide and its monodealkylated metabolite. *J Pharm Sci* 63: 1684, 1974.
69. Lima JJ, Haughey DB, Leier CV: Disopyramide pharmacokinetics and bioavailability following the simultaneous administration of disopyramide and ^{14}C-disopyramide. *J Pharmacokinet Biopharm* 12: 289, 1984.
70. Cunningham JL, Shen DD, Shudo I, et al: The effect of non-linear disposition kinetics on the systemic availability of disopyramide. *Br J Clin Pharmacol* 5: 343, 1978.
71. Haughey DB, Lima JJ: Influence of concentration-dependent protein binding on serum concentrations and urinary excretion of disopyramide and its metabolite following oral administration. *Biopharm Drug Dispos* 4: 103, 1983.
72. Karin A, Schubert EN, Burns TS, et al: Disopyramide plasma concentrations following single and multiple doses of the immediate- and controlled-release capsules. *Angiology* 34: 375, 1983.
73. Giacomini KM, Swezey SE, Turner-Tamiyasu K, et al: The effect of saturable binding to plasma proteins on the pharmacokinetic properties of disopyramide. *J Pharmacokinet Biopharm* 10: 1, 1982.
74. Aitio M-L: Plasma concentrations and protein binding of disopyramide and mono-N-dealkyldisopyramide during chronic oral disopyramide therapy. *Br J Clin Pharmacol* 11: 369, 1981.
75. Roberto P, Vitaliano B, Donatella P, et al: Disopyramide pharmacokinetics in the elderly after single oral administration. *Pharmacol Res Commun* 20: 1025, 1988.

76. Bonde J, Pedersen LE, Bodtker S, et al: The influence of age and smoking on the elimination of disopyramide. *Br J Clin Pharmacol* 20: 453, 1985.
77. Shen DD, Cunningham JL, Shudo I, et al: Disposition kinetics of disopyramide in patients with renal insufficiency. *Biopharm Drug Dispos* 1: 133, 1980.
78. Braun J, Sorgel F, Gluth WP, et al: Does alpha$_1$-acid glycoprotein reduce the unbound metabolic clearance of disopyramide in patients with renal impairment? *Eur J Clin Pharmacol* 35: 313, 1987.
79. Sevka MJ, Matthews SJ, Nightingale CH, et al: Disopyramide hemodialysis and kinetics in patients requiring long-term hemodialysis. *Clin Pharmacol Ther* 29: 322, 1981.
80. Bonde J, Graudal NA, Pedersen LE, et al: Kinetics of disopyramide in decreased hepatic function. *Eur J Clin Pharmacol* 31: 73, 1986.
81. Aitio M-L, Vuorenmaa T: Enhanced metabolism and diminished efficacy of disopyramide by enzyme induction? *Br J Clin Pharmacol* 9: 149, 1980.
82. Nightingale J, Nappi JM: Effect of phenytoin on serum disopyramide concentrations. *Clin Pharm* 6: 46, 1987.
83. Aitio M-L, Mansury L, Tala E, et al: The effect of enzyme induction on the metabolism of disopyramide. *Br J Clin Pharmacol* 11: 279, 1981.
84. Kapil RP, Axelson JE, Mansfield, IL, et al: Disopyramide pharmacokinetics and metabolism: effect of inducers. *Br J Clin Pharmacol* 24: 781, 1987.
85. Lima JJ, Wenzke SC, Boudoulas H: Antiarrhythmic activity and unbound concentrations of disopyramide enantiomers in patients. *Ther Drug Monitor* 12: 23, 1990.
86. Giacomini KM, Cox BM, Blaschke TF: Comparative anticholinergic potencies of R and S disopyramide in longitudinal muscle strips from guinea pig ileum. *Life Sci* 27: 1191, 1980.
87. Pollick C, Giacomini KM, Blaschke TF, et al: The cardiac effects of d-and l-disopyramide in normal subjects: a noninvasive study. *Circulation* 66: 447, 1982.
88. Huet M, LeLorier J, Pomier G, et al: Bioavailability of lidocaine in normal volunteers and cirrhotic patients. *Clin Pharmacol Ther* 25: 229, 1979 (abstr).
89. Rowland M, Thomson PD, Guichard A, et al: Disposition kinetics of lidocaine in normal subjects. *Ann NY Acad Sci* 179: 383, 1971.
90. Benowitz NL, Meister W: Clinical pharmacokinetics of lignocaine. *Clin Pharmacokinet* 3: 177, 1978.
91. Abernethy DR, Greenblatt DJ: Impairment of lidocaine clearance in elderly male subjects. *J Cardiovasc Pharmacol* 5: 1093, 1983.
92. Routledge PA, Barchausky A, Bjornsson TD, et al: Lidocaine plasma protein binding. *Clin Pharmacol Ther* 27: 347, 1980.
93. Thomson PD, Melmon KL, Richardson JA, et al: Lidocaine pharmacokinetics in advanced heart failure, liver disease and renal failure in humans. *Ann Intern Med* 78: 499, 1973.
94. Keenaghan JB, Boyes RN: The tissue distribution, metabolism and excretion of lidocaine in rats, guinea pigs, dogs and man. *J Pharmacol Exp Ther* 180: 454, 1972.
95. Bennett PN, Aarons LJ, Bending MR, et al: Pharmacokinetics of lidocaine and its deethylated metabolite: dose and time dependency studies in man. *J Pharmacokinet Biopharm* 10: 265, 1982.
96. Thomson AH, Elliott HL, Kelman AW, et al: The pharmacokinetics and pharmacodynamics for lignocaine and MEGX in healthy subjects. *J Pharmacokinet Biopharm* 15: 101, 1987.
97. Davison R, Parker M, Atkinson AJ: Excessive serum lidocaine levels during maintenance infusions: mechanisms and prevention. *Am Heart* J 104: 203, 1982.
98. Collinsworth KA, Strong JM, Atkinson AJ, et al: Pharmacokinetics and metabolism of lidocaine in patients with renal failure. *Clin Pharmacol Ther* 18: 59, 1975.
99. Strong JM, Mayfield DE, Atkinson AJ, et al: Pharmacological activity, metabolism, and pharmacokinetics of glycinexylidide. *Clin Pharmacol Ther* 17: 184, 1975.
100. Suzuki T, Fujita S, Kawai R: Precursor-metabolite interaction in the metabolism of lidocaine. *J Pharm Sci* 73: 136, 1984.
101. Abernethy DR, Greenblatt DJ: Lidocaine disposition in obesity. *Am J Cardiol* 53: 1183, 1984.

102. Baciewicz AM, Baciewicz FA: Effect of cimetidine and ranitidine on cardiovascular drugs. *Am Heart J* 118: 114, 1989.
103. Ochs HR, Carstens G, Greenblatt DJ: Reduction in lidocaine clearance during continuous infusion and by coadministration of propranolol. *N Engl J Med* 303: 373, 1980.
104. Bax NDS, Tucker GT, Lennard MS, et al: The impairment of lignocaine clearance by propranolol—major contribution from enzyme inhibition. *Br J Clin Pharmacol* 19: 597, 1985.
105. Miners JO, Wing LMH, Lillywhite KJ, et al: Failure of "therapeutic" doses of B-adrenoreceptor antagonists to alter the disposition of tolbutamide and lignocaine. *Br J Clin Pharmacol* 18: 853, 1984.
106. Svendsen TL, Tango M, Waldorff S, et al: Effects of propranolol and pindolol on plasma lignocaine clearance in man. *Br J Clin Pharmacol* 13: 223S, 1982.
107. Pieper JA, Wyamn MG, Goldreyer BN, et al: Lidocaine toxicity: effects of total versus free lidocaine concentration. *Circulation* 62(suppl III): 181, 1980 (abstr).
108. Lalka D, Meyer MB, Duce BR, et al: Kinetics of the oral antiarrhythmic lidocaine congener, tocainide. *Clin Pharmacol Ther* 19: 757, 1976.
109. Graffner C, Conradson T-B, Hofvendahl S, et al: Tocainide kinetics after intravenous and oral administration in healthy subjects and in patients with acute myocardial infarction. *Clin Pharmacol Ther* 27: 64, 1980.
110. Elvin AT, Keenaghan JB, Byrnes EW, et al: Tocainide conjugation in humans: novel biotransformation pathway for a primary amine. *J Pharm Sci* 69: 47, 1980.
111. Wiegers U, Hanrath P, Kuck KH, et al: Pharmacokinetics of tocainide in patients with renal dysfunction and during hemodialysis. *Eur J Clin Pharmacol* 24: 503, 1983.
112. Oltmanns D, Pottage D, Endell W: Pharmacokinetics of tocainide in patients with combined hepatic and renal dysfunction. *Eur J Clin Pharmacol* 25: 787, 1983.
113. Mohiuddin SM, Esterbrooks D, Hilleman DE, et al: Tocainide kinetics in congestive heart failure. *Clin Pharmacol Ther* 34: 596, 1983.
114. MacMahon B, Bakshi M, Branagan P, et al: Pharmacokinetics and hemodynamic effects of tocainide in patients with acute myocardial infarction complicated by left ventricular failure. *Br J Clin Pharmacol* 19: 429, 1985.
115. Rice TL, Patterson JH, Celestin C, et al: Influence of rifampin on tocainide pharmacokinetics in humans. *Clin Pharm* 8: 200, 1989.
116. Sheldon RS, Cannon NJ, Nies AS, et al: Sterospecific interaction of tocainide with cardiac sodium channel. *Mol Pharmacol* 33: 327, 1988.
117. Edgar B, Heggelund A, Johansson L, et al: The pharmacokinetics of R- and S-tocainide in healthy subjects. *Br J Clin Pharmacol* 17: 216P, 1984.
118. Campbell NPS, Kelly JG, Adgey AAJ, et al: Mexiletine in normal volunteers. *Br J Clin Pharmacol* 6: 372, 1978.
119. Grech-Belanger O, Barbeau G, Kishka P, et al: Pharmacokinetics of mexiletine in the elderly. *J Clin Pharmacol* 29: 311, 1989.
120. Haselbarth V, Doevendans JE, Wolf M: Kinetics and bioavailability of mexiletine in healthy subjects. *Clin Pharmacol Ther* 29: 729, 1981.
121. Pentikainen PJ, Halinen MO, Helin MJ: Pharmacokinetics of intravenous mexiletine in patients with acute myocardial infarction. *J Cardiovasc Pharmacol* 6: 1, 1984.
122. Beckett AH, Chidomer EC: The distribution, metabolism and excretion of mexiletine in man. *Postgrad Med J* 53(suppl 1): 60, 1977.
123. Latini R, Maggioni AP, Cavalli A: Therapeutic drug monitoring of antiarrhythmic drugs. Rationale and current status. *Clin Pharmacokinet* 18: 91, 1990.
124. Nitsch J, Steinbeck G, Luderitz B: Increase in mexiletine plasma levels due to delayed hepatic metabolism in patients with chronic liver disease. *Eur Heart J* 4: 810, 1983.
125. Leahy EB, Giardina EGV, Bigger JT: Effect of ventricular failure on steady state kinetics of mexiletine (abstr). *Clin Res* 28: 239A, 1980.
126. El Allaf D, Henrard L, Crochelet L, et al: Pharmacokinetics of mexiletine in renal insufficiency. *Br J Clin Pharmacol* 14: 431, 1982.

127. Wang T, Wuellner D, Woosley RL, et al: Pharmacokinetics and nondialyzability of mexiletine in renal failure. *Clin Pharmacol Ther* 37: 649, 1985.
128. Wing LMH, Meffin PJ, Grygiel JJ, et al: The effect of metoclopramide and atropine on the absorption of orally administered mexiletine. *Br J Clin Pharmacol* 9: 505, 1980.
129. Herzog P, Holtermuller KH, Kasper W, et al: Absorption of mexiletine after treatment with gastric antacids. *Br J Clin Pharmacol* 14: 746, 1982.
130. Pentikainen PJ, Koivula IH, Hiltunen HA: Effect of rifampicin treatment on the kinetics of mexiletine. *Eur J Clin Pharmacol* 23: 261, 1982.
131. Begg EJ, Chinwah PM, Webb C, et al: Enhanced metabolism of mexiletine after phenytoin administration. *Br J Clin Pharmacol* 14: 219, 1982.
132. Grech-Belanger O, Gilbert M, Turgeon J, et al: Effect of cigarette smoking on mexiletine kinetics. *Clin Pharmacol Ther* 37: 638, 1985.
133. Loi CM, Vestal RE: Effect of mexiletine on theophylline metabolism. *Clin Pharmacol Ther* 47: 130, 1990 (abstr).
134. Hill RJ, Duff HJ, Sheldon RS: Determinants of stereospecific binding of type I antiarrhythmic drugs to cardiac sodium channels. *Mol Pharmacol* 34: 659, 1988.
135. Fenster PE, Kern KB: Mexiletine in refractory ventricular arrhythmias. *Clin Pharmacol Ther* 34: 777, 1983.
136. Campbell NPS, Kelly JG, Shanks RG, et al: Mexiletine in the management of ventricular dysrhythmias. *Lancet* 2: 404, 1973.
137. Howrie DL, Pieniaszek HJ, Fogoros RN, et al: Disposition of moricizine (ethmozine) in healthy subjects after oral administration of radiolabelled drug. *Eur J Clin Pharmacol* 32: 607, 1987.
138. Woosley RL, Morganroth J, Fogoros RN, et al: Pharmacokinetics of moricizine HCl. *Am J Cardiol* 60: 35F, 1987.
139. Biollaz J, Shaheen O, Wood AJJ: Cimetidine inhibition of ethmozine metabolism. *Clin Pharmacol Ther* 37: 665, 1985.
140. McQuinn RL, Quarfoth GJ, Johnson JD, et al: Biotransformation elimination of 14C-flecainide acetate in humans. *Drug Metab Dispos* 12: 414, 1984.
141. Conard GJ, Ober RE: Metabolism of flecainide. *Am J Cardiol* 53: 41B, 1984.
142. Guehler J, Gornick CC, Tobler G, et al: Electrophysiologic effects of flecainide acetate and its major metabolites in the canine heart. *Am J Cardiol* 55: 807, 1985.
143. Roden DM, Woosley RL: Drug therapy: flecainide. *N Engl J Med* 315: 36, 1986.
144. Franciosa JA, Wilen M, Weeks CE, et al: Pharmacokinetics and hemodynamic effects of flecainide in patients with chronic low output heart failure. *J Am Coll Cardiol* 1: 699, 1983.
145. Weeks CE, Conard GJ, Kvam DC, et al: The effect of flecainide acetate, a new antiarrhythmic, on plasma digoxin levels. *J Clin Pharmacol* 26: 27, 1986.
146. Lewis GP, Holtzman JL: Interaction of flecainide with digoxin and propranolol. *Am J Cardiol* 53: 52B, 1984.
147. Tjandra Maga TB, Verbesselt R, Van Hecken A, et al: Oral flecainide elimination kinetics: effects of cimetidine. *Circulation* 68: III-416, 1983.
148. Shea P, Lai R, Kim SS, et al: Flecainide and amiodarone interaction. *J Am Coll Cardiol* 7: 1127, 1986.
149. Morganroth J, Anderson J, Gentzkow GD: Classification by type of ventricular arrhythmia predicts frequency of adverse cardiac events from flecainide. *J Am Coll Cardiol* 8: 607, 1986.
150. Fontaine G, Frank R, Tonet JL: Association amiodarone-flecainide dans le traitement des troubles du rythme ventriculaires graves. *Arch Mal Coeur* 76: 1218, 1983.
151. Frabetti L, Marchesini B, Capucci A, et al: Antiarrhythmic efficacy of propafenone: evaluation of effective plasma levels following single and multiple doses. *Eur J Clin Pharmacol* 30: 685, 1986.
152. Product information: Rythmol (propafenone hydrochloride), in *Physician's Desk Reference*. Montvale, NJ, Medical Economic Co. 1991, p. 1153.
153. Siddoway LA, Thompson KA, McAllister CB, et al: Polymorphism of propafenone metabolism in man: clinical and pharmacokinetic consequences. *Circulation* 75: 785, 1987.

154. Lee PJT, Yee Y, Dorian P, et al: Influence of hepatic dysfunction on the pharmacokinetics of propafenone. *Clin Pharmacol Ther* 27: 4, 1987.
155. Burgess E, Duff H, Wilkes P: Propafenone disposition in renal insufficiency and renal failure. *J Clin Pharmacol* 29: 2, 1989.
156. Nolan PE, Marcus FI, Erstad BL, et al: Effects of coadministration of propafenone on the pharmacokinetics of digoxin in healthy volunteer subjects. *J Clin Pharmacol* 29: 6, 1989.
157. Singh BH, Venkatesh N, Nademanee K, et al: The historical development, cellular electrophysiology and pharmacology of amiodarone. *Prog Cardiovasc Dis* 31: 249, 1989.
158. Holt DW, Tucker GT, Jackson PR, et al: Amiodarone pharmacokinetics. *Am Heart J* 106: 840, 1983.
159. Herre JM, Sauve MJ, Malone P, et al: Long-term results of amiodarone therapy in patients with recurrent sustained ventricular tachycardia or ventricular fibrillation. *J Am Coll Cardiol* 13: 442, 1989.
160. Harris L, Hind CRK, McKenna WJ: Renal elimination of amiodarone and its desethyl metabolite. *Postgrad Med J* 59: 440, 1983.
161. Rotmensch HH, Belhassen B, Swanson BN, et al: Steady-state serum amiodarone concentrations: relationships with antiarrhythmic efficacy and toxicity. *Ann Intern Med* 101: 462, 1984.
162. Torres V, Tepper D, Flowers D, et al: QT prolongation and the antiarrhythmic efficacy of amiodarone. *J Am Coll Cardiol* 7: 142, 1986.
163. Pollack PT, Sharma AD, Carruthers SG: Correlation of amiodarone dosage, heart rate, QT interval and corneal microdeposits with serum amiodarone and desethylamiodarone concentrations. *Am J Cardiol* 64: 1138, 1989.
164. Kerin NZ, Blevins RD, Benaderet D, et al: Relation of serum reverse T3 to amiodarone antiarrhythmic efficacy and toxicity. *Am J Cardiol* 57: 128, 1986.
165. Lesko LJ: Pharmacokinetic drug interactions with amiodarone. *Clin Pharmacokinet* 16: 130, 1989.
166. Nolan PE, Marcus FI, Karol MD, et al: Effect of phenytoin on the clinical pharmacokinetics of amiodarone. *J Clin Pharmacol* 30: 1112, 1990.
167. Vrobel TR, Miller PE, Mostow ND, et al: A general overview of amiodarone toxicity: its prevention, detection, and management. *Prog Cardiovasc Dis* 31: 393, 1989.
168. Boura ALA, Green AF: The actions of bretylium: Adrenergic neuron blocking and other effects. *Br J Pharmacol* 14: 536, 1959.
169. Garrett ER, Green JR Jr, Bialer M: Bretylium pharmacokinetics and bioavailabilities in man with various doses and modes of administration. *Biopharm Drug Disposition* 3: 129, 1982.
170. Narange PK, Adir J, Josselson J, et al: Pharmacokinetics of bretylium in renal insufficiency. *N Engl J Med* 300: 1390, 1974.
171. Standards and guidelines for cardiopulmonary resuscitation (CPR) and emergency cardiac care (ECC). *JAMA* 255: 2843, 1986.
172. Reele S, Woosley RL, Oates JA: Pharmacologic reversal of the hypotensive effect that complicates therapy with bretylium. *Circulation* 1158: 962, 1978.
173. Product Information, Lyphomed, Rosemont, 1989.
174. Conradson TBG, Dixon CMS, Clarke B, et al: Cardiovascular effects of infused adenosine in man: potentiation by dipyridamole. *Acta Physiol Scand* 129: 387, 1987.
175. Moser GH, Schrader J: Half-life of adenosine in human blood. Effects of dipyridamole. *Pflugers Arch* 407: S37, 1986.
176. Evoniuk G, Von Borstel RW, Wurtman RJ: Antagonism of the cardiovascular effects of adenosine by caffeine or 8-(p-sulfophenyl) theophylline. *J Pharmacol Exp Ther* 240: 428, 1987.
177. Garratt CJ, Antoniou A, Griffin MJ, et al: Use of intravenous adenosine in sinus rhythm as a diagnostic test for latent preexcitation. *Am J Cardiol* 65: 868, 1990.
178. Belhassen B, Pelleg A, Shoshani D, et al: Atrial fibrillation induced by adenosine triphosphate. *Am J Cardiol* 53: 1405, 1984.
179. DiMarco JP, Sellers TD, Lerman BB, et al: Diagnostic and therapeutic use of adenosine in patients with supraventricular tachyarrhythmias. *J Am Coll Cardiol* 6: 417, 1985.
180. Saito D, Ueeda M, Abe Y, et al: Treatment of paroxysmal supraventricular tachycardia with intravenous adenosine. *Br Heart J* 55: 291, 1986.

CHAPTER

7

DIGOXIN

Paul E. Nolan, Jr.
Arshag D. Mooradian

Digitalis glycosides have been used in clinical medicine for over 200 years.[1] Despite current disagreement regarding the therapeutic benefit of these compounds, digitalis remains a commonly prescribed medication particularly in the elderly.[2] The intent of this chapter is to review the mechanism of action of digitalis, the alterations in the pharmacokinetics of digoxin which occur with advanced age, and the pharmacokinetic and pharmacodynamic interactions of other drugs with digoxin and to discuss the controversial role of digoxin in contemporary clinical practice. In addition, this review will include a brief discussion of newer inotropic agents.

MECHANISMS OF ACTION OF DIGITALIS GLYCOSIDES

Digitalis binds to and inhibits magnesium- and adenosine triphosphate (ATP)-dependent sodium- and potassium-activated adenosine triphosphatase (NaK-ATPase).[1] Consequently sodium accumulates intracellularly and is subsequently exchanged for extracellular calcium. The influx of calcium then triggers the release of calcium stored by the sarcoplasmic reticulum. This released calcium binds to troponin C and permits an interaction between actin and myosin and thus the generation of mechanical force. Digitalis may also increase intracellular entry of calcium via the slow calcium channels. In addition, digitalis stimulates the release and blocks reuptake of norepinephrine. These combined events result in the establishment of a positive inotropic action for digitalis.

The aged left atrial and ventricular myocardium may be more responsive to the inotropic actions of digitalis than the cardiac muscle of young adults.[3] Clinically this is evidenced by an increase in the ejection fraction of elderly patients (mean age: 84 years; range: 74 to 90) with congestive heart failure (CHF) at relatively low serum digoxin concentrations ranging from 0.4 to 1.0 ng/mL.[4]

Digitalis also demonstrates therapeutically important electrophysiologic actions.[1] An increase in vagal tone is the predominant effect of digitalis at subtoxic doses. This produces both a slowing in conduction and an increased refractoriness in the atrioventricular (AV) node and junctional tissues and ultimately a decrease in the ventricular rate. Direct effects of digitalis may also play a role in mediating these electrophysiologic actions. Following single intravenous bolus doses of digoxin to patients with ischemic heart disease, the effect on AV conduction precedes the appearance of its positive inotropic effects.[5]

PHARMACOKINETICS OF DIGOXIN IN THE ELDERLY

Absorption

The absolute bioavailability of digoxin tablets in elderly patients (76 percent) is similar to younger patients (84 percent) (Table 7-1).[6] Interpatient variability in the elderly (bioavailability range: 51 to 111 percent) is also not significantly different from younger patients (range: 60 to 110 percent). However, the rate of digoxin absorption is slower in the elderly, thereby prolonging attainment of peak plasma digoxin concentrations.

Administration of the encapsulated solution of digoxin to cardiac patients enhances the absolute bioavailability.[7] However, the use of the digoxin capsule in patients does not significantly diminish the interpatient variability in absorption.[8]

Table 7-1 Summary of the pharmacokinetics of digoxin in the elderly

Pharmacokinetic parameter	Value in elderly
Absolute bioavailability	76%[a] (range 51–111%)
Volume of distribution (Vβ)	194 L[a] (range 129-314 L)
Volume of distribution (Vβ) corrected for weight	4.1 L/kg (range 2.2-9.0 L/kg)
Protein binding	Not determined but would not be anticipated to vary much from 25 ± 4.5%[b] reported in young, normal subjects
Elimination half-life	69 h[a] (range 31–132 h)
Total body clearance	0.8 mL/min/kg[a] (range 0.4–1.5 mL/min/kg)

[a] Data obtained from Ref. 6.
[b] Data obtained from Ref. 14.

Distribution

The volume of distribution of digoxin in the elderly (mean: 194 L; range: 129 to 314 L) is significantly diminished relative to younger patients (mean: 339 L; range: 246 to 485 L).[6] When the volume of distribution is corrected for body weight, there is a trend toward a difference between elderly (4.1 ± 0.9 L/kg) and young individuals (5.3 ± 0.6 L/kg). As skeletal muscle serves as a major reservoir for digoxin,[9] the reduction in the volume of distribution may reflect a decrease in muscle mass frequently observed in elderly individuals.[10] In addition, renal failure diminishes the volume of distribution of digoxin.[11] Therefore, age-related reductions in renal function[12] may also contribute to the decrease in the volume of distribution of digoxin in the elderly.

In plasma, digoxin binds to albumin.[13] The plasma protein binding of digoxin in normal subjects is 25 ± 4.5 percent.[14] Although the protein binding of digoxin has not been determined in the elderly, clinically important differences from younger individuals would not be anticipated due to the relatively small amount of digoxin which binds to circulating albumin.

Elimination

The half-life of digoxin in elderly patients averages 69 h and ranges from 31 to 132 h.[6] Corresponding values in younger patients are 38 h and 30 to 51 h, respectively. As digoxin is principally eliminated by the kidneys via both glomerular filtration and renal tubular secretion,[15] the prolongation in half-life in the elderly with a normal serum creatinine most likely reflects age-associated reductions in the renal filtration and secretion of digoxin.[16]

Total body clearance of digoxin is also decreased in the elderly.[6] The mean total body clearance in elderly patients (0.8 mL/min/kg) is approximately 50 percent of that in younger patients (1.7 mL/min/kg). Therefore, on average, the daily dose of digoxin in the elderly should be 50 percent of that in younger patients in order to achieve similar serum digoxin concentrations.

Effects of Concurrent Disease States on Digoxin Pharmacokinetics

Several disease states which are often seen in the elderly can modify the pharmacokinetics of digoxin. Both hyper- and hypothyroidism have been shown to alter the distribution and elimination of digoxin.[17] Relative to the euthyroid state, patients with hyperthyroidism had an increased renal clearance and reduced volume of distribution of digoxin. Contrariwise, patients with hypothyroidism demonstrated a diminished renal clearance and expanded volume of distribution of digoxin. The half-life of digoxin among euthyroid, hyperthyroid, and hypothyroid patients was similar, however. Based on these findings, doses of digoxin on average may have to be increased at least 75 percent for patients with hyperthyroidism and decreased as much as 40 percent for individuals with hypothyroidism. However, other investigators did not describe any consistent abnormality in either the renal or nonrenal clearance of digoxin in patients with either hyper- or hypothyroidism.[18] Therefore, monitoring of serum digoxin concentrations is advisable when designing dosage regimens for patients with either hyper- or hypothyroidism.

Renal dysfunction decreases the elimination of digoxin.[11] Both glomerular filtration and renal tubular secretion deteriorate as a consequence of aging.[12] Creatinine clearance is positively correlated with total body clearance of digoxin.[14] Therefore, to estimate dosage requirements for digoxin in the elderly, creatinine clearance can be estimated by the method of Cockcroft and Gault[19]:

$$CL_{cr} = \frac{(140 - \text{age})\ \text{wt}}{72 \times P_{cr}}$$

where CL_{cr} is the calculated creatinine clearance in milliliters per minute; age is in years; wt is the actual body weight in kilograms; and P_{cr} is the patient's actual serum creatinine. If the patient is female, the above equation must be multiplied by 0.85. Total body clearance of digoxin (CL_t) can then be approximated by multiplying CL_{cr} by 1.303 (i.e., the renal clearance of digoxin) and then adding 20 mL/min (i.e., the nonrenal clearance of digoxin)[14,20]: $CL_t = (1.303 \times CL_{cr}) + 20$ mL/min.

The maintenance dose of digoxin can be calculated after deciding the target steady-state serum concentration of digoxin as follows:

$$C_{ss} = \frac{F \times \text{dose}}{CL_t \times \tau}$$

where C_{ss} is the targeted steady-state concentration of digoxin in nanograms per milliliter (i.e., 1.0 to 1.5 ng/mL); F is the bioavailability of the prescribed dosage form of digoxin (i.e., 0.75 for digoxin tablets and 1.0 for digoxin capsules); dose is the total daily dose in nanograms; CL_t is the total body clearance of digoxin in milliliters per minute; and τ is the dosing interval of digoxin expressed in minutes (i.e., 1440 min = 1 day).

Exercise may induce a reduction in serum digoxin concentrations in the elderly.[21] Exercise increases the uptake of digoxin into skeletal muscle, thereby decreasing serum concentrations. Therefore, knowledge of a patient's physical activity is potentially important when interpreting serum digoxin levels.

DIGOXIN TOXICITY IN THE ELDERLY

The elderly remain at risk for digoxin toxicity. A recent retrospective analysis of 219 patients discharged with the presumptive diagnosis of digoxin intoxication indicates that the mean age of these patients was 75 ± 11 years.[22] Of the 43 patients with definite intoxication, 42 (98 percent) had serum digoxin concentrations in excess of 2 ng/mL. Gastrointestinal adverse effects were the most prominent noncardiac adverse effects. Atrioventricular nodal and sinus nodal conduction or rhythm disturbances were the predominant cardiac side effects.

Interestingly, the incidence of digoxin intoxication may be declining. This is evidenced by another component of the recent retrospective analysis.[22] Only 4 of 563 inpatients (0.7 percent) prescribed digoxin for heart failure could be classified as definitely intoxicated. The diagnosis could not be excluded in another 16 (3 percent) patients. One possible explanation for this reduced toxicity is the frequency at which serum digoxin concentrations of less than 1.0 ng/mL are observed in the elderly.[23]

Some elderly patients may present with neuropsychiatric symptoms of digoxin intoxication. These symptoms can manifest at digoxin serum concentrations either within or exceeding the conventional therapeutic range.[24] Digoxin is distributed into the choroid plexus[25,26] and cerebrospinal fluid.[27] Perhaps brain tissue, which contains large amounts of NaK-ATPase,[25] becomes more sensitive to the effects of digitalis with advanced age in accordance with cardiac tissue.[3]

DRUG INTERACTIONS WITH DIGOXIN

Elderly patients taking digoxin are frequently receiving additional medications.[28] Several of these other drugs may potentially interact with digoxin, causing clinically significant changes in the pharmacokinetics and/or pharmacodynamics of digoxin (Table 7-2).

The absorption of digoxin may be altered by a number of other drugs.[29] Most of these agents decrease digoxin absorption and include antacids, kaolin-pectin, the bile sequestrants cholestyramine and colestipol, dietary bran fiber, activated charcoal, some chemotherapeutic regimens, and sulfasalazine, neomycin, and aminosalicylic acid. Either avoiding concurrent administration of most of these other drugs or prescribing digoxin capsules may minimize the reduction in absorption. On the other hand, erythromycin and tetracycline may increase the bioavailability of digoxin. Erythromycin and tetracycline modify the enteric flora which facilitate the metabolism of digoxin to inactive reduction products in 10 to 15 percent of patients taking digoxin. Substitution of digoxin capsules for tablets can minimize the risk of enhanced bioavailability by these antibiotics in this subgroup of patients.

Several drugs, including selected antiarrhythmics, calcium channel blocking agents, and diuretics, significantly change the disposition of digoxin.[29] Quinidine decreases total body clearance, renal and nonrenal clearance, and the volume of distribution of digoxin. These effects result in a two- to threefold increase in digoxin serum concentrations. Elderly patients may demonstrate a higher incidence of digoxin-related adverse effects during combined treatment with digoxin and quinidine. Therefore, in general, doses of digoxin should be halved when quinidine therapy is initiated.

Amiodarone decreases the total body clearance of digoxin by diminishing both

Table 7-2 Drug interactions with digoxin

Drugs	Interaction	Recommendation
Antiarrhythmic agents		
Quinidine	Decreases total body clearance, renal clearance, nonrenal clearance, and volume of distribution of digoxin	Lower loading and maintenance doses of digoxin by 50% and monitor serum digoxin concentration
Amiodarone	Decreases total body clearance, renal clearance, and nonrenal clearance of digoxin	Lower maintenance dose of digoxin by 50% and monitor serum digoxin concentration
Propafenone	Decreases total body clearance, nonrenal clearance, and volume of distribution of digoxin	Lower loading and maintenance doses of digoxin by 25% and monitor serum digoxin concentration
Calcium channel blocking drugs		
Verapamil	Decreases total body clearance of digoxin	Lower maintenance dose of digoxin by 25% and monitor serum digoxin concentration
Diltiazem, nifedipine	May decrease elimination of digoxin	Monitor serum digoxin concentration
Miscellaneous agents		
Antacids, kaolin-pectin, colestipol, cholestyramine	Decrease absorption of digoxin	Administer digoxin at least 1-2 h before these agents and monitor serum digoxin concentration
Neomycin, cancer chemotherapy, sulfasalazine, aminosalicylic acid	Decrease absorption of digoxin	Monitor serum digoxin concentration
Erythromycin, tetracycline	May increase absorption of digoxin in 10-15% of patients	Monitor serum digoxin concentration; may substitute digoxin capsule formulation for this patient subgroup
Indomethicin, ibuprofen, diclofenac	May decrease elimination of digoxin	Monitor serum digoxin concentration
Rifampin	May increase elimination of digoxin	Monitor serum digoxin concentration; may need to increase dose of digoxin

renal and nonrenal clearance.[29] Amiodarone may also enhance the bioavailability of digoxin. Digoxin toxicity as evidenced by bradycardia or delays in AV nodal conduction may occur with concurrent use of digoxin and amiodarone. Digoxin doses should be decreased by 50 percent when amiodarone is coadministered.

Propafenone reduces the total body clearance of digoxin probably by decreasing the nonrenal clearance and volume of distribution of digoxin.[30] In patients coadministered digoxin and propafenone, a decrease in heart rate frequently accompanies the increase in serum digoxin concentrations.[31] Prior to initiation of propafenone, the dose of digoxin can be decreased by 25 percent.

Of the currently available calcium channel blocking drugs, verapamil most consistently elevates serum digoxin concentrations.[29] Total body clearance of digoxin decreases 20 to 30 percent following administration of verapamil, and therefore, doses of digoxin can be decreased an average of 25 percent during concomitant verapamil therapy. Conflicting information exists regarding the effects of diltiazem and nifedipine on the pharmacokinetics of digoxin.[29] Monitoring of serum digoxin concentrations should be used to guide digoxin dosing during concurrent treatment with these two agents. Isradipine, nicardipine, and nitrendipine appear unlikely to produce clinically important changes in the pharmacokinetics of digoxin.[29]

Spironolactone may increase serum digoxin concentrations by decreasing renal and perhaps nonrenal clearance of digoxin by as much as 25 percent.[29] However, the risk of digoxin toxicity may not be enhanced by spironolactone. Spironolactone and its metabolites may also falsely elevate serum digoxin concentrations because of cross-reactivity with digoxin-binding antibodies in some commercial radioimmunoassay kits.

Other miscellaneous pharmacokinetic drug interactions with digoxin include reported increases in serum digoxin concentrations with coadministration of the nonsteroidal anti-inflammatory agents indomethacin, ibuprofen, and diclofenac.[29] Contrariwise, concurrent treatment with rifampin induces hepatic metabolism of digoxin and may decrease serum digoxin concentrations by approximately 50 percent in patients with chronic renal failure.[32] This finding suggests that nonrenal elimination of digoxin is relatively significant in this patient subgroup.

MONITORING SERUM DIGOXIN CONCENTRATIONS

Digoxin fulfills several criteria which support the monitoring of serum digoxin concentrations[33]: (1) digoxin possesses a low toxic-to-therapeutic ratio; (2) there is a poor correlation between the dose of digoxin and serum digoxin concentrations; and (3) there is difficulty in distinguishing between signs and symptoms of digoxin toxicity and those of the disease being treated.

When monitoring serum digoxin concentrations, blood samples should be obtained at or near attainment of pharmacokinetic steady state. For an elderly patient with a normal serum creatinine, the average time to pharmacokinetic steady state is approximately 15 days (range: 5 to 25 days) based upon the findings of Cusack and coworkers.[6] Blood samples should be acquired no sooner than 6 h following the previous dose because of the long distribution time of the drug.[33] However, it may be more pragmatic to delay sampling until just prior to the next scheduled dose. Possible indications for measuring serum digoxin concentrations include (1) establishing an initial relationship between the maintenance dose of digoxin and the corresponding serum level; (2) following the addition of a drug known or suspected to pharmacokinetically interact with digoxin; (3) during a change in a physiologic parameter known or suspected to alter the pharmacokinetics of digoxin, such as renal function; (4) following a substitution in the dosage form of digoxin; (5) to assist in the diagnosis of digoxin toxicity; (6) to evaluate either a poor response to initial therapy or a decline in response following early therapeutic success; and (7) to assess patient compliance. In addition, routine assessment of serum digoxin concentrations in elderly patients may be useful because the elderly constitute a patient subgroup in whom dosage requirements for digoxin are especially unpredictable.[34]

When evaluating serum digoxin concentrations, it is important for the clinician to be cognizant of the assay procedure. Both metabolites of digoxin and endogenous digoxin-like immunoreactive substances (DLISs) may cross-react with the antibodies used in immunoassays.[35] Metabolites of digoxin may accumulate in patients with renal impairment. DLISs have been found in digoxin-free sera of pregnant women, neonates, uremic patients, umbilical cord specimens, and patients with hepatic disease. Recent findings indicate that a monoclonal antibody assay and a radioimmunoassay incorporating a double antibody system are most specific for quantifying serum digoxin concentrations.[35]

THERAPEUTIC USES OF DIGOXIN

Based upon its inotropic actions, digoxin is prescribed for patients with chronic CHF secondary to predominant systolic dysfunction.[1] However, controversy surrounding the use of digoxin for CHF exists for several reasons: (1) the lack of a controlled trial exhibiting an improvement in mortality due to digoxin alone; (2) the lack of clinical deterioration following the withdrawal of maintenance digoxin in a majority of patients with CHF and sinus rhythm; (3) the risk of digoxin toxicity; and (4) the demonstrated positive effects of vasodilatory drugs on both mortality and functional status in patients with CHF.[36] However, in the latter situation, patients are frequently also taking digoxin and diuretics.

Various clinical, hemodynamic, and exercise effects of digoxin in CHF have been evaluated. Almost 40 percent of patients with CHF and atrial fibrillation clinically deteriorated following discontinuation of digoxin.[37] However, in another study, only 2 of 49 patients with CHF and sinus rhythm had increased symptoms of CHF after digoxin was discontinued.[38] Digoxin significantly improved resting left ventricular ejection fraction an average of 9 percent in elderly patients with

CHF.[4] Resting left ventricular ejection fraction was also significantly increased by digoxin in a multicenter comparison with captopril and placebo.[39] However, in a more recent crossover comparison, digoxin did not increase resting left ventricular ejection fraction.[40] Digoxin significantly enhanced treadmill exercise duration in a multicenter trial with milrinone and placebo.[41] Nonetheless, in another investigation digoxin did not improve mean peak oxygen consumption, a measure of maximal aerobic capacity, despite significantly increasing peak exercise ejection fraction.[40]

Reasons for the discrepant observations in the above investigations are not always apparent. Certainly the diagnostic and/or etiologic heterogeneity of the patient populations studied is one possible explanation.[42] For example, patients with CHF secondary to diastolic dysfunction would not be anticipated to demonstrate significant salutary effects from digoxin. A recent meta-analysis of several digoxin trials suggests that only one of nine patients with CHF and sinus rhythm may derive clinically important improvement from digoxin and that predictors of benefit include severity and duration of CHF and the presence of a third heart sound.[43] Although the presence of a third heart sound may not necessarily predict benefit such as an increase in resting ejection fraction,[4] the severity of CHF as determined by exercise testing may correlate with digoxin-enhanced improvements in maximal aerobic capacity.[40] Baseline aerobic capacities below 15 mL/kg/min may identify a subgroup of patients with CHF who are likely to benefit from maintenance digoxin therapy.[40]

Because of its negative chronotropic and dromotropic effects, digoxin is also utilized in the management of atrial fibrillation or flutter with a rapid ventricular response but without ventricular preexcitation.[1] However, increases in sympathetic activity may readily negate the ventricular rate-slowing effects of digoxin, which are principally mediated by an increase in vagal tone. Profibrillatory vagotonic effects of digoxin include a shortening of the atrial refractory period and an increase in the dispersion of refractoriness.[44] Beta-adrenergic antagonists and the calcium channel blocking drugs verapamil and diltiazem, either used alone or concurrently with digoxin in the management of chronic atrial fibrillation, frequently reduce resting and exercise ventricular rates better than digoxin alone.[45] In addition, if urgent rate control is indicated, intravenous beta-adrenergic blockade or calcium channel blockade may be superior to digoxin.[44] However, beta-adrenergic antagonists and calcium channel blocking drugs either used alone or in combination with digoxin do not generally improve exercise duration relative to digoxin monotherapy.[45] Lastly, careful withdrawal of digoxin from a patient receiving concomitant digoxin and an atrial antiarrhythmic drug for recurrent, refractory paroxysmal atrial fibrillation may occasionally result in a significant decline in the paroxysms.[44]

In an uncontrolled study of recent-onset atrial fibrillation, conversion to sinus rhythm was accomplished in 32 of 47 episodes within 8 h of administration of IV digoxin.[46] However, in a more recent trial, orally administered digoxin was no different than placebo in converting recent-onset atrial fibrillation to sinus rhythm.[47] The latter study demonstrated that spontaneous reversion to sinus rhythm frequently occurs in patients with recent-onset atrial fibrillation.

In summary, digoxin may be useful in treating small numbers of selected patients in sinus rhythm with CHF primarily due to systolic dysfunction. These patients are likely to have more severe CHF as determined by clinical signs and symptoms or by exercise testing. Patients with CHF and atrial fibrillation also appear to be candidates for maintenance digoxin. The results of an ongoing, 6-year placebo-controlled trial jointly funded by Burroughs Wellcome, NHLBI, and the Veterans Administration will hopefully determine digoxin's effect on mortality secondary to CHF. For patients with chronic atrial fibrillation unaccompanied by CHF, the beta-adrenergic antagonists verapamil or diltiazem, administered alone or in combination with digoxin, may be preferable to digoxin monotherapy in controlling either resting or exercise heart rates.

NEWER INOTROPIC AGENTS

The past decade has resulted in the development and clinical testing of a variety of inotropic agents for patients with CHF.[48] Most of these drugs exert their positive inotropic effects by increasing intracellular cyclic adenosine monophosphate (AMP). These agents principally include beta-adrenergic and dopaminergic agonists as well as phosphodiesterase inhibitors.

Most long-term, double-blind investigations with beta-adrenergic agonists fail to demonstrate sustained improvements in symptoms, ventricular performance, or exercise tolerance.[48] However, a recent study with xamoterol, a partial β_1-receptor agonist, suggests that this agent is potentially beneficial in the management of mild to moderate chronic CHF.[49] Xamoterol significantly improves exercise performance relative to digoxin. In addition, symptoms of CHF are significantly improved by xamoterol in comparison to placebo. Despite these encouraging findings, the administration of xamoterol to patients with severe CHF results in an increase in mortality relative to placebo.[50] Consequently, the use of xamoterol has been restricted to the treatment of patients with mild CHF.[51]

Ibopamine is a dopaminergic agonist which holds some promise for treating CHF.[52] Ibopamine is a prodrug which is converted to *N*-methyldopamine, which exerts a positive inotropic effect by binding to cardiac β_1 receptors and a vasodilatory effect through binding to peripheral dopamine-1 receptors.[48] During short-term administration, ibopamine appears equivalent to digoxin in improving exercise tolerance.[52] Nonetheless, long-term studies with ibopamine are needed to further assess its role in the management of CHF.

The presently available literature suggests that phosphodiesterase inhibitors fail to demonstrate prolonged improvements in symptoms, hemodynamics, or exercise tolerance.[41,53] Furthermore, both milrinone and enoximone may be detrimental in terms of patient survival when administered over several months.[41,53] The use of phosphodiesterase inhibitors appears to be limited to the acute management of decompensated cardiac failure.

REFERENCES

1. Smith TW: Digitalis. Mechanisms of action and clinical use. *N Engl J Med* 318:358-365, 1988.
2. Papadakis MA, Massie BM: Appropriateness of digoxin use in medical outpatients. *Am J Med* 85:365-368, 1988.
3. Katano Y, Kennedy RH, Stemmer PM, et al: Aging and digitalis sensitivity of cardiac muscle in rats. *Eur J Pharmacol* 113:167-178, 1985.
4. Ware JA, Snow E, Luchi JM, Luchi RJ: Effect of digoxin on ejection fraction in elderly patients with congestive heart failure. *J Am Geriatr Soc* 32:631-635, 1984.
5. Powell AC, Horowitz JD, Hasin Y, et al: Acute myocardial uptake of digoxin in humans: correlation with hemodynamic and electrocardiographic effects. *J Am Coll Cardiol* 15:1238-1247, 1990.
6. Cusack B, Kelly J, O'Malley K, et al: Digoxin in the elderly: pharmacokinetic consequences of old age. *Clin Pharmacol Ther* 25:772-776, 1979.
7. Astorri E, Bianchi G, LaCanna G, et al: Bioavailability and related heart function index of digoxin capsules and tablets in cardiac patients. *J Pharm Sci* 68:104-106, 1979.
8. Johnson BJ, Lindenbaum J, Budnitz E, Marwaha R: Variability of steady-state digoxin kinetics during administration of tablets or capsules. *Clin Pharmacol Ther* 39:306-312, 1986.
9. Doherty JE, Perkins HW, Flanigan WJ: The distribution and concentration of tritiated digoxin in human tissues. *Ann Intern Med* 66:116-124, 1967.
10. Forbes GB, Reina JC: Adult lean body mass declines with age: some longitudinal observations. *Metabolism* 19:653-663, 1970.
11. Aronson JK: Clinical pharmacokinetics of cardiac glycosides in patients with renal dysfunction. *Clin Pharmacokinet* 8:155-178, 1983.
12. Meyer BR, Bellucci A: Renal function in the elderly. *Cardiol Clin* 4:227-234, 1986.
13. Evered DC: The binding of digoxin by the serum proteins. *Eur J Pharmacol* 18:236-244, 1972.
14. Koup JR, Jusko WJ, Elwood CM, Kohli RK: Digoxin pharmacokinetics: role of renal failure in dosage regimen design. *Clin Pharmacol Ther* 18:9-21, 1975.
15. Steiness E: Renal tubular secretion of digoxin. *Circulation* 50:103-107, 1974.
16. Ewy GA, Kapadia GG, Yao L, et al: Digoxin metabolism in the elderly. *Circulation* 39:449-453, 1969.
17. Doherty JE, Perkins WH: Digoxin metabolism in hypo- and hyperthyroidism. Studies with tritiated digoxin in thyroid disease. *Ann Intern Med* 64:489-507, 1966.
18. Lawrence JR, Sumner DJ, Kalk WJ, et al: Digoxin kinetics in patients with thyroid dysfunction. *Clin Pharmacol Ther* 22:7-13, 1977.
19. Luke DR, Halstenson CE, Opsahl JA, Matzke GR: Validity of creatinine clearance estimates in the assessment of renal function. *Clin Pharmacol Ther* 48: 503-508, 1990.
20. Jones WN, Perrier D, Trinca CE, et al: Evaluation of various methods of digoxin dosing. *J Clin Pharmacol* 22:543-550, 1982.
21. Meghee S, Mooney C, Deshmukh AA, et al: Prescribing digoxin in geriatric units: exercise and redistribution of drug. *J Clin Pharm Ther* 12:415-418, 1987.
22. Mahdyoon H, Battilana G, Rosman H, et al: The evolving pattern of digoxin intoxication: observations at a large urban hospital from 1980 to 1988. *Am Heart J* 120:1189-1194, 1990.
23. Nolan L, Kenny R, O'Malley K: The need for reassessment of digoxin prescribing for the elderly. *Br J Clin Pharmacol* 27:367-370, 1989.
24. Eisendrath SJ, Sweeney MA: Toxic neuropsychiatric effects of digoxin at therapeutic serum concentrations. *Am J Psychiatr* 144:506-507, 1987.
25. Andersson KE, Bertler A, Wettrell G: Post-mortem distribution and tissue concentrations of digoxin in infants and adults. *Acta Paediatr Scand* 64:497-504, 1975.
26. Krakauer R, Steiness E: Digoxin concentration in choroid plexus, brain, and myocardium in old age. *Clin Pharmacol Ther* 24:454-458, 1978.

27. Gayes JM, Greenblatt DJ, Lloyd BL, et al: Cerebrospinal fluid digoxin concentrations in humans. *J Clin Pharmacol* 18:16-20, 1978.
28. Weedle PB, Poston JW, Parish PA: The use of digoxin in 55 residential homes for elderly people. *Postgrad Med J* 64:292-296, 1988.
29. Rodin SM, Johnson BF: Pharmacokinetic interactions with digitalis. *Clin Pharmacokinet* 15:227-244, 1988.
30. Nolan PE, Marcus FI, Erstad BL, et al: Effects of coadministration of propafenone on the pharmacokinetics of digoxin in healthy volunteer subjects. *J Clin Pharmacol* 29:46-52, 1989.
31. Calvo MV, Martin-Suarez A, Luengo CM, et al: Interaction between digoxin and propafenone. *Ther Drug Monitor* 11:10-15, 1989.
32. Gault H, Longerich L, Dawe M, Fine A: Digoxin-rifampin interaction. *Clin Pharmacol Ther* 26:750-754, 1984.
33. Aronson JK. Indications for the measurement of plasma digoxin concentrations. *Drugs* 26:230-242, 1983.
34. Dobbs RJ, O'Neill CJA, Deshmukh AA, et al: Serum concentration monitoring of cardiac glycosides. How helpful is it for adjusting dosage regimens? *Clin Pharmacokinet* 20:175-193, 1991.
35. Mojaverian P, Green PJ, Jhangiania RK, Chase GD: Digoxin-like immuoreactive substance: monoclonal and polyclonal RIA and FPIA compared. *J Pharmaceut Biomed Anal* 7:585-592, 1989.
36. Mulrow CD, Mulrow JP, Linn WD, et al: Relative efficacy of vasodilator therapy in chronic congestive heart failure. *JAMA* 259:3422-3426, 1988.
37. Bowman K: Digoxin and the geriatric in-patient. *Acta Med Scand* 214:353-360, 1983.
38. Davies RF: Reduced exercise tolerance after digoxin withdrawal in class II-III heart failure. *Circulation* 78(suppl 2):53, 1988.
39. The Captopril-Digoxin Multicenter Research Group. Comparative effects of therapy with captopril and digoxin in patients with mild to moderate heart failure. *JAMA* 259:539-544, 1988.
40. Fleg JL, Rothfeld B, Gottlieb SH, Wright J: Effect of maintenance digoxin therapy on aerobic performance and exercise left ventricular function in mild to moderate heart failure due to coronary artery disease: a randomized, placebo-controlled, crossover trial. *J Am Coll Cardiol* 17: 743-751, 1991.
41. DiBianco R, Shabetai R, Kostuk W, et al: A comparison of oral milrinone, digoxin, and their combination in the treatment of patients with chronic heart failure. *N Engl J Med* 320:677-683, 1989.
42. Marantz PR, Alderman MH, Tobin JN: Diagnostic heterogeneity in clinical trials for congestive heart failure. *Ann Intern Med* 109:55-61, 1988.
43. Jaeschke R, Oxman AD, Guyatt GH: To what extent do congestive heart failure patients in sinus rhythm benefit from digoxin therapy? A systematic overview and meta-analysis. *Am J Med* 88:279-286, 1990.
44. Falk RH, Leavitt JI: Digoxin for atrial fibrillation: a drug whose time has gone? *Ann Intern Med* 114:573-575, 1991.
45. Zoble RG, Brewington J, Olukotun AY, Gore R: Comparative effects of nadolol-digoxin combination therapy and digoxin monotherapy for chronic atrial fibrillation. *Am J Cardiol* 60:39D-45D, 1987.
46. Weiner P, Bassan MM, Jarchovsky J, et al: Clinical course of acute atrial fibrillation treated with rapid digitalization. *Am Heart J* 105: 223-227, 1983.
47. Falk RH, Knowlton AA, Bernard SA, et al: Digoxin for converting recent-onset atrial fibrillation to sinus rhythm. *Ann Intern Med* 106:503-506, 1987.
48. Packer M: Vasodilator and inotropic drugs for the treatment of chronic heart failure: distinguishing hype from hope. *J Am Coll Cardiol* 12:1299-1317, 1988.
49. The German and Austrian Xamoterol Study Group. Double-blind placebo-controlled comparison of digoxin and xamoterol in chronic heart failure. *Lancet* 1:489-493, 1988.
50. The Xamoterol in Severe Heart Failure Study Group. Xamoterol in severe heart failure. *Lancet* 336:1-6, 1990.

51. Virk SJS, Qiang F, Anfilogoff NH, et al: Acute and chronic hemodynamic effects of xamoterol in mild to moderate congestive heart failure. *Am J Cardiol* 67:48C–54C, 1991.
52. Alicandri C, Fariello R, Boni E, et al: Ibopamine vs. digoxin in chronic heart failure: a double-blind, crossover study. *J Cardiovasc Pharmacol* 14(suppl 8):S77–S82, 1989.
53. Uretsky BF, Jessup M, Konstam MA, et al: Multicenter trial of oral enoximone in patients with moderate to moderately severe congestive heart failure. *Circulation* 82:774–780, 1990.

CHAPTER

8

ANXIOLYTIC DRUGS AND SEDATIVE-HYPNOTIC AGENTS

Martha P. Fankhauser

OVERVIEW OF ANXIETY

Anxiety is the most common symptom that people experience during their lifetime.[1,2] Anxiety exists not only as a symptom but as a disorder when a certain cluster of symptoms occur together.[3] The *Diagnostic Statistical Manual of Mental Disorders, Third Edition Revised* (DSM-III-R) has several diagnostic criterias for different anxiety syndromes (Table 8-1).[4] The clinical manifestations of anxiety are numerous, and symptoms often overlap with other psychiatric disorders, physical illnesses, and drug/alcohol abuse.[5-8] Anxiety usually consists of both psychic and motor/somatic symptoms (Table 8-2). The most common psychic symptoms include worrying, apprehension, anticipation, uncertainty, tension, fear, and sleep disturbances. Common somatic sensations include sweating, tachycardia, heart palpitations, headache, dry mouth, diarrhea, and gastrointestinal distress.[5,9]

Most people accept a certain degree of anxiety or stress as part of normal daily living, but the elderly may find the anxiety states distressing and incapacitating. The elderly are particularly vulnerable to significant changes and losses during the later years of life (e.g., loss of friends and loved ones, loneliness, medical illnesses, retirement, financial stability, dependency on others, institutionalization, mobility, dementia, loss of control over decisions, and the prospect of dying).[1,3,5,10,11] These stressors may be especially difficult for elderly patients if there is an underlying physical disorder, depression, cognitive dysfunction, or lack of social networks.[5,12]

Approximately 10 to 15 percent of elderly people seek medical treatment

Table 8-1 Types of anxiety disorders (DSM-III-R)

I. Phobic disorders
Agoraphobia: fear of places or situations where help may not be available with avoidance behavior.
Social phobia: fear of situations where the person may do something humiliating or embarrassing.
Simple phobia: excessive and unreasonable fear of an object or situation.

II. Panic disorder
Discrete panic attacks with intense fear (with at least four associated autonomic/motor symptoms); either four attacks within a 4-week period or one or more attacks followed by a month with fear of having another panic attack.
With agoraphobia: avoidance of places or situations.
Without agoraphobia: no avoidance behavior.

III. Obsessive compulsive disorder
Recurrent and persistent ideas and thoughts and repetitive, purposeful behaviors that cause marked distress and consume more than an hour a day.

IV. Posttraumatic stress disorder
Persistent reexperiencing of a traumatic event by flashbacks or nightmares; associated with increased arousal, avoidance behavior, and numbing.

V. Generalized anxiety disorder
An unrealistic or excessive anxiety or worry about two or more life circumstances (with symptoms of motor tension, autonomic hyperactivity, and vigilance/scanning) for 6 months or longer.

VI. Atypical anxiety disorder
Does not meet diagnostic criteria for another anxiety disorder.

VII. Adjustment disorders
Maladaptive reactions to a psychosocial stressor that occurs within 3 months of the stressor(s) and lasts no longer than 6 months.
With anxious mood: prominent anxiety symptoms.
With mixed emotional features: anxiety and depressive symptoms.

VIII. Organic mental disorder
Organic anxiety syndrome: recurrent panic attacks or generalized anxiety that is related to an organic cause.

because of anxiety symptoms.[11] The cause of anxiety varies and requires a complete evaluation to determine if symptoms are related to an anxiety disorder or depression, induced by a physical illness or medications, or a normal response to stress.[3,6] An accurate diagnosis is essential since there are a wide variety of pharmacologic and nonpharmacologic treatment approaches. Several anxiety disorders are considered chronic (e.g., panic disorder, obsessive compulsive disorder), and patients may suffer a lifetime with symptoms and impairment if not properly treated. Elderly patients should not be treated solely with medications. Reassurance, stress reduction techniques, environmental changes, and individual, group, or family therapy are often helpful in reducing anxiety. These nonpharmacologic approaches should be tried first or used in conjunction with pharmacologic treatments.[11] Elderly patients may be more difficult to manage with medications. They are particularly vulnerable to adverse central nervous system (CNS) effects (e.g., drowsiness, memory impairment, disorientation, motor incoordination) that are common with sedative-hypnotic agents.[13,14]

Although anxiety is a common emotion and experienced in all life stages, it is

Table 8-2 Common symptoms of anxiety

Psychic
Fearfulness
Apprehension, anticipation, or worry
Tension or feeling uptight
Anger or hostility
Difficulty concentrating
Difficulty making decisions
Irritability or impatience
Feeling detached or floating sensation
Depersonalization or derealization
Feeling out of control
Preoccupation with certain thoughts or ideas
Recurrent dreams or nightmares
Fear of dying or going insane
Motor or somatic
Headache
Trouble swallowing
Shortness of breath or difficulty breathing
Excessive sweating or flushing
Dry mouth
Frequent urination
Trembling or shakiness
Clumsiness or poor motor control
Muscle twitching
Nausea or stomach upset
Diarrhea or irritable bowel syndrome
Weakness or fatigue
Inability to relax
Difficulty falling or staying asleep
Faintness or dizziness
Hot flashes or chills
Tingling or numbness in parts of body
Palpitations or increased heart rate
Chest pain, pressure, or discomfort
Exaggerated startle response

poorly defined and studied in the elderly.[5,10] Anxiety symptoms overlap with numerous medical conditions, so the elderly may manifest anxiety differently than younger patients. Cognitive changes such as poor attention and concentration/memory impairment are associated with anxiety and depressive states and may be more common in the elderly. The memory problems and difficulty with making decisions under high anxiety states may be misdiagnosed as part of normal aging or dementia.

Elderly patients may not complain of the psychic or mental distress of anxiety but rather may focus on physical or somatic symptoms. These physical symptoms of anxiety may be misdiagnosed as a medical condition and improperly treated with medications that are not effective for the underlying anxiety disorder. Elderly patients may also self-treat with alcohol or other drugs that may mask an anxiety disorder.[7,15]

EPIDEMIOLOGY OF ANXIETY

Epidemiologic studies show that anxiety disorders as a group are the most common psychiatric disorders in the United States, followed by alcoholism and substance abuse.[8] It is estimated that 15 to 20 percent of the population experience an anxiety disorder in their lifetime.[16,17] Anxiety disorders are approximately eight times more prevalent than major depression in the elderly.[18]

Prevalence rates for anxiety disorders in elderly patients range from 5 to 68 percent depending on the population studied.[10,18,19] Some of the variables that influence prevalence rates are sex, age, race, marital status, education, medical conditions, living situation, degree of independence, cognitive abilities, and hearing loss.[5] Epidemiology studies indicate that most anxiety syndromes begin early in life (e.g., phobic disorders during childhood and into the twenties, onset of panic disorder by the thirties).[20] Patients with mixed anxiety and depressive syndromes may have an earlier onset of the disorder than patients with depression alone.

The 6-month and lifetime prevalence rates for different anxiety disorders in persons aged 65 or higher are listed in Table 8-3. The Epidemiologic Catchment Area Study found that the prevalence rates were lower in older adults (> 65) than in middle-aged adults (45 to 64).[17] These rates may not be accurate due to underreporting of anxiety in the elderly. Several studies have reported higher anxiety rates in elderly females as compared to elderly males.[18,21]

PATHOPHYSIOLOGY

The exact etiology of different anxiety disorders is not known, but several theories have been investigated. The most studied hypothesis involves the dysfunction of the autonomic nervous system with either an increased sensitivity or overreactivity

Table 8-3 Prevalence rates (%) of anxiety disorders in a community sample of elderly patients (epidemiologic catchment area study) prevalence rates for > 65 years

	Six months, %	Lifetime, %
Simple phobia	9.63	16.10
Social phobia	1.37	2.64
Agoraphobia	5.22	8.44
Panic disorder	0.04	0.29
Obsessive compulsive disorder	1.54	1.98
Generalized anxiety disorder	1.90	4.60

Source: Adapted from Ref. 18.

of norepinephrine release and changes in receptor sensitivity. Patients with panic disorder have hyperactivity of the noradrenergic system (part of the sympathetic nervous system) that is involved in the fight-or-flight response. The noradrenergic system is mediated by the locus coeruleus (LC) in the brain stem, which contains the majority of norepinephrine neurons and is involved in anxiety states and in acute fear responses.[22] The LC has widespread projections to the limbic system that regulates arousal and emotional states. Medications that stimulate LC activity (e.g., sodium lactate, CO_2, caffeine, isoproterenol, yohimbine) can precipitate a panic attack in patients with panic disorder but not in normal subjects.[23] Panic disorder patients are extremely sensitive to over-the-counter cold preparations that contain sympathomimetic agents (e.g., phenylpropanolamine, pseudoephedrine, caffeine). Thus, these agents should be avoided.[24] Medications that inhibit LC activity (e.g., antidepressants and benzodiazepines) have antipanic activity. Panic disorder patients also have asymmetry of blood flow in the limbic area on positron emission tomography (PET) scans[25] and a high genetic risk for the disorder (i.e., 45 percent for monozygotic twins versus 15 percent for dizygotic twins).[26]

Posttraumatic stress disorder (PTSD) is also associated with hyperactivity of the noradrenergic system (due to an initial depletion and then a hypersensitivity of the system over time).[27] PTSD patients have exaggerated responsiveness to mild stimuli that cause flashbacks, nightmares, increased heart rate, respiratory rate, galvanic skin response, and dysfunction of rapid eye movement (REM) sleep activity.[27]

Gamma-aminobutyric acid (GABA), the major inhibitory neurotransmitter system in the CNS, is involved in arousal and anxiety states.[28] $GABA_B$ acts as a inhibitory neurotransmitter in the limbic system, which is important for modulating arousal and survival behavior. GABA receptors (along with benzodiazepine receptors) are found throughout the CNS (e.g., brainstem, cerebellum, hippocampus, cortex, and spinal cord).[22] At least two types of GABA receptors have been identified: $GABA_A$ receptors are coupled to chloride channels; $GABA_B$ receptors are coupled to calcium ions and possibly cyclic adenosine monophosphate (cAMP).[22] Benzodiazepine receptors are closely linked to $GABA_A$ receptors and help to augment the inhibitory activity of the GABA system by opening chloride channels. Benzodiazepines increase the affinity of the $GABA_A$ receptor to GABA that causes influx of chloride ions and hyperpolarization of the neuron.[22] The augmentation of GABA activity inhibits the release of other neurotransmitters (e.g., norepinephrine, serotonin, and dopamine).[22] There is some evidence that changes in GABA activity, receptor binding, or changes in the secondary messenger system may be related to different anxiety states.[28]

The serotonergic system is probably involved in obsessive compulsive disorder (OCD), but there are inconsistent results with other anxiety disorders.[28] Some hypothesize that OCD is caused by a deficit or dysfunction in the serotonin system.[29] PET scans of OCD patients have shown increased brain metabolic activity in the frontal lobes (right orbital frontal area), caudate nucleus, and cingulate gyrus that contain serotonin neurons. The "hyperfunctioning" of this brain serotonin loop could be responsible for the repetitive obsessions and compulsions associated with OCD.[29] OCD has been effectively treated with serotonergic agents (e.g., clomipramine, fluoxetine) that cause a down-regulation of the serotonin system over time. The serotonin may also be involved with generalized anxiety states. Buspirone, an anxiolytic used in generalized anxiety disorder (GAD), is thought to act as a partial 5-HT_{1A} receptor agonist. The significance of the different serotonin receptor subtypes is currently under investigation.

There have been few controlled studies investigating the biologic changes in anxious elderly patients. Some of the changes observed with normal aging are similar to those observed in anxiety disorders.[28] During normal aging, there appears to be a reduced transmission of neuronal activity in the brain which may be related to the amount and activity of various neurotransmitters, changes in receptor sensitivity, and feedback regulation between neurons.[30] Studies performed with adrenergic markers (e.g., plasma catecholamines, metabolites of norepinephrine, $alpha_2$- and beta-adrenergic receptor activity, and monoamine oxidase activity) suggest that there is a decline in noradrenergic function and activity with increasing age.[28] There is either no change or a decrease in serotonin (5-HT) functioning in the elderly [i.e., decrease in response to 5-HT challenge tests, decrease in peripheral 5-HT markers, decrease in central 5-HT levels, increase in cerebrospinal fluid (CSF) 5-hydroxyindoleacetic acid levels, and a decrease in 5-HT_1 receptor levels].[28] Studies in elderly patients have shown either no change or a reduction in central GABA levels and receptor levels.[28] Further studies are needed to determine the significance of noradrenergic, serotonergic, and GABA changes during aging and their relationship to different anxiety disorders. (For a more complete review of neurobiologic changes observed in anxiety and aging studies, see Ref. 28.)

ORGANIC CAUSES OF ANXIETY

Since the onset of anxiety disorders usually occurs before the age of 40, a new onset of anxiety or panic (without a situational stressor) may indicate a possible organic etiology. Many medical illnesses, medications, and psychiatric disorders are associated with anxietylike symptoms (Table 8-4). Anxiety symptoms are particularly prominent in cardiovascular, pulmonary, metabolic, and endocrine diseases as well as in drug-induced states.[11,31-34] Some of the most common causes of anxiety symptoms include hyperthyroidism, hypoglycemia, angina, arrhythmias, mitral valve prolapse, vertigo, chronic obstructive pulmonary disease, pulmonary embolism, caffeinism, theophylline, sympathomimetics, akathisia from antipsychotics, and withdrawal from sedative hypnotics or alcohol. Several psychiatric disorders have anxiety as part of the symptomatology (e.g., depression, mania, schizophrenia, delirium, dementia, and other organic mental disorders).

Table 8-4 Organic causes of anxiety

Medical illnesses

- Cardiac
  - Angina
  - Arrhythmias
  - Congestive heart failure
  - Hypertension
  - Myocardial infarction
  - Syncope
  - Mitral valve prolapse
- Respiratory
  - Asthma
  - Chronic obstructive pulmonary disease
  - Hypoxia
  - Pulmonary edema
  - Pulmonary embolus
  - Pneumonia
- Endocrine
  - Hypo- and hyperthyroidism
  - Hypo- and hyperadrenalism
  - Hyperparathyroidism
  - Menopause
  - Premenstrual syndrome
- Secreting tumors
  - Carcinoid
  - Pheochromocytoma
  - Insulinoma
- Metabolic
  - Hyperkalemia
  - Hypocalcemia
  - Hypoglycemia
- Gastrointestinal
  - Ulcers
  - Irritable bowel syndrome
- Anemias
  - Vitamin B_{12} deficiency
  - Folate acid deficiency
- Immunologic
  - Systemic lupus erythematosus
  - Anaphylaxis
  - Acquired immunodeficiency syndrome
- Neurologic
  - Essential tremor
  - Intracranial tumors
  - Encephalopathies
  - Multiple sclerosis
  - Parkinson's disease
  - Postconcussion syndrome
  - Poststroke syndrome
  - Seizure disorders (temporal lobe epilepsy)
  - Vertigo

Psychiatric illnesses

- Alzheimer's disease
- Depression
- Organic brain disease
- Schizophrenia
- Agitation associated with psychosis

Sensory impairment

- Hearing loss
- Visual disturbances
- Sensory deprivation

Medications

- Bronchodilators
  - Albuterol
  - Isoproterenol
  - Metaproterenol
- Sympathomimetics
  - Ephedrine
  - Pseudoephedrine
  - Phenylpropanolamine
  - Phenylephrine
  - Epinephrine
- Psychostimulants
  - Amphetamines
  - Cocaine
  - Methylphenidate
- Xanthine derivatives
  - Theophylline
  - Aminophylline
  - Caffeine
- Antidepressants
  - Desipramine
  - Protriptyline
  - Fluoxetine
  - Bupropion
  - Tranylcypromine
- Neuroleptic-induced akathisia
  - Haloperidol
  - Fluphenazine
  - Thiothixene
  - Perphenazine
  - Metoclopramide
- Withdrawal states
  - Benzodiazepines, especially short acting
  - Alcohol
  - Nicotine
- Hallucinogens
  - Phencyclidine
  - Lysergic acid
  - Marijuana

(*Continues*)

Table 8-4 (*continued*) Organic causes of anxiety

Antihypertensives
Guanethidine
Methyldopa
Reserpine
Toxicity
Salicylates
Digitalis
Anticholinergic
Dietary
Caffeinism
Monosodium glutamate
Tyramine
Refined sugar
Chocolate
Vitamin deficiency
Thiamine
Niacin
B_{12}
Folic acid

Source: Adapted from Refs. 31, 32, 44.

ANXIETY AND DEPRESSION

There is a significant overlap in clinical symptoms for anxiety and affective disorders. Thus both anxiety and depression may coexist in a majority of elderly patients.[2,6,35-37] A comparison of symptoms associated with anxiety and affective disorders is found in Table 8-5 and biologic responses are presented in Table 8-6. Some believe that anxiety and affective disorders are part of a continuum and that patients exhibit different diagnoses over time.[20] Others believe anxiety and depression are two distinct illnesses that share similar symptoms.[8,38,39] If anxiety disorders are not recognized and treated appropriately, many patients may later develop major depression (or secondary depression).[11,20] Studies have reported that 21 to 91 percent of patients with panic disorder, generalized anxiety disorder, and agoraphobia meet criteria for major depression.[8,40] Approximately 50 to 80 percent of patients with major depression exhibit anxiety symptoms,[40-42] whereas 20 to 65 percent of anxious patients become depressed in their lifetime.[22]

MORBIDITY AND MORTALITY OF ANXIETY DISORDERS

There is little information about morbidity and mortality rates of different anxiety states in the elderly.[43] Because anxiety, depression, and alcoholism often occur together (comorbidity rates of 30 to 50 percent), there may be an increased risk of morbidity in geriatric patients.[8,20,40] Anxious patients with depression (compared

Table 8-5 Symptoms associated with anxiety and affective disorders

	GAD	PD	PbD	PTSD	MD
Difficulty concentrating	+			+	+
Irritability	+			+	+
Fatigue/lack of energy	+				+
Appetite disturbances	+				+
Difficulty falling/staying asleep	+			+	+
Apprehension/worrying	+	+	+		
Phobic avoidance behavior			+	+	
Fear of being in places or situations			+	+	
Hypervigilance	+			+	
Exaggerated startle response	+			+	
Reexperiencing traumatic event (flashbacks/nightmares)				+	
Motor tension					
Twitching/shaky	+				
Muscle tension	+				
Restlessness	+				
Fatigability	+				
Autonomic hyperactivity					
Breathing difficulty	+	+			
Tremor	+	+			
Palpitations	+	+			
Hot or cold spells	+	+			
Faintness/dizziness	+	+			
Sweating/cold hands	+	+			
Nausea/abdominal distress	+	+			
Dry mouth	+				
Frequent urination	+				
Trouble swallowing	+				
Choking		+			
Numbness/paresthesias		+			
Chest pain/discomfort		+			
Depersonalization		+			
Derealization		+			
Fear of another attack		+			
Fear of dying		+			
Depressed mood; sad/blue/down					+
Excessive sleeping					+
Early morning awakening					+
Feeling worse in the morning					+
Psychomotor retardation					+
Hopeless/helpless					+
Worthlessness/guilt feelings					+
Loss of interest in usual activities				+	
Inability to experience pleasure				+	+
Thoughts of suicide or death		+			+

GAD = generalized anxiety disorder; PD = panic disorder; PbD = phobic disorder; PTSD = posttraumatic stress disorder; MD = major depression.

Source: Adapted from Refs. 8, 36, 37, 44.

Table 8-6 Biologic overlap between affective and anxiety disorders

Test	MD	PD	OCD	GAD	Phobia
Heart rate (increased)	+	+		+	+
Catecholamines (increased)	+	+		+	+
Dexamethasone suppression test (nonsuppression)	+	?	?		
TSH response to thyrotropin-releasing hormone (blunted)	+	+			
Lactate infusion (panic attack)		+			
Yohimbine infusion (panic attack)		+			?
REM latency (decreased)	+		+		
Genetic risk	+	+	+		?

MD = major depression; PD = panic disorder; OCD = obsessive compulsive disorder; GAD = generalized anxiety disorder.

Source: Adapted from Ref. 37.

to patients with a primary anxiety disorder) have a greater impairment in functioning and a poorer outcome.[8,39,40] Untreated panic disorder patients usually have significant impairment in functioning and are more likely to be financially dependent on others.[44,45] Patients with panic attacks (compared to other psychiatric disorders) have an increased risk of suicide ideation and attempts.[44,46,47] Between 40 and 90 percent of panic disorder patients become depressed during their lifetime.[39] Patients with both depression and high anxiety levels (panic attacks) have an increased risk of suicide within 1 year.[42,47]

Anxious elderly patients have an increase in urinary epinephrine and heart rate when under stress and a delayed return to baseline parameters.[3,10] Patients with significant anxiety states (e.g., panic disorder) have elevated catecholamines and increased heart rate, which may increase their morbidity risk of cardiovascular disease.[6,48] Further studies are needed to determine if chronic hyperarousal states negatively impact other medical illnesses (e.g., cardiovascular, endocrine, immune functioning) and result in increased morbidity and mortality.

EVALUATION

The clinical presentation of anxiety disorders in the elderly can be confusing since anxiety symptoms are associated with numerous psychiatric disorders.[20,49] Anxiety disorders may not be easily recognized in the elderly. Thus, they are at a high risk for misdiagnosis and improper treatment.[22] There are no laboratory tests available to diagnosis anxiety. Instead the diagnosis is based on identifying specific symptoms and determining the course and history of the illness (e.g., age of onset, family history). A thorough physical examination and laboratory testing should be used to rule out medical or drug-induced causes of anxiety (Table 8-4).[31] Polypharmacy is common in the elderly, so a complete medication history (prescribed and over the counter) helps to determine underlying medical illnesses and somatic complaints that are being self-treated.[1,14] Elderly patients should be asked about alcohol and substance abuse since these disorders often overlap with anxiety and depressive states.[7,8,39]

Elderly patients usually first come to their primary care physician with anxiety complaints and do not seek out psychiatric care from the mental health sector.[5,17] It is estimated that only 25 percent of patients with generalized anxiety disorder receive treatment, and many patients suffer several years before they seek treatment.[22] Elderly patients may not admit to having a psychiatric disorder and would rather discuss physical symptoms. There is a tendency for elderly patients to attribute physical symptoms to aging or to a medical illness. Thus they may deny or underreport anxiety symptoms.[31] Elderly patients with numerous somatic complaints may be misdiagnosed as having hypochondriasis (the fear or preoccupation of having a serious disease) or a somatization disorder (the recurrence of multiple somatic complaints without any established medical illness).[2,32]

Physicians may need to refer some patients to a psychiatrist or psychologist when there is doubt about the diagnosis or treatment. Psychometric testing (e.g., mental status exam, personality assessment to determine characterlogical traits, and ruling out other psychiatric disorders such as depression) is often essential in making an accurate diagnosis.

CLINICAL PRESENTATION OF ANXIETY DISORDERS

The anxiety disorders listed in the DSM-III-R (Table 8-1) consist of anxiety states (i.e., GAD, panic disorder, OCD, PTSD) and phobic disorders [i.e., social phobia, simple phobia, and agoraphobia (with or without panic attacks)].[4] The anxiety disorders are differentiated by either a free-floating state (unfocused) or one focused on avoiding a particular situation, activity, or object (phobias). If the anxiety state occurs suddenly and is associated with intense fear and physical symptoms, these discrete episodes are called panic attacks. *Panic disorder* often occurs with avoidance behavior (or agoraphobia). *Generalized anxiety disorder* is characterized by a chronic and excessive worry and anxiety symptoms which are present for at least 6 months. *Obsessive compulsive disorder* is characterized by either obsessive or persistent thoughts or ideas or by compulsive or repetitive behaviors. *Posttraumatic stress disorder* occurs in response to a severe stressful event and is characterized by reexperiencing the traumatic event by recurrent and intrusive thoughts of the event or by recurrent dreams or nightmares. There are three different types of phobic disorders. *Agoraphobia* is a fear of being alone or in a public place where escape could be difficult or there may be no help. *Social phobia* is an irrational fear and desire to avoid situations where the person may be exposed to scrutiny by others and fears that they may do something that would be embarrassing or humiliating. *Simple phobia* is a persistent and irrational fear and desire to avoid a specific object or situation.

Of the DSM-III-R anxiety disorders, OCD and panic disorder rarely begin later in life, so are usually not seen in the elderly unless the disorder has continued from early adulthood. Phobic disorders and GAD are more common in the elderly and may be associated with increased isolation, physical illnesses, financial difficulties, worrying about safety, and fears of social situations. Although GAD and phobic disorders are common in elderly patients, other anxiety states such as agitation, situational anxiety, and adjustment disorder with anxious mood are probably even more prevalent.

Agitation

Agitation is not recognized as a type of anxiety-related syndrome in the DSM-III-R, but it is a common symptom in the elderly.[49,50] Agitation is characterized by a combination of irritability, restlessness, inability to communicate or perform specific tasks, and confusion which may lead to aggressive behavior. Agitation is often associated with dementia, mood disorders, and toxic states.[49] Irritability, agitation, and aggression may be an early sign of an underlying organic mental disorder (e.g., medication-induced, drug withdrawal, medical illness).[51] Because elderly patients often receive medications that affect the CNS, medications should always be suspected as causing agitation.[6]

Agitated-anxious behaviors and insomnia are frequently observed in elderly demented patients.[10,31,49,50] Verbal and physical aggression are common in nursing home patients and typically occur in the late afternoon or evening (called *sundowning*). Explosive rage or violent behavior may occur in geriatric patients with brain lesions or after diffuse CNS damage.[51] The pharmacologic treatment of agitation (or aggression) depends on the severity and if it is an acute or chronic problem. The acute management of aggression usually requires rapid tranquilization with a sedative agent such as a benzodiazepine (e.g., lorazepam 1 to 2 mg PO or IM or 0.5 to 1 mg IV) or an antipsychotic (e.g., haloperidol 1 mg PO or 0.5 mg IV or IM) given alone or in combination every 1 to 2 h until sedation occurs.[51] Although antipsychotics are frequently used for treating agitation in the elderly, the higher potency agents are more likely to cause akathisia (motor restlessness and pacing), which can make the underlying agitation worse. In some patients, benzodiazepines may exacerbate clinical symptoms because of disinhibition or cause further impairment in cognition and reasoning.[1] Pharmacologic treatments for chronic management of aggression or severe agitation include antipsychotics, beta blockers, lithium, carbamazepine, and buspirone.[51-54]

Situational Anxiety

The most common anxiety state is a *situational anxiety*, which occurs in response to a stressful situation or experience. This type of anxiety "state" is short-lived and is considered a normal emotional response to stress. Examples of situations that may provoke an acute anxiety state include visiting a physician or dentist, being hospitalized, flying in an airplane, being interviewed or questioned by an authority figure, learning how to operate mechanical or electrical appliances, driving an unfamiliar car, waiting in lines or in traffic, involvement in an accident, and traveling in a new city or country. Although adults of all ages may have situational anxiety, the elderly may have more difficulty in coping with novel situations and experiences due to more anticipation and worrying, poorer coping skills, and cognitive dysfunction. Elderly patients under high anxiety states may have a deterioration in cognition and motor performance.[10,14] Situational anxiety is a primary cause of insomnia and sleep disturbances, which are common complaints in the elderly.[55]

Because the anxiety state is usually brief, pharmacologic therapy is not needed or recommended unless the reaction causes significant distress or if there is a disruption in functioning. Relaxation techniques, behavioral therapy, or cognitive training should be tried first, particularly if elderly patients have recurrent exposure to situational stressors (or if they develop a simple or social phobia). Beta blockers can be used in acute anxiety-provoking situations. However, they are contraindicated in patients with diabetes, heart failure, or asthma.[1] Benzodiazepines work rapidly to decrease anticipation but may disinhibit older patients or cause fatigue, gait disturbances, and confusion. If benzodiazepines are tried, they should be used in lower doses and for short-term or intermittent therapy.[1] Buspirone, monoamine oxidase inhibitors (MAOIs), and tricyclic antidepressants are also beneficial in the treatment of anxiety, but because they have a slower onset of action, they may not be useful in acute situational anxiety states.

Adjustment Disorder with Anxious Mood

An adjustment disorder with anxious mood lasts longer than situational anxiety (but no longer than 6 months) and usually occurs after a major life event. There is little epidemiologic information about the incidence or prevalence of adjustment disorders in elderly patients. Adjustment disorders are probably the most common psychiatric diagnosis made in medically ill patients.[56] The adjustment diagnostic category is frequently used when elderly patients are hospitalized in medical or psychiatric facilities or if there is an identifiable stressor preceding the psychologic reaction.

The DSM-III-R diagnostic criteria for adjustment disorder with anxious mood requires that the anxiety symptoms occur within 3 months of the onset of the stressor, cause social and/or occupational impairment, and last no longer than 6 months.[57] Patients with symptoms of both anxiety and depression are diagnosed as an adjustment disorder with mixed emotional features. If depression is more prominent, then a diagnosis of adjustment disorder with depressed mood is used. All patients with adjustment disorders should be closely monitored for the future development of a major depression episode (when depressive symptoms last for more than 2 weeks) or a GAD (when anxiety symptoms persist for more than 6 months).

Adjustment disorder with anxious or depressed mood is frequently found in the elderly since they are more likely to have significant life changes, personal crises, and losses than are younger adults.[12,56] Significant stressful life events include moving to a new location, developing a medical illness (even if it is not life threatening or disabling), long-term hospitalization, chronic illness or pain, illness or death of a family member, marital discord, separation or divorce, financial problems, or retirement.[1,56] Elderly patients may possibly have multiple psychosocial stressors occurring at the same time.

It is difficult to predict individual vulnerability to stressors since some people have better coping skills and social support systems.[53] Also the severity of the stressor does not necessarily predict the expected intensity of the adjustment reaction. Patients with a previous history of adjustment disorders or prolonged psychologic reactions to stressful situations may be at increased risk for having difficulties with major life events.

The preferred first-line treatment for adjustment disorder with anxious mood is education and counseling, relaxation training, cognitive/behavioral therapies, and development of new and better coping strategies.[56] Elderly patients may benefit from weekly or biweekly counseling or supportive group therapy.[56] Other approaches such as relaxation training, stress reduction classes, development of new hobbies, or regular exercise programs should be encouraged. Lifestyle changes (e.g., cessation of smoking, reduction in alcohol and caffeine consumption, proper nutrition, and good sleep hygiene) are important and recommended for all patients.

Patients with incapacitating anxiety symptoms may need brief pharmacologic intervention with a short-acting benzodiazepine (e.g., lorazepam, alprazolam, oxazepam). Benzodiazepines are the most widely prescribed agents and are safe and effective when used for short-term treatment (i.e., 1 to 4 weeks). Although the benzodiazepines can be used prn, it may be better to prescribe a low dose on a regular schedule and to gradually taper the dose when the patient is stabilized.[56] Buspirone, a nonbenzodiazepine, is also beneficial for anxiety but may take several weeks before full therapeutic effect is observed.

Those patients with more chronic anxiety or mixed anxiety-depression may benefit from an antidepressant trial (e.g., nortriptyline, desipramine, fluoxetine, bupropion, trazodone), but it takes several weeks before full therapeutic benefit occurs. Beta-adrenergic blockers (e.g., propranolol, atenolol) are effective in low doses for reducing the autonomic hyperactivity or somatic complaints of anxiety (e.g., tachycardia, tremor) but may cause bradycardia, hypotension, and depression at higher doses.[56] For patients with a significant problem with insomnia or sleep disturbances, a brief treatment with a short-acting hypnotic benzodiazepine (e.g., triazolam, temazepam, estazolam) may be used. Antihistamines (e.g., diphenhydramine or hydroxyzine) or a sedative antidepressant (e.g., trazodone, imipramine, doxepin) can be used for short-term management of acute anxiety and insomnia. The nonaddicting agents are preferred for patients with a history of alcohol or substance abuse.

Generalized Anxiety Disorder

Generalized anxiety disorder (GAD) is characterized by a continuous and chronic anxiety state with persistent worrying about two or more life circumstances that lasts for at least 6 months.[22] Because the duration of symptoms was increased in the DSM-III-R from 1 month to 6 months, fewer patients may fit this diagnostic criteria and instead meet the diagnosis of adjustment disorder with anxious mood. The GAD diagnostic requires that 6 of 18 symptoms listed under categories of motor tension, autonomic hyperactivity, vigilance, and scanning must be present. The GAD criteria do not take into account that elderly patients have more physical illnesses and symptoms that are part of the normal aging process (e.g., muscle aches, feeling shaky, easily fatigued, frequent urination, shortness of breath, trouble falling asleep and staying asleep).[10] Elderly patients that have multiple somatic complaints may self-medicate with alcohol or other medications that can confuse the clinical presentation. All organic anxiety states should be ruled out (e.g., caffeinism, CNS stimulants, hyperthyroidism, vertigo), since these are often the cause of chronic "organic" anxiety symptoms.

The prevalence rate of GAD in the elderly is not known, but estimates of 1 month to 1 year prevalence rates are 2 to 6 percent in adults.[22] GAD usually begins early in life (i.e., teens, early twenties or thirties) after a stressful life event and tends to have a chronic course with periodic exacerbations of symptoms secondary to psychosocial stressors. Although elderly patients may not remember the onset of anxiety in early life, most have a lifelong history of anxiety.

GAD may be a "trait" anxiety disorder with fluctuations in the severity of the disorder over time.[58] Patients with GAD may overly react to stressful life events and have exaggerated anticipation and excessive worrying (apprehensive expectation) about normal life circumstances. GAD patients often develop a major depression or panic disorder during their lifetime. Frequently both anxiety and depression coexist, so it may be difficult to determine whether anxiety or depression is the major disorder (Table 8-5).[8,10,37]

Because GAD is often a chronic disease, every effort should be made to reduce symptoms to a manageable level. Nonpharmacologic approaches listed under "situational anxiety" are effective for patients with mild symptoms associated with psychosocial stressors (e.g., supportive counseling, psychotherapy, relaxation, biofeedback, meditation, exercise, and stress management). These techniques and therapies are beneficial for lessening the chronic anxiety state so that pharmacologic treatments are only used as needed during significant stressful situations.

Pharmacologic treatment for GAD is indicated only when symptoms are severe or persistent. Medications should be used for short-term therapy (2 to 6 months) and combined with the nonpharmacologic treatment approaches. Every attempt should be made to taper and discontinue medications so that patients do not become dependent on antianxiety agents. Patients need to be educated about the fluctuating course of the illness and how to manage acute situational anxiety with minimal medication intervention. Anxiolytics should help reduce the anticipatory anxiety so that patients can concentrate on learning more effective coping skills or relaxation techniques.

Anxiety syndromes are primarily treated with three general classes of medications: benzodiazepines, azapironones (buspirone), and antidepressants (tricyclic antidepressants and MAOIs). The antidepressant medications will be briefly reviewed and are discussed in detail in Chap. 15. The molecular structures for the benzodiazepines and buspirone are shown in Fig. 8-1.

Benzodiazepines Benzodiazepines are the most widely prescribed class of psychotropic agents in the United States and are extensively used in the elderly (range from 17 to 50 percent).[13,14,22] Approximately 11 percent of the population takes a benzodiazepine during the year, and up to one-third of patients receive them for longer than a year.[22]

Benzodiazepines have been shown to be superior to placebo in numerous clinical trials.[14,31] They are effective as anxiolytics, muscle relaxants, hypnotics, and anticonvulsants and for alcohol withdrawal. Benzodiazepines are effective for GAD to decrease anticipatory anxiety (at relatively low doses), but at higher doses, they may cause significant CNS and respiratory depression.[59] Acute toxicity is associated with disinhibition, psychomotor disturbances, incoordination, falling, and impaired concentration/memory.[11] Chronic dosing also causes cognitive impairment that may be confused as dementia or depression.

The benzodiazepines are divided into two groups based on half-life (short- or

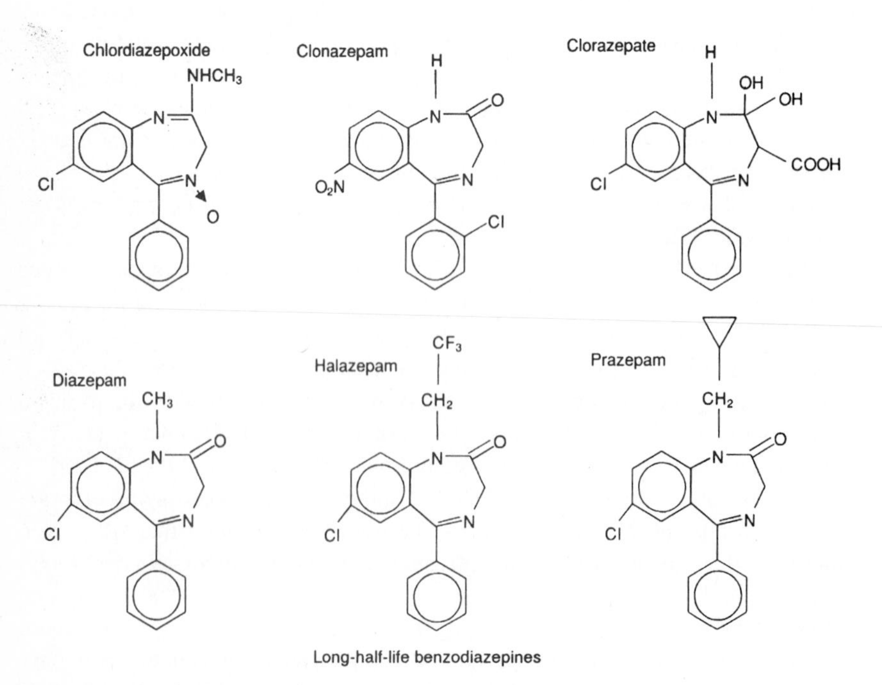

Figure 8-1 Chemical structures for benzodiazepines and buspirone.

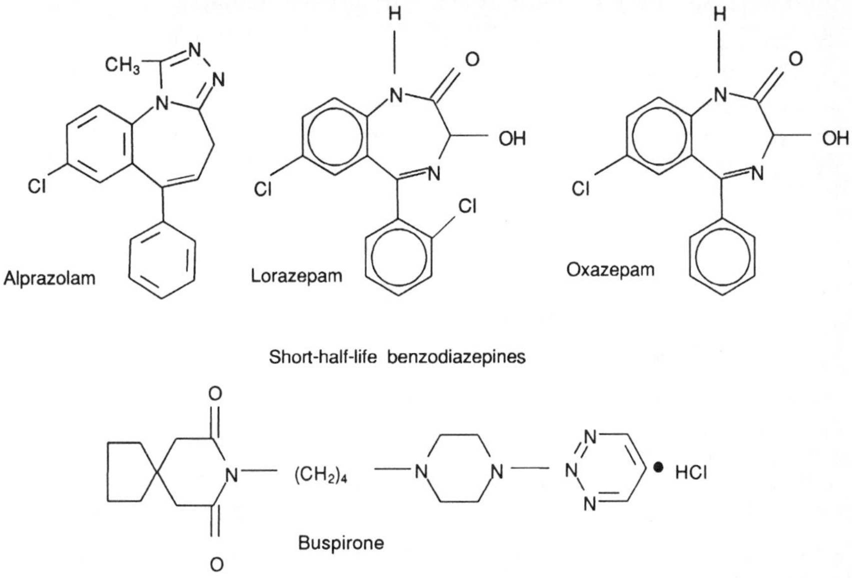

CH_3 N N N Cl Alprazolam

H N O OH N Cl Cl Lorazepam

H N O OH N Cl Oxazepam

Short-half-life benzodiazepines

O N — $(CH_2)_4$ — N N — N N N • HCl O

Buspirone

Figure 8-1 (*Continued*)

Table 8-7 Drugs used in the treatment of generalized anxiety disorder

Generic	Brand name	Approximate dose equivalents, mg	Dosage range, mg/day	
			Adult	Elderly
Benzodiazepine				
Short-acting				
Alprazolam	Xanax	0.5	0.25 - 2.0	0.125 - 1.0
Lorazepam	Ativan[a]	1	1 - 4	0.5 - 2
Oxazepam	Serax[a]	15	10 - 60	10 - 30
Long-acting				
Chlordiazepoxide	Librium[a]	10	10 - 100	5 - 30
Clorazepate	Tranxene	7.5	15 - 60	7.5 - 15
Diazepam	Valium[a]	5	5 - 30	2 - 10
Halazepam	Paxipam	20	20 - 120	20 - 40
Prazepam	Centrax	10	20 - 60	10 - 15
Azaspirodecanedione				
Buspirone	BuSpar	—	15 - 60	15 - 45

[a]Available generic.

Table 8-8 Pharmacokinetic differences of benzodiazepines

Generic	(Trade)	Half-life h Parent	Metabolite	Lipid solubility	Indication
Midazolam	(Versed)	1-4	—	High	Preanesthetic
Triazolam	(Halcion)	2-6	—	—	Hypnotic
Oxazepam	(Serax)	5-15	—	Moderate	Antianxiety
Alprazolam	(Xanax)	8-15	—	Moderate	Antianxiety, antipanic
Temazepam	(Restoril)	8-20	5-15[a]	Moderate	Hypnotic
Estazolam	(ProSom)	8-24	—	Moderate	Hypnotic
Lorazepam	(Ativan)	10-20	—	Moderate	Antianxiety
Chlordiazepoxide	(Librium)	10-30	40-200[a-c]	Moderate	Antianxiety
Diazepam	(Valium)	20-50	40-200[a,c]	High	Antianxiety
Clonazepam	(Klonopin)	18-50	—	Low	Anticonvulsant, antipanic[d]
Flurazepam	(Dalmane)	1-2	50-200[e]	High	Hypnotic
Quazepam	(Doral)	20-40	50-200[e]	High	Hypnotic
Clorazepate	(Tranxene, Azene)	20-50	40-200[a,c]	High	Antianxiety
Prazepam	(Centrax)	20-50	40-200[a,c]	Low	Antianxiety
Halazepam	(Paxipam)	14	40-200[a,c]	Low	Antianxiety

[a]Oxazepam.
[b]Desmethylchlordiazepoxide, demoxepam.
[c]Desmethyldiazepam.
[d]Not FDA approved.
[e]Desalkylflurazepam.
Source: Adapted from Refs. 2, 13, 22, 31, 101.

long-acting) and oral potency in milligrams (high or low potency). For a comparison of dosing and pharmacokinetic differences see Tables 8-7 and 8-8. The shorter-acting agents are not metabolized in the liver to active metabolites but are conjugated to glucuronide and then eliminated in the urine.[31] The two anxiolytic benzodiazepines in this category are lorazepam and oxazepam. Neither drug has a problem with accumulation after chronic dosing, and their half-life is minimally affected by liver dysfunction or by changes in metabolism that occur with aging. Although alprazolam is considered a short-acting agent, it does have a number of minor metabolites and its half-life increases with age (e.g., 11 h in young males and 19 h in elderly males).[31] Alprazolam is currently the most widely prescribed benzodiazepine in the United States and accounts for 25 percent of all benzodiazepine prescriptions.[60]

Due to the short half-lives of lorazepam, oxazepam, and alprazolam, these agents must be administered two to four times daily for continuous coverage of anxiety symptoms. If they are not administered on a regular schedule, there may be a breakthrough of symptoms between doses.[61] The shorter-acting benzodiazepines have more problems with withdrawal reactions if abruptly stopped after long-term treatment, particularly the higher potency agents like alprazolam and lorazepam. The higher-potency agents may bind more tightly to the benzodiazepine receptor and are more likely to cause severe withdrawal syndromes if the drug is abruptly discontinued.[11,62] Of the shorter-acting agents, only lorazepam is available parenterally (IM or IV) and is frequently used when oral dosing is impossible (e.g., acute agitation, seizures). Although all the short-acting agents are effective in the treatment of anxiety, oxazepam (a short-acting, low-potency agent) may be the preferred anxiolytic in elderly patients.[14,34]

The longer-acting anxiolytic benzodiazepines (diazepam, chlordiazepoxide, clorazepate, prazepam, halazepam) have a longer duration of action due to their active metabolites. All of the long-half-life benzodiazepines require oxidation. Then they are conjugated to form glucuronide metabolites that are renally excreted. Diazepam, clorazepate, prazepam, and halazepam are all metabolized to oxazepam and to desmethyldiazepam (which has a half-life of 100 to 200 h in the elderly). Clorazepate and prazepam are prodrugs and are not active until they are biotransformed to desmethyldiazepam in the stomach (clorazepate) or liver (prazepam). Chlordiazepoxide is metabolized to desmethylchlordiazepoxide, demoxepam, oxazepam, and desmethyldiazepam. The mean half-lives of the longer acting agents are significantly increased with advancing age or with liver dysfunction.[13,31] Elderly patients taking longer-acting benzodiazepines (>24 h) have an increased risk of falls and hip fractures in comparison to patients on short-acting agents.[63] For this reason, the dose of long-acting agents should be increased gradually (no sooner than once every 7 to 14 days), since it takes several weeks to achieve steady-state serum concentrations. Some long-half-life benzodiazepines can be administered once a day (or possibly every other day).[31] There are fewer problems with withdrawal reactions when the longer-acting agent is abruptly stopped due to more gradual tapering of the drug from the body.

Benzodiazepines have a propensity to cause physical dependence, abuse, and withdrawal after chronic treatment.[61] Patients with a history of alcohol or drug abuse are at increased risk for dependence and withdrawal problems, and so should not receive benzodiazepines.[58,61] There is some evidence that elderly medical patients do not abuse benzodiazepines and actually take less than is prescribed.[59] But there are some elderly patients who become psychologically dependent and reluctant to discontinue the medications.[11]

Benzodiazepines can cause withdrawal reactions after abrupt discontinuation after chronic dosing.[61] Patients taking a benzodiazepine for longer than 8 months are five times more likely to experience a withdrawal syndrome than those taking the drug for less than 1 month. Thus, patients should not receive benzodiazepines for longer than 6 months without an attempt to discontinue the medication.[58] There is some clinical evidence that discontinuation of benzodiazepines may be more difficult in older patients,[14] but others have found no difference in tapering or withdrawal problems compared to younger patients.[64] Patients should be monitored for the reemergence of the original anxiety symptoms (or rebound anxiety) and withdrawal symptoms during benzodiazepine discontinuation.[61] Short-half-life agents produce withdrawal symptoms within 1 to 2 days, whereas there is a delay in the onset of symptoms with long-half-life agents (e.g., 3 to 5 days). The withdrawal syndrome may be uncomfortable for several days (e.g., increased blood pressure, pulse and respiration rate, sweating, tremors, muscle weakness/aching, nervousness, decreased appetite, insomnia, tinnitus, perceptual distortions), but the symptoms gradually subside over several weeks.[62] Severe withdrawal symptoms are more pronounced and may be life threatening (e.g., delirium, psychosis, visual and auditory hallucinations, depersonalization, hyperthermia, and seizures). Seizures are more common after high-dose, long-term treatment or with concomitant drugs that lower the seizure threshold.[61]

Patients exhibiting any withdrawal symptoms should be closely monitored, particularly patients taking high doses for a long period of time. The higher potency, short-half-life benzodiazepines (e.g., alprazolam and lorazepam) may have more problems and need to be tapered more gradually to avoid a serious withdrawal syndrome.[58,61,62] There is some evidence that doses may be rapidly lowered by 50 percent during the first week, but the second 50 percent reduction requires a longer and more gradual reduction over 4 to 8 weeks (e.g., one-eighth reduction every 4 to 7 days).[62] Patients on short-half-life benzodiazepines who do not tolerate the gradual tapering method may benefit from switching to a long-half-life agent (e.g., switching alprazolam to clonazepam or diazepam), then tapering off the long-half-life agent.[62] Some recommend that a higher equivalent dose of the long-half-life benzodiazepine may be required for a successful substitution.[62] Carbamazepine in doses of 200 to 800 mg/day has also been used to prevent benzodiazepine withdrawal and to rapidly taper patients off of alprazolam.[62] Preliminary results in small numbers of patients indicate that concomitant use of imipramine or buspirone may also be useful in benzodiazepine discontinuation and help to prevent the reemergence of anxiety symptoms.[62]

At higher doses, benzodiazepines can interfere with memory and concentration and impair psychomotor functioning, particularly if combined with alcohol or other sedative-hypnotics.[61,65,66] Elderly subjects may be more sensitive to drowsiness and CNS depression with benzodiazepines. Thus they should be maintained on the lowest possible dose to treat the anxiety disorder.[14,37] Anterograde amnesia (the inability to learn new information) has been reported with several benzodiazepines (e.g., triazolam, diazepam).[67] The amnestic effect appears to be worse with higher doses (due to sedation) and with higher lipophilic agents (more rapid onset of activity).[31,66] The benzodiazepines may cause impairment of delayed recall but not immediate recall of information.[31] In some extremely anxious patients, benzodiazepines may actually improve recall and memory.[31]

A recent study comparing the cognitive performance of elderly subjects on buspirone versus alprazolam reported that alprazolam (0.25 mg tid) had minimal effect on memory, psychomotor speed, and vigilance on the first day and no effects after repeated doses up to 14 days. With repeated doses, there may be a tolerance to adverse effects on cognitive and motor performance.[66] (For a complete review on cognitive and performance studies with benzodiazepines in the elderly, see Ref.

66.) There is an increased potential for sedative effects and memory impairment during the initiation of therapy. Thus, elderly patients should be started on the lowest possible dose (one-third to one-half the recommended adult dose). If any deterioration of cognition or motor coordination occurs (e.g., impaired driving skills), the dose should be lowered or discontinued.[14]

Benzodiazepines may have an increased risk of causing disinhibition and dyscontrol (e.g., aggressive outbursts, hostility, irritability, agitation) in elderly demented patients.[1,11,68] Patients should be closely monitored for impairment of neurologic functioning and worsening of behaviors when placed on benzodiazepines.

Although benzodiazepines are considered to cause less respiratory depression than barbiturates, they may cause suppression of respiration at higher doses.[31] Patients with chronic obstructive pulmonary disease, bronchitis, emphysema, or sleep apnea may be highly susceptible to the respiratory depressant effect and should probably not receive benzodiazepines unless closely monitored.[1] If a benzodiazepine is tried, the short-half-life agents (e.g., lorazepam, oxazepam, or alprazolam) are considered first line in patients with lung disease.

Benzodiazepines should be prescribed at the lowest therapeutic dose (preferably a short-half-life, low-potency agent) for the briefest period of time to treat the GAD.[11] Long-term therapy should only be used if there is a definite psychiatric indication (e.g., panic disorder) and if there is frequent monitoring of clinical efficacy and safety. Benzodiazepines are generally not considered as effective antidepressants. The exception to this is alprazolam, which may down-regulate beta-adrenergic receptors (like antidepressants) and may be useful in higher doses for treating depression with or without anxiety symptoms.[39] Alprazolam is not approved by the Federal Drug Administration (FDA) as an antidepressant, so it should be reserved for anxiety disorders or possibly for mixed anxiety-depressive conditions.

Buspirone Buspirone (BuSpar), an azapirone, has been shown to be as effective as benzodiazepines in the treatment of GAD.[11] Buspirone is a partial agonist of the presynaptic and postsynaptic 5-HT_{1A} receptors. It may also down-regulate postsynaptic 5-HT_2 receptors, similar to antidepressants. Azapirones are thought to normalize serotonergic functioning by increasing serotonin activity in depression and decreasing serotonin activity in anxiety.[69] In addition to the serotonergic effects, buspirone may act as a mixed dopamine agonist at the postsynaptic receptor and as an antagonist at both the presynaptic autoreceptor and postsynaptic dopamine receptor sites. The exact effect on dopaminergic neurotransmission is still under investigation. In higher doses (i.e., up to 90 mg/day) buspirone may have antidepressant activity[70,71] and decrease agitation in elderly demented patients.[54] Buspirone has a delayed onset of activity and may take 1 or 2 weeks before anxiolytic effects occur and up to 3 or 4 weeks for full clinical effect.

Buspirone has not been extensively studied in elderly patients; however, many elderly patients participated in clinical trials, and no unusual adverse effects were identified nor was modification in dosing required. Buspirone is rapidly and completely absorbed from the gastrointestinal (GI) tract and has extensive first-pass hepatic metabolism (only about 4 percent of the drug reaches systemic circulation after oral administration). Buspirone is extensively distributed in the body and is 95 percent bound to plasma proteins. The elimination half-life of buspirone is approximately 2 to 4 h (range of 2 to 11 h) and may be prolonged in patients with renal impairment (anuria) or with hepatic dysfunction (cirrhosis). Buspirone has several metabolites and the major metabolite, 1-pyrimidinylpiperazine (1-PP), may have some anxiolytic activity.

For the treatment of anxiety in the elderly, buspirone is dosed at 5 mg three times daily, and after several weeks, the dose may be increased by 5 mg/day every 2 to 4 days up to 20 to 30 mg/day. The maximum recommended daily dose is 60 mg/day. Although there are no confirmed guidelines, the dose of buspirone should be reduced by 25 to 50 percent in patients with renal or hepatic impairment. Buspirone is not effective prn and so must be dosed regularly for therapeutic effect. In doses of 15 mg/day, the most common adverse effects are gastric complaints, nausea, vomiting, dizziness, drowsiness, headache, miosis, sleep disturbances, and fatigue.[72,73] There is some evidence that elderly patients may have more problems tolerating buspirone's adverse effects than younger adults.

Buspirone appears to be well tolerated in elderly patients (e.g., it is nonsedating, has minimal cardiovascular effects, does not cause respiratory depression, does not impair cognitive or psychomotor performance, and does not potentiate the effects of alcohol or other CNS depressants). Buspirone, in doses of 15 mg/day, has no effect on memory, attention/concentration, and psychomotor function in normal elderly subjects.[65] It has a large margin of safety and is safe in overdoses (no deaths have been reported in humans either due to intentional or accidental overdosage). Buspirone has no apparent abuse potential, it does not cause a withdrawal syndrome when the medication is abruptly discontinued, and there is no evidence of tolerance after long-term treatment. Buspirone is not cross tolerant with benzodiazepines and so will not prevent a benzodiazepine withdrawal syndrome.[31] If a patient is switched from a benzodiazepine to buspirone, it may be best to start concurrent buspirone therapy for several weeks. Then the benzodiazepine should be gradually withdrawn to avoid an abstinence syndrome.

Antidepressants Tricyclic antidepressants (TCAs) are also beneficial in GAD, especially if patients have depressive symptoms or if they require long-term treatment.[22,39,58] Elderly patients may have difficulty tolerating the sedative and anticholinergic side effects of the tertiary amine TCAs (e.g., amitriptyline, imipramine, and doxepin). Secondary amine agents (e.g., desipramine and nortriptyline) are better tolerated because of less sedative and anticholinergic side effects. The newer antidepressants (e.g., fluoxetine, bupropion, and sertraline) have less anticholinergic and cardiovascular effects but may cause overstimulation (e.g., insomnia, nervousness, tremor, agitation) and make anxiety symptoms worse. For a more complete description of antidepressants, see Chap. 15.

Panic Disorder with or without Agoraphobia

The characteristic feature of the panic disorder (PD) is a "panic attack" (a discrete period of intense fear and autonomic discharge that lasts several minutes to an hour and is not expected or triggered by the attention of others). The intensity of the attacks usually peaks by 10 min and tapers off within 60 min. Elderly patients who develop a late-onset PD may think they are experiencing a myocardial infarction or transient ischemic attack and seek emergency treatment.[44] The diagnosis of PD is usually made after the individual has experienced several panic attacks and there are no positive laboratory tests. Symptoms of panic attacks resemble other medical conditions (e.g., myocardial infarction, mitral valve prolapse, angina, hypertension, hyperthyroidism, seizure disorders, asthma), so these conditions should be excluded before making the diagnosis.[44,74] Several pharmacologic agents and exogenous factors may precipitate panic attacks so patients should be closely evaluated for any possible cause of organic PD.[34]

The onset of PD usually begins in the twenties (rarely before age 12 or after age 40) and is more common in women.[44,74] There is a high genetic risk for PD and the illness may run in families.[46] The lifetime prevalence of recurrent panic attacks may be as high as 3 to 4 percent, although the Epidemiologic Catchment Area study reported that 1.5 percent of the adult population has a PD.[44,75] PD is approximately twice as common in the 25-to-44 age group than in the over-65 age group.[75]

The DSM-III-R diagnostic criteria for PD requires that patients must have either four panic attacks within a 4-week period or one or more attacks followed by at least a month of persistent fear of having another attack.[4] The panic attacks usually involve intense apprehension coupled with physical symptoms (e.g., palpitations, chest pain, shortness of breath, choking sensation, dizziness, and faintness). Most patients with PD develop agoraphobia (the fear of being in places or situations from which escape might be difficult or embarrassing). PD patients have significant anticipatory anxiety that they will have another attack. Thus they develop avoidance behaviors (e.g., restrict travel by bus, train, or car and avoid elevators, shopping malls, and public places). Patients with agoraphobia usually become housebound and incapacitated for several years before they seek treatment.[12]

Nonpharmacologic approaches for PD include reassurance, patient education, supportive psychotherapy, cognitive behavioral therapy, relaxation, exercise, breathing retraining, imagery, and hypnosis.[74] The treatment of phobias requires real-life exposure to the phobic stimulus with a gradual desensitization program. These nonpharmacologic therapies may be sufficient for some selected patients, but usually combination therapy with medications is most beneficial.

Pharmacologic treatments of PD include the benzodiazepines (e.g., alprazolam, clonazepam), the TCAs (e.g., imipramine, desipramine, nortriptyline), and MAOIs (e.g., phenelzine and tranylcypromine; Table 8-9). Although most of these agents are effective in treating PD, there is a major difference in onset of action and side effects. Most of these medications will block panic attacks, but some patients require behavioral therapy to treat the phobia. Therapy of approxi-

Table 8-9 Drugs used in the treatment of panic disorder

Class/generic	Brand name	Antipanic dosage range, mg/day[a] Adult	Elderly
Heterocyclic antidepressants			
Tricyclic antidepressants			
Imipramine	Tofranil	125-300	50-150
Nortriptyline	Pamelor	50-150	25-75
Newer antidepressants			
Fluoxetine	Prozac	5-80	5-40
Monoamine oxidase inhibitors			
Phenelzine	Nardil	45-90	30-60
Benzodiazepines			
Alprazolam	Xanax[b]	4-8	1.5-6
Clonazepam	Klonopin	3-6	1-4

[a]Estimated dosing ranges for adults and elderly.
[b]FDA approved for panic disorder.

mately one-third of PD patients who respond to treatment can be tapered off after 6 months, one-third may need a longer treatment to achieve a complete remission, and the other third of patients may need to be treated indefinitely.[74] Patients may relapse after medications are discontinued, and they should be reassured that this is expected with a chronic illness and is not a personal shortcoming.[58]

Heterocyclic antidepressants Of the TCAs, imipramine has been the most widely studied and prescribed agent for PD. Although other heterocyclic antidepressants may have antipanic effect, more clinical trials are needed to determine efficacy and dosing recommendations. Imipramine is usually started with doses of 10 to 25 mg/day in younger adults, but for elderly patients, doses should be low (e.g., 5 to 10 mg at bedtime, increased by 10 to 20 mg/day every 3 days as tolerated until 75 to 100 mg/day). Very little information is available about the use of antipanic agents in the elderly and if they respond differently than younger patients. Most younger patients require at least 150 mg/day of imipramine, but some may not respond until doses of 200 to 300 mg/day are reached, whereas other patients may respond to very low doses.[76,77]

There are several adverse effects associated with TCAs which may limit their clinical use (see Chap. 15 for more detailed information). PD patients often become overstimulated from antidepressants (particularly desipramine, fluoxetine) and complain of insomnia, irritability, jitteriness, and increased energy. Patients who experience the stimulatory side effects may need lower doses or require the addition of a benzodiazepine or beta-blocking agent until the stimulation subsides with continued use.[78] Approximately 30 percent of patients discontinue treatment because of adverse effects.[24] The new nontricyclic agents such as trazodone and bupropion may not be as effective for PD according to early efficacy studies.[79] Fluoxetine, a serotonin-selective antidepressant, may be effective in PDs but can cause overstimulation like imipramine and so should be started with low doses (5 to 10 mg/day) and gradually titrated up to 20 to 40 mg/day.[80]

MAOIs are usually reserved as a second or third choice or if the TCA is not tolerated or effective. Phenelzine in doses of up to 90 mg/day has been shown to be effective in PD in younger adults.[76] Although tranylcypromine has been prescribed for PD, its efficacy has not been well studied. MAOIs are stimulating and may cause insomnia (particularly tranylcypromine) and so should be started at a low dose and gradually titrated upward over 1 to 2 weeks. Phenelzine is usually started at 15 mg/day and increased by 15 mg/day every 3 to 4 days until 45 to 60 mg/day is reached.

MAOIs cause several adverse effects and require avoidance of foods and beverages that may decrease patient compliance and acceptance (see Chap. 15). Some of the most bothersome side effects include postural hypotension, weight gain, and sexual dysfunction.[24] Because of dietary and drug restrictions (avoidance of foods and beverages high in tyramine and CNS stimulants or sympathomimetics due to increased risk of a hypertensive crises), only the most compliant and reliable patient should receive MAOIs. If a patient has previously been receiving a TCA, there should be a 2-week washout before the MAOI is started to avoid a potential drug interaction. Because of the long half-life of fluoxetine, a 5-to-6-week washout is recommended before the MAOI is started.[24]

Both imipramine and phenelzine usually take 3 to 5 weeks to stop panic attacks and up to 6 to 10 weeks to improve phobic avoidance behaviors.[24,81] Once patients are stabilized on an antidepressant, the dose may be gradually lowered to a maintenance dose (e.g., decrease by 10 to 25 mg imipramine every month) until the reemergence of anxiety or panic symptoms. PD patients should be kept on the lowest maintenance dose that controls symptoms for approximately 6 months.[58] At this time, a discontinuation trial should be attempted. Dosing reduction schedules should be done gradually (e.g., 10 to 25 mg imipramine every 2 to 4 weeks). If symptoms reemerge, then the dose may be increased and continued for another 6 to 12 months.[76] Because PD is often a chronic illness, some patients may need to take antipanic medications indefinitely.

Benzodiazepines Alprazolam, a triazolobenzodiazepine, is widely accepted for the treatment of both GAD and PD. Alprazolam in higher doses (up to 8 mg/day) has documented efficacy in the treatment of PD and was recently approved by the FDA for this indication. Although some patients respond to lower doses of alprazolam (1 to 2 mg/day), most patients require higher doses (3 to 6 mg/day).[82] Other benzodiazepines (e.g., clonazepam, lorazepam, and diazepam) may also have antipanic properties in higher doses but require further studies to determine efficacy. Alprazolam has an advantage of working faster than TCAs and MAOIs (e.g., antipanic and antiphobic effect has been reported within the first week or two of treatment).[82-84] Because alprazolam has a short half-life, it should be given three or four times a day. There have been problems with breakthrough panic (or interdose rebound), so regular dosing is required.

Clonazepam, an anticonvulsant, has been shown to be effective for PD in higher doses. It has an advantage of having a longer half-life (20 to 50 h), so it can be administered once or twice daily.[85] Patients who cannot be stabilized on alprazolam due to interdose panic attacks can be switched to clonazepam (dosing equivalence is approximately 0.5 to 1 mg clonazepam equals 1 mg alprazolam). Clonazepam may have a higher risk of causing depression and sedation than alprazolam.[86] Higher doses of benzodiazepines have a potential to impair memory, concentration, alertness, and motor coordination and should be closely monitored in the elderly. These agents should be used cautiously in patients with depression or in those with a history of alcohol or drug abuse.[77]

Alprazolam or clonazepam dosing should initially be low and gradually increased over 3 to 4 weeks as tolerated until clinical response (e.g., alprazolam 0.25 mg tid and increased by 0.25 mg every 2 to 4 days up to 3 mg/day; clonazepam 0.25 mg bid and increased by 0.25 every 3 to 4 days up to 2 mg/day).[85] Side effects such as sedation, drowsiness, ataxia, faintness, dizziness, and fatigue usually are lessened by lowering the dose, dividing the dose, giving the larger portion of dose at bedtime, or giving the dose with food.[87] Tolerance to the side effects usually occurs after a few days, so patients should be instructed not to increase the dose until they tolerate the side effects. Some patients may go through several dosage plateaus before an ideal dose is obtained.[82]

There are few studies assessing the long-term efficacy and safety of benzodiazepines in PD. Initial reports suggest there is no tolerance to therapeutic effects for alprazolam after 8 months of therapy.[74] The most frequently reported side effects with long-term alprazolam treatment include changes in libido, weight loss, headache, and depressed mood.[74]

Benzodiazepines may cause dependence and withdrawal, especially after high-dose, long-term use.[24] Therefore, discontinuation of alprazolam (or clonazepam) should be done gradually over 4 to 24 weeks (approximately 0.25 to 0.5 mg/week) to avoid rebound panic attacks and withdrawal symptoms.[85] Some patients on higher doses of alprazolam may take up to 8 weeks to totally discontinue the medication and may still experience some mild-to-moderate symptoms with the slow taper method.[88]

Obsessive Compulsive Disorder

Obsessive compulsive disorder (OCD) is characterized by ritualistic behavior that helps to reduce anxiety or other distressing symptoms which are triggered by an obsessional thought. Although the onset of OCD is very rare after the age of 50, patients may not present for treatment until they are older.[29,89] Patients with OCD may not admit to their symptoms. Thus they do not seek medical treatment until they have the disorder for many years. OCD is considered a chronic disorder that may never completely respond to treatment.[58,90] OCD has a high comorbidity with other disorders (e.g., generalized anxiety, panic attacks, major depression, Tourette's syndrome, schizophrenia, anorexia).[29]

The lifetime prevalence of OCD may be as high as 2 to 3 percent of the population and is frequently associated with depression.[74] One-third of OCD cases begin by the age of 15 and continue throughout adulthood.[78] OCD patients have a very high relapse rate if treatment is discontinued and rarely respond to placebo treatment. OCD is sometimes confused with obsessive compulsive personality disorder, which begins in early adulthood and has a pervasive pattern of perfectionism and inflexibility but does not interfere with the patient's functioning, as does OCD.

There are several subtypes of OCD (e.g., cleaning rituals, checking compulsions, placing objects in a certain order, obsessive thoughts only, obsessional slowness, or mixed rituals).[29] The most common obsessions involve thoughts of contamination (with cleaning or washing rituals), doubts (with checking behavior), and thoughts of violence.[12,29] Patients with compulsive rituals usually have obsessional thoughts which cause a great deal of anxiety. Because of health concerns, elderly patients often have obsessional fears of having an illness (e.g., cancer, AIDS) and seek medical treatment.[89]

Patients with OCD should be educated about the disorder and receive supportive therapy since it is extremely distressing to the patient and family. Behavioral therapy (based on teaching the patient how to alter or control compulsive rituals) may be more effective in reducing compulsive behaviors than obsessions.[90] Patients are exposed to stimuli that cause the obsessional fears (either in real life or by imagination) so that the fear and distress are decreased with continued exposure and the person tries to decrease the ritualistic behaviors.[90]

Patients with obsessive thoughts only or with both obsessions and compulsions should be given a trial of antidepressant medication. Combined behavioral therapy and pharmacotherapy is usually recommended for most patients. Although numerous antidepressants have been reported to be useful in treating OCD (e.g., imipramine, amitriptyline, doxepin, trazodone, fluoxetine, fluvoxamine, phenelzine, tranylcypromine, lithium carbonate), only clomipramine has been approved by the FDA for OCD in the United States.

Clomipramine, a tricyclic antidepressant, is very similar to imipramine (except for a chlorine atom in the 3 position), but it has significantly more serotonergic activity.[90] Clomipramine has prominent side effects (e.g., anticholinergic effects, orthostatic hypotension, tachycardia, muscle twitches, tremor, fatigue, and weight gain) which may not be tolerated by elderly patients. It also causes sexual disturbances (anorgasmia or delayed ejaculation) and has an increased risk of seizures at higher doses. Initial dosing of clomipramine is 25 mg/day, with gradual dosing increases of 25 to 50 mg/day up to 200 to 250 mg/day.[91]

Because of clomipramine's adverse effects, it may not be the drug of choice for elderly patients. Fluoxetine, a highly serotonergic antidepressant, has been shown to be effective in several uncontrolled and controlled OCD studies.[91] Fluoxetine is started at 10 to 20 mg in the morning (due to overstimulation and insomnia) and gradually increased by 10 to 20 mg every 3 to 4 days up to doses of

60 to 80 mg/day.[91] Side effects commonly reported with fluoxetine are nausea, weight loss, headache, anxiety, insomnia, and inhibited orgasm.[90] Fluoxetine also causes inhibition of liver enzyme metabolism that may increase serum levels of other medications (e.g., tricyclic antidepressants). Initial improvement may be evident by 4 to 8 weeks, but an adequate trial usually takes 10 to 12 weeks.[89] Clinical improvement of OCD is usually defined as a partial reduction in symptoms (e.g., 50 percent reduction).[91] Patients who have an adequate response at higher doses may be tried on a lower dose for maintenance therapy.

OCD patients with psychotic symptoms may respond to antipsychotic agents (e.g., pimozide) along with clomipramine or fluoxetine, but these should be avoided unless the symptoms are severe.[89] Patients with significant anxiety symptoms may benefit from an augmenting trial of a benzodiazepine or buspirone. Buspirone has been shown to augment the effects of fluoxetine in an open OCD trial[90] and was equally effective as clomipramine for the acute treatment of OCD (in doses of 60 mg/day) in a preliminary clinical trial.[92] Clonazepam, a benzodiazepine that may affect serotonergic transmission, may have antiobsessional properties according to preliminary open studies. L-Tryptophan (a serotonin precursor) in doses of 6 g/day has been used as an augmenting agent with clomipramine, but it is currently unavailable due to problems with an eosinophilia-myalgia syndrome.[89,90] Lithium in doses of 600 to 900 mg/day has been used as an adjunctive treatment to increase serotonin transmission and may be effective in some patients.[90,91] Patients who are refractory to standard treatments (and depressed) may respond to electroconvulsive therapy (ECT).[89] Only the most severe and treatment-resistant OCD patients should consider psychosurgery.[89] Although psychosurgery is reserved for severe cases, it may cause 80 percent improvement in OCD symptoms.[90]

Social Phobias

Social phobias are characterized by an exaggerated fear of being scrutinized or evaluated by others that results in avoidance of specific social situations.[93] There are two different subtypes of social phobias (i.e., specific or generalized), and both may interfere with social and occupational functioning.[93] A specific social phobia is isolated to a performance type of fear with accompanying avoidance behavior (e.g., fear of urinating in a public toilet, writing a check, eating in the presence of others, musical performance, or public speaking).[93] The generalized phobia is more widespread (e.g., difficulty with authority figures, dating strangers, or socializing with new people). Social phobias usually begin in childhood or adolescence and may follow a chronic course with concomitant generalized anxiety or panic attacks.[93]

The prevalence of social phobia is approximately 1.2 to 2 percent of the general population.[93] The Epidemiologic Catchment Area Study reported a 6-month prevalence rate of 1.5 to 2.6 percent for women and 0.9 to 1.7 percent for men.[16] Patients with social phobias frequently use alcohol to self-treat their fears, and alcohol dependence has a 20 percent comorbidity rate.[94]

Elderly patients with a social phobia may have significant anticipation or fear of one or more situations along with symptoms of anxiety (e.g., tremor, tachycardia, sweating). This often leads to an avoidance behavior and impairment of social functioning (e.g., not going out of the home, avoiding social events). Treatment of this disorder will usually require both psychologic treatments (to reduce avoidance behavior and negative cognition) and pharmacologic agents (to reduce the anticipatory and phobic anxiety).[93]

Nonpharmacologic treatment approaches include exposure therapy, cognitive therapy, and social skills training.[95] Pharmacologic treatments include beta blockers (propranolol, atenolol), MAOIs (phenelzine), and benzodiazepines (alprazolam and clonazepam). Beta blockers are better for the pretreatment of a specific feared situation. A single dose of a beta blocker taken 45 to 60 min prior to a specific performance situation (e.g., public speaking) has demonstrated benefit in younger adults, but no studies have been performed in elderly patients to determine safety and efficacy. Caution should be used in the elderly, since high doses of beta blockers may lower blood pressure and pulse and result in weakness, fatigue, and memory difficulties. Beta blockers should not be used in elderly patients with asthma, diabetes, CHF, or significant bradycardia. A trial of a beta blocker should be done to determine the best dose that eliminates the physical symptoms of anxiety without causing significant reductions in heart rate (below 60 beats/min) or blood pressure. Therapeutic effects are usually observed with 5 to 10 mg of propranolol one to four times a day.[96] Patients with more generalized social phobia may benefit from the daily use of a more cardioselective beta blocker (e.g., atenolol 50 to 100 mg/day).[96]

Phenelzine has been studied for phobic disorder and appears to be more effective than atenolol for the generalized type of disorder.[97] Phenelzine is usually prescribed 15 mg two to three times daily and increased up to 45 to 90 mg/day depending on clinical response.[93] Benzodiazepines such as alprazolam and clonazepam may also be effective for social phobias and can be taken either as needed (prior to the phobic situation) or on a daily basis if the symptoms are severe. The therapeutic effects of benzodiazepines are usually evident very rapidly or within the first week of treatment. Open studies with fluoxetine and buspirone indicate clinical efficacy in social phobia.[98]

Long-term studies have not been performed in elderly patients to determine the best treatment or therapeutic dose range for social phobias. Patients may require different trials of medications to determine which agent produces the best benefit with minimal adverse effects.

Posttraumatic Stress Disorder

Posttraumatic stress disorder (PTSD) may develop at any age after the exposure to a traumatic event (outside the normal range of life experiences). There is little information about age differences in the clinical presentation or causes of PTSD. PTSD is characterized by reexperiencing the event along with increased autonomic arousal and persistent avoidance behavior or numbing of responsiveness. Examples of PTSD situations include a natural disaster, war, automobile accident, rape, sexual abuse, house fire, or burglary.[12] Often there is severe psychologic distress if the person is exposed to a situation that resembles the traumatic event. Patients often exhibit sleep disturbances (nightmares), irritability, explosive outbursts, social withdrawal, and high levels of anxiety and somatic complaints. The lifetime prevalence rate of PTSD is approximately 1 percent and up to 15 percent of people may experience PTSD after a severe traumatic event.[99] PTSD has a high comorbidity risk of depression, phobias, PD, and alcohol and substance abuse.[27]

There are few controlled studies of pharmacologic treatment of PTSD.[27] Several antidepressants have shown clinical improvement of PTSD symptoms (e.g., desipramine, doxepin, imipramine, amitriptyline, phenelzine).[27] PTSD patients with depression or panic attacks may benefit from a 6-to-8-week antidepressant trial to assess clinical response. Although the pharmacologic agents often decrease the hyperarousal state, the avoidance and withdrawal behaviors usually respond poorly to medications.[27] Education, supportive group therapy, psychotherapy, and relaxation techniques and/or biofeedback can be helpful in some patients.

Other agents that may be effective either alone or in combination with an antidepressant are clonidine or propranolol. Both agents reduce adrenergic activity resulting in a decrease in intrusive dreams, recollections, sleep disturbance, startle response, and increased vigilance in PTSD patients.[27] Propranolol is dosed 10 to 20 mg tid and increased gradually every 3 days to avoid hypotension (systolic pressure less than 90) or bradycardia (pulse rate less than 50). Clonidine dosing is approximately 0.05 to 0.1 mg bid, increased gradually to 0.6 mg/day in divided doses. Common adverse effects occurring with clonidine include drowsiness, dry mouth, constipation, dizziness, headache, and fatigue. Usually these adverse effects decrease with continued therapy or may be relieved by a reduction in dose. Beta blockers may also be used to pretreat PTSD patients prior to reexposure to a situation that reminds them of the traumatic event, similar to the social phobic situation.

Agents used for bipolar disorder (carbamazepine, valproate, and lithium) and PD (alprazolam and clonazepam) have also shown to improve anger, dreams, flashbacks, and startle response in PTSD.[27] Benzodiazepines should be used with caution in patients with alcohol or substance abuse. Nonaddicting anxiolytics such as buspirone may be effective as an augmenting agent for patients with generalized anxiety. PTSD patients frequently complain of sleep disturbances, so sedating antihistamines, antidepressants (e.g., trazodone), or short-acting benzodiazepine hypnotic agents may be helpful for initiating and maintaining sleep.

Simple Phobia

A phobia is an excessive, unreasonable, and persistent fear of a specific object, activity, or situation that results in avoidance behavior. The most common simple phobias are fears of flying, heights, animals (dogs, cats, mice, snakes), insects (bees, spiders), lightning, thunderstorms, and elevators.[12] As long as the person avoids the circumstance or situation, there is little distress. But if there is a chance of experiencing the situation, the person has anticipatory anxiety (e.g., fear, insomnia) and becomes increasingly anxious and distressed until the situation is finished.

Simple phobias are very common with lifetime prevalence rates of 4 percent for men and 9 percent for women,[75] but these rates may be higher in elderly patients.[18] Although most simple phobias begin in childhood and dissipate with age, some people continue to have long-standing phobias. Elderly patients may develop new fears with advancing age which are related to novel situations or poor coping skills.

Most simple phobias can be treated by gradually exposing the person to the feared situation (desensitization) through an exposure program. Some patients may require pretreatment prior to the feared situation (e.g., a benzodiazepine or beta-blocker taken 1 to 2 h before flying) and repeated if needed. Exposure therapy to the phobic situation (along with education and group support) is the recommended treatment for social phobias.

Sleep Disorder

Insomnia is a common complaint in the elderly and is characterized by a problem initiating or maintaining sleep or feeling unrested after an adequate amount of sleep.[55,100] The DSM-III-R diagnosis of insomnia requires that the sleep disturbance occurs at least three times a week for at least a month and results in daytime fatigue, irritability, or impaired daytime functioning.[100] Insomnia is associated with medical disorders (e.g., acute and chronic pain, arthritis, fever, nocturia, dyspnea, sleep apnea), stimulating medications (e.g., over-the-counter decongestants, caffeine, theophylline, amphetamines), and drug/alcohol abuse.[34,55,100,101] For this reason, elderly patients are at increased risk of sleep disturbances. It is estimated that although the elderly only represent 11 to 12 percent of the population, they receive 35 to 40 percent of hypnotic agents.[55,101] (For a more complete description of differential diagnosis and changes in sleep with aging, see Refs. 55, 100, 101.)

A complete evaluation is essential to determine the cause of insomnia so that the actual cause of sleeplessness is treated first.[101] A list of common medical/psychiatric disorders, situations, and medications associated with causing insomnia is found in Table 8-10. Nonpharmacologic treatment approaches (Table 8-11) should be tried first. When pharmacologic treatment is indicated, only short-term therapy should be used. Hypnotics should never be routinely prescribed for insomnia, particularly in hospitals or long-care institutions, since sleep disturbances are usually transient and do not require chronic treatment.[5]

The best hypnotic agent for the elderly should be relatively short-acting (to avoid morning hangover, drowsiness, ataxia) and have minimal effect on sleep stages.[34] A list of commonly prescribed medications used to treat insomnia is found in Table 8-12. Older hypnotics (e.g., barbiturates, glutethimide) suppress REM sleep after chronic use and cause significant REM rebound upon discontinuation. Longer-acting benzodiazepines that accumulate after chronic dosing (flurazepam, quazepam) have an increased risk of causing daytime sedation, ataxia, delirium, and falls with fractures.[63,101]

Table 8-10 Situations, medical and psychiatric disorders, and medications associated with causing insomnia

Medical illnesses
Pain (arthritis, headache)
Nocturia
Hypo- or hyperthyroidism
Angina
Duodenal or peptic ulcer
Congestive heart failure
Sleep disorders
Sleep apnea
Nocturnal myoclonus
Restless leg syndrome
Sleep-wake schedule changes (jet lag, night shifts)
Night terrors or nightmares
Dream anxiety attacks
Psychiatric disorders
Schizophrenia
Depression
Mania
Anxiety (PTSD, GAD, panic, adjustment disorder)
Sleep environment/hygiene
Noise
Temperatures above 24°C
Hunger
Overeating
Medications
Stimulants (sympathomimetics, cold preparations)
Caffeine
Nicotine
Alcohol
Sedative-hypnotic withdrawal
Antidepressants (TCAs, MAOIs, fluoxetine, bupropion)
Situational stressors
Recent travel
Marital difficulties
Financial worries
Bereavement

When prescribing hypnotics in elderly patients, the dose should be initiated one-half to one-third of doses recommended for adults and gradually increased as needed to avoid adverse CNS effects.[101] Patients should not receive chronic hypnotic therapy due to increased risks of dependence, tolerance, and abuse. Patients with chronic insomnia should be closely evaluated for symptoms of depression, a chronic anxiety disorder, or a primary sleep disorder (such as sleep apnea or nocturnal myoclonus).[55,100]

Benzodiazepines in higher doses are effective as hypnotics (even those marketed as anxiolytics), but there are differences in onset of activity (secondary to

Table 8-11 Nonpharmacologic aids for sleep

1. Go to bed and arise at the same time each day.
2. Avoid daytime naps.
3. Maintain a comfortable temperature in the bedroom and use it primarily for sleeping.
4. Exercise regularly (preferably in the afternoon and not at night).
5. Avoid eating a large meal before bedtime (light snack is better).
6. Avoid excessive caffeine, alcohol, or nicotine.
7. Engage in pleasant or relaxing activities prior to sleep (warm bath, sex, light reading).
8. Restrict fluids in the evening (if a problem with nocturia).
9. Avoid taking medications that are stimulating in the late afternoon or evening (take earlier in the day).
10. Control nighttime pain.

Source: Adapted from Refs. 100, 101.

Table 8-12 Medications used to treat insomnia

Class/generic	Brand name	Dosage for elderly, mg, at bedtime
Chloral hydrate	Noctec	500-2000
Antihistamine		
Diphenhydramine	Benadryl	25-50
Hydroxyzine	Vistaril/Atarax	25-50
Benzodiazepines		
Short-acting		
Oxazepam	Serax	10-30
Lorazepam	Ativan	0.5-2
Alprazolam	Xanax	0.25-1
Triazolam	Halcion	0.125-0.25
Temazepam	Restoril	15-30
Estazolam	ProSom	0.5-2
Long-acting		
Flurazepam	Dalmane	15-30
Quazepam	Doral	7.5-15
Sedating antidepressants		
Trazodone	Desyrel	25-75
Amitriptyline	Elavil	25-50
Doxepin	Sinequan	25-50

Source: Adapted from Refs. 100, 101.

absorption and lipophilic properties) and duration of action (secondary to elimination half-life and active metabolites).[55,101,102,103] Highly lipid-soluble benzodiazepines (e.g., diazepam) are rapidly absorbed and rapidly cross the blood-brain barrier to cause clinical effects within 15 to 30 min. The less lipid-soluble agents (e.g., lorazepam, oxazepam, temazepam) diffuse into the brain less extensively and less rapidly and have a delayed onset of action (45 to 90 min). Thus, these agents must be administered 1 to 2 h before bedtime so that the sedation occurs at the desired time to initiate sleep.[100]

A comparison of pharmacokinetic differences between hypnotic agents is listed in Table 8-8.[102] Agents such as estazolam, temazepam, lorazepam, and oxazepam have short to intermediate half-lives (5 to 24 h) and cause less daytime sedation or hangover effect. The longer-half-life agents (flurazepam or quazepam) require liver metabolism (hydroxylation or *N*-dealkylation) and have active desalkyl metabolites with half-lives up to 100 to 200 h in the elderly. The higher-potency benzodiazepines (alprazolam, estazolam, triazolam) are oxidized to relatively minor metabolites with short half-lives and are quickly inactivated by glucuronidation in the liver.[102-103]

The shorter-half-life benzodiazepines are the best choice for the elderly. The most commonly prescribed hypnotic in the United States is triazolam (an ultrashort half-life) that requires 1.5 h to reach peak serum levels and has a half-life of 2.5 to 4.5 h.[55,102] Although triazolam is very effective for initiating sleep, its half-life is so short that it does not work well for patients with early morning awakening or sleep continuity disturbances. Older patients frequently complain of early morning awakening or difficulty falling back to sleep if they awake during the night.[55] It also has more problems with causing anterograde amnesia, delirium, paradoxical reactions, agitation, psychosis, and nightmares than longer-acting benzodiazepines.[55,103] Because these adverse effects are associated with higher doses of triazolam, elderly patients should not receive more than 0.125 mg and rarely should doses greater than 0.25 mg be used.

Temazepam has a short to intermediate half-life (8 to 10 h) and is eliminated by glucuronide conjugation (with a minor active metabolite).[55] It has a slower onset of absorption and delayed onset of action and so must be taken 1 to 2 h before bedtime. Dosing in the elderly should be 15 mg at bedtime since higher doses have increased risks of residual daytime sedation.[55]

Estazolam (a new triazolobenzodiazepine hypnotic) is rapidly absorbed and has an intermediate duration of action (6 to 8 h).[55] Estazolam is metabolized to two minor active metabolites and has a half-life of 12 to 15 h in younger adults. It may have advantages over other hypnotic benzodiazepines since it works as rapidly as triazolam and flurazepam but has a long half-life to help maintain sleep without causing residual daytime sedation.[55]

Although flurazepam and quazepam are effective hypnotics and have a rapid onset of activity (due to the rapid conversion to the active desalkyl metabolite), their half-life is too long for elderly patients.[100] Flurazepam and other long-acting agents such as diazepam and quazepam have increased risk of daytime sedation, impairment of cognition, and psychomotor functioning at higher doses.[55] These agents should be started at lower doses (e.g., 15 mg flurazepam, 2 mg diazepam, 7.5 mg quazepam) and be used cautiously in the elderly.

The abrupt discontinuation of hypnotic benzodiazepines can cause a withdrawal syndrome, which can be a problem in the elderly.[103] Agents with short half-lives cause a more rapid and severe withdrawal syndrome than long-half-life agents. Short-half-life agents should be tapered gradually over several days, whereas long-half-life agents are usually eliminated gradually after abrupt discontinuance and have less rebound and withdrawal phenomena (although there have been reports of withdrawal reactions after stopping flurazepam).[103]

Other nonbenzodiazepine agents used for sleep include antihistamines, chloral hydrate, sedating antidepressants, and L-tryptophan.[101] Since L-tryptophan was taken off the market, it is no longer available as a "natural" sleeping medication. In higher doses, antihistamines (diphenhydramine and hydroxyzine) may cause significant anticholinergic side effects, memory impairment, and delirium. Several over-the-counter sleep aids contain antihistamines, and elderly patients frequently self-medicate with these or alcohol. Diphenhydramine in doses of 50 mg has been shown to be as effective as 15 mg temazepam in elderly patients, although both agents may cause daytime hypersomnolence.[104]

Chloral hydrate is frequently used as a short-term hypnotic in the elderly since it has less effect on daytime sedation and sleep states.[100] Chloral hydrate is rapidly metabolized to trichloroethanol, which causes a rapid hypnotic effect (and has a half-life of approximately 8 h).[105] Chloral hydrate can displace acidic drugs (such as warfarin and phenytoin) from protein-binding sites. Chloral hydrate induces hepatic microsomal enzyme activity that can cause changes in hepatic clearance of other medications. Higher doses (greater than 1.0 g) can cause CNS depression and confusion, so chloral hydrate should be used cautiously in the elderly. The most common adverse effect is gastric irritation or GI upset.[105]

Sedative antidepressants (e.g., trazodone, imipramine, doxepin, and amitriptyline) are also beneficial for sleep induction due to sedation from antihistamine and alpha-adrenergic blockade side effects. Doses of 25 to 50 mg doxepin or amitriptyline have been used for insomnia in nondepressed patients, which is lower than the doses required for the treatment of depression. Trazodone has an advantage over tricyclic antidepressants of not causing anticholinergic or cardiovascular adverse effects and may minimally affect sleep states.[106] A bedtime dose of trazodone (25 to 75 mg) has been used with MAOIs and fluoxetine to counteract acute insomnia and sleep disturbances.[107] Although sedating antidepressants are not approved for the treatment of insomnia in nondepressed patients, they may have a place in therapy for the anxious-depressed patient or for patients with a past drug or alcohol history. Further studies are needed with antidepressants to determine long-term safety and efficacy in elderly patients.

CONSIDERATIONS IN PRESCRIBING ANXIOLYTICS AND HYPNOTICS IN THE ELDERLY

Pharmacokinetic Changes with Aging

There are numerous physiologic changes that occur with aging that may affect the pharmacokinetics of anxiolytics (e.g., changes in absorption, distribution, protein binding, hepatic metabolism, and renal excretion). Elderly patients usually have an increase in total body fat that increases the volume of distribution of highly lipid soluble drugs.[55] There is also a reduction in serum albumin in elderly patients that can result in more free active drug in medications that are highly protein-bound.[55] Hepatic function is very important in the elimination of anxiolytics, particularly the long-half-life agents that have active metabolites. Liver disease or a reduction in hepatic blood flow can result in significant reduction in clearance of these benzodiazepines and can produce CNS toxicity if doses are not reduced.[1] The hepatic cytochrome P-450 activity decreases with age. Thus desmethylation is reduced and can result in higher levels of the parent compound. There is also decreases of oxidation, hydroxylation, and *N*-dealkylation with aging, particularly in men.[1,55] Additionally, the glomerular filtration rate and renal blood flow decline with age, which results in decreased excretion of medications that are primarily renally excreted.[1,55] Thus, the elderly are at an increased risk of toxicity from most psychotropic agents unless the dose is adjusted downward. (For a more detailed description of pharmacokinetic and pharmacodynamic differences in the elderly, see Refs. 2, 13, 31, 55, 59 and Chap. 3.)

Use of Older Antianxiety Agents

Before the widespread use of benzodiazepines, barbiturates (Seconal, Nembutal), meprobamate (Miltown, Equanil), glutethimide (Doriden), methyprylon (Noludar), and ethchlorvynol (Placidyl) were commonly used anxiolytic or hypnotic agents. Because of the significant problem with REM sleep deprivation and rebound, increases of hepatic microsomal enzymes, tolerance, physical dependence, and life-threatening withdrawal symptoms, none of these agents should be used today.[1,2,31,105] Antipsychotics were also used to treat anxiety in the past but should not be used because of increased risks of causing tardive dyskinesia.[31]

Combination of Antidepressants and Anxiolytics

Although benzodiazepines and buspirone are the most prescribed agents for anxiety disorders, antidepressants are being used more commonly as first-line agents for PD and OCD and in patients with mixed depression and anxiety. Since antidepressants take several weeks before therapeutic effects occur, low doses of a short-half-life benzodiazepine (e.g., oxazepam, alprazolam, lorazepam) can be added initially and gradually discontinued as the symptoms subside.[31] Whenever depression is suspected, an antidepressant drug therapy should be tried first. In cases of mixed anxiety-depression, combination therapy of an antidepressant and antianxiety agent may be warranted.

Drug Interactions with Anxiolytics

Short-half-life benzodiazepines (with no active metabolites) and buspirone have relatively few drug interactions and can be administered safely with other medications. The longer-acting benzodiazepines have more kinetic interactions secondary

Table 8-13 Drug interactions with anxiolytics

Long-acting benzodiazepines (BNZ) (e.g., diazepam, chlordiazepoxide, clorazepate, halazepam, prazepam, flurazepam)	
Cimetidine (Tagamet)	Increase BNZ blood levels
Valproic acid	Displace diazepam from plasma protein binding and may inhibit metabolism
Phenytoin (Dilantin)	May increase phenytoin blood levels
Digoxin (Lanoxin)	May increase digoxin blood levels with diazepam
Disulfiram (Antabuse)	Increase BNZ blood levels
Antacids	Slow BNZ absorption; decrease clorazepate metabolism
Food	Slow BNZ absorption
Alcohol	Increase diazepam blood levels; potentiate CNS depressant effects

to changes in liver metabolism (Table 8-13).[108] Concomitant administration of other sedatives and hypnotics or alcohol potentiates CNS depression with all benzodiazepines but not with buspirone.

REFERENCES

1. Shader RI, Greenblatt DJ: Management of anxiety in the elderly: the balance between therapeutic and adverse effects. *J Clin Psychiatry* 43:8-18, 1982.
2. Treatment of anxiety, in Salzman C (ed): *Clinical Geriatric Psychopharmacology*. New York, McGraw-Hill, 1984, pp 132-148.
3. Ruskin PE: Anxiety and somatoform disorders, in Bienenfeld D (ed): *Verwoerdt's Clinical Geropsychiatry*, 3d ed. Baltimore, Williams & Wilkins, 1990, pp 137-163.
4. Anxiety Disorders (or Anxiety and Phobic Neuroses), American Psychiatric Association: *Diagnostic and Statistical Manual of Mental Disorders*, 3d ed, rev. Washington, District of Columbia, American Psychiatric Association, 1987, pp 235-253.
5. Gurian BS, Miner JH: Clinical presentation of anxiety in the elderly, in Salzman C, Lebowitz BD (eds): *Anxiety in the Elderly, Treatment and Research*. New York, Springer, 1991, pp 31-44.
6. Fogelson D, Bystrictsky A, Sussman N: Interrelationships between major depression and the anxiety disorders: clinical relevance. *Psychiatr Ann* 18:158-167, 1988.
7. Liptzin B: Masked anxiety—alcohol and drug use, in Salzman C, Lebowitz BD (eds): *Anxiety in the Elderly, Treatment and Research*. New York, Springer, 1991, pp 87-101.
8. Clayton PJ: The comorbidity factor establishing the primary diagnosis in patients with mixed symptoms of anxiety and depression. *J Clin Psychiatry* 51:35-39, 1990.
9. Klerman GL: Classifying anxiety—the new nosology, in Fawcett J (ed): *Anxiety in the Elderly in Contemporary Psychiatry*. Chicago, Pragmaton Publications, 1983, pp 7-10.
10. Shamoian CA: What is anxiety in the elderly? in Salzman C, Lebowitz BD (eds): *Anxiety in the Elderly, Treatment and Research*. New York, Springer, 1991, pp 3-15.
11. Salzman C: Anxiety in the elderly: treatment strategies. *J Clin Psychiatry* 51:18-21, 1990.
12. Turnbull JM: Anxiety and physical illness in the elderly. *J Clin Psychiatry* 50(11, suppl):40-45, 1989.
13. Cutler NR, Narang PK: Implications of dosing tricyclic antidepressants and benzodiazepines in geriatrics. *Psychiatr Clin North Am* 7:845-861, 1984.
14. Salzman C: Pharmacologic treatment of the anxious elderly patient, in Salzman C, Lebowitz

BD (eds): *Anxiety in the Elderly, Treatment and Research*. New York, Springer, 1991, pp 149–173.
15. Atkinson JH Jr, Schuckit MA: Geriatric alcohol and drug misuse and abuse. *Adv Subst Abuse* 3:195–237, 1983.
16. Myers JK, Weissman MM, Tischler GL, et al: Six-month prevalence of psychiatric disorders in three communities: 1980–1982. *Arch Gen Psychiatry* 41:959–967, 1984.
17. Blazer D, George LK, Hughes D: The epidemiology of anxiety disorders: an age comparison, in Salzman C, Lebowitz BD (eds): *Anxiety in the Elderly, Treatment and Research*. New York, Springer, 1991, pp 17–30.
18. Regier DA, Boyd JH, Burke JD, et al: One-month prevalence of mental disorders in the United States based on five epidemiologic catchment area sites. *Arch Gen Psychiatry* 45:977–986, 1988.
19. Rapp SR, Parisi SA, Walsh DA: Psychological dysfunction and physical health among elderly medical inpatients. *J Consul Clin Psychol* 56:851–855, 1988.
20. Alexopoulos GS: Anxiety and depression in the elderly, in Salzman C, Lebowitz BD (eds): *Anxiety in the Elderly, Treatment and Research*. New York, Springer, 1991, pp 63–77.
21. Himmelfarb S, Murrell SA: Prevalence and correlates of anxiety symptoms in older adults. *J Psychol* 116:159–167, 1984.
22. Dubvosky SL: Generalized anxiety disorder: new concepts and psychopharmacologic therapies. *J Clin Psychiatry* 51(1, suppl):3–10, 1990.
23. Judd FK, Burrows GD, Norman TR: The biological basis of anxiety: an overview. *J Affect Disord* 9:271–284, 1985.
24. Hayes PE: Treatment of panic disorder. *J Pharm Pract* 3:233–240, 1990.
25. Reiman EM, Raichle ME, Robins E, et al: The application of positron emission tomography to the study of panic disorder. *Am J Psychiatry* 143:469–477, 1986.
26. Weissman MM: The epidemiology of anxiety disorders: rates, risks and familial patterns. *J Psychiatr Res* 22(1, suppl):99–114, 1988.
27. Silver JM, Sandberg DP, Hales RE: New approaches in the pharmacotherapy of posttraumatic stress disorder. *J Clin Psychiatry* 51(10, suppl):33–38, 1990.
28. Sunderland T, Lawlor BA, Martinez RA, Molchan SE: Anxiety in the elderly: neurobiological and clinical interface, in Salzman C, Lebowitz BD (eds): *Anxiety in the Elderly, Treatment and Research*. New York, Springer, 1991, pp 105–129.
29. Rapoport JL: The waking nightmare: an overview of obsessive compulsive disorder. *J Clin Psychiatry* 51(11, suppl):25–28, 1990.
30. Neurotransmission in the aging central nervous system, in Salzman C (ed): *Clinical Geriatric Psychopharmacology*. New York, McGraw-Hill, 1984, pp 18–31.
31. Anxiety disorders of old age, in Jenike MA (ed): *Geriatric Psychiatry and Psychopharmacology: A Clinical Approach*. Chicago, Year Book Medical Publishers, 1989, pp 248–271.
32. Cohen GD: Anxiety and general medical disorders, in Salzman C, Lebowitz BD (eds): *Anxiety in the Elderly, Treatment and Research*. New York, Springer, 1991, pp 47–62.
33. Cassem EH: Depression and anxiety secondary to medical illness. *Psychiatr Clin North Am* 13:597–612, 1990.
34. Roy-Bryne PP, Uhde TW: Exogenous factors in panic disorder: clinical and research implications. *J Clin Psychiatry* 49:56–61, 1988.
35. Kendler KS, Health AC, Martin WG, et al: Symptoms of anxiety and symptoms of depression: same genes, different environments? *Arch Gen Psychiatry* 122:451–457, 1987.
36. Stavrakaki C, Vargo B: The relationship of anxiety and depression: a review of the literature. *Br J Psychiatry* 149:7–16, 1986.
37. Coplan JD, Gorman JM: Treatment of anxiety disorder in patients with mood disorders. *J Clin Psychiatry* 51(10, suppl):9–13, 1990.
38. Paul SM: Anxiety and depression: a common neurobiological substrate? *J Clin Psychiatry* 49:13–16, 1988.

39. Dubovsky SL: Understanding and treating depression in anxious patients. *J Clin Psychiatry* 51(10, suppl):3-8, 1990.
40. Wetzler S, Katz MM: Problems with the differentiation of anxiety and depression. *J Psychiatr Res* 23:1-12, 1989.
41. Schatzberg AF, Samson JA, Rothschild AJ, et al: Depression secondary to anxiety: findings from the McLean Hospital Depression Research Facility. *Psychiatr Clin North Am* 13:633-649, 1990.
42. Fawcett J: Targeting treatment in patients with mixed symptoms of anxiety and depression. *J Clin Psychiatry* 51(11, suppl):40-43, 1990.
43. Lader M: Differential diagnosis of anxiety in the elderly. *J Clin Psychiatry* 43:4-7, 1982.
44. Weissman MM: The hidden patient: unrecognized panic disorder. *J Clin Psychiatry* 51(11, suppl):5-8, 1990.
45. Markowitz JS, Weissman MM, Ouellette R, et al: Quality of life in panic disorder. *Arch Gen Psychiatry* 46:984-992, 1989.
46. Weissman MM, Klerman GL, Markowitz JS, Ouellette R: Suicidal ideation and suicide attempts in panic disorder and attacks. *N Engl J Med* 321:1209-1214, 1989.
47. Fawcett J: Predictions of early suicide: identification and appropriate intervention. *J Clin Psychiatry* 49(10, suppl):7-8, 1988.
48. Coryell W, Noyes R, Clancy J: Excess mortality in panic disorder: a comparison with unipolar depression. *Arch Gen Psychiatry* 39:701-703, 1982.
49. Yesavage JA, Taylor B: Anxiety and dementia, in Salzman C, Lebowitz BD (eds): *Anxiety in the Elderly, Treatment and Research.* New York, Springer, 1991, pp 79-85.
50. Salzman C: Treatment of agitation, anxiety, and depression in dementia. *Psychopharmacol Bull* 24:49-53, 1988.
51. Yudofsky SC, Silver JM, Hales RE: Pharmacologic management of aggression in the elderly. *J Clin Psychiatry* 51(10, suppl):22-28, 1990.
52. Barnes R, Raskind M: Strategies for diagnosing and treating agitation in the aging. *Geriatrics* 35:111-119, 1980.
53. Greendyke RM, Kanter RR, Schuster DB, et al: Propranolol treatment of assaultive patients with organic brain disease. *J Nerv Ment Dis* 174:290-294, 1986.
54. Colenda CC: Buspirone in the treatment of agitated demented patients. *Lancet* 1:1169, 1988.
55. Gottlieb GL: Sleep disorders and their management: special considerations in the elderly. *Am J Med* 88(3A, suppl)29S-33S, 1990.
56. Schatzberg AF: Anxiety and adjustment disorder: a treatment approach. *J Clin Psychiatry* 51:20-24, 1990.
57. Adjustment Disorder, American Psychiatric Association: *Diagnostic and Statistical Manual of Mental Disorders*, 3d ed, rev. Washington, District of Columbia, American Psychiatric Association, 1987, pp 329-331.
58. Gorman JM, Papp LA: Chronic anxiety: deciding the length of treatment. *J Clin Psychiatry* 51(1, suppl):11-15, 1990.
59. Greenblatt DJ, Shader RI: Benzodiazepines in the elderly: pharmacokinetics and drug sensitivity, in Salzman C, Lebowitz BD (eds): *Anxiety in the Elderly, Treatment and Research.* New York, Springer, 1991, pp 131-145.
60. Sussman N, Chou JCY: Current issues in benzodiazepine use for anxiety disorders. *Psychiatr Ann* 18:139-145, 1988.
61. Salzman C: The APA Task Force Report on Benzodiazepine Dependence, Toxicity, and Abuse. *Am J Psychiatry* 148:151-152, 1991.
62. Rickels K, Case WG, Schweizer E, et al: Benzodiazepine dependence: management of discontinuation. *Psychopharmacol Bull* 26:63-68, 1990.
63. Ray WA, Griffin MR, Schaffner W: Psychotropic drug use and the risk of hip fracture. *N Engl J Med* 316:363-369, 1987.
64. Scheizer E, Case WG, Rickels K: Benzodiazepine dependence and withdrawal in elderly patients. *Am J Psychiatry* 146:529-531, 1989.

65. Hart RP, Colenda CC, Hamer RM: Effects of buspirone and alprazolam on cognitive performance of normal elderly subjects. *Am J Psychiatry* 148:73–77, 1991.
66. Pomara N, Deptula D, Singh R, Monroy CA: Cognitive toxicity of benzodiazepines in the elderly, in Salzman C, Lebowitz BD (eds): *Anxiety in the Elderly, Treatment and Research.* New York, Springer, 1991, pp 175–214.
67. Scharf MB, Fletcher K, Graham JD: Comparative amnestic effects of benzodiazepine hypnotic agents. *J Clin Psychiatry* 49:134–137, 1988.
68. Dietch JT, Jennings RK: Aggressive dyscontrol in patients treated with benzodiazepines. *J Clin Psychiatry* 49:184–188, 1988.
69. Eison MS: Azapirones: clinical uses of serotonin partial agonists. *Fam Pract Recertification* 11(9, suppl):8–16, 1989.
70. Robinson DS, Alms DR, Shrotriya RC, et al: Serotonergic anxiolytics and treatment of depression. *Psychopathology* 22(1, suppl):27–36, 1989.
71. Rickels K, Amsterdam JD, Clary C, et al: Buspirone in major depression: a controlled study. *J Clin Psychiatry* 52:34–38, 1991.
72. Napoliello MJ: An interium multicentre report on 677 anxious geriatric outpatients treated with buspirone. *Br J Clin Pract* 40:71–73, 1986.
73. Robinson D, Napoliello MJ, Schenk J: The safety and usefulness of buspirone as an anxiolytic drug in elderly versus young patients. *Clin Ther* 10:740–746, 1988.
74. Burrows GD: Managing long-term therapy for panic disorder. *J Clin Psychiatry* 51(11, suppl):9–12, 1990.
75. Robins LN, Helzer JE, Weissman MM, et al: Lifetime prevalence of specific psychiatric disorders in three sites. *Arch Gen Psychiatry* 41:949–958, 1984.
76. Noyes R, Perry P: Maintenance treatment with antidepressants in panic disorder. *J Clin Psychiatry* 51(12, suppl):24–30, 1990.
77. Ballenger JC: Pharmacotherapy of panic disorders. *J Clin Psychiatry* 47:27–32, 1986.
78. Pohl R, Yeragani VK, Balan R, et al: The jitteriness syndrome in panic disorder patients treated with antidepressants. *J Clin Psychiatry* 49:100–104, 1988.
79. Liebowitz MR: Antidepressants in panic disorder. *Br J Psychiatry* 155(6, suppl):46–52, 1989.
80. Schneier FR, Liebowitz MR, Davie SO, et al: Fluoxetine in panic disorder. *J Clin Psychopharmacol* 10:119–121, 1990.
81. Charney DS, Woods SW, Goodman WK, et al: Drug treatment of panic disorder: the comparative efficacy of imipramine, alprazolam, and trazodone. *J Clin Psychiatry* 47:580–586, 1986.
82. Ballenger JC, Burrows GD, DuPont RL, et al: Alprazolam in panic disorder and agoraphobia: results from a multicenter trial, I. Efficacy in short-term treatment. *Arch Gen Psychiatry* 45:413–422, 1988.
83. Sheehan DV: Benzodiazepines in panic disorder and agoraphobia. *J Affect Disord* 13:169–181, 1987.
84. Chouinard G, Annable L, Fontaine R, et al: Alprazolam in the treatment of generalized anxiety and panic disorders: a double-blind placebo-controlled study. *Psychopharmacology* 77:229–233, 1982.
85. Davidson JRT: Continuation treatment of panic disorder with high-potency benzodiazepines. *J Clin Psychiatry* 51(12, suppl):31–37, 1990.
86. Pollack MH, Rosenbaum J: Benzodiazepines in panic-related disorders. *J Anxiety Disord* 2:95–107, 1988.
87. Noyes R, Dupont RL, Pecknold JC, et al: Alprazolam in panic disorder and agoraphobia: results from a multicenter trial, II: patient acceptance, side effects, and safety. *Arch Gen Psychiatry* 45:423–428, 1988.
88. Pecknold JC, Swinson RP, Kuch K, et al: Alprazolam in panic disorder and agoraphobia: results from a multicenter trial, III: discontinuation effects. *Arch Gen Psychiatry* 45:429–436, 1988.
89. Jenike MA: Obsessive-compulsive disorders in the elderly, in Jenike MA (ed): *Geriatric Psychiatry and Psychopharmacology. A Clinical Approach.* Chicago, Year Book Medical Publishers, 1989, pp 339–362.

90. Greist JH: Treating the anxiety: therapeutic options in obsessive compulsive disorder. *J Clin Psychiatry* 51(11, suppl):29-34, 1990.
91. Insel TR: New pharmacologic approaches to obsessive compulsive disorder. *J Clin Psychiatry* 5(10, suppl):47-51, 1990.
92. Pato MT, Pigott TA, Hill JL, et al: Controlled comparison of buspirone and clomipramine in obsessive-compulsive disorder. *Am J Psychiatry* 148:127-129, 1991.
93. Agras WS: Treatment of social phobias. *J Clin Psychiatry* 51(10, suppl):52-55, 1990.
94. Schneier FR, Martin LY, Liebowitz RM, et al: Alcohol abuse in social phobia. *J Anxiety Disord* 3:15-23, 1989.
95. Heimberg RG, Barlow DH: Psychosocial treatments for social phobia. *Psychosomatics* 29:27-37, 1988.
96. Gorman JM, Gorman LK: Drug treatment of social phobia. *J Affect Disord* 13:183-192, 1987.
97. Liebowitz MR, Gorman JM, Fyer AJ, et al: Pharmacotherapy of social phobia: an interium report of a placebo-controlled comparison of phenelzine and atenolol. *J Clin Psychiatry* 49:252-257, 1988.
98. Liebowitz MR, Schneier FR, Hollander E, et al: Treatment of social phobia with drugs other than benzodiazepines. *J Clin Psychiatry* 52[11, suppl]: 10-15, 1991.
99. Helzer JE, Robins LN, McCvoy L: Post-traumatic stress disorder in the general population: findings of the Epidemiologic Catchment Area Survey. *N Engl J Med* 317:1630-1634, 1987.
100. Jenike MA: Sleep disorders in the elderly, in Jenike MA (ed): *Geriatric Psychiatry and Psychopharmacology, a Clinical Approach.* Chicago, Year Book Medical Publishers, 1989, pp 272-288.
101. Moran MG, Thompson TL, Nies AS: Sleep disorders in the elderly. *Am J Psychiatry* 145:1369-1378, 1988.
102. Greenblatt DJ: Benzodiazepine hypnotics: sorting the pharmacokinetic facts. *J Clin Psychiatry* 52 (9, suppl): 4-10, 1991.
103. Mendels J: Criteria for selection of appropiate benzodiazepine hypnotic therapy. *J. Clin Psychiatry* 52 (9, suppl): 42-46, 1991.
104. Mueleman JR, Nelson RC, Clark RL Jr: Evaluation of temazepam and diphenhydramine as hypnotics in a nursing-home population. *Drug Intell Clin Pharm* 21:716-720, 1987.
105. Regestein QR: Treatment of insomnia in the elderly, in Salzman C (ed): *Clinical Geriatric Psychopharmacology.* New York, McGraw-Hill, 1984, pp 149-170.
106. Ware JC, Pittard JT: Increased deep sleep after trazodone use: a double blind placebo-controlled study in healthy young adults. *J Clin Psychiatry* 51(9,suppl):18-22, 1990.
107. Jacobson FM: Low-dose trazodone as a hypnotic in patients with MAOIs and other psychotropics: a pilot study. *J Clin Psychiatry* 51:298-302, 1990.
108. Tatro DS (ed): Drug Interaction Facts. St. Louis, J. B. Lippincott Co., 1991.

CHAPTER

9

PAIN CONTROL

Mark Holdsworth
Walter B. Forman

As the population ages, the need for better control of pain also assumes greater importance. The elder person is subject to the development of two broad categories of diseases associated with pain: degenerative arthritis and cancer. It has been estimated that over 80 percent of individuals over 65 years of age will suffer from arthritis pain.[1] In addition, over 60 percent of the common malignancies occur in persons over the age of 65.[2] Mortality data indicate that persons age 55 and older account for the majority of deaths due to lung, colon and rectum, breast, and prostate cancers.[3] Since these malignancies are the leading causes of cancer mortality and are very likely to be quite painful in the later stages due to their predilection for pain-sensitive structures (e.g., periosteum), the elderly are the age group most likely to experience cancer pain. Therefore, the need to understand the clinical pharmacology and the proper use of analgesics in the elderly is of vital importance. It is suggested that the reader review Chap. 20 for the current therapy of arthritis. This chapter focuses primarily on chronic cancer pain. Pain management in the postoperative setting is also discussed, as the elderly may frequently be candidates for surgical procedures.

Opioid agents, although available almost since the earliest description of pain management and known to be effective, have been clouded in a veil of mystery because of their abuse by society. The history of opioid use and abuse is reviewed by Grossman.[4] Therefore, the clinician must also be aware of the various social issues involved in their administration. Recent works of Cleeland[5] and others[6] have begun to "lift the veil," allowing for a rational approach to the care of individuals with chronic, particularly cancer, pain. The many factors they list as contributors to poor management of pain include opioidophobia (an irrational fear of these agents) and attitudes of patients, friends, and families toward addiction and toxicity. Max,[7] in his article on analgesic treatment, advances the hypothesis that education alone will not change behavior in regard to prescribing patterns. He suggests that practice patterns, patient attitudes toward pain, and pain assessment techniques must be altered if we are to overcome the poor outcomes in pain management noted in surveys of many of our leading health care facilities.[8,9] Thus, at a time when our understanding of the spinal opiate receptor systems is being clarified[10] and numerous technologic advances in drug delivery are taking place, our efforts to change society's preconceived notions about pain and its treatment remain a unique challenge. In order to adequately treat pain, the caregiver must believe that the patient is in pain.

With this as background, the reader should, after reading this chapter, gain an expanded knowledge of the role of opioid therapy in the elderly with either acute postoperative pain or chronic cancer pain.

CLINICAL PHARMACOLOGY

Systemic Administration

The opioids are classified as either agonists, mixed agonist-antagonists, or antagonists (Table 9-1). The agonists are classified chemically as phenanthrenes, phenylpiperidines, or diphenylheptanes. A majority of the opioid agonists are phenanthrenes. However, despite the vastly different structures of the phenylpiperidines and the diphenylheptanes, these agents exert qualitatively similar effects on the opiate receptors. These agents are strong agonists to the opiate mu receptors. Table 9-2 provides a list of the main opiate receptors and the agonists and antagonists that bind to them. The consequences of agonist binding to these receptors are as follows: mu—analgesia, respiratory depression, miosis, decreased gastrointestinal motility, and euphoria; kappa—analgesia, dysphoria, and psychotomimetic effects; sigma—uncertain in humans. These receptors are often found on presynaptic nerve terminals, where they cause a decreased release of excitatory neurotransmitters.[11] The exact distributions of each of these receptors, their subtypes, as well as other yet-to-be-discovered receptors and their roles in spinal and supraspinal analgesia will require a great deal of further investigation.

Certain agonists are commonly formulated into combinations with acetaminophen or aspirin (Table 9-3). Maximal doses of these combination products are determined by the dose-limiting toxicities of these latter agents. Thus, their use in these combinations results in a ceiling dose. This ceiling dose is not observed when noncombination products (e.g., morphine) are utilized.[12] Therefore, there is limited experience with higher doses of the agonists in these combination products.

The mixed agonist-antagonists behave as competitive antagonists to the opiate receptors. These agents are agonists to the kappa opiate receptors responsible for

Table 9-1 Narcotic analgesics

Opioid agonists	Equianalgesic dose, mg	
Phenanthrenes	Oral (rectal)	Parenteral
Codeine	200	130
Hydrocodone	30	—
Hydromorphone	7.5 (3)	1.5
Levorphanol	4	2
Morphine	30 (30)	10
Oxycodone	30	—
Phenylpiperidines		
Alfentanil	—	0.6
Fentanyl	—	0.1
Meperidine	300	75
Sufentanil	—	0.02
Diphenylheptanes		
Methadone	20	10
Propoxyphene	180	—

Mixed Agonists/Antagonists	Partial agonists
Butorphanol	Buprenorphine
Nalbuphine	
Pentazocine	

Antagonists
Naloxone
Naltrexone

Table 9-2 Opiate receptors

	Receptor type		
Agent	Mu	Sigma	Kappa
Morphine-like agonists	+++	+	+
Pentazocine	–	NA	++
Butorphanol	–	NA	++
Buprenorphine	P	NA	–
Naloxone	–	–	–

Note: + = agonist; – = antagonist; P = partial agonist; NA = data inadequate.

Source: Adapted from Jaffe JH, Martin WR: Opioid analgesics and antagonists, in: Gilman AG, Rall TW, Nies AS, Taylor P (eds): *The Pharmacological Basis of Therapeutics.* New York,

Table 9-3 Narcotic fomulations

Agent	Oral	Parenteral, mg/mL
Alfentanil	—	0.5/1
Codeine	15, 30, 60 mg	30/1, 60/1
Fentanyl	—	0.05/1 Transdermal: 25, 50, 75, 100 μg
Hydromorphone	1, 2, 3, 4 mg	1/1, 2/1, 3/1, 4/1, 10/1
Levorphanol	2 mg	2/1
Meperidine	Syrup: 50 mg/5 mL Tablets: 50, 100 mg	10/1, 25/1, 50/1, 75/1, 100/1
Methadone	Solution: 5/5, 10/5, 10/10, 10/1 mg/mL Tablets: 5, 10 mg	10/1
Morphine	Solution: 10/5, 20/5 20/1 mg/mL Tablets: 10, 15, 30 mg SR tablets: 15, 30 60, 100 mg	1/1, 2/1, 3/1, 4/1, 5/1, 8/1, 10/1, 15/1 Preservative-free: 0.5/1
Sufentanil	—	0.05/1

Oral combinations

Opioids	Acetaminophen, mg		Aspirin, mg		Other
Codeine					
12 mg/5 mL	120				alcohol 7%
1-60 mg	97-650	and/or	230-389		
Hydrocodone					
2.5-7.5 mg	120-750	or	224-500		
Meperidine					
25-50 mg	300			or	promethazine 25 mg
Oxycodone					
2.25-5 mg	300-500	or	325		
Propoxyphene					
32-100 mg	325-389				

spinal analgesia and either have antagonist properties or minimal effect on mu receptors. These agents produce a flat dose-response curve, which creates a ceiling effect.[13] Also, both butorphanol and pentazocine possess affinity for the sigma opiate receptors which are responsible for dysphoria, hallucinations, and vasomotor effects. Buprenorphine functions as a partial agonist for the mu and kappa receptors.

It occupies the receptor but does not fully activate it. This agent also results in a much flatter dose-response curve when compared with the opioid agonists.[13]

The literature contains several reports which document differences in the pharmacokinetics and/or pharmacodynamics of certain opioids in the elderly population. A majority of these clinical pharmacology studies to determine differences versus younger age groups have examined the pure opiate agonists. Whether appreciable differences in potency or toxicity exist in the elderly population for the opiate agonist combinations products, the agonist-antagonists or the antagonists will require further study. Since the combination opiate agonists are indicated for mild-to-moderate pain and their initial dosing is therefore usually modest, these agents are less likely to result in toxicity. However, since these agents are frequently utilized, pharmacokinetic-pharmacodynamic studies would be valuable to document any differences which may exist in the elderly.

Studies by both Belleville[14] and Kaiko[15] reported an increased analgesia with morphine in the elderly population. In both studies, it was demonstrated that despite no differences in initial pain intensity between age groups, elderly patients obtained considerably greater pain relief than younger patients administered the same morphine dose. It was also shown by Kaiko that the elderly achieved greater pain relief at an 8-mg dose than the younger patients could achieve when given twice this dose. These observed differences appeared to be primarily related to the duration of action, as 72 percent of the youngest patients were again in pain 4 h after a dose versus 29 percent of the oldest patients. Also of interest in this study was an apparent continuum of increasing analgesia with increasing age across four age groups. These studies, however, did not determine whether these differences were due to changes in pharmacokinetics and/or alterations in sensitivity. It is also unknown if these differences, which were observed in the acute postoperative setting, are at all predictive of any differences in the chronic pain situation.

A study performed by Owen et al[16] examined the pharmacokinetics of morphine in young versus elderly patients. These investigators discovered a smaller volume of distribution at steady state, a shorter elimination half-life, and a reduced plasma clearance in the elderly. These data might explain the previously observed pharmacodynamic differences in the elderly. However, they reported much higher clearance values than those determined by prior investigators.[17,18] In addition, these investigators utilized two different morphine assays and did not report which patient samples were quantitated by which assay. Another group of investigators found no appreciable differences in the pharmacokinetics of morphine between young and old patients.[19]

When examining morphine pharmacokinetics, it must be kept in mind that differences in morphine metabolite concentrations need also be considered. It has been shown that patients with reduced renal function accumulate morphine-6-ucuronide.[20,21] Also, morphine-6-glucuronide has proven to be a potent analgesic itself in humans and appears to be comparable to that of the parent compound.[22] Since plasma morphine-6-glucuronide concentrations exceed parent drug concentrations after single-dose studies of both intravenous and especially oral morphine,[23] it is quite possible that this metabolite may account for a significant amount of the analgesia during therapy with morphine. Therefore, pharmacokinetic studies attempting to explain differences in the elderly which fail to consider morphine-6-glucuronide concentrations may be invalid. To date, a rigorous trial has yet to be performed to document differences in morphine-6-glucuronide concentrations in young versus elderly patients. Such differences are quite likely given the dependence of morphine-6-glucuronide excretion on renal function and the known decrease in renal function which occurs in the elderly.

Morphine absorption does not appear different in the elderly population. A recent study by Baillie et al[24] discovered no significant difference in the oral bioavailability of morphine solution or sustained release tablets between young and elderly patients. Therefore, the commonly utilized method of reducing the dose by a third when switching from oral to parenteral morphine is recommended for the elderly as well.

At least two trials have examined the influence of aging on the elimination of meperidine. Holmberg et al[25] demonstrated a decreased plasma clearance of meperidine and normeperidine in the elderly. Further study of this agent demonstrated that these lower clearance values in the elderly for meperidine appeared to be due to decreased metabolic clearance, while for normeperidine it was due to a decreased creatinine clearance.[26]

No well-designed trials exist to demonstrate differences in the analgesic effect or plasma concentrations of methadone between young and elderly patients. Recent work by Inturrisi et al[27] determined marked interpatient variability in the methadone concentration required for pain relief in a group of cancer patients, some of whom were elderly. Of some interest is that the lowest concentration providing adequate analgesia occurred in one of the elderly patients. One trial did demonstrate a significant correlation of increasing plasma methadone half-life and patient age.[28] However, this trial found no correlation between the minimum analgesic blood concentration and patient age. These investigators also determined that patient age only accounted for a small percentage of the variance in duration of analgesia.

Fentanyl and one of its derivatives, alfentanil, have also been examined for pharmacokinetic differences in the elderly population. Bentley et al[29] demonstrated longer elimination half-lives and lower clearance values in older patients. Unfortunately, their sampling duration was for a shorter period of time than the half-life which they calculated. Thus, their estimate of half-life may have been subject to considerable error. Other researchers examining fentanyl pharmacokinetics in a similar group of elderly surgical patients did not discover any effects of age on plasma concentrations despite a 24-h sampling time.[30] This lack of age-related changes in fentanyl pharmacokinetics has also been demonstrated by Cartwright et al[31] in patients ranging in age from 39 to 72 years.

One recent trial compared alfentanil pharmacokinetics in elderly versus young patients and volunteers.[32] These researchers observed lower clearance values in both groups of elderly than in the young patients and volunteers. Again, their sampling duration was also less than their calculated half-lives for some of their patients. Of some interest, they observed greater variance in the pharmacokinetics in younger patients than in the elderly, suggesting a more predictive dose-response relationship in older patients.

Recently, Scott and Stanski[33] examined whether the elderly require decreased dosages of fentanyl and alfentanil in comparison to younger patients. They also sought to determine whether any alterations in dose requirements were related to changes in pharmacokinetics and/or pharmacodynamics. To measure narcotic effect, they examined for changes in electroencephalogram (EEG) frequencies. They determined that for both fentanyl and alfentanil, pharmacokinetics did not appear to be influenced by the patient's age. However, they did observe that elderly patients displayed an increased brain sensitivity to both agents. Although it remains to be proven whether these EEG changes are related to or predictive of analgesia, the range of serum concentrations producing EEG slowing was within what is considered the therapeutic range for these agents. The authors postulated that the increased sensitivity which they observed in the elderly may be due to differences in the number of opioid receptors, differences in opioid receptor binding, or increased translation of binding into effect.

The above findings suggest that narcotic analgesic dosing regimens for the elderly should be designed to achieve lower serum concentrations and that dose increases should be made cautiously. However, large clinical trials do not exist to document that the elderly typically require lower narcotic doses or smaller dose increases. Also, these experimental findings may not apply to the chronic pain situation, where increasing pain and/or tolerance are probably more important dosage determinants than may be patient age. To determine whether the elderly are truly candidates for lower opioid doses for acute and chronic pain, large-scale surveys of analgesic efficacy and dosage requirements for different patient age groups need to be performed.

CLINICAL APPLICATIONS

General Concepts

The opioids discussed in this section are listed in Table 9-1. Although the mixed agonist-antagonists were discussed in the pharmacology section, they are not covered in this section. These agents were produced in an attempt to develop drugs with analgesic properties but without many of the adverse effects and the potential for dependence and addiction associated with the opiates. However, analgesia with these agents may be difficult to achieve due to the dose-limiting psychotomimetic effects of many of these agents and/or the potential for increased opiate antagonist activity as the dose is increased. Also, these agents may precipitate withdrawal symptoms in patients who have been receiving opiate agonists. These agents appear to have either no or limited usefulness in patients with pain (especially chronic pain) and are best avoided. The variety of agonists available are more than adequate to care for all situations and can be used interchangeably when their relative potency is considered.

There are some general issues that must be dealt with prior to beginning a discussion of opioid use in either the acute or chronic situation. When used in patients with pain, these drugs can lead to physical dependence. Patients receiving opioids for a period of time cannot be abruptly discontinued from the drug lest they develop the classic withdrawal syndrome (drenching sweats, abdominal cramps, malaise, and a dread fear). However, physical dependence is not addiction. Addiction occurs when an individual habitually uses a substance for its psychologic effects. Eventually, tolerance occurs in this situation, leading to increasing consumption. These individuals will also develop physical dependence, thus obscuring the difference between physical dependence and addiction. In patients receiving opioids who do not have a past history of substance abuse, addiction is exceedingly rare.[34] The withdrawal syndrome can be avoided by tapering the opioids over a few days to a week, depending upon the dose. In general a 25-percent reduction every other day will be adequate to avoid the withdrawal syndrome. Tolerance is thought to occur when the dose of the opioid must be increased in order to control pain, due to a decreased sensitivity or number of the opiate receptors. Tolerance does not appear to be a problem for the majority of patients (elderly included)[35-37] and is virtually impossible to separate from the situation where a patient is requiring increasing dosages due to disease progression. Since patients may interpret a withdrawal syndrome (with abrupt discontinuation) or tolerance (with increasing dosage requirements) as signs of addiction, the need for patient counseling to alleviate patient apprehension is vital to establish an effective analgesic plan.

Whenever analgesic therapy in any group of patients is indicated, an adequate medication history is very important. This may be especially true in the elderly. In a survey of analgesic use by the elderly, the Iowa 65+ Study found that 72.3 percent was obtained without prescription, 14.4 percent of women and 10.5 percent of men were taking two or more analgesics, and 6.4 percent of women and 11.3 percent of men were taking both prescription and nonprescription drugs.[38] Toxicity, particularly in the elderly, can be anticipated in this situation. Therefore, it is important to take an adequate analgesic history with particular reference to use of friends' or relatives' medications and to nonprescription agents, including traditional or folk remedies.

Postoperative Pain

Studies have demonstrated the inadequate control of postoperative pain in the elderly.[39,40] The reasons for poor pain management include many of the factors already discussed.

Since for many elderly patients, acute pain will be just the beginning of a long arduous course of therapy leading to chronic pain (i.e., a breast biopsy followed by surgery, radiation therapy, etc.), careful attention to pain control during the acute phases of treatment will make the patient less apprehensive and more confident in the practitioner's abilities to control the most feared aspect of chronic pain—unremitting pain.[41]

The technique of intramuscular opioid administered on as-needed basis (prn) has been shown to lead to inadequate pain control as well as being associated with fluctuation in serum concentrations of the analgesic drug. The prn dosing is associated with increased toxicity such as hypoventilation, confusion, and sedation.[42,43] Meperidine is probably the most popular analgesic in the postoperative setting. When administered over a period of time, especially in the elderly with compromised renal function, it may lead to severe central nervous system toxicity manifested by twitching and seizures due to accumulation of the metabolite, normeperidine.[44] Meperidine should be avoided in the elderly, particularly for chronic administration.

Patient-controlled analgesia (PCA) with intravenous infusion of opioids has been found to be effective in even the frail elderly.[45] A review of the various devices and dosing regimens for PCA is available by Barkas and Duafala.[46] Further discussion can be found in the section dealing with the treatment of chronic pain. While this approach allows patients to better titrate the therapy to their analgesic needs, PCA probably offers no real advantages over diligent nursing care with frequent patient assessment. For the elderly, as with younger patients, rapidly titratable agents such as morphine and hydromorphone appear to be most useful in this setting.

Spinal Administration

Over the past decade, the spinal route of opioid administration has gained considerable popularity for the management of both acute and chronic pain conditions. Both epidural and intrathecal routes of administration have been utilized. The rationale of these routes of administration is to maximize analgesia and minimize the adverse effects of systemically administered opiates.[47] Since the elderly may be especially prone to certain opiate side effects (e.g., somnolence, constipation), spinal administration may be especially advantageous in this age group, since the incidence of these adverse effects appears to be reduced by this route. Table 9-4 lists the possible adverse effects of spinal opioid administration.

Table 9-4 Adverse effects of spinal opiate administration

Constipation
Drowsiness
Nausea/vomiting
Pruritus
Spinal pain following injection
Sweating
Urinary retention

One study has questioned the empirical advantages that the spinal route may offer to the elderly population. Klinck et al[48] performed a controlled trial to compare the analgesia and adverse effects of morphine administered epidurally versus intramuscularly in a group of elderly patients. Although sedation was reduced in patients receiving morphine via the epidural route, postoperative respiratory mechanics were not improved and one patient developed delayed respiratory depression.

Morphine appears to be the drug of choice for spinal administration. Although analgesia is somewhat delayed with epidural morphine administration, any respiratory depression that is encountered may be reversed with systemic naloxone administration without loss of analgesia.[49] Attempts to circumvent respiratory depression with naloxone in patients receiving epidural fentanyl have resulted in a decrease in analgesia, due to high naloxone infusion required versus that necessary for epidural morphine.[50] It may be that the more lipid-soluble opiates such as fentanyl are more difficult to manage by this route of administration.

One Swedish nationwide survey has examined the adverse effects of spinally administered opiates.[51] This study reported 22 cases of respiratory depression secondary to epidural morphine from 84 anesthesia departments responding. Of these 22 cases, 10/22 were greater than 70 years of age and 18/22 were greater than 60 years old. It was not reported whether other adverse effects such as severe pruritus or urinary retention were more common in the elderly population or whether the elderly were overrepresented in this survey. Whether the incidence of respiratory depression from epidural morphine is more common in the elderly is not yet known. Since this trial surveyed anesthesia departments, patients with acute pain were primarily examined. Adverse effect patterns in the chronic pain population treated by this route may be different. Indeed, a recent trial did not demonstrate the side effects of urinary retention, pruritus, or respiratory depression in a group of pain patients receiving chronic epidural morphine therapy, many of whom were elderly.[52] Waldman[53] reviewed the current data for the use of this technique in the treatment of cancer pain.

At least one trial examining pharmacokinetic disposition of epidural morphine in the cerebrospinal fluid (CSF) reported a relationship of increasing concentrations with age.[54] Unfortunately, the age range for this study was only 22 to 53 years, and large interindividual variations in CSF concentrations were present. Also, CSF concentrations of epidurally administered morphine do not appear to be directly related to analgesia[52,55] and may be influenced by many factors, including injection site (e.g., thoracic, lumbar) and injection volume.[56]

Two trials examining epidural morphine analgesia have discovered some age-related differences. Ready et al[57] reported considerable age-related patient variability in dosage requirements in women undergoing abdominal hysterectomy. They demonstrated a decreased dosage requirement with age. The significance of this positive correlation is questionable, however, since older patients were initiated on lower dosages. This may have influenced the total dose which these patients received, especially if patients were not offered frequent dosage adjustments. Moore et al[58] studied two groups of patients, age greater than 65 years or age less than 50, undergoing major abdominal surgery. All patients were given an equivalent dose of epidural morphine based on body weight. Postoperatively, significantly more young patients required supplementary analgesia. It was also observed that the older patients obtained a significantly longer duration of analgesia, similar to prior studies of systemically administered opiates. There were no differences in adverse effects between the two groups. These investigators found no differences in plasma morphine concentrations between the two groups, suggesting that differences in systemic absorption were not responsible for the differences observed.

One final issue which should be mentioned in relation to spinal administration of opiates is that of the preservatives in the parenteral preparations. Both phenol and formaldehyde, present in significant concentrations in some commercial preparations of parenteral morphine, have been shown to cause both disorientation and mental confusion.[59] Although a preservative-free morphine preparation is commercially available, its potency (1 mg/mL) limits its usefulness in chronic dosing situations. However, other more potent morphine preparations which are preserved with chlorbutanol or a low concentration of sodium bisulfite (0.1%) have not been shown to cause toxicity. Thus these latter preparations, further diluted if necessary with a preservative-free solution of 0.9% sodium chloride, are the preparations of choice when high doses or chronic dosing are required.

Thus, at present both epidural and intrathecal administration of morphine appear to be safe and effective in the elderly population. Spinal administration may offer advantages, especially when systemic toxicity is problematic. While the elderly may require lower starting and maintenance doses in the acute postoperative setting, dosage reductions may not be necessary in the treatment of chronic pain.

Chronic Pain: General Concepts

This discussion follows the guidelines established by the World Health Organization (WHO) in its "pain ladder" approach (Fig. 9-1).[60] The following principles apply:

1. The oral route is always the approach of first choice, since it will be effective in the majority of patients[61] and allows for greater patient independence in analgesic administration.
2. The ladder should be "climbed" quickly (the patient should not be allowed to have unrelieved pain, point 7 notwithstanding), i.e., the patient should not languish on the bottom rung of the ladder when smaller doses of a more potent agent will be more effective and in general less toxic.
3. The type of pain that is best relieved by opioids is nociceptive in type, and for pain of neuropathic nature (e.g., postherpetic, nerve compression, brachial plexopathy) characterized as burning, shooting, electricity, or piercing, an adjuvant agent is usually required.[62]
4. Analgesics are to be administered on around-the-clock schedules and never

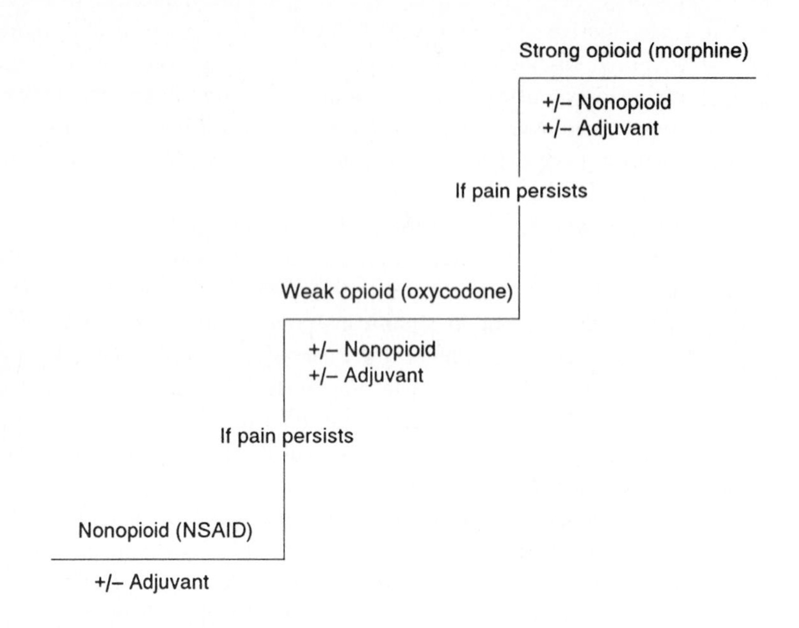

Figure 9-1 WHO analgesic ladder for cancer pain. (From *Cancer Pain Relief*, World Health Organization, Geneva, Switzerland, 1987, pp 1-73.)

prn. Once a stable dose of short acting oral opioid is established, a conversion to a sustained release preparation can be made.[63,64]

5. Careful attention to the conversion between opioids or different routes of administration must be observed (Table 9-1).
6. A simple approach to assessing pain must be at hand and familiar to the clinician.[65] For example the visual analog scale (VAS) can be used in most patients to determine the severity of pain.
7. A general empiric rule in the elderly is start low and go slow. Dosage increases, when indicated, are in general approximately 25 to 30 percent increases in the total daily dose rather than the typical 40 to 50 percent dose increases provided to younger patients. This is not to say that larger increases cannot be made in the elderly if pain is severe and unresponsive to smaller adjustments.

Oral Route

Table 9-2 lists the commonly utilized opioid preparations available. These agents can be added to the regimen if the patients' pain is unrelieved by acetaminophen or nonsteroidal anti-inflammatory drugs (NSAIDs) at the first step of the WHO ladder. If the patient has moderate pain at presentation, pain which interferes with activities and especially sleep, the use of a combination opioid-acetaminophen or aspirin product is appropriate. The use of propoxyphene, whose metabolite norpropoxyphene causes seizures, must be prescribed with caution in the elderly because this metabolite is mainly excreted renally.[66] If at this point pain of moderate-to-severe intensity is still present despite consuming greater than 12 dosage units per day, one can consider the patient no longer responsive to these agents. It is important at this juncture not to switch to an alternative drug of the same variety (i.e., a different combination opioid), but to convert to a noncombination opioid agonist.[67] Although it has been suggested to use one-half of the calculated conversion dose in the elderly,[68] since the patient has been receiving an opioid without relief, the standard conversion to a short-acting pure agonist can be initiated with careful observation.

Morphine sulfate is the preferred drug at this stage. It is convenient to use and easy to administer since it is available in a variety of formulations. Also, due to its short half-life, it can be rapidly titrated in a given patient (including the elderly). Additional benefits of morphine for the elderly include allowing the patient and family to become familiar with one product, which the dispensing pharmacist can have available in its various formulations. Also, employing a single agent simplifies the medication schedule in a group of patients who are often subjected to polypharmacy and have difficulty with complex dosing regimens.[69] The recommended oral morphine initiation dose for a patient with unrelieved pain currently receiving 12 dosage units of a combination opioid product (as described above) is 10 mg every 4 h. In addition, a "rescue dose," calculated as one-half of the every 4-h scheduled dose (i.e., 5 mg for this example) should be offered to the patient every 2 to 3 h to allow for coverage of breakthrough pain. Rescue dosing, the method of supplemental analgesia during the course of long-acting analgesic therapy, has been advocated both on an empiric and scientific basis.[70,71]

To initiate therapy, the use of the liquid morphine preparation (20 mg/mL) is recommended. One can utilize this product over a wide dose range, and it may be administered through a feeding tube in patients who cannot swallow.[72] Its small dosage volume will also allow masking of any unpleasant taste by combining it with a large volume of a favorite beverage. Other short-acting opioids are available. Although hydromorphone is an effective drug, it has the unfortunate problem of being one of the more desirable "street drugs." For the elderly, who, e.g., might be vulnerable to robbery, this drug may represent a distinct source of unneeded problems if used in its oral preparation. In addition, there is no sustained release preparation available. Meperidine, as mentioned above, should not be considered as a desirable agent for any purpose in the elderly because of central nervous system toxicity. Given the long plasma half-life of methadone of 9 to 87 h,[28] its use as a first-line analgesic should also be discouraged due to difficulty in titration to an effective dose and the potential for dangerous accumulation, resulting in excess sedation and respiratory depression.[73,74] An additional product which should be discouraged is the Brompton's mixture. This combination of morphine, cocaine, alcohol, and often other ingredients offers no advantages over morphine alone[75] and may result in bothersome psychotomimetic effects with increasing doses. If a short-acting agent (e.g., morphine, hydromorphone) is used for initial titration, the patient can usually be stabilized on a given dose in 2 to 3 days. It should also be noted that this initial titration to an effective dose may be performed at home. Once the patient has been stabilized on a dosing schedule, sustained-release morphine can be introduced. It has the advantage in the elderly of needing less frequent dosing (8 to 12 h), which is advantageous in those in whom forgetfulness is a problem. It also allows for less interruption of an already disturbed sleep pattern. In the elderly patient, rather than a milligram-for-milligram conversion, we recommend that 75 percent of the short-acting dose be administered initially. Here dose adjustment, i.e., rescue dosing, is critical. Without the understanding of rescue dosing, the relief of pain will in all likelihood not be successful. This approach is especially useful in the elderly, since it can provide actual objective evidence of the amount of the dosage increase which the patient may require. Rescue dosing can and should be used to adjust the fixed-dose regimen.[76] As a general rule, when a patient is consuming four or more rescue doses per day, the maintenance dose should be increased. As an example, a patient receiving 60 mg of sustained-release morphine every 12 h who has consumed four 10-mg rescue doses should have his or her dosage increased to 90 mg every 12 h. At this time, the rescue doses should also be increased to 15 mg every 2 to 3 h as needed. Although this is a 50 percent increase in the total daily dosage, the patient has already demonstrated the need for the majority of this dosage increase through the consumption of rescue doses.

The elderly are particularly prone to somnolence early in the course of opioid treatment. Sedation will usually pass in a few days after starting treatment (many patients will be in a state of sleep deprivation, due to physical exhaustion from previously unrelieved pain). However, if sedation is severe and does not improve, the dose should be decreased by approximately 50 percent. As a general rule, if the patient can be easily aroused, then the patient may continue to receive opioids. The concern about respiratory depression is such that many patients receive inadequate pain relief. However, as demonstrated by Walsh,[77] even in patients with chronic obstructive pulmonary disease, neither P_{CO_2} nor P_{O_2} were affected by chronic oral morphine administration.

Opioid-induced constipation must be treated early in the elderly. Since decreased frequency of bowel movements is a common complaint in the elderly, one needs to have the patient record both frequency and character of stool when they are receiving opioids.[78] It is best to initiate laxatives early in the course of opiate therapy, in order to prevent severe constipation from occurring. A stool softener (e.g., docusate) to decrease stool hardness and a stimulant cathartic (e.g., senna)[79] to increase colonic motility should be used in doses that correct the situation. Lactulose and other osmotic cathartics may also be helpful when used in combination. Bulking agents such as psyllium are usually not effective alone in opioid-induced constipation, and they do not appear to be as useful in combination as are the osmotic agents. A realistic goal to achieve is a bowel movement at least every other day. There are no controlled trials examining the treatment of constipation during opioid therapy in the elderly or in the chronic pain population.

Another adverse effect which may occur is that of opioid-induced nausea/vomiting. Estimates as to the incidence of this complication vary but may approach or exceed 15 percent of patients.[11] This situation may resolve on its own but usually does not. While a phenothiazine (e.g., prochlorperazine) or agents useful for motion sickness may alleviate the nausea/vomiting temporarily, they do not remove the stimulus. In addition, patients may object to chronic use of these agents due to the additional adverse effects which they may experience. No scientific evidence exists to document the most effective means of eliminating this side effect. It appears from experience that it may often be managed by either converting the patient to an alternate opioid of a different chemical structure or changing the route of administration (e.g., oral to parenteral continuous infusion).

Miscellaneous Routes

When the oral route is no longer possible, what options are available to continue pain control in the elderly?

Rectal Although considered to be the alternate of choice when the oral route is no longer possible, many patients and caregivers have an aversion to this route, particularly in the elderly. How many children are willing to use rectal medication for their parent or grandparent? If this route is used, dosing is approximately 1 : 1 that of the oral dose.[80]

Parenteral: intramuscular This route is to be avoided. It not only is painful, particularly in frail elderly, but as stated above, the sporadic absorption leads to very difficult pain management. As demonstrated by Rutter et al,[81] examining this route in comparison with continuous intravenous administration, almost a fourfold increase in morphine dose is required. This situation may lead to toxicity as well as inadequate analgesia in the elderly.

Intravenous and subcutaneous The use of continuous infusion (CI) of opioids has found considerable success in the chronic administration of these agents.[35,36] Although considerable information is available regarding intravenous infusion in the elderly, little data are available regarding the subcutaneous administration in the elderly. The following situations indicate the need for CI:

1. When oral medication cannot be tolerated or adequately absorbed.
2. When the oral route becomes impractical due to very large oral dosage requirements.
3. Where rescue dosing requires such frequent administration that it becomes impractical for caregivers to provide.

4. When it is necessary to allow for rapid titration to effective analgesia in patients with severe pain.
5. When it is necessary to provide continuous relief in the terminally ill who have been stabilized on an intermittent dosing parenteral regimen.

The useful agents for this approach include the following:

Morphine This is again the agent of choice for reasons mentioned earlier. Although there is probably only minimal risk, the health care worker should be aware of the reported somnolence observed secondary to morphine infusion due to the preservative chlorbutanol.[82] This is likely a complication with very high morphine doses, although no data are available in the elderly. When morphine administration becomes difficult due to volume considerations (e.g., subcutaneous route), then one of the following agents should be considered.

Hydromorphone This agent is particularly useful in this setting because it has a high potency-solubility ratio, making it the ideal agent for subcutaneous infusion.

Fentanyl This agent is of even greater potency than hydromorphone and is also very useful for subcutaneous infusions, especially when infusion volume constraints are present.

Reviews by Coyle,[83] Portenoy,[84] and Payne[85] are thorough in describing the technique of CI. The addition of PCA[86] may make the combination the most effective treatment of chronic pain in the elderly, although studies are lacking. The use of PCA in combination with CI will allow for rapid dosage titration, analogous to the use of rescue doses in patients receiving oral opioids. As with oral rescue doses, use of rescue doses via PCA and the resultant titration should follow the same principles (i.e., a 25 to 50-percent increase in the daily CI dose should be made when four or more PCA doses are delivered in a day). The PCA dose should be equivalent to one-half of the hourly opioid dose and be set with approximately a 2-h lockout.

Spinal The use of CI may also be applied to spinal administration. No trials exist at this time comparing bolus administration with CI for the spinal route. It is therefore unclear whether either route is preferable in terms of adverse effects or the development of tolerance. The usual dosing interval for bolus administration via the spinal route is 8 to 12 h,[87-88] which is considerably longer than the 4-h interval required for parenteral bolus dosing. When converting a patient from the parenteral to the epidural route, the total daily epidural dose should be reduced to approximately 10 percent of the daily parenteral dose. The conversion for parenteral to intrathecal is approximately 1 percent of the daily parenteral dose. It has been demonstrated that the efficacy and safety of opioids administered either via the intrathecal or epidural route can be maintained for months if necessary.[47,52,87,88]

Transdermal Administration

Fentanyl has been formulated as a transdermal patch. The advantages for this system include all of those discussed for the CI route in addition to the simplicity of not requiring a needle. An excellent review by Enck[89] suggests good patient acceptance of this formulation. Although the vast majority of studies have examined its safety and efficacy in the postoperative setting,[90-93] the first patch to be marketed was approved only for chronic pain. Due to the absorption-rate-limited pharmacokinetics of this patch,[94] characterized by slow absorption and a long terminal half-life, rapid dosage titration is difficult. A few trials have had some limited clinical experience with this delivery system in elderly patients.[91,92,95] It has not yet been determined whether the elderly may have a different absorption profile, since no comparative trials have been performed to examine differences in the pharmacokinetics of transdermal fentanyl between young versus elderly patients. This may be of some importance, since chronic pain patients would require a dosage conversion from their prior narcotic regimen when being switched to a transdermal fentanyl system. If elderly patients did display altered absorption pharmacokinetics, either toxicity or decreased efficacy could result. Percutaneous absorption may increase, decrease, or remain unchanged with age, depending upon the site of application, the agent applied, and other factors.[96] Thus, absorption from such transdermal systems may indeed be different in the elderly.

Adjuvant Analgesics

In addition to the opioid analgesics, several classes of drugs are also useful adjuncts. These adjunct agents are especially useful in the treatment of cancer pain. Especially useful adjunct agents include the NSAIDs, the corticosteroids, the heterocyclic antidepressants, and the diphosphonates.

The NSAIDs have proven to increase analgesia above that achievable with the opioid alone.[97,98] Whether this same analgesia could be achieved with a larger opioid dose is currently unknown. These agents appear to be especially useful in patients with skeletal metastases, due to their antiprostaglandin effect, which may decrease pain mediation in areas of bony metastases.[99-101]

One report has recently questioned the safety of these agents in patients with reduced renal function, such as the elderly.[102] However, since patients who developed worsening renal function in this trial had rather substantial renal dysfunction to begin with, it does not appear that their results are applicable to the entire elderly population. Additional data exist to demonstrate the safety of NSAIDs in the elderly population.[103]

When skeletal metastases are no longer responsive to NSAIDs, a corticosteroid or a biphosphonate (e.g., etidronate) may be indicated.[104-106] It is currently unclear which of these two classes of agents is most efficacious as no comparative trials have been performed. It is also unknown whether either of these agents offers more advantages in the elderly in terms of their side-effect profile. The biphosphonates to date have been almost totally devoid of adverse effects. However, there are also few if any reports documenting considerable side effects for the corticosteroids when used in terminal malignancy.

The heterocyclic antidepressants are also widely used for pain relief, especially when there is a burning or shooting component to the pain. As yet, no controlled trials exist to determine their efficacy, although anecdotal reports suggest it.[107,108] Recent evidence suggests that their efficacy may be due to an alteration in morphine pharmacokinetics.[109]

It appears that these four classes of agents may offer advantages to cancer patients, especially those with either bone pain or a shooting/burning pain component. It is as yet unknown whether the elderly population may require altered dosing of these agents.

Nonmalignant Pain

It is apparent that for this type of pain, the medical needs of the patient are often outweighed by the societal pressure to regulate these agents and reserve them for acute pain or terminal patients. However, a study of 38 patients with nonmalignant pain demonstrated that 60 percent of patients treated with opioids achieved a level of pain relief which allowed them to function.[110] Many of these patients were maintained on these agents for many months without developing significant tolerance or other complications. In addition, a recent review by Portenoy[111] identifies multiple studies which demonstrate the value of opioids in a variety of nonmalignant pain syndromes. Thus, the future may hold promise for patients with intractable chronic pain of nonmalignant origin. These patients are quite possibly the most undertreated group of chronic pain patients due to the concerns regarding addiction and tolerance with long-term administration.

SUMMARY

The elderly are clearly a population for which analgesia is of vital importance. Despite some gaps in our knowledge of how this age group may differ from others in their metabolism and or sensitivity to the opioids, the available data and clinical experience suggest that these agents may be used safely in this patient population provided they are dosed appropriately and dosage increases are performed in a logical stepwise manner. It does not appear that there is a lack of analgesics or special techniques available to safely treat the elderly patient with pain. However, evidence suggests that patients in pain often receive inadequate analgesia. Given the greater likelihood of pain in elderly patients, this translates into inadequate analgesia for many of the elderly. The impediments to effective analgesia in these patients may lie in such areas as inadequate assessment and improper utilization of available techniques. Improved knowledge of the proper use of available opioid agonists by clinicians and a more diligent approach to pain management may improve this situation, although these changes may require a considerable period of time. Recent success with the opioids in patients with nonmalignant pain may help to spur a change in the prescribing practices of these agents. The title of a recent editorial by Melzack[112] may sum it up best: "The Tragedy of Needless Pain."

REFERENCES

1. Davis MA: Epidemiology of osteoarthritis. *Clin Geriatr Med* 4: 241-255, 1988.
2. Daut RL, Cleeland CS: The prevalence and severity of pain in cancer. *Cancer* 50:1913-1918, 1982.
3. Boring CC, Squires TS, Tong T: *Cancer Statistics, 1991, CA* 41:19-36, 1991.
4. Grossman A: Opioid peptides and pain, in Mann RD (ed): *The History of the Management of Pain.* Park Ridge, Parthenon Publishing Group, 1988, pp 127-141.
5. Cleeland CS: Barriers to the management of cancer pain. *Oncology* 1:19-27, 1987.
6. Hill CS, Fields WS (eds): Drug treatment of cancer pain in a drug oriented society. *Adv Pain Res Ther* 11:1-353, 1989.
7. Max MB: Improving outcome of analgesia treatment: Is education enough. *Ann Intern Med* 113:885-889, 1990.
8. Donovan M, Dillon P, McGuire L: Incidence and characteristics of pain in a sample of medical-surgical inpatients. *Pain* 30:69-87, 1987.
9. Marks RM, Sacher EJ: Undertreatment of medical inpatients with narcotic analgesics. *Ann Intern Med* 38:173-181, 1973.
10. Sabbe ME, Yaksh TL: Pharmacology of spinal opioids. *J Pain Symptom Manag* 5:191-203, 1990.
11. Jaffe JH, Martin WR: Opioid analgesics and antagonists, in Gilman AG, Rall TW, Nies AS, Taylor P (eds): *The Pharmacological Basis of Therapeutics.* New York, Pergamon, 1990, pp 486-493.
12. Foley KM: Controversies in cancer pain. *Cancer* 63:2257-2265, 1989.
13. Lipman AG: Clinically relevant differences among the opioid analgesics. *Am J Hosp Pharm* 47 (1, suppl 1): S7-13, 1990.
14. Belleville JW, Forrest WH, Miller E, Brown BW: Influence of age on pain relief from analgesics; a study of postoperative patients. *JAMA* 217:1835-1841, 1971.
15. Kaiko RF: Age and morphine analgesia in cancer patients with postoperative pain. *Clin Pharmacol Ther* 28:823-826, 1980.
16. Owen JA, Sitar DS, Berger L, et al: Age-related morphine kinetics. *Clin Pharmacol Ther* 34:364-368, 1983.
17. Sawe J, Dahlstrom B, Paalzow L, Rane A: Morphine kinetics in cancer patients. *Clin Pharmacol Ther* 30:629-635, 1981.
18. Stanski DR, Greenblatt DJ, Lowenstein E: The kinetics of intravenous and intramuscular morphine. *Clin Pharmacol Ther* 24:52-59, 1978.
19. Berkowitz BA, Ngai SH, Yang JC, et al: The disposition of morphine in surgical patients. *Clin Pharmacol Ther* 17:629-635, 1975.
20. Osborne R, Joel S, Slevin M: Morphine intoxication in renal failure: the role of morphine-6-glucuronide. *Br Med J* 293:1101, 1986.
21. Peterson GM, Randall CTC, Paterson J: Plasma levels of morphine and morphine glucuronides in the treatment of cancer pain: relationship to renal function and route of administration. *Eur J Clin Pharmacol* 38:121-124, 1990.
22. Osborne R, Joel S, Trew D, Slevin M: Analgesic activity of morphine-6-glucuronide. *Lancet* I:828, 1988.
23. Osborne R, Joel S, Trew D, Slevin M: Morphine and metabolite behavior after different routes of morphine administration: demonstration of the importance of the active metabolite morphine-6-glucuronide. *Clin Pharmacol Ther* 47:12-19, 1990.

24. Baillie SP, Bateman DN, Coates PE, Woodhouse KW: Age and the pharmacokinetics of morphine. *Age Ageing* 18:258–262, 1989.
25. Holmberg L, Odar-Cederlof I, Boreus LO, et al: Comparative disposition of pethidine and norpethidine in old and young patients. *Eur J Clin Pharmacol* 22:175–179, 1982.
26. Boreus LO, Odar-Cederlof I, Bondesson U, et al: Elimination of meperidine and its metabolites in old patients compared to young patients. *Adv Pain Res Ther* 8:167–169, 1986.
27. Inturrisi CE, Portenoy RK, Max MB, et al: Pharmacokinetic-pharmacodynamic relationships of methadone infusions in patients with cancer pain. *Clin Pharmacol Ther* 47:565–577, 1990.
28. Gourlay GK, Wilson PR, Glynn CJ: Pharmacodynamics and pharmacokinetics of methadone during the perioperative period. *Anesthesiology* 57:458–467, 1982.
29. Bentley JB, Borel JD, Nenad RE, Gillespie TJ: Age and fentanyl pharmacokinetics. *Anesth Analg* 61:968–971, 1982.
30. Hudson RJ, Thomson IR, Cannon JE, et al: Pharmacokinetics of fentanyl in patients undergoing abdominal aortic surgery. *Anesthesiology* 64:334–338, 1986.
31. Cartwright P, Prys-Roberts C, Gill K, et al: Ventilatory depression related to plasma fentanyl concentrations during and after anesthesia in humans. *Anesth Analg* 62:966–974, 1983.
32. Sitar DS, Duke PC, Benthuysen JL, et al: Aging and alfentanil disposition in healthy volunteers and surgical patients. *Can J Anaesth* 2:149–154, 1989.
33. Scott JC, Stanski DR: Decreased fentanyl and alfentanil dose requirements with age. A simultaneous pharmacokinetic and pharmacodynamic evaluation. *J Pharmacol Exp Ther* 240:159–166, 1987.
34. Porter J, Jick H: Addiction rare in patients treated with narcotics. *N Engl J Med* 302:123, 1980.
35. Kerr IG, Sone M, DeAngelis C, et al: Continuous narcotic infusion with patient-controlled analgesia for chronic cancer pain in outpatients. *Ann Intern Med* 108:554–557, 1988.
36. Stuart GJ, Davey EB, Sight SE: Continuous intravenous morphine infusions for terminal pain control: a retrospective review. *DICP Ann Pharmacother* 20:968–972, 1986.
37. Brescia FJ, Walsh M, Savarese JJ, Kaiko RF: A study of controlled-release oral morphine (MS Contin) in an advanced cancer hospital. *J Pain Symptom Manag* 2:193–198, 1987.
38. Chrischilles EA, Lemke JH, Wallace RB, Drube GA: Prevalence and characteristics of multiple analgesic use in an elderly study group. *J Am Geriatr Soc* 38:979–984, 1990.
39. Portenoy RK, Kanner RM: Patterns of analgesic prescription and consumption in a university-affiliated community hospital. *Arch Intern Med* 145:439–441, 1985.
40. Pernik MS: *A Calculus of Suffering*. New York, Columbia University Press, 1985, pp 238–239.
41. Levin DN, Cleeland CS, Dar R: Public attitudes toward cancer pain. *Cancer* 56:2337–2339, 1985.
42. Rice JRA, Browne RA, Davis C, et al: Variations in the disposition of morphine after IM injection in surgical patients. *Br J Anaesth* 50:1125–1129, 1978.
43. Austin KL, Stapleton JV, Mather LE: Multiple intramuscular injections: a major source of variability in analgesic response to meperidine. *Pain* 8:47–62, 1980.
44. Kaiko RF, Foley KM, Grabinsli PY, et al: Central nervous system excitatory effects of meperidine in cancer patients. *Ann Neurol* 13:180–185, 1983.
45. Egbert MD, Parks LH, Short LM, Burnett ML: Randomized trial of postoperative patient-controlled analgesia versus intramuscular narcotics in frail elderly men. *Arch Intern Med* 150:1897–1903, 1990.
46. Barkas G, Duafala ME: Advances in cancer pain management: a review of patient-controlled analgesia. *J Pain Symptom Manag* 3:150–160, 1988.
47. Ventafridda V, Spoldi E, Caraceni A, DeConno F: Intraspinal morphine for cancer pain. *Acta Anaesthiol Scand* 31 (suppl 85):47–53, 1987.
48. Klinck JR, Lindop MJ: Epidural morphine in the elderly. A controlled trial after upper abdominal surgery. *Anaesthesia* 37:907–912, 1982.
49. Korbon GA, James DJ, Verlander JM, et al: Intramuscular naloxone reverses the side effects of epidural morphine while preserving analgesia. *Reg Anesth* 10:16–20, 1985.
50. Gueneron JP, Ecoffey C, Carli P, et al: Effect of naloxone infusion on analgesia and respiratory depression after epidural fentanyl. *Anesth Analg* 67:35–38, 1989.

51. Gustafsson LL, Schildt B, Jacobsen K: Adverse effects of extradural and intrathecal opiates: report of a nationwide survery in Sweden. *Br J Anaesth* 54:479–485, 1982.
52. Samuelsson H, Nordberg G, Hedner T, Lindquist J: CSF and plasma morphine concentrations in cancer patients during chronic epidural morphine therapy and its relation to pain relief. *Pain* 30:303–310, 1987.
53. Waldman SD: The role of spinal opioids in the management of cancer pain. *J Pain Symptom Manag* 5:163–168, 1990.
54. Gustafsson LL, Grell AM, Garle M, et al: Kinetics of morphine in cerebrospinal fluid after epidural administration. *Acta Anaesthesiol Scand* 28:535–539, 1984.
55. Sjöström S, Hartvig P, Persson MP, Tamsen A: Pharmacokinetics of epidural morphine and meperidine in humans. *Anesthesiology* 67:877–888, 1987.
56. Nordberg G, Hansdottir V, Kvist L, et al: Pharmacokinetics of different epidural sites of morphine administration. *Eur J Clin Pharmacol* 33:499–504, 1987.
57. Ready LB, Chadwick HS, Ross B: Age predicts effective epidural morphine dose after abdominal hysterectomy. *Anesth Analg* 66:1215–1218, 1987.
58. Moore AK, Vilderman S, Lubenskyi W, et al: Differences in epidural morphine requirements between elderly and young patients after abdominal surgery. *Anesth Analg* 70:316–20, 1990.
59. DuPen SL, Ramsey D, Chin S: Chronic epidural morphine and preservative-induced injury. *Anesthesiology* 67:987–988, 1987.
60. Cancer Pain Relief, World Health Organization. Geneva, World Health Organization, 1986, pp 1–73.
61. Ventafridda J, Tamburini M, Caraccni A, et al: A validation study of the WHO method for cancer pain relief. *Cancer* 59:850–857, 1987.
62. Swerdlow M: Anticonvulsant drugs and chronic pain. *Clin Neuropharmacol* 7:51–82, 1987.
63. Ventafridda V, Saita L, Bartetta L, et al: Clinical observation on controlled-release morphine in cancer pain. *J Pain Symptom Manag* 4:124–129, 1989.
64. Thrillwell MP, Sloan PA, Maroun JA, et al: Pharmacokinetics and clinical efficacy of oral morphine solution and controlled-release morphine tablets in cancer patients. *Cancer* 63:2275–2283, 1989.
65. Cleeland CS: Assessment of pain in cancer, in Foley KM, et al (eds): *Advances in Pain Research and Therapy.* New York, Raven, 1990, pp. 47–55.
66. Gibson TP, Giacomini KM, Briggs WA, et al: Propoxyphene and norpropoxyphene plasma concentrations in the anephric patient. *Clin Pharmacol Ther* 27:665–679, 1980.
67. Hill CS: Guidelines for treatment of cancer pain: final report of Texas Cancer Council's Work Group on Pain Control in Cancer. Austin, Texas Cancer Plan, 1990, p 8.
68. Kaiko RF, Wallenstein SL, Rogers AG, et al: Narcotics in the elderly. *Med Clin North Am* 66:1079–1089, 1983.
69. Nolan L, O'Malley K: Prescribing for the elderly, Parts 1, 2. *J Am Geriatr Soc* 36:142–149, 245–254, 1988.
70. Savarese JJ, Thomas GB, Homesley H, Hill CS: Rescue factor: a design for evaluating long-acting analgesics. *Clin Pharm Ther* 43:376–380, 1988.
71. Foley KM, Inturrisi CE: Analgesic drug therapy in cancer pain: principles and practices. *Med Clin North Am* 71:207–232, 1987.
72. Pitorak EF, Kraus JC: Pain control with sublingual morphine. *Am J Hospice Care* 4:39–41, 1987.
73. Ettinger DS, Vitale PJ, Trump DL: Important clinical pharmacologic considerations in the use of methadone in cancer patients. *Can Treat Rep* 63:457–459, 1979.
74. Symonds P: Methadone and the elderly. *Br Med J* 1:512, 1977.
75. Melzack R, Mount BM, Gordon JM: The Brompton Mixture versus morphine solution given orally: effects on pain. *Can Med Assoc J* 120:435–438, 1979.
76. Portenoy RK, Hagen NR: Breakthrough pain: definition, characteristics and prevalence. *Pain* 41:273–282, 1990.
77. Walsh TD: Control of pain and other symptoms in advanced cancer. *Oncology* 1:5–9, 1987.

78. Sykes NP: Methods of assessment of bowel function in patients with advanced cancer. *Pall Med* 4:287–293, 1990.
79. Izard MW, Ellison FS: Treatment of drug induced constipation with a purified senna derivative. *Conn Med* 26:589–592, 1962.
80. Twycross RG, Lack SA: *Therapeutics in Terminal Cancer.* London, Pitman 1984, p 166.
81. Rutter PC, Murphy F, Dudley HAF: Morphine: controlled trial of different methods of administration for postoperative pain relief. *Br Med J* 280:12–13, 1980.
82. DeChristoforo R, Corden BJ, Hood JC, et al: High-dose morphine infusion complicated by chlorobutanol-induced somnolence. *Ann Intern Med* 98:335–336, 1983.
83. Coyle N, Mauskop A, Maggard J, Foley K: Continuous subcutaneous infusions of opiates in cancer patients with pain. *ONF* 13:53–57, 1986.
84. Portenoy RK: Continuous infusion of opioid drugs in the treatment of cancer pain. *J Pain Symptom Manag* 1:223–228, 1986.
85. Payne R: Novel routes of opioid administration, in Hill CS, Fields WD (eds): *Advances in Pain Research.* New York, Raven, 1989, pp 319–338.
86. Swanson G, Smith J, Bulich R, et al: Patient-controlled analgesia for chronic cancer pain in the ambulatory setting: a report of 117 patients. *J Clin Oncol* 7:1903–1908, 1989.
87. DuPen SL, Peterson DG, Bogosian AC, et al: A new permanent exteriorized epidural catheter for narcotic self-administration to control cancer pain. *Cancer* 59:986–993, 1987.
88. Brazenor GA: Long term intrathecal administration of morphine: a comparison of bolus injection via reservoir with continuous infusion by implanted pump. *Neurosurgery* 21:484–491, 1987.
89. Enck RE: Transdermal narcotics for pain control. *Am J Hosp Pall Care* 7:15–17, 1990.
90. Caplan RA, Ready LB, Oden RV, et al: Transdermal fentanyl for postoperative pain management; a double-blind placebo study. *JAMA* 261:1036–1039, 1989.
91. Holley FO, Steennis CV: Postoperative analgesia with fentanyl: pharmacokinetics and pharmacodynamics of constant-rate I.V. and transdermal delivery. *Br J Anaesth* 60:608–613, 1988.
92. Duthie DJR, Rowbotham DJ, Wyld R, et al: Plasma fentanyl concentrations during transdermal delivery of fentanyl to surgical patients. *Br J Anaesth* 60:614–618, 1988.
93. Plezia PM, Kramer TH, Linford J, Hameroff SR: Transdermal fentanyl: pharmacokinetics and preliminary clinical evaluation. *Pharmacotherapy* 9:2–9, 1989.
94. Varvel JR, Shafer SL, Hwang SS, et al: Absorption characteristics of transdermally administered fentanyl. *Anesthesiology* 70:928–934, 1989.
95. Miser AW, Narang PK, Dothage JA, et al: Transdermal fentanyl for pain control in patients with cancer. *Pain* 37:15–21, 1989.
96. Roskos KV, Guy RH, Maibach HI: Percutaneous absorption in the aged. *Dermatol Clin* 4:455–465, 1986.
97. Weingart WA, Sorkness CA, Earhart RH: Analgesia with oral narcotics and added ibuprofen in cancer patients. *Clin Pharm* 4:53–58, 1985.
98. Ferrer-Brechner T, Ganz P: Combination therapy with ibuprofen and methadone for chronic cancer pain. *Am J Med* 7:78–83, 1984.
99. Galasko CS, Bennett A: Relationship of bone destruction in skeletal metastases to osteoclast activation and prostaglandins. *Nature* 263:508–510, 1976.
100. Powles TJ, Clark SA, Easty DM, et al: The inhibition by aspirin and indomethacin of osteolytic tumor deposits and hypercalcaemia in rats with Walter tumor, and its possible application to human breast cancer. *Br J Cancer* 28:316–321, 1973.
101. Powles TJ, Dowsett M, Easty GC, et al: Breast-cancer osteolysis, bone metastases, and anti-osteolytic effect of aspirin. *Lancet* I:608–610, 1976.
102. Whelton A, Stout RL, Spillman PS, Klassen DK: Renal effects of ibuprofen, piroxicam, and sulindac in patients with asymptomatic renal failure. A prospective, randomized, crossover comparison. *Ann Intern Med* 112:568–576, 1990.
103. Cummings DM, Amadio P, Nettler S, et al: Office-based evaluation of renal function in elderly patients receiving nonsteroidal anti-inflammatory drugs. *J Am Board Fam Pract* 1:77–80, 1988.

104. Adami S, Mian M: Clodronate therapy of metastatic bone disease in patients with prostatic carcinoma. *Recent Results Cancer Res* 116:67–72, 1989.
105. Carey PO, Lippert MC: Treatment of painful prostatic bone metastases with oral etidronate disodium. *Urology* 32:403–407, 1988.
106. Bruera E, Roca E, Cedaro L, et al: action of oral methylprednisolone in terminal cancer patients: A prospective randomized double-blind study. *Cancer Treat Rep* 69:751–754, 1985.
107. Kocher R: The use of psychotropic drugs in the treatment of cancer pain. *Recent Results Cancer Res* 89:118–126, 1984.
108. Magni G, Conlon P, Arsie D: Tricyclic antidepressants in the treatment of cancer pain: a review. *Pharmacopsychiatry* 20:160–164, 1987.
109. Ventafridda V, Ripamonti C, DeConno F, et al: Antidepressants increase bioavailability of morphine in cancer patients. *Lancet* I:1204, 1987.
110. Portenoy RK, Foley KM: Chronic use of opioid analgesics in non-malignant pain. *Pain* 25:171–186, 1986.
111. Portenoy RK: Chronic opioid therapy in non-malignant pain. *J Pain Symptom Manag* 5:S46–62, 1990.
112. Melzack R: The tragedy of needless pain. *Sci Am* 262:27–33, 1990.

CHAPTER

10

HEADACHE

Michael D. Katz

Headache is a common complaint of the elderly.[1-3] Acute and chronic headache syndromes often result in frequent physicians' visits and the use of multiple medications. Headache, while often thought to be an affliction of industrialized society, dates back at least to the Sumerian era. Roman writings from the second century describe the aura of migraine, and the Greek physician Galen described a variety of headache syndromes in the second century. Numerous famous individuals in history have suffered from headache, including Queen Mary Tudor, Freud, Thomas Jefferson, and Ulysses Grant.[4]

EPIDEMIOLOGY

At least 65 percent of patients over age 65 complain of at least occasional headache, and up to 20 percent of the elderly complain of frequent headache.[5] However, various studies report very different incidences of headache in the population studied. The Dunedin Program, a study which used annual questionnaires to screen elderly people for undetected medical disorders, reported a headache incidence of 13.9 percent in 1927 women and 6.5 percent in 1040 men.[6]

Solomon et al[7] studied the demographics of headache in 359 patients over the age of 65 years. Elderly patients comprised 4 percent of the total headache population studied, suggesting that headache is less common in the elderly than in the younger population. While other studies also have shown a lower incidence of headache in the elderly,[4] the elderly seek medical attention for headache more often than the young. In Solomon's study,[7] the average age of older headache sufferers was 73.5 years, with 66 percent of patients being female. The most common causes of headache included tension, migraine, temporal arteritis, and mixed (Table 10-1).

Table 10-1 Prevalence of primary headache in 423 elderly patients

Type	Total, %	Male, %	Female, %	Mean age
Tension	27	35	65	73.9
Migraine	15	41	59	75.9
Temporal arteritis	15	30	70	73.7
Mixed	14	32	68	68.1
Cluster	4	72	28	71.8
Other	25	24	76	74.8

Source: Adapted from Ref. 7.

Elderly patients with headache often had multiple medical problems and were receiving several medications. Hale et al[8] found no correlation between age and incidence of headache in a population of 92 elderly patients with headache. These authors found that elderly patients with headache often have multiple symptomatic complaints, such as temporary loss of vision, brief loss of speech, brief loss of the use of an arm or leg, paresthesias and symptoms of depression. Patients with underlying arthritis, peptic ulcer disease, and angina more frequently complained of headache.

Patients with headache often are treated with multiple medications. In a study of 500 patients[9] with a primary headache disorder (9 percent were over the age of 55 years), patients were receiving three to five drugs per patient.

CLASSIFICATION OF HEADACHE

The most recent classification and diagnostic criteria for headache disorders was published by the International Headache Society in 1988.[10,11] These criteria are outlined in Table 10-2.

GENERAL APPROACH TO THE PATIENT

It may be difficult to ascertain the cause of headache in an elderly patient based on history alone. The most important effort should be, of course, to identify patients who have a potentially life-threatening disorder associated with headache, such as cerebrovascular disease, brain tumor, subdural hematoma, and temporal arteritis. Usually benign headaches have been present for some time. A new-onset, severe headache or one that becomes progressively worse in severity deserves special attention. The presence of focal neurologic deficits or constitutional symptoms should be cause for initiation of a full diagnostic evaluation. In addition to the neurologic examination and vital signs, special attention should be given to the

Table 10-2 Classification of primary headache disorders

Migraine
Migraine without aura
Migraine with aura
Ophthalmoplegic migraine
Retinal migraine
Complications of migraine
Tension-type headache
Episodic
Chronic
Cluster headache and chronic paroxysmal hemicrania
Miscellaneous headaches unassociated with structural lesion
Idiopathic stabbing headache
External compression headache
Cold stimulus headache
Benign cough headache
Benign exertional headache
Headache associated with sexual activity

Source: Adapted from Refs. 10, 11.

cervical spine, carotid and temporal arteries, temporomandibular joints, teeth, and ocular pressure. In the elderly, a complete blood count (CBC) and erythrocyte sedimentation rate (ESR) should be included as screens for temporal arteritis.[3]

HEADACHE SYNDROMES

While certain headache syndromes have similar features in the young and elderly, some disorders, such as cerebrovascular disease and temporal arteritis, are much more common in the elderly. This section will review the most common headache syndromes with features characteristic or unique to the elderly emphasized. More information can be found in several recent reviews.[1-3,12-17]

Migraine

In the elderly, 10 to 25 percent of headaches are due to migraine. While the onset of migraine after the age of 50 is unusual,[2] up to 50 percent[3] of patients who have had migraine may continue to have attacks as they age. It is not clear why the incidence of migraine decreases in the elderly. With aging,[2] there may be a reduced ability of cerebral arteries to dilate and constrict in response to the triggering events of migraine. Hormonal changes that precipitate migraine in younger women no longer occur after menopause. Potential changes in neurotransmitter levels with aging also could alter the incidence of attacks.

Signs and symptoms The signs and symptoms of acute migraine,[1,2,12,17,18] in the elderly are similar to those in younger patients. Nausea and vomiting, photophobia, phonophobia, throbbing pain, and scalp tenderness are characteristic. Prodromal symptoms such as a visual aura will continue to be present. However, new onset of aura in a patient without previous auras should indicate the possibility of an additional neurologic problem.[1] The signs, symptoms, diagnosis, and pathophysiology of migraine are described in more detail in several excellent reviews.[12,17,19] Many now feel that serotonin plays a major role in the pathophysiology of migraine. Release of serotonin as well as prostaglandins and norepinephrine causes vasoconstriction. Subsequent depletion of serotonin and other neurotransmitters is thought to result in vasodilation and pain. The underlying causes and mechanism for the initial neurotransmitter release are not well understood.

Some patients may have migraine equivalents, that is, episodes of transient neurologic deficits or dysfunction without headache in a patient with a previous history of migraine.[2] These episodes may include scintillating scotoma, homonymous hemianopsia, aphasia, paresthesias, dysarthria, hemiplegia, vertigo, transient global amnesia, mood disorders, and cardiac arrhythmias. In the elderly, it may be quite difficult to distinguish these migraine equivalents from transient ischemic attacks (TIAs). The relatively slow progression of visual and other symptoms over 5 to 30 min and the persistence of visual symptoms with the eyes closed are thought to be helpful distinguishing characteristics suggesting the presence of migraine.

Therapy The treatment of migraine is separated into treating or aborting the acute attack and chronic, preventative therapy. Because of the importance of serotonin in the pathophysiology of migraine, the effect of various antimigraine drugs on serotonin and its receptors has been studied.[12,15,16,20-23] Many of the commonly used antimigraine agents have effects on serotonin. At least three general types of serotonin (5-HT) receptors[21-23] exist: 5-HT_1, 5-HT_2, and 5-HT_3. In addition, the 5-HT_1 receptor has at least three subtypes. Acute relief of migraine is thought to be mediated by drugs that are 5-HT_{1a} or 5-HT_{1D} agonists, while prophylactic relief may be mediated by 5-HT_2 or 5-HT_{1C} antagonists.[21] The effects mediated by the various 5-HT receptors are listed in Table 10-3.

Acute treatment[1,2,12,15-17,20] The time-honored treatment for acute migraine is ergotamine, and in fact, pain relief after administration of ergot is considered a diagnostic hallmark of migraine. During an acute attack, ergotamine may be more effective if administered rectally (60 percent efficacy) or by injection (70 to 80 percent), since oral absorption (40 to 50 percent efficacy) may be erratic and incomplete.[24] Ergot alkaloids have both α-blocking and α-agonist effects and inhibit the reuptake of serotonin and norepinephrine. Dihydroergotamine (DHE) is given only by injection and may have less peripheral arterial vasoconstrictive effects than ergotamine.[20] The efficacy of ergot alkaloids in acute migraine is thought to be related primarily to their vasoconstrictive properties. Caffeine appears to enhance the efficacy of ergotamine by potentiating vasoconstriction and

Table 10-3 Classification of serotonin receptors

Receptor	Effects mediated	Agonist	Antagonist
5-HT_{1A}	Basilar artery constriction Neuronal inhibition	Ergotamine Methysergide	Methiothepin
5-HT_{1D}	Cranial vasoconstriction	Ergotamine Sumatriptan Amitriptyline Propranolol Nifedipine	
5-HT_2	Vasoconstriction Small muscle contraction Platelet aggregation	Methysergide Amitriptyline Cyproheptadine Verapamil Nifedipine	Lisuride
5-HT_3	Emesis CNS excitation		Ondansetron Metoclopramide

Source: Adapted from Refs. 21, 23.

enhancing the gastrointestinal (GI) absorption of the ergotamine.[12] Table 10-4 lists the drugs and doses used in the treatment of migraine. Intractable migraine has been successfully treated with intravenous (IV) DHE and metoclopramide.[20] Because DHE is not water soluble, it should not be diluted prior to injection. Common adverse effects of ergotamine include nausea and vomiting, abdominal cramping, paresthesias, cold extremities, and rebound headache.

Because of its vasoconstrictive properties, the use of ergotamine may be especially harmful in the elderly. Ergot alkaloids have the potential for reducing cerebral blood flow and could precipitate a stroke in a patient with hemiplegic migraine or associated cerebrovascular disease. Ergotamine-induced peripheral vasoconstriction could increase the incidence of angina, precipitate a myocardial infarction, or worsen symptoms of intermittent claudication. Ergotamine should not be used in patients with coronary artery disease, peripheral vascular disease, renal insufficiency, and liver disease. In addition, the drug is best avoided in patients with hypertension. Ergotamine should not be used for chronic, preventative therapy.

Isometheptene mucate, a component of the commercial product Midrin (isometheptene 65 mg, dichloralphenazone 100 mg, acetaminophen 325 mg), may be a safer alternative to ergot alkaloids in the elderly.[2,20] This agent, an α-agonist, has been shown to be effective in the treatment of mild to moderate acute migraine. The dichloralphenazone is a chloral hydrate derivative and may provide some sedation. Isometheptene may be more effective if administered with 650 mg aspirin or a nonsteroidal anti-inflammatory drug (NSAID). However, this agent also is a

Table 10-4 Drugs used in the treatment of migraine

Drug	Dose	Precautions
	Acute attack	
Ergotamine (oral)	1 mg, may repeat in 30–60 min, maximum 3–4 mg/attack	Avoid in elderly
Dihydroergotamine (IV)	0.25–0.5 mg, with prochlorperazine or metoclopramide, may repeat in 30 min	Avoid in elderly
Isometheptene (oral, Midrin)	1–2 capsules, may repeat in 30–60 min, maximum 4–5 capsules	Similar adverse effects as ergot, CNS depression
Naproxen sodium (oral)	825 mg, then 275 mg in 30 min	Sodium retention, renal toxicity, gastropathy, bleeding
Chlorpromazine (oral, rectal, IV)	0.1 mg/kg every 15 min 3 times	Avoid in elderly; hypotension
Prochlorperazine (IV)	10 mg	Extrapyramidal effects
Sumatriptan (SQ)	6–8 mg, may repeat in 60 min	Possible EKG changes
	Prophylaxis	
Beta blockers		
Propranolol	20–40 mg tid, titrate up to 320–360 mg/day	Avoid in CHF, asthma, COPD
Nadolol	20 mg/day, titrate up to 160–320 mg/day	
Metoprolol	25 mg bid, titrate up to 100–200 mg/day	
Methysergide	2 mg/day, titrate up to maximum of 8 mg/day; 6 months on, 1 month off	Avoid in elderly; retroperitoneal fibrosis
Antidepressants		
Amitriptyline	25 mg/day, titrate up to maximum of 75–100 mg/day	Avoid amitriptyline in elderly; sedation, hypotension, anticholinergic
Nortriptyline	25 mg/day, titrate up to maximum 75 mg/day	
Doxepin	25 mg/day, titrate up to maximum 100 mg/day	

Table 10-4 ***(continued)*** **Drugs used in the treatment of migraine**

Drug	Dose	Precautions
Calcium blockers		
Verapamil	80 mg bid, titrate up to maximum 480 mg/day	May worsen CHF, constipation, conduction abnormalities
Nifedipine	10 mg tid, titrate to maximum 60 mg tid	May cause hypotension, edema, reflex tachycardia
Diltiazem	30 mg bid, titrate up to maximum 90 mg tid	
Nonsteroidals		
Naproxen	375-500 mg bid	Adjunctive therapy, Na retention, renal toxicity, gastropathy, bleeding
Ibuprofen	400-600 mg qid	

Note: IV = intravenous; SQ = subcutaneous; CHF = congestive heart failure; COPD = chronic obstructive pulmonary disease.

vasoconstrictor and shares the same contraindications as ergotamine. Isometheptene is given as two capsules at the onset of headache followed by one to two capsules every 30 to 60 min up to a maximum of five capsules.

Analgesics and NSAIDs also have been used in the acute treatment of migraine.[20] Patients with severe pain may have rapid, though temporary, relief with a narcotic analgesic. Routine use of narcotics in these patients should be avoided due to the risk of narcotic dependence. The precautions discussed in Chap. 9 regarding the use of narcotics in the elderly must be considered. Since platelet aggregation and release and prostaglandins appear to play a role in the pathophysiology of acute migraine, the use of NSAIDs has some rationale. Aspirin has been used for migraine for over 100 years. Of the newer NSAIDs, naproxen has been the agent most studied in migraine. The potential adverse effects of NSAIDs in the elderly must be considered. However, agents such as naproxen probably are safer in this population than ergotamine. Combination products such as Fiorinal (aspirin, acetaminophen, butalbital) are best avoided. The administration of metoclopramide may enhance the effect of NSAIDs in migraine by speeding their GI absorption.[20] However, the potential for extrapyramidal effects due to metoclopramide, especially in elderly patients with renal insufficiency, must be considered.

Phenothiazines and other antiemetics are commonly given during an acute migraine attack. In addition to their obvious effects in relieving nausea, certain of these agents, including chlorpromazine and prochlorperazine,[20,25,26] also appear to be effective in treating migraine itself. The potential extrapyramidal and cardiovascular effects of these agents in the elderly must be considered, however.

The newest class of agents used in the acute treatment of migraine are serotonin agonists.[21-23] Serotonin appears to have a central role in the pathophysiology of migraine, and the intravenous administration of serotonin precursors can alleviate migraine attacks. Sumatriptan is the first agent of this class to be studied. This agent[23] binds to 5-HT_{1d} receptors, thus avoiding the vasoconstrictive effects of 5-HT_2 stimulation. Sumatriptan is usually given by subcutaneous injection in doses of 6 to 8 mg. The pharmacokinetics and clinical efficacy of sumatriptan in the elderly have not been studied. However, the clinical efficacy of this agent appears quite promising. In a study[27] of 639 patients randomized to sumatriptan or placebo, 86 to 92 percent of patients who received 6 to 8 mg sumatriptan had improvement after 120 min versus 37 percent in the placebo group. Cady et al[28] found similar results in 1104 patients with acute migraine. Thus far, adverse effects associated with sumatriptan appear to be mild and include pain with injection, feeling of warmth, dizziness, vertigo, malaise, and fatigue. However, one study[27] found 6 patients who developed EKG changes (PR prolongation, PVC, T-wave changes) after receiving sumatriptan. The role of sumatriptan in acute migraine therapy is unclear, especially in the elderly. In the studies published, few, if any, of the patients were over the age of 65. However, based on placebo-controlled trials, sumatriptan appears to be as effective as ergotamine and is probably safer in the elderly population. Patients with preexisting heart disease should receive sumatriptan with caution. As with any new drug, the possibility of unexpected adverse reactions must always be considered.

Preventative therapy[1,2,12,15-17,20,29] The use of preventative therapy for migraine is based upon the frequency of acute attacks, inability to tolerate acute therapy, ineffectiveness of acute therapy, and impact of migraine on quality of life.[12,17] In general, more than four acute attacks per month warrant preventative therapy. A variety of agents have been used for chronic prophylaxis. Prophylaxis should be initiated with a single drug at low dose, with a gradual increase in dose as tolerated by the patient. Once effective stabilization has been achieved, the medication should be continued for 6 months and then slowly tapered to assess continued need for the therapy.

Beta blockers are the most widely used class of agents for migraine prophylaxis. The antimigraine mechanism[12,17] of beta blockers is not clear. The relative increase in α-adrenergic tone induced by beta blockade may prevent migraine-induced carotid vasodilation. In addition, beta blockers have been shown to bind to central nervous system (CNS) 5-HT_1 receptors. Propranolol has been the most extensively studied beta blocker for migraine. A recent meta-analysis of 53 published studies[30] found that propranolol reduces migraine activity by 44 to 65 percent. The oldest patient in these trials was 44 years old. Other beta blockers, including nadolol, metoprolol, and timolol, appear to be as effective as propranolol. Agents with intrinsic sympathomimetic activity such as pindolol as well as acebutolol, oxprenolol, and alprenolol are less effective than propranolol.[21]

The relative efficacy of beta blockers for migraine in the elderly is not known. The precautions for the use of these agents in the elderly must be considered. In general, beta blockers should be avoided in patients with congestive heart failure, reactive airways disease, cardiac conduction abnormalities, and depression or sleep disorders.

Methysergide,[12,15,17] a lysergic acid derivative related to the ergot alkaloids, has been used in migraine prophylaxis since 1959. This agent is a peripheral antagonist of serotonin and has no intrinsic vasoconstrictor effects. Methysergide may reduce the pain-producing effects of serotonin on vessel walls and alter vessel constriction and dilation induced by migraine. In most studies, 60 to 70 percent of patients with migraine treated with methysergide will have a decreased incidence of acute attacks.[12,17] The initial dose of methysergide is 2 mg daily, with the maximum daily dose 8 mg. At least 40 to 50 percent of patients will have some adverse effect from methysergide, such as nausea and vomiting, abdominal discomfort, muscle cramps, leg cramps, paresthesias, and edema. Less commonly, methysergide therapy is associated with first-dose hallucinations, limb ischemia, and worsening angina. The most severe adverse effect of methysergide is retroperitoneal, cardiac, and pulmonary fibrosis. The incidence of fibrotic reactions is approximately 1 percent of patients treated continuously, and the effects are reversible when the drug is discontinued. Signs and symptoms may include hydronephrosis, heart murmurs, chest pain, pleural effusion, and dysphagia. The risk of fibrosis is minimized by administering methysergide for 6-month periods followed by a 1-month drug-free period. It is not known whether the elderly are at greater risk of these fibrotic reactions. Because of the potentially severe adverse effects associated with this agent and the availability of other effective agents, methysergide is best avoided in the elderly. Other serotonin antagonists such as cyproheptadine may be effective,[12,17] though anticholinergic side effects would be a major limitation of this agent in the elderly.

Calcium channel blockers[15,17] are relatively new agents used in migraine prophylaxis. These drugs may act by blocking arterial vasoconstriction with resulting rebound dilation, inhibiting serotonin uptake and release and augmenting cerebral blood flow. Verapamil, diltiazem, nifedipine, nimodipine, and flunarizine have been found effective in migraine prophylaxis. Though verapamil is the most commonly used calcium blocker for migraine, agents such as nimodipine that are relatively selective for cerebral vessels may be more effective. An initial verapamil dose of 80 mg two to three times daily is then titrated to 160 mg three to four times daily. Sustained-release preparations may be more convenient for patients and improve long-term compliance. The onset of antimigraine efficacy of the agents may be delayed for 2 to 4 weeks. The adverse effects of the calcium blockers are somewhat agent specific and are discussed in detail in Chap. 5. Verapamil should be avoided in patients with congestive heart failure and cardiac conduction abnormalities, while nifedipine is especially likely to cause orthostatic hypotension and pedal edema. The relative efficacy and safety of calcium blockers for migraine in the elderly is not known. As a class, however, the calcium blockers are widely used in the elderly. Of the available agents, diltiazem may be the best tolerated calcium blocker in the elderly.

Antidepressants,[12,17] including amitriptyline, nortriptyline, doxepin, and the monoamine oxidase (MAO) inhibitor phenelzine are effective in migraine prophylaxis. The antimigraine effects of these agents probably are related to their actions on central serotonin receptors. Daily doses of amitriptyline 25 to 150 mg, nortriptyline 25 to 75 mg, and doxepin 25 to 150 mg have been used. The potential adverse effects of antidepressants in the elderly are discussed extensively in Chap. 15. Amitriptyline is best avoided in the elderly due to its strong anticholinergic effects and propensity to cause cardiovascular problems. Whether the more specific serotonin-altering antidepressants trazadone and fluoxetine are effective for migraine prophylaxis remains to be seen. While the MAO inhibitor phenelzine is effective in migraine prophylaxis, the potential complications of this agent make it a less attractive agent for this patient population.

Nonsteroidal anti-inflammatory agents[2,17] have been used in migraine prophylaxis. These agents inhibit platelet serotonin release and inhibit mediator-induced inflammation. Naproxen, ketoprofen, fenoprofen, flurbiprofen, and mefenamic acid have been studied with demonstrated efficacy. The NSAIDs may be combined with other prophylactic agents in patients who do not have an adequate response to the first agent. The adverse effects of the NSAIDs are discussed in Chap. 20. Because of the risk of NSAID-induced gastropathy in the elderly, these agents should be reserved for elderly patients who do not respond to less toxic agents.

A variety of miscellaneous agents have been used in migraine prophylaxis. In general, the evidence to support the efficacy of these agents is less than for the previous agents. Other drugs that have been used include the angiotensin-converting enzyme (ACE) inhibitors, valproic acid, *s*-adenosylmethionine, opiate antagonists, and fish oil.[12,15,17] The potential efficacy of serotonin agonists such as sumatriptan for migraine prophylaxis is unknown.

The greatest amount of efficacy data for migraine prophylaxis exists for the beta blockers, calcium blockers, methysergide, and antidepressants. In the elderly, the choice of a specific agent must be based on coexisting illnesses such as lung or heart disease that could contraindicate the use of a specific drug class. No matter what agent is chosen, the initial drug dose should be low and titrated very slowly. Drugs with relatively short half-lives should be chosen in the elderly patient who may have decreased renal and hepatic drug clearance. The elderly patient must be monitored closely for the development of adverse drug reactions.

Tension Headache

Tension headache is a common symptom in the elderly.[1,2] Solomon et al[7] found that tension headache was the single most common type of headache in elderly patients, occurring in 27 percent of the population studied. However, few patients with tension headache have the onset of symptoms past the age of 60 years.[31] Tension headache can be acute or chronic, with the chronic type occurring for more than 15 days per month for at least 6 months.[31] The pain of tension headache is characteristically described as a steady, bandlike global ache. While the headache may occasionally be unilateral, nausea and vomiting and photophobia do not occur, and the headache usually does not limit daily activities. While the cause of acute tension headache may be obvious in a patient enduring a stressful event, the cause of chronic headache may be obscure. Possible causes include depression, sleep disorders, cervical spine disease, ocular pathology, and dental disease.[1,2,17,31] Patients with a chronic, daily headache should receive a diagnostic evaluation to rule out mass lesions, metabolic disorders, and other systemic diseases.

The pathophysiology of tension headache is not clear. While acute tension headache is associated with increased scalp and neck muscle contraction, electromyographic studies do not indicate that chronic headache is associated with excessive muscle contraction either during or between attacks.[32] Alterations in serotonin and histamine have been seen in patients with tension headache.[2]

Acute tension headache is best treated by local heat, nonnarcotic analgesics, and stress reduction. The treatment of chronic tension headache[1,2,12,31] is more difficult. A secondary cause, such as depression, should be sought since therapy of the underlying disorder likely will relieve the headache. In general, potentially addicting drugs such as benzodiazepines, narcotics, and muscle relaxants should be avoided in patients with chronic tension headache. In most studies,[2,12,31] antidepressants (such as nortriptyline and doxepin) or beta blockers (such as propranolol and nadolol) are effective in the treatment of chronic headache. Antidepressants are effective even in those patients who are not depressed.[12] Non-drug therapy such as biofeedback and relaxation techniques also may be effective in these patients. Other agents that have been used include calcium blockers, NSAIDs, clonidine, phenothiazines, lithium, and anticonvulsants.[2,12,31] These agents appear to be less effective than antidepressants and beta blockers but may be useful in refractory cases.

Cluster Headache

Cluster headache[1,2,12,17,33] is a severe, stereotypical disorder that can begin at any age. Cluster headache that begins after age 60 is seen more commonly in women, although overall, cluster headache is much more common in men. Of elderly patients with headache, cluster headache comprises only 4 percent of patients.[7] In the elderly, it is important to differentiate cluster headache from temporal arteritis, since the symptoms may be somewhat similar. Cluster headache can be episodic or chronic. Most cluster headaches are short-lived, lasting from 15 to 120 min. Most attacks are similar, with unilateral pain beginning in or around the eye, progressing to excruciating pain involving the whole side of the head. Ipsilateral rhinorrhea, tearing, and nasal congestion accompany the pain 50 percent of the time, and miosis and ptosis occur in 30 percent.[12] Generally, patients suffer one to three attacks per day, often at night, with the average cluster period lasting 2 months. Alcohol, nitroglycerine, and histamine will induce an attack during a cluster but not between cluster periods.[12]

The pathophysiology of cluster headache is probably similar to migraine, with release of neurotransmitters such as serotonin altering vascular tone.[33]

The treatment of acute attacks[1,2,12,33] can include analgesics, ergot alkaloids, and oxygen. During the cluster period, alcohol and vasodilating drugs must be avoided. Inhalation of 100 % oxygen at a rate of 6 to 7 L/min for 15 min may be very effective.[12,33] Immersion of the hands in ice water may cause cerebral vasoconstriction and relieve pain but also could precipitate angina in an elderly patient with coronary artery disease. In one study,[34] sumatriptan was much more effective than placebo in acute cluster headache, causing an improvement of headache within 15 min in 74 percent of patients treated. Corticosteroids may occasionally abort an acute attack.[33]

For preventative therapy,[1,2,12,33] a variety of agents have been used with some success. Lithium[33] is probably the most frequently used agent, given initially at a dose of 300 to 600 mg daily. The dose is titrated to achieve a steady-state serum concentration of 0.6 to 1.2 meq/L. Since lithium is excreted renally and has many drug interactions and adverse effects, it must be used in the elderly with great caution. The use of lithium is discussed in Chap. 15. While methysergide is often considered a second-line agent to lithium in cluster headache, this agent is best avoided in the elderly. Prophylactic ergotamine, while effective, also should be avoided in this patient population.

Corticosteroids[12,33] have been effective in patients who do not respond to lithium. Prednisone 40 to 60 mg daily is given as an initial dose, with pain relief beginning in 8 to 12 h and peaking in 2 to 3 days. After stabilization of symptoms, the steroid dose is rapidly tapered over a period of 2 to 4 weeks. Other prophylactic agents[12,33] advocated such as beta blockers, antidepressants, antihistamines, calcium blockers, and chlorpromazine have not been well studied in cluster headache. However, one comparative trial[35] found verapamil and lithium to be equal in efficacy, but fewer adverse effects were seen in patients treated with verapamil.

Temporal (Giant-Cell) Arteritis

Temporal arteritis (TA)[1-3] is a systemic disease involving inflammation of cranial arteries. This disorder is virtually always seen in patients over 50 years of age. Headache is the most common complaint of patients with TA, and up to 15 percent of elderly patients who seek medical attention for headache will have TA.[7] The headache occurs only in the temples in 25 to 50 percent of patients, though pain can occur anywhere in the scalp. The pain may be continuous or intermittent and may be characterized as aching, throbbing, or burning. Patients may complain of scalp tenderness over inflamed arteries, fever, weight loss, jaw pain, polymyalgia rheumatica, and sweating. Since any arterial bed can be involved, symptoms of aortitis and coronary, mesenteric, hepatic, and renal arteritis as well as involvement of the vasa nervorum may be seen.

Sudden loss of vision is the most feared and most serious complication and is due to optic nerve and retinal ischemia. Permanent blindness will occur if the disorder is not treated rapidly and aggressively.[2] Stroke may occur as well.

The treatment of temporal arteritis[2] is discussed in Chap. 20. Corticosteroids are the mainstay of therapy and very effective. Because temporal arteritis is a disease of the elderly with headache as its most common symptom, any patient over the age of 50 with a new onset or progressively worsening headache should be evaluated for this disorder.

Cerebrovascular Disease

Cerebrovascular disease, including hemorrhage, infarcts, and TIAs, is commonly associated with headache. Portenoy et al[36] found that 34 percent of 215 patients with a cerebrovascular event complained of headache, and 60 percent of the time, the headache preceded the neurologic event. Headache was most frequently associated with parenchymal hemorrhage (57 percent) followed by TIA (36 percent) and infarcts (17 to 29 percent). Gorelick et al[37] found headache to be a frequent accompaniment of ischemic and hemorrhagic events, with headache and vomiting predictive of the presence of subarachnoid hemorrhage. An explosive or extremely severe headache is especially suggestive of a hemorrhagic event or presence of a Berry aneurysm. There is no specific therapy for the headache associated with cerebrovascular disease.[1,2] Narcotics should be avoided, since their use may cloud subsequent neurologic examinations. Except in TIA, NSAIDs should be avoided, since their antiplatelet effect could worsen a hemorrhagic event.

Hypertension

Though hypertension is commonly thought to be associated with headache, a diastolic blood pressure of <110 mmHg should not be considered a cause of headache.[1,11] Blood pressure above this level may cause bilateral, throbbing pain, and acute, severe elevations of blood pressure may cause intracerebral vasospasm and hypertensive encephalopathy. Hypertensive encephalopathy must be treated as a medical emergency with intensive care unit monitoring and intravenous antihypertensives such as nitroprusside.

Brain Tumor

Brain tumors are associated with headache in 60 percent of patients with tumors, and headache is the presenting symptom in 30 percent.[1] The headache is typically severe on rising and may awaken the person from sleep. Nausea and vomiting, altered mental status, and focal neurologic deficits are often present. While papilledema may be present, its absence does not eliminate the presence of a mass lesion or increased intracranial pressure. Corticosteroid therapy will often markedly improve symptoms within 24 h.

Metabolic Disorders

Several metabolic disorders are associated with headache,[1,11] and these disorders are more common in the elderly. Carbon dioxide narcosis in patients with severe obstructive pulmonary disease is often associated with a dull, diffuse headache. Morning headaches may be suggestive of sleep apnea. Patients with chronic renal failure receiving hemodialysis may develop headaches after dialysis. Diabetes mellitus may be associated with headache that is usually associated with hypoglycemia.[38] Virtually any systemic illness or febrile condition can be associated with headache.

Drug-related Headache

It is now well recognized that a variety of drugs can provoke headache.[39-43] These drugs may be given for non-headache conditions, but headache is also associated with excessive use of symptomatic agents in the treatment of primary headache disorders.

Askmark et al[40] have reported on 10,506 cases of drug-induced headache from five countries between 1972 and 1987. This study included unclassified headache, drug-induced migraine, and drug-induced intracranial hypertension. Drugs commonly associated with a nonspecific type of headache include NSAIDs such as indomethacin, nifedipine, H-2 blockers, vasodilators (nitrates, ACE inhibitors), and estrogens. Dietary supplements such as aspartame[44] and caffeine withdrawal[45] also have been associated with headache. Drug-related migraine was most commonly associated with H-2 blockers and oral contraceptives. Table 10-5 lists some of the common drugs associated with headache. Any patient with headache should have an evaluation of the drug regimen. A temporal relationship between onset of headache and initiation of a new agent should suggest drug-induced headache.

Table 10-5 Drugs that may cause headache

Indomethacin	Nitrates
Piroxicam	Captopril
Diclofenac	Methyldopa
Nifedipine	Estrogens
Cimetidine	Oral contraceptives
Ranitidine	Danazol
Atenolol	Isotretinoin
Metoprolol	Terfenadine
Propranolol	Ergotamine
Trimethoprim-sulfamethoxazole	Excessive analgesic use
Metronidazole	

Source: Adapted from Refs. 39, 40.

Antiheadache medications also can be associated with chronic, persistent headache.[39,41-43] These are patients with a primary headache disorder who are using excessive amounts of symptomatic medications such as acetaminophen, aspirin, butalbital, and ergotamine in various combinations. This analgesic rebound headache will often improve with discontinuance of the offending medications.[41-43] The mechanism for these drug-induced headaches is not known.

It is clear that patients who ingest large amounts of these medications may develop worsening headache symptoms. Patients whose headache disorder appears to be worsening or refractory to treatment need to have their medication use evaluated. Strict limits for analgesic use should be set at the initiation of therapy. The initiation of prophylactic therapy may reduce the need for analgesic medications.

FACIAL PAIN SYNDROMES

Trigeminal Neuralgia

Trigeminal neuralgia (tic douloureux)[1-3,12,46,47] is a disorder of severe, episodic facial pain whose onset is most common in the sixth and seventh decades. The disorder occurs more frequently in women. The pain occurs spontaneously but can often be initiated by stimulation of trigger zones around the mouth, nose, or eyes. The pain comes in attacks of sharp, lancinating, recurrent jabs lasting only seconds. After a number of paroxysms of pain, symptoms usually improve. The diagnosis of trigeminal neuralgia usually is obvious. While thought to be idiopathic in most cases, the disorder can be associated with cerebellopontine angle tumors and multiple sclerosis. A closely related disorder is glossopharyngeal neuralgia in which the pain is referred to the oropharynx or ear. The etiology of trigeminal neuralgia is not known.

Medical therapy[1-3,46] for trigeminal neuralgia is usually efficacious, and surgical therapy should be reserved for those patients who are truly refractory to drug therapy. Carbamazepine is the most effective therapy for trigeminal neuralgia. The dose of this agent must be initiated at a low level (100 mg daily) with slow upward titration to improve tolerance of the medication. Phenytoin and clonazepam also have been used, but their effectiveness is less than that of carbamazepine. The use of these anticonvulsant medications is discussed in detail in Chap. 13.

Baclofen, a gamma-aminobutyric acid-mimetic agent (GABA), has been used with some success in trigeminal neuralgia.[1,47] However, this drug can cause CNS depression, especially in the elderly and those with renal failure. Also, acute withdrawal of baclofen may precipitate hallucinations and seizures.[1,47] Other agents that have been used include sodium valproate and oxcarbazine, an investigational carbamazepine derivative. In patients who fail medical therapy, radiofrequency rhizotomy or surgical procedures may be indicated.

Postherpetic Neuralgia

Postherpetic neuralgia[2,4,48] is defined as pain persisting for 1 month after a herpes zoster eruption. The overall incidence of postherpetic neuralgia is reported to be 10 to 15 percent, but in the elderly, the reported incidence is as high as 50 to 75 percent.[2] Approximately 25 percent of cases of herpes zoster occur in the trigeminal dermatomes, usually the first division. During the acute infection, nerve ganglion hemorrhagic inflammation is followed by scarring of myelinated nerve fibers. Postherpetic neuralgia is characterized by chronic, persistent, deep-seated pain and hyperesthesia to sensory stimuli. The pain is often described as burning or tingling, and lancinating pain can be induced by external stimulation.[2,4]

Therapy of acute herpes zoster with corticosteroids appears to reduce the frequency of postherpetic neuralgia.[2,49] Acyclovir has not been consistently effective in reducing the incidence of postherpetic neuralgia.

Antidepressants have been the most extensively used agents in the treatment of postherpetic neuralgia. Amitriptyline in doses of 10 to 150 mg daily produces some pain relief in 47 to 78 percent of patients.[2,50,51] Topical capsaicin cream also may provide some pain relief for these patients.[48] Capsaicin is thought to relieve pain by releasing and then depleting substance P. The cream is applied four to five times daily after the acute lesions have healed. The burning sensation produced by application of the cream can be minimized by pretreatment application of topical lidocaine. Because local depletion of substance P is delayed, maximum pain relief may not occur for 4 to 6 weeks.[48] Treatment with nerve blocks, ethyl chloride spray, epidural injections, and transcutaneous electrical stimulation (TENS) have been without consistent benefit.

CONCLUSION

Headache is a common complaint in the elderly. Because the causes of headache may be somewhat different in the elderly due to the frequency of cerebrovascular disease and temporal arteritis in this population, these patients should be approached differently than younger patients with headache. Headache due to a secondary cause such as temporal arteritis may reflect a serious disorder that could respond dramatically to specific therapy for the underlying disorder.

The specific therapy of elderly patients with primary headache disorders must be based primarily on clinical judgment and patient-specific factors. Studies that evaluate therapeutic regimens for disorders such as migraine and tension headache rarely, if ever, include elderly subjects. Therefore, the safety and efficacy of most headache treatments in the elderly are not known. However, following the basic principles of drug use in the elderly will aid the clinician in avoiding severe drug-related morbidity. The patient's underlying medical problems and organ function must be considered so that drugs that could adversely effect these problems may be avoided. Liver and renal function must be considered since drugs are cleared from the body by these routes. Choosing drugs with short half-lives may minimize the risk of drug accumulation and subsequent toxicity. Since the elderly are often receiving multiple medications, the potential for drug-drug interactions must always be kept in mind. When therapy is initiated in the elderly, low doses should be used with very slow dosage titration. Elderly patients must be monitored closely for adverse drug reactions, and the patient must be observed for unusual drug reactions. Given these principles, the clinician managing a patient with headache can provide maximum therapeutic efficacy with the least risk of drug-related morbidity.

Patient education also is an important consideration in patients who may receive multiple, potentially toxic medications. In a study of 100 patients[52] with headache, some over the age of 60 years, 52 percent of the patients were found to be noncompliant with the medication regimen. Reasons for noncompliance included use of nonprescription medications in lieu of prescribed agents, overuse or abuse of analgesics, missed doses of prophylactic agents, ineffectiveness, adverse effects, and cost. Patients must be instructed regarding the efficacy of the agents given and the importance of proper compliance. Compliance issues are discussed in detail in Chap. 4.

REFERENCES

1. Kaminski HJ, Ruff RL: Treatment of the elderly patient with headache or trigeminal neuralgia. *Drugs Aging* 1: 48-56, 1991.
2. Baumel B, Eisner LS: Diagnosis and treatment of headache in the elderly. *Med Clin North Am* 75: 661-675, 1991.
3. Hammerstad JP: Headache and facial pain, in Cassel CK, Walsh JR (eds): *Geriatric Medicine*. New York, Springer-Verlag, 1984, pp 61-70.
4. Ziegler DK: Headache. Public health problem. *Neurol Clin* 8: 781-791, 1990.
5. Cook NR, Evans DA, Funkenstein HH, et al: Correlates of headache in a population-based cohort of elderly. *Arch Neurol* 46: 1338-1344, 1989.
6. Hale WE, Perkins LL, May FE, et al: Symptom prevalence in the elderly. *J Am Geriatr Soc* 34: 333-340, 1986.
7. Solomon GD, Kunkel RS, Frame J: Demographics of headache in the elderly. *Headache* 30: 273-276, 1990.
8. Hale WE, May FE, Marks RG, et al: Headache in the elderly: an evaluation of risk factors. *Headache* 27: 272-276, 1987.
9. Scarani G, Beghi E, Tognoni G: Pharmacological treatment of primary headache: analysis of current practice from a drug utilization study. *Headache* 27: 345-350, 1987.
10. Olesen J: The classification and diagnosis of headache disorders. *Neurol Clin* 8: 793-799, 1990.
11. Headache Classification Committee of the International Headache Society: Classification and diagnostic criteria for headache disorders, cranial neuralgias and facial pain. *Cephalalgia* 7(suppl 8): 1-96, 1988.
12. Repschlaeger BJ, McPherson MA: Classification, mechanisms and management of headache. *Clin Pharm* 3: 139-152, 1984.
13. Vestal RE: Treatment of headache and trigeminal neuralgia in the elderly, in Vestal RE (ed): *Drug Treatment in the Elderly*. Sydney, ADIS Health Science Press, 1984, pp 213-220.

14. Thomas TL: Headache and facial pain, in Pathy MJ, Finucane P (eds): *Geriatric Medicine: Problems and Practice*. New York, Springer-Verlag, 1989, pp 33-43.
15. Solomon GD: Pharmacology and use of headache medications. *Cleveland Clin J Med* 57: 627-635, 1990.
16. Fromm GH: Clinical pharmacology of drugs used to treat head and face pain. *Neurol Clin* 8: 143-151, 1990.
17. Saper JR: Chronic headache syndromes. *Neurol Clin* 7: 387-412, 1989.
18. Campbell JK: Manifestations of migraine. *Neurol Clin* 8: 841-855, 1990.
19. Moskowitz MA: Basic mechanisms in vascular headache. *Neurol Clin* 8: 801-815, 1990.
20. Raskin NH: Modern pharmacotherapy of migraine. *Neurol Clin* 8: 857-865, 1990.
21. Peroutka SJ: Developments in 5-hydroxytriptamine receptor pharmacology in migraine. *Neurol Clin* 8: 829-839, 1990.
22. Lance JW: A concept of migraine and the search for the ideal headache drug. *Headache* 30(suppl 1): 17-23, 1990.
23. Humphrey PA, Feniuk W, Perren MJ: Anti-migraine drugs in development. Advances in serotonin receptor pharmacology. *Headache* 30(suppl 1) : 12-16, 1990.
24. Graham JR: Migraine headache: diagnosis and management. *Headache* 19: 133-141, 1979.
25. Jones J, Sklar D, Dougherty J, et al: Randomized double-blind trial of intravenous prochlorperazine for the treatment of acute headache. *JAMA* 261: 1174-1176, 1989.
26. Lane PL: Comparative efficacy of chlorpromazine and meperidine with dimenhydrinate in migraine headache. *Ann Emerg Med* 18: 360-365, 1989.
27. Subcutaneous Sumatriptan International Study Group: Treatment of migraine attacks with sumatriptan. *N Engl J Med* 325: 316-321, 1991.
28. Cady RK, Wendt JK, Kirchner JR, et al: Treatment of acute migraine with subcutaneous sumatriptan. *JAMA* 265: 2831-2835, 1991.
29. Peroutka SJ: The pharmacology of current anti-migraine drugs. *Headache* 30(suppl 1) : 5-11, 1990.
30. Holroyd KA, Penzien DB, Cordingley GE: Propranolol in the management of recurrent migraine: a meta-analytic review. *Headache* 31: 333-340, 1991.
31. Saper JR: Daily chronic headache. *Neurol Clin* 8: 891-901, 1990.
32. Pikoff H: Is the muscular model of headache still viable? A review of conflicting data. *Headache* 24: 186-198, 1984.
33. Mathew NT: Advances in cluster headache. *Neurol Clin* 8: 867-890, 1990.
34. Sumatriptan Cluster Headache Study Group: Treatment of acute cluster headache with sumatriptan. *N Engl J Med* 325: 322-326, 1991.
35. Bussone G, Leone M, Peccarisi C, et al: Double blind comparison of lithium and verapamil in cluster headache prophylaxis. *Headache* 30: 411-417, 1990.
36. Portenoy RK, Abisi TJ, Lipton RB, et al: Headache in cerebrovascular disease. *Stroke* 15: 1009-1012, 1984.
37. Gorelick PB, Hier DB, Caplan LR, Langenberg P: Headache in acute cerebrovascular disease. *Neurology* 36: 1445-1450, 1986.
38. Martins I, Blau JN: Headaches in insulin-dependent diabetic patients. *Headache* 29: 660-663, 1989.
39. Mathew NT: Drug-induced headache. *Neurol Clin* 8: 903-912, 1990.
40. Askmark H, Lundberg PO, Olsson S: Drug-related headache. *Headache* 29: 441-444, 1989.
41. Baumgartner C, Wessely P, Bingol C, et al: Long-term prognosis of analgesic withdrawal in patients with drug-induced headaches. *Headache* 29: 510-514, 1989.
42. Diener HC, Dichgans J, Scholz E, et al: Analgesic-induced chronic headache: long-term results of withdrawal therapy. *J Neurol* 236: 9-14, 1989.
43. Mathew NT, Kurman R, Perez F: Drug-induced refractory headache—Clinical features and management. *Headache* 30: 634-638, 1990.
44. Lipton RB, Newman LC, Cohen JS, Solomon S: Aspartame as a dietary trigger of headache. *Headache* 29: 90-92, 1989.
45. Smith R: Caffeine withdrawal headache. *J Clin Pharm Ther* 12: 53-57, 1987.

46. Solomon S, Lipton RB: Facial pain. *Neurol Clin* 8: 913-928, 1990.
47. Fromm GH: Trigeminal neuralgia. *Neurol Clin* 7: 305-319, 1989.
48. Watson CN: Post-herpetic neuralgia. *Neurol Clin* 7: 231-248, 1989.
49. Keczkes K, Basheer AM: Do corticosteroids prevent post-herpetic neuralgia? *Br J Dermatol* 102: 551-555, 1980.
50. Max MB, Schafer SC, Culnane M, et al: Amitriptyline, but not lorazepam, relieves post-herpetic neuralgia. *Neurology* 38: 1427-1432, 1988.
51. Watson CP, Evans RJ, Reed K, et al: Amitriptyline vs. placebo in postherpetic neuralgia. *Neurology* 32: 670-673, 1982.
52. Packard RC, O'Connell P: Medication compliance among headache patients. *Headache* 26: 416-419, 1986.

CHAPTER

11

PHARMACOLOGIC THERAPY OF INCONTINENCE

Kathleen Yochum
John T. Boyer
Michael D. Katz

Incontinence, the involuntary loss of urine leading to social or hygienic problems, is a major difficulty for the elderly. In the community at large the prevalence is likely to be as high as 30 percent in the elderly during a 12-month period.[1] In the nursing home as many as 50 percent of residents suffer from incontinence on a regular basis.[2] The cost of this problem is enormous, both to the patient and to society. Embarrassment, depression, painful dermatitis, cutaneous ulceration, and infections are a source of suffering, morbidity, and mortality to the individual. Estimates for the direct health care costs relating to urinary incontinence are over $10 billion annually.[3]

Age alone is the major risk factor for the development of incontinence; however, numerous medical conditions (all of which are increased in the elderly) are contributing factors. Frailty, immobility, stroke, dementia, and complications of drug therapy are associated with incontinence.

ANATOMY

The collection and storage of urine has been well summarized by Rubin.[4] The bladder body or detrusor consists of an interlacing meshwork of smooth muscle. At the bladder trigon, a triangular area is bordered laterally by ureterovesical junctions and inferiorally by the urethral meatus. Superficially the trigon has a thin layer of smooth muscle that is continuous with the ureters. In the deep layers the muscles of the trigon are indistinguishable from the detrusor. In the bladder neck of the male there is a proximal smooth muscle sphincter which is not present in the female. A true external sphincter is present in both sexes and is believed to be responsible for maintaining continence between normal voidings. Most importantly, the fibrous and elastic tissues at the bladder neck contribute to the mechanical closure of the urethra and are positioned above the pelvic floor in such a way as to ensure that pressure transmission during rises of intraabdominal pressure closes off the urethra by equaling the pressure there with the pressure that is placed upon the bladder.

Neural control of these structures involves four loops: (1) cortical thalamic and cerebellar centers, (2) the primary reflex arc linking bladder sensation to brain stem motor neurons, (3) a loop allowing passive relaxation of the pelvic floor during bladder filling, and (4) a conscious control over pelvic floor muscles and sphincters. Thus a distended bladder leads to detrusor contractions (loop 2) which must be inhibited in higher centers (loop 1) while further filling of the bladder causes pelvic muscle relaxation (loop 3) and awareness of the urge to void appears (loop 4).

Although not yet fully understood, localization of the adrenergic and cholinergic receptors has done much to clarify normal voiding physiology and provide the basis for understanding the effects of drug therapy (Fig. 11-1). The α-adrenergic

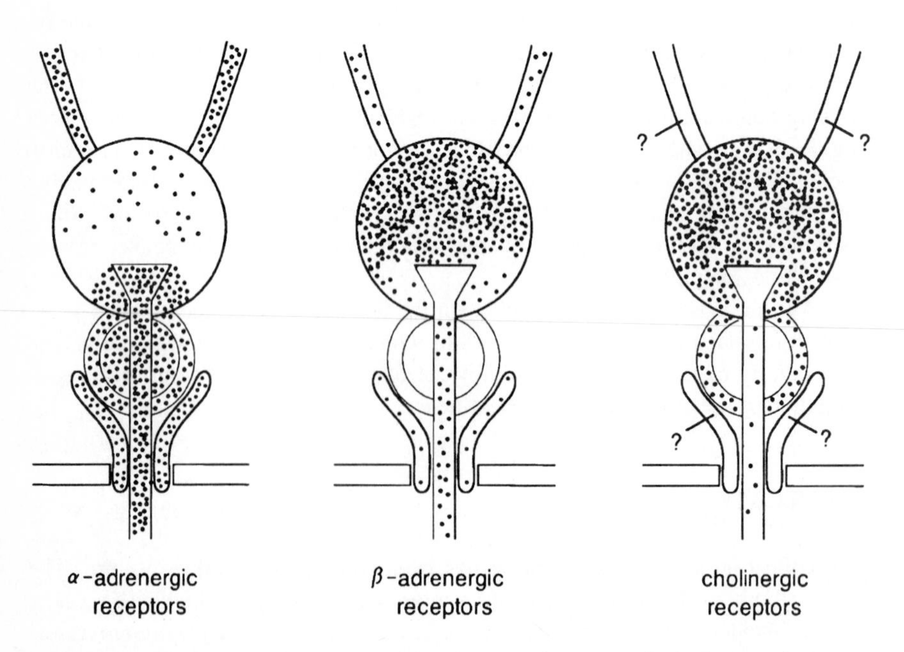

Figure 11-1 Distribution and relative densities of autonomic receptors in the human urinary tract. (Adapted from Ref. 4.)

(primarily α_1) receptors are located at the bladder outlet and along the urethra, which increase urethral resistance upon stimulation. The β-adrenergic (primarily β_2) receptors occur throughout the remainder of the bladder and cause relaxation when stimulated. Cholinergic receptors are found throughout the bladder and urethra and mediate contractions of the detrusor. Bladder filling can thus be viewed as a sympathetic nervous system activity in which there is increased urethral resistance at the same time the bladder is in the relaxed state. On the other hand, voiding is essentially a parasympathetic activity following inhibition of sympathetic activity and stimulation of bladder contractions.

NORMAL FUNCTION AND PATHOPHYSIOLOGY

Continence depends upon maintaining bladder pressure below urethral pressure.[5] Intraabdominal pressure, bladder filling, and detrusor tone effect the former, while urethral smooth muscle tone, urethral mucosal thickness, and maintenance of the posterior urethrovesical angle (which may be altered by traumatic tears during childbirth, the presence of tumors, etc.) are important factors affecting the latter. The process of aging itself alters the function of bladder mechanisms and may contribute to the development of incontinence: decreases have been reported in bladder capacity, the ability to postpone voiding, urethral and bladder compliance, maximal urethral closure pressure, and urinary flow rate; while increases have been described in postvoid residual volume and the prevalence of uninhibited detrusor contractions.[6] In fact, development of incontinence in the elderly is likely to be precipitated by factors from outside the lower urinary tract.[6]

TYPES OF INCONTINENCE[7,8]

According to the National Institutes of Health (NIH) Conference on Urinary Incontinence, "the most commonly encountered clinical forms of urinary incontinence in adults are stress incontinence, urge incontinence, overflow incontinence and a mixed form of incontinence"[7] (Table 11-1).[4] An additional type of incontinence known as functional incontinence is not due to abnormalities in function of the lower urinary tract and is found in individuals with such severe mobility or cognitive impairment that they either cannot or do not toilet when appropriate. Most importantly, transient or reversible causes of incontinence should initially be ruled out. Resnick's[6] mnemonic DIAPPERS [*d*elirium and *d*ementia; *i*nfections; *a*trophic vaginitis; *p*sychological causes (depression); *p*harmacologic agents; *e*ndocrinologic problems; *r*estricted mobility; *s*tool impaction] summarizes the transient or reversible causes of incontinence. Table 11-2 summarizes the medications that may contribute to incontinence.[9]

Table 11-1 Basic types and causes of established urinary incontinence

	Stress	Urge	Overflow	Functional
Definition	Involuntary loss of urine from increased abdominal pressure	Leakage of urine secondary to inability to delay voiding after sensing an urge	Leakage of urine from mechanical forces on an overdistended bladder	Leakage of urine associated with inability to toilet due to cognitive, psychologic, or physical factors
Common causes	Lax pelvic floor or weak sphincter	Detrusor instability of infection, stones, tumors, CNS disease	Obstruction, neuropathy, detrusor-sphincter dyssynergy	Dementia, psychosis, regression, depression

Source: Adapted from Ref. 4.

Table 11-2 Medications contributing to incontinence

Type	Possible mechanism	Clues to diagnosis
Anticholinergic	Detrusor relaxation, high residual volume	Hesitancy, straining to void, overflow incontinence
Diuretics	Increased urine volume	Polyuria, frequency, urgency
Sedatives	Sedation, obtundation	Confusion, delirium
Antipsychotics	Sedation, anticholinergic effects; bradykinesia, rigidity	Same as for anticholinergic; inability to toilet secondary to immobility
Tricyclics and narcotics	Anticholinergic, sedation, confusion	Same as for anticholinergic, sedatives
Alpha-adrenergic blockers	Decreased urethral resistance	Stress incontinence
Alpha-adrenergic agonists	Increased urethral resistance	Same as for anticholinergic
Calcium channel blockers	Detrusor relaxation, increased residual urine	Same as for anticholinergic
Alcohol	Increased urinary volume, sedation, altered mental status	Urgency, frequency, nocturia, sedation, confusion, immobility

Source: Adapted from Ref. 9.

Stress Incontinence

In this case the word *stress* is confined in its meaning entirely to physical stresses such as coughing, sneezing, laughing, lifting, and other causes of increased intra-abdominal pressure such as that which occurs when leaning over to tie one's shoes. Usually, urinary leakage occurs in small amounts, mostly during daytime activities and seldom at night. It is confined almost entirely to women or the occasional male following prostate surgery. The cause is usually anatomic change in the pelvic floor muscles or less commonly to the urethral sphincter itself.

Urge Incontinence

Urge incontinence is the most common cause of incontinence in the elderly. It is characterized by leakage of relatively large amounts of urine a few seconds to a few minutes following the warning sensations of a desire to void. The usual situation involves detrusor overactivity of unknown cause in otherwise healthy individuals leading to bladder contractions that override voluntary central inhibition. A similar mechanism is found less commonly as a result of central nervous lesions such as stroke, dementia, or demyelinating disease.

Mixed Incontinence

Frequently older patients, and especially older women, have a mixture of both stress and urge incontinence. Successful evaluation of this form of incontinence frequently requires urodynamic studies.

Overflow Incontinence

Overflow incontinence occurs when a markedly distended bladder overcomes the resistance of the urethral sphincter leading to leakage of small amounts of urine sometimes almost constantly. It is a relatively uncommon cause of incontinence in the elderly and it is the most difficult to manage. The residual urine volume is high and the bladder distention easily recognizable by palpation on physical examination. Bladder neck obstruction from prostatic hypertrophy is a common cause in men and loss of bladder tone from neurologic disorder is a cause in both sexes.

MEDICAL MANAGEMENT OF URINARY INCONTINENCE: BEHAVIORAL METHOD

Before drug therapy is considered, behavioral techniques should be considered and are generally the more important aspect of care. A discussion of these forms of therapy is beyond the purpose of this chapter, and the reader is referred to review articles cited in the References.[10-12] Burgio[12] noted an 88 percent reduction in urge incontinence in patients after utilizing education and biofeedback training in pelvic muscle exercises in which the patients learn to contract and strengthen the voluntary urethral sphincter while voluntarily inhibiting detrusor contractions. Learning to circumvent certain conditioned reflexes leading to urge incontinence has also been successful. With regard to stress incontinence, pelvic muscle exercises have resulted in benefit to women from 20 to 90 percent, but design and criteria for improvement differ among the various studies.[7]

TREATMENT OF INCONTINENCE: PHARMACOLOGIC METHODS

Urinary incontinence has received relatively little attention from the pharmaceutical industry. No effective new drug for urinary incontinence has been introduced in the United States for over 20 years, and most drugs employed for incontinence were originally developed for some other use. Further, most studies of the effects of drugs on incontinence do not include large numbers of older patients. Therefore, extrapolation of the information available to one's 85-year-old patient must be undertaken with caution. Finally, as with all other drug use in the elderly, *the physician is well advised to start with lower doses than those usually recommended by the manufacturer and proceed with caution*, taking into consideration the effects of decreased kidney and liver function, underlying medical conditions, and altered body composition that are common in such individuals. Unfortunately, because most of the agents used in the treatment of incontinence have been available for many years, little pharmacokinetic data exist to describe the absorption, distribution, duration of effect, and clearance in any patient population, including the elderly.

Wein[3,14] has divided drugs which have been used to treat incontinence into those which decrease bladder contractility and those which increase outlet resistance.

Agents Which Decrease Bladder Contractility

Anticholinergic agents Discovery that inability to void is an important side effect of the use of anticholinergic drugs such as atropine in men was an observation that predicted the later finding that bladder contraction could be caused by stimulation of cholinergic receptors of the bladder. Anticholinergic drugs were an obvious choice for the treatment of bladder irritability or detrusor overactivity. Because parasympathetic activity is a primary stimulus of bladder smooth muscle contraction, anticholinergic agents will depress involuntary bladder contraction of any etiology. The use of agents such as atropine or propantheline is reliably associated with decreased urinary frequency, increased bladder capacity, and decrease in urge incontinence.[14] However, the classic side effects of anticholinergic drugs, including confusion, dizziness, constipation, blurred vision, and tachycardia are frequent and poorly tolerated in the vulnerable elderly. Nevertheless, propantheline is still considered a valuable drug for treatment of bladder overactivity, usually in doses of 15 to 30 mg every 4 to 6 h. Poor oral absorption can be minimized by administration one-half hour before meals. There seems to be little advantage of propantheline over related antimuscarinic agents such as glycopyrrolate or hyoscyamine.[14] Likewise, anticholinergic drugs which are effective ganglionic blocking agents such as methantheline show little advantage over those which are purely antimuscarinic.

Bladder relaxant drugs These agents are capable of causing smooth muscle relaxation through a mechanism that is metabolically beyond the reaction of the neuroreceptor. However, all of those for which success has been claimed in treating urinary incontinence also possess anticholinergic qualities as well as local anesthetic properties. It may well be that the favorable reactions reported are due to the anticholinergic effects more than the direct smooth muscle relaxing effects.

Oxybutynin chloride has been described as a moderately potent anticholinergic agent with strong smooth muscle relaxant and local anesthetic activity. This drug has been used to treat both the overactive bladder of common urge incontinence as well as to treat the uninhibited detrusor contractions in patients with neurogenic bladder dysfunction.[14] Studies have also shown superiority of oxybutynin over placebo in middle-aged and "young-old" patients (usually considered to be between 65 and 75 years of age).[15-17] In contrast, two studies performed among institutionalized elderly found oxybutynin less effective than placebo.[18,19] In addition, oxybutynin has been compared to propantheline.[20] In 23 women with detrusor instability, 14 reported subjective improvement with oxybutynin compared with 11 treated with propantheline. Both agents demonstrated significant cystometric improvement, with oxybutynin demonstrating a greater increase in the maximum cystometric capacity. Dry mouth, dry skin, and constipation were common complaints among patients in the various studies. In our clinical experience with elderly patients treated with oxybutynin, starting cautiously with doses of 2.5 mg twice daily and gradually increasing to three times daily has been better tolerated than using the recommended 5-mg dose. Adverse effects seen with oxybutynin are primarily anticholinergic in nature.

Dicyclomine hydrochloride This drug also possesses both anticholinergic and muscle relaxant properties but is much less well studied. A dose of 20 to 30 mg three times daily is often necessary. Side effects, like those of oxybutynin, are generally those of all anticholinergic drugs.[14]

Flavoxate hydrochloride This agent also has both anticholinergic and smooth muscle relaxing properties as well as local analgesic properties. Doses of 100 to 200 mg three or four times daily are suggested, though some studies have shown this agent to be no more effective than placebo in the treatment of detrusor overactivity or hyperreflexia in the elderly.[14]

Calcium antagonists Since calcium has a role in the contraction of both striated and smooth muscle, considerable interest in this category of drugs has been generated. Nifedipine inhibits contraction induced by several mechanisms in human bladder smooth muscle.[14] Terolidine, a drug not yet approved in the United States, has both calcium antagonist and anticholinergic effect.[21] This agent is well absorbed from the gastrointestinal tract. In healthy volunteers, the elimination half-life of terolidine averages 60 h, while in the elderly, the half-life is approximately 130 h. While most of the drug is metabolized, both total and renal terolidine clearance are decreased in the elderly. Given the same dose as younger patients, elderly patients receiving terolidine achieve steady-state serum concentrations twice that of younger patients.[21] A variety of studies have compared terolidine to placebo and other pharmacologic agents. Terolidine has consistently proved superior to placebo in the treatment of detrusor instability. When compared to emepronium, an anticholinergic agent, terolidine demonstrated greater subjective and objective improvement. In a large study comparing terolidine to flavoxate, terolidine was the more effective agent.[21] Side effects seen with terolidine are more common with higher doses and are primarily anticholinergic in nature. Dry mouth, blurred vision, and tremor are the most common complaints. Recently, several cases of cardiac arrhythmias, including torsades de pointes, have been reported in patients receiving terolidine. The relationship between the drug and these arrythmias is not clear and is currently undergoing evaluation. Other cardiovascular effects seen with other calcium antagonists have not been seen with terolidine. The usual dose of terolidine is 25 mg twice daily. However, given the known pharmacokinetics of this agent in the elderly, a starting dose of 12.5 to 25 mg once daily may be more reasonable in this population. The common side effects which are sometimes seen with calcium antagonists have not been reported in clinical studies. While it is not clear what place in therapy terolidine will have, its main advantage may be less toxicity as compared to the anticholinergic and smooth muscle relaxant agents. However, the risk of cardiac arrhythmias with terolidine therapy must be clarified prior to recommending this agent for widespread use in the elderly.

Prostaglandin inhibitors While drugs such as the nonsteroidal anti-inflammatory agents have been heralded for their potential use in treating detrusor instability, in fact, only meager evidence exists for their effectiveness.[14] Because of the risk of gastropathy and renal dysfunction associated with these agents in the elderly, the prostaglandin inhibitors should not be used unless future studies demonstrate clear efficacy in the treatment of incontinence.

Beta-adrenergic agonists The presence of beta receptors in the bladder has prompted attempts to increase bladder capacity with beta-adrenergic agonist agents. In animals, beta-$_2$ stimulation causes significant relaxation of the bladder body. In 15 women with urge incontinence,[22] 14 claimed a beneficial effect with terbutaline 5 mg three times daily. However, tremor and tachycardia were common adverse effects. There are no studies comparing beta agonists to other agents in the treatment of incontinence.

Tricyclic antidepressants These agents have a variety of pharmacologic actions, including anticholinergic activity, blockade of the reuptake of norepinephrine and serotonin, central sedation, histamine receptor (both H_1 and H_2) antagonism, and blockade of peripheral alpha-adrenergic receptors.[14] Imipramine, which has been most studied, also has a direct relaxant effect on bladder smooth muscle. In one study,[23] 6 of 10 elderly patients with detrusor instability became continent with imipramine therapy. Doxepin also has been studied but was no more effective than placebo in one report.[14] Whether other antidepressants are effective in the treatment of incontinence is not known.

A tricyclic antidepressant agent such as imipramine may be useful in the incontinent patient with depression. In general, low doses of these agents should be used in the elderly due to the prolonged drug clearance and increased risk of adverse effects. A starting dose of imipramine 10–20 mg at bedtime is reasonable, with the dose cautiously increased on a weekly basis. Tricyclic antidepressants have a variety of potentially severe adverse effects. Orthostatic hypotension is an especially severe problem with a documented increase in the risk of falls and hip fracture associated with the use of antidepressants in the elderly.[24] The reader is referred to Chap. 15 for a complete discussion of the adverse effects of these agents.

Drugs Which Modify Bladder Outlet Incompetence

When urine loss occurs because of incompetence of the urethral sphincters, it is usually associated with symptoms of stress incontinence. Drug treatment of this condition is based on the fact that the outlet area has an abundance of alpha-adrenergic receptors which, when stimulated, increase resistance to urine leakage. It also depends on "mucosal seal" (the absence of mucosal atrophy) which, in turn, is dependent on estrogenic stimulation.

Alpha-adrenergic agonists All of the agents in this class of drugs have well-known side effects including blood pressure elevation, anxiety, insomnia, tremor, headache, palpitations, and cardiac arrhythmias. The seriousness of these side effects is, of course, even greater in the elderly. Surgical and mechanical restructuring is often to be preferred and is generally more successful than drug therapy. Still, large numbers of individuals exist for whom surgery is not an option, and a cautious trial of these drugs may be warranted. Ephedrine, pseudoephedrine, and phenylpropanolamine have been shown to have beneficial effects in patients with minimal to moderate stress incontinence.[14] While phenylpropanolamine hydrochloride appears to be equally effective while causing less central stimulation, recent reports have emphasized the potential severe complications associated with phenylpropanolamine use.[14]

Imipramine Discussed above for the treatment of bladder overreactivity by virtue of its anticholinergic effect, imipramine was also noted to possess an alpha-adrenergic effect due to reuptake inhibition and would therefore be a rational drug to use in stress incontinence. Indeed, one study has shown both subjective and objective improvement for a majority of women who received imipramine for stress incontinence.[14]

Beta-adrenergic antagonists Theoretically, beta blockers could cause a relative increase in alpha-adrenergic activity, thereby increasing urethral resistance. While one study has shown propranolol to be effective in the treatment of stress incontinence, the risk of cardiac toxicity and bronchospasm may outweigh the potential utility of these agents for incontinence in the elderly.[14]

Estrogens The urethra and trigon areas of the bladder are stimulated by estrogen therapy, and one of the most remarkable findings in women who develop incontinence is the frequent association of severe atrophic vaginitis and urethritis. While estrogen receptors have been identified in the human female urethra, it has also been suggested that estrogen therapy may induce proliferation of alpha-adrenergic receptors of the bladder,[25] and increased responsiveness to alpha-adrenergic drugs has been claimed following the use of estrogens.[14] Most reports in the literature show a positive effect of estrogen therapy on various kinds of incontinence. However, relatively few studies have been randomized or placebo controlled. Oral as well as intravaginal and percutaneous estrogen administration has been reported to be effective. Cardozo[26] has summarized conclusions regarding estrogen from controlled studies to date:

1. "There have been very few appropriate placebo-controlled studies using subjective and objective parameters for assessment—so more are urgently needed.
2. "Estrogen replacement apparently alleviates urgency, urge incontinence, frequency, nocturia and dysuria.
3. "There is no conclusive evidence that estrogen even improves (let alone cures) stress incontinence."

Recent data requiring substantiation, however, indicate that phenylpropanolamine and estrogen have been successfully combined to treat stress incontinence when there was response to neither drug alone.

While the use of estrogen therapy in the elderly has been controversial in the past, increasingly geriatricians prescribe estrogens in order to minimize osteoporosis, fractures, and cardiovascular disease. The preponderance of evidence seems to indicate that serious problems with breast or genital cancer are relatively small compared to the benefit of the estrogens. Thus the added advantage of minimizing the likelihood of urge incontinence and perhaps sensitizing local tissues for the treatment of stress incontinence with alpha-adrenergic drugs offers encouragement to the use of estrogens for the elderly in general and for the incontinent elderly in particular. The decision to use estrogen in the elderly is highly individual, however, usually because patients are reluctant to tolerate side effects such as breast swelling or intermittent vaginal bleeding. Estrogens may be administered orally, vaginally, or percutaneously, both in cyclic or continual administration, with or without progesterone. A discussion of estrogen administration is beyond the scope of this review and the reader is referred to Chaps. 18 and 19.

Treatment of Bladder Outlet Obstruction and Overflow Incontinence

These syndromes of difficulty in bladder emptying are fortunately rare, for medical management has relatively little to offer.

An underactive detrusor which leads to bladder distention and overflow incontinence may be reversible when secondary to drugs, especially postoperative. Otherwise it represents a serious neurologic disorder such as diabetic neuropathy or paraplegia. The parasympathomimetic agents carbachol and bethanechol, which can be shown to cause bladder contraction in normal animals and man, have almost no clinical usefulness in overflow incontinence.

In the bladder outlet obstruction of prostatic hypertrophy the alpha-adrenergic antagonist phenoxybenzamine and prazosin have been found to relieve obstructive symptoms of outlet obstruction.[9] While antidepressant drugs with peripheral α-adrenergic blocking activity theoretically should be effective in these patients, the anticholinergic activity of these drugs would likely worsen bladder outlet obstruction.

SUMMARY

Most incontinence can be improved or cured and drug therapy, while often not primary therapy, is an excellent adjunct. Careful diagnosis is critical. Patient education, pelvic muscle exercises, behavioral therapy, and mechanical aids (pessary) are essential components of the medical approach. Oxybutynin is a reasonable first-line agent to treat urge incontinence, although imipramine might be preferred in the presence of depression. Terolidine is a promising agent that may become widely used if it is marketed in the United States. Most patients with stress incontinence will wish to have surgery, but phenylpropanolamine and estrogen may also be of value.

REFERENCES

1. Herzog AR, Fultz N: Prevalence and incidence of urinary incontinence in community-dwelling populations. *J Am Geriatr Soc* 38: 273–281, 1990.

2. Mohide EA: The prevalence and scope of urinary incontinence. *Clin Geriatr Med* 2: 639-655, 1986.
3. Hu TW: Impact of urinary incontinence on health care costs. *J Am Geriatr Soc* 38: 292-295, 1990.
4. Rubin C: Urinary incontinence in the elderly. *Am J Med Sci* 299: 131-147, 1990.
5. Williams ME, Pannill FC: Urinary incontinence in the elderly: physiology, pathophysiology, diagnosis and treatment. *Ann Intern Med* 97: 895-907, 1982.
6. Resnick NM, Yalla SV: Management of urinary incontinence in the elderly. *N Engl J Med* 313: 800-805, 1985.
7. Anonymous: Urinary incontinence in the elderly. NIH Consensus Development Conference. *J Am Geriatr Soc* 38: 265-272, 1990.
8. DuBeau CE, Resnick NM: Evaluation of the causes and severity of geriatric incontinence. *Urol Clin North Am* 18: 243-256, 1991.
9. Pannill FC: Practical management of urinary incontinence. *Med Clin North Am* 73: 1423-1439, 1989.
10. Fantl JA, Wyman JF, Hawkins SW, Hadley EC: Bladder training in the management of lower urinary tract dysfunction in women. A review. *J Am Geriatr Soc* 38: 329-332, 1990.
11. Wells TJ: Pelvic (floor) muscle exercises. *J Am Geriatr Soc* 38: 333-337, 1990.
12. Burgio KL, Engel BT: Biofeedback-assisted behavioral training for elderly men and women. *J Am Geriatr Soc* 38: 338-340, 1990.
13. Wein AJ: Pharmacologic treatment of incontinence. *J Am Geriatr Soc* 38: 317-325, 1990.
14. Wein AJ: Practical uropharmacology. *Urol Clin North Am* 18: 269-281, 1991.
15. Moisey CU, Stephenson TP, Brendeler CB: The urodynamic and subjective results of treatment of detrusor instability with oxybutynin chloride. *Br J Urol* 52: 472-475, 1980.
16. Moore KH, Hay DM, Imrie AE, et al: Oxybutynin hydrochloride (3 mg) in the treatment of idiopathic detrusor instability. *Br J Urol* 66: 479-485, 1990.
17. Tapp AJS, Cardozo D, Versi E, Cooper D: The treatment of detrusor instability in post-menopausal women with oxybutynin chloride: a double-blind placebo-controlled study. *Br J Obstet Gynecol* 97: 521-526, 1990.
18. Zorzitto ML, Holliday PJ, Jewett AS, et al: Oxybutynin chloride for geriatric urinary dysfunction: a double-blind placebo-controlled study. *Age Ageing* 18: 195-200, 1989.
19. Ouslander JG, Blaustein J, Connor A, Pitt A: Habit training and oxybutynin for incontinence in nursing home patients in a placebo-controlled trial. *J Am Geriatr Soc* 36: 40-46, 1988.
20. Holmes DM, Monty FJ, Stanton SL: Oxybutynin versus propantheline in the management of detrusor instability: a patient-regulated variable dose trial. *J Obstet Gynecol* 96: 607-610, 1989.
21. Langtry HD, McTavish D: Terolidine. A review of its pharmacological properties and therapeutic use in the treatment of urinary incontinence. *Drugs* 40: 748-761, 1990.
22. Lindholm P, Lose G: Terbutaline (Bricanyl) in the treatment of female urge incontinence. *Urol Int* 41: 158-160, 1986.
23. Castleden CM, George CF, Renwick AG, et al: Imipramine: a possible alternative to current therapy for urinary incontinence in the elderly. *J Urol* 125: 318-320, 1981.
24. Ray WA, Griffin MR, Schaffner W, et al: Psychotropic drug use and the risk of hip fracture. *N Engl J Med* 316: 363-369, 1988.
25. Beisland HO, Fossberg E, Moer A, Sander S: Urethral sphincteric insufficiency in postmenopausal females. Treatment with phenylpropanolamine and estriol separately and in combination. *Urol Int* 39: 211-216, 1984.
26. Cardozo L: Role of estrogen in the treatment of female urinary incontinence. *J Am Geriatr Soc* 38: 326-328, 1990.

CHAPTER

12

IMPOTENCE

Thomas H. Stanisic
George E. Francisco

Impotence is the inability to attain and/or sustain an erection rigid enough to penetrate and have sexual intercourse. Although disturbances of libido, orgasm, or ejaculation are related disorders, we exclude them from consideration herein, except as they might be secondary to impotence as a primary problem. Isolated episodes of erectile dysfunction, often associated with fatigue, preoccupation, or anxiety, are commonplace in most men's lives and of little concern. When erectile failure persists over a sustained period of several months, however, most would consider it a clinical disorder warranting evaluation and possible treatment.

The precise prevalence of impotence, by any definition, is difficult to ascertain, but Kinsey et al[1] report an incidence of 1.9 percent at age 40 and 25 percent at age 65. Incidence of this disorder is certainly age dependent, and in high-risk subpopulations, i.e., elderly diabetic patients, the incidence approaches 50 percent.[2] Clearly impotence is an extremely common problem in the geriatric population with substantial adverse effects on the well-being of many in this group.

Today the elderly male is more likely than ever before to seek attention for sexual dysfunction. Lowered inhibitions regarding discussion of sexual matters and increased coverage in the media have improved the patient's education. Recent improvements in technology and understanding of the pathophysiology of erectile dysfunction now allow the medical community to accurately identify causative factors and to offer effective treatment to most impotent males. The improved general health status in the elderly population today allows this group to take advantage of this increased awareness and improved treatment capacity.

In most instances, the impotent male's initial interface with the health care system is a primary practitioner. We provide this chapter as a hopefully practical compact resource of information regarding erectile physiology and the diagnosis and treatment of the impotent male.

ANATOMY AND PHYSIOLOGY OF ERECTION

The end organs of penile erection are the corpora cavernosa, which are parallel and paired in the pendulous distal penis but bifurcate beneath the pubis and subsequently course along the medial aspects of the ischial rami in the perineum. Distally, the corpus spongiosum lies beneath them and surrounds the urethra beneath the genitourinary diaphragm. Each corpus consists of lacunar spaces lined by endothelium and separated by trabeculae made of smooth muscle and fibrous tissue. The interior of the two corpora intercommunicate through the intracorporal septum allowing for free spread of injected drugs and/or infections from one corpus to another. Each corpus is covered by a tough fibrous sheath, the tunica albuginea, which limits expansion and pressurizes the corpus as blood accumulates within during sexual excitation. The hypogastric-internal pudendal arterial axis supplies blood to the corpora through the paired terminal cavernosal arteries, which give rise to helicine arteries that fill the lacunae directly. Venous drainage is initially via venules located just beneath the tunica albuginea which, because of this location, are easily compressible against the fibrous covering as the lacunar spaces deep to them expand and fill with blood during erection (Fig. 12-1). Venous drainage is ultimately via the deep and superficial dorsal veins distally and the crural veins and cavernosa veins proximally. The controlling mechanisms of penile erection are contraction and relaxation of the arteriolar and trabecular smooth muscle within the penis. With erection, the smooth muscle in the arterial walls and trabeculae relaxes, lowering peripheral resistance; blood flow subsequently increases logarithmically when compared to the resting state. As these lacunae fill, the intracorporal pressure rises, compressing the peripheral intracorporal venules against the tunica albuginea and inhibits venous return (Fig. 12-1). Eventually, as intracorporal pressure approaches systolic pressure, blood flow into the penis diminishes to maintain a steady state of turgidity. To initiate detumescence, the smooth muscle in the lacunar walls contracts with climax or other stimuli to expel blood from the lacunae. As the corpora depressurize, arterial inflow further decreases to the resting state.[3] Interference with the erectile mechanism by exogenous agents may result in impotence, but on the other hand, the erectile mechanism can also be purposely manipulated pharmacologically to effectively treat impotence.

Peripheral penile innervation is via T11-L2 sympathetics and S2-4 somatic and parasympathetic nerves.[4] At a microscopic level, adrenergic nerves constrict corporal smooth muscle while cholinergic nerves relax it, as do nonadrenergic, noncholinergic neurotransmitters not yet identified or precisely characterized. Other factors, which probably derive from an endothelial source, are also involved in ways currently not well understood.

Even when this structural-functional framework is intact, an appropriate

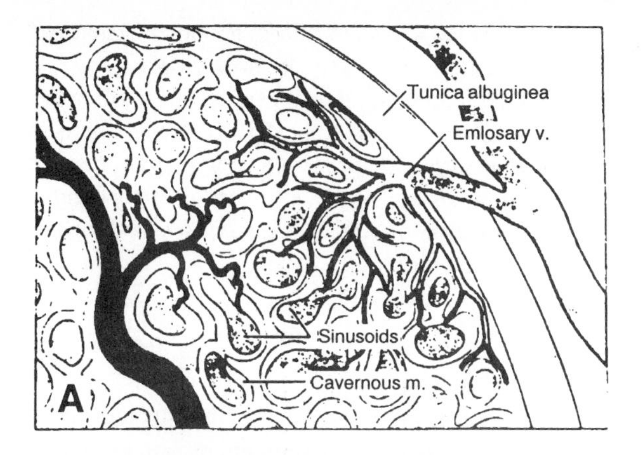

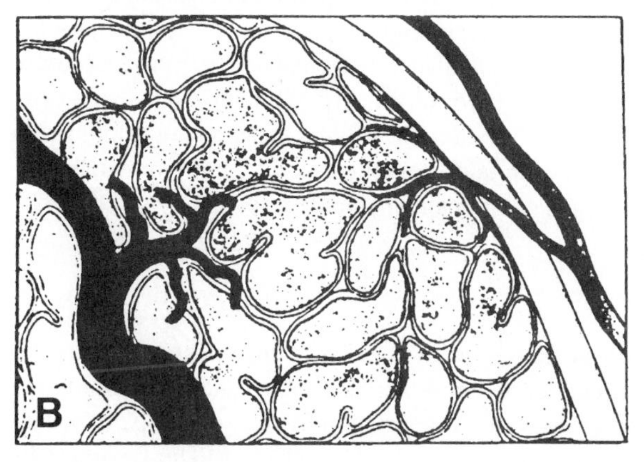

Figure 12-1 *A*. In the flaccid state the arteries, arterioles, and sinusoids are contracted. The intersinusoidal and subtunical venular plexuses are open with free flow to the emissary veins. *B*. In the erect state the muscles of the sinusoidal wall and the arterioles relax, allowing maximal flow to fill the now-compliant sinusoidal spaces. The small venules are compressed between the sinusoids. The larger intermediary venules are sandwiched and compressed between the distended sinusoidal wall, and the noncompliant tunica albuginea thus restricts the venous flow to a minimum. [From Lue TF: Male sexual dysfunction, in Lue TF, McClure RD (eds): *Contemporary Management of Impotence and Infertility*. Baltimore, Williams & Wilkins, 1982. Reprinted with permission.]

hormonal environment is necessary for optimum sexual function. With aging, both free and total serum testosterone levels fall progressively, paralleling the decline in sexual interest and the need for greater stimulation for climax generally observed in older men.[5] However, the relationship between testosterone, sexual interest, performance, and erectile capacity is not completely straightforward. When testicular androgens are completely withdrawn, libido and erectile capacity are generally diminished, but many castrates can maintain normal sexual functioning. In impotent hypogonadal men, androgen replacement will often enhance libido and restore erectile response to external stimuli. The precise mechanism and molecular site of action of testicular androgens in the erectile process are unknown.

When all these factors are operative, erections result not only from sexual stimulation but also at night during rapid eye movement (REM) sleep. When all physical aspects of the erectile mechanisms are in order, a healthy postadolescent male will have three to five erectile episodes each night, each lasting 20 to 40 min. This nocturnal activity explains the erection that many men awaken with in the morning and at night when they get up to void.

ETIOLOGY

It is useful to take a structured approach to the initial interview of the impotent male. As detailed later, during this session one forms an important impression as to how much of the patient's problem may be psychologic or physical. To explore possible physical causes, we use the standard medical history format in which past or present disease entities, surgical procedures and/or physically traumatic events, and drug intake are systematically catalogued. Each of these three areas is then examined in detail to determine whether factors in question might affect the hormonal, neurologic, vascular, or penile end organ component of erectile response.

Diseases Causing Impotence

Endocrine Endocrine factors are rare causes of impotence. Primary testicular failure is the most common endocrine cause and can be secondary to childhood mumps orchitis, Klinefelter's syndrome, past cryptorchidism, or rarely, exposure to environmental toxins like radiation or cancer chemotherapy. The Leydig cells are quite resistant to most toxic insults. Deficient gonadotrophins do occasionally cause secondary gonadal failure, either congenitally or secondary to pituitary tumor or idiopathic pituitary dysfunction. More common is hyperprolactinemia, either secondary to pituitary adenoma or simple idiopathic hypersecretion. When this occurs, serum luteinizing hormone (LH) levels are lowered as is serum testosterone, and generally both the hyperprolactinemia and the diminished serum testosterone must be treated to restore sexual function. Hyperthyroidism and Cushing's disease can also alter the pituitary gonadal axis, causing impotence which will respond to case-specific intervention.[5]

Neurologic Trauma and multiple sclerosis are the most common causes of central neurologic lesions resulting in impotence. The degree of sexual impairment associated with these is a function of the extent and location of the lesion. Large lesions completely transsecting the cord clearly isolate psychologic stimuli from the neuroeffector end organ. Men with upper cord and incomplete lesions maintain erectile function more commonly than do those with lower cord or complete lesions.[6] Lumbar disc disease and peripheral neuropathy associated with alcoholism, diabetes, or other metabolic factors commonly affect the lower somatic neurons, sympathetics, and sensory fibers, thus adversely impacting on erectile function.

Vascular Any disease associated with accelerated atherosclerosis will result in an increased incidence of impotence. Upon examination many impotent men discovered to have arterial impairment as the cause of their dysfunction have associated diabetes, hyperlipidemias, and/or hypertension. In untreated hypertension, the incidence of impotence is reported as 8 to 20 percent in various studies.[7] Unfortunately medication used to treat the disease often makes matters worse sexually. One investigator reports that venous leakage is present in 75 percent of impotent men who have normal neural and hormonal function. The incidence does not seem to rise with age,[8] suggesting that the relatively high incidence of vascular impotence seen in older men is principally due to atherosclerosis and associated diminished arterial capacity to overcome venous leakage that may have been present in most men for some time.

Penile Peyronie's disease is a fibrotic process of the tunica albuginea of unknown cause which produces pain and curvature with erection. Its course is generally self-limited. Erectile dysfunction can result from psychologic factors associated with "self-consciousness" regarding the deformity and pain. However, organic impairment is also possible in some afflicted men, probably on the basis of venous leakage.[9] In evaluating impotent men with Peyronie's disease using duplex ultrasound, one may note good erections proximal to the plaque of scar tissue but a flaccid penis distally, associated with normal arterial flow throughout the entire length of the phallus. This suggests a localized venous leak as a causative factor.

Surgical Causes of Impotence

Endocrine As mentioned above, pharmacologic or surgical castration will generally diminish libido and erectile capacity in most men, but a minority (18 percent) will still maintain sexual capability and interest.[10]

Neurologic Sexual complications of anterior lumbar fusion occur in less than 1 percent of cases, but lumbar sympathectomy in older men causes impotence in 50 percent.[11] Rectal surgery causes impotence of a mixed neurovascular nature and frequently is a function of patient age and extent of dissection. The rate of impotence is 15 percent in young men after abdominal perineal resection but almost 100 percent in men over 70. The neurovascular bundle to the corpora lies just lateral to the rectum and is undoubtedly damaged during radical removal of that structure. External beam radiotherapy for prostatic cancer produces impotence in 41 to 84 percent of men treated, presumably secondary to damage to both nerves and blood vessels in the area of the prostate. These structures are readily visualized surgically and run at 3 o'clock and 9 o'clock in the membranous urethra and at 5 o'clock and 7 o'clock in the prostate. During radical retropubic prostatectomy for cancer, these can be avoided, and as a result, this commonly performed procedure causes impotence in less than half the patients so treated. Some individuals report rates as low as 15 percent. Radical cystoprostatectomy can also now be performed with preservation of potency in 50 to 60 percent of patients treated.[12] While impotence after transurethral prostatectomy for benign disease is unusual (less than 5 percent), increased awareness of the location of the neurovascular bundle should make cautery injury to this structure during transurethral surgery a truly rare event.

Vascular In the past, 25 percent of men undergoing aortoiliac surgery became impotent. Recent awareness of the importance of sparing the hypogastric nerves and establishing iliac flow without disturbing collaterals has reduced this figure markedly. Renal transplantation has been associated with a high impotence rate in the past, in part secondary to accelerated small-vessel disease associated with chronic renal failure and hypertension but also due to surgical technical factors like end-to-end anastomosis of the hypogastric artery to the allograft. Use of an end-to-side anastomosis to the external iliac artery should improve this. Perineal trauma (straddle injury) can thrombose the internal pudendal or penile arteries directly causing impotence. Pelvic fracture frequently produces impotence[13] probably secondary to combined neurovascular trauma.

Drugs Causing Impotence

The incidence of sexual dysfunction increases dramatically with age, especially after age 60. Unfortunately so does the use of prescription medications, many of which cause or contribute to loss of libido, impotence, or problems with ejaculation. Virtually any drug which affects the autonomic nervous system can cause sexual dysfunction. Other known mechanisms include elevation of serum prolactin levels, antiandrogenic effects, production of central nervous system (CNS) depression, and drug-induced changes in vascular flow. It may be difficult to distinguish drug-induced sexual dysfunction from the effects of depression or disease, especially since many drugs have a relatively low incidence of such side effects. Therefore, it is imperative to determine a time relationship between when a drug was initiated and when the problem(s) arose. The length of time the patient has been taking the medication is also important, since impotence is more often associated with chronic rather than acute administration of the drug. It is not surprising that the drugs most commonly implicated in causing sexual dysfunction are those which patients take chronically, i.e., antihypertensives, psychotropics and other drugs affecting the CNS, and gastrointestinal agents. Fortunately most problems are reversible upon reducing the dose of the medication or discontinuing the offending agent.

Antihypertensives Of the seven classes of antihypertensive agents, diuretics and beta-adrenergic blocking agents have received the most attention with regard to their potential for causing sexual dysfunction.[14,15] In the case of thiazides, this is due primarily to their widespread use. The thiazides are reported to cause decreased libido, erectile dysfunction, and ejaculatory failure in 4 to 36 percent of males. Erectile and ejaculatory problems have been linked to a reduction in peripheral vascular resistance, which causes shunting of blood away from the penis.[16] Most of these studies have utilized relatively large doses of hydrochlorothiazide (50 to 100 mg/day), sometimes in combination with other drugs known to produce sexual dysfunction. There is a lack of information on the incidence of impotence in males receiving a daily dose of 12.5 to 25 mg of hydrochlorothiazide, the currently recommended dosage for elderly hypertensives. Since it is estimated that 8 to 20 percent of untreated hypertensive males are impotent upon initial diagnosis and since the incidence of both hypertension and impotence increases with increasing age, it is currently felt that the incidence of impotence associated with thiazides is rare in the elderly.[17]

On the other hand, spironolactone, with a steroidlike chemical structure, has antiandrogen activity and produces impotence, gynecomastia, and decreased libido. The effects on erection are dose related—30 percent of men taking 400 mg/day exhibit impotence, whereas impotence is seen much less often in patients taking 50 to 100 mg/day.[16] The overall incidence of impotence in males taking spironolactone alone ranges from 4 to 30 percent.[17]

The beta-adrenergic blocking agents (beta blockers) include propranolol, metoprolol, atenolol, acebutolol, nadolol, pindolol, timolol, penbutolol, and labetalol. While impotence can occur with any of the beta blockers, propranolol produces the highest incidence, up to 28 percent in men taking greater than 320 mg/day.[16] Although the exact mechanism by which propranolol produces impotence is unknown, it is probably related to the drug's lipid solubility and subsequent ability to cross the blood-brain barrier. This suggests that impotence with propranolol may be due to a central beta-receptor blockade. Impotence occurs rarely (usually <2 percent) from those beta blockers that are cardioselective. However, the occurrence and degree of impotence is directly related to the dose of the particular agent. Even ocular administration of timolol for glaucoma has been known to cause erectile dysfunction.[16] It should also be noted that priapism has been reported with the use of beta blockers, particularly labetalol.[17]

Centrally acting antihypertensives include methyldopa, clonidine, guanabenz, and guanfacine. Impotence has been reported more frequently and ejaculatory dysfunction less frequently than with peripherally acting agents. Clearly methyldopa and clonidine produce the highest incidence of sexual dysfunction in males. In studies where patients received 1 to 3 g/day of methyldopa, impotence was reported 2 to 80 percent of the time, with an average of 20 to 30 percent.[16,17] The occurrence may be higher than with other agents because methyldopa produces CNS sedation and depression plus an increase in serum prolactin concentrations.[18,19] With clonidine, impotence has been reported in 10 to 24 percent of patients receiving 0.2 to 0.8 mg/day.[14,16] Other studies have reported an incidence approaching 70 percent, but these patients were also receiving diuretics or had diseases associated with sexual dysfunction.[16] In patients taking guanabenz or guanfacine, impotence has been reported in less than 1 percent.

The class of peripherally acting antihypertensives includes reserpine, guanethidine, guanadrel, prazosin, and terazosin. While these drugs produce more problems with ejaculation than impotence, guanethidine and reserpine have been associated with many cases of erectile failure. Since these drugs are usually prescribed in combination with diuretics, it is not surprising that impotence occurs in 4 to 100 percent of patients receiving guanethidine and in 11 to 33 percent of patients on reserpine.[16,17] Many cases of impotence from these agents have been attributed to psychogenic causes, e.g., depression over ejaculatory dysfunction. Moreover, depression associated with higher doses of reserpine may contribute to the incidence of erectile failure. The other peripherally acting agents have an incidence of erectile dysfunction less than 2 percent. There is one study in which guanadrel was associated with an 8 percent incidence of impotence; however, most of these patients were also taking 50 to 100 mg of hydrochlorothiazide per day.[20]

The direct vasodilators hydralazine and minoxidil have a low incidence of producing sexual dysfunction. There have been only scattered case reports of impotence resulting from hydralazine in doses of 35 to 50 mg/day[18] and no cases of erectile dysfunction reported with minoxidil. Similarly, the angiotensin converting enzyme (ACE) inhibitors (captopril, enalapril, lisinopril) have not been associated with significant occurrence of impotence. Of the calcium channel blockers (nifedipine, verapamil, diltiazem, nicardipine), only verapamil has been reported to cause impotence, and there are only scattered reports to substantiate this.[16,21] Antipsychotics, tricyclic antidepressants, antianxiety agents, narcotics, and other drugs which alter the CNS can produce impotence by their sedative properties, effects on neurotransmitters, or their effects on the autonomic nervous system, i.e., anticholinergic or sympatholytic effects. Sexual dysfunction is often a manifestation of the particular condition these drugs are used to treat. Therefore, it is often difficult to distinguish between drug- and disease-induced causes of impotence.

Antipsychotics These drugs include the phenothiazines and butyrophenones. Depending on the particular agent and its dose, impotence may be insignificant or a major side effect. The antipsychotics may cause sexual dysfunction by a central antidopaminergic effect, an alpha-antagonist action, a release of prolactin, anticholinergic activity, or sedation.[17] Thioridazine has been reported to cause impotence in 2 to 44 percent of patients. It is also the most potent inhibitor of ejaculation (49 percent) based on its alpha-blocking properties. Fluphenazine has also been reported to be a frequent cause of impotence (65 to 75 percent) in alcoholics.[16] Other antipsychotics, including chlorpromazine, fluphenazine, haloperidol, and thiothixene, have generated only rare case reports of impotence.[17] It is noteworthy that most cases of impotence associated with the antipsychotics tend to occur within 24 h of initiating therapy and improve quickly when the drug is discontinued.[16]

Antidepressants Tricyclic antidepressants probably induce impotence by their sedative or anticholinergic properties or by their inhibition of the reuptake of norepinephrine or serotonin. Amitriptyline, protriptyline, and desipramine have generated only scattered case reports of sexual dysfunction.[17] It is ironic that imipramine has been cited for causing impotence, since it has been used to treat retrograde ejaculation in diabetics. Nontricyclics include doxepin, amoxapine, trazodone, maprotiline, buproprion, and fluoxetine. There is one study where 8 of 19 patients receiving amoxapine developed sexual dysfunction, decreased libido, impotence, or painful/absent ejaculation, although these side effects cleared in several patients during therapy.[16,17] Trazodone is well known to cause priapism in patients. The other drugs have been implicated only sporadically in causing erectile failure.

Lithium Several studies have concluded that lithium causes impotence in 3 to 20 percent of patients[16,17] probably by decreasing central dopamine activity. Other documentation is found in several individual case reports. However, since increased sexuality can be one of the manifestations of mania, it is often difficult to assess whether decreased sexual function is a predictable result of drug therapy or a side effect of the drug itself.

Antianxiety drugs Benzodiazepines generally depress the limbic system and the reticular formation of the brain stem. Theoretically this can lead to decreased libido.[18] Diazepam has often been implicated in causing various types of sexual dysfunction, although it is unclear whether the dysfunction is caused by the drug or the anxiety state itself. There have been only scattered case reports of other benzodiazepines causing impotence.

Drugs of abuse Acute ingestion of alcohol or narcotics has been linked to impotence, and chronic ingestion of alcohol, cocaine, amphetamines, or narcotics has been associated with various types of sexual dysfunction. Moreover, inhaled nicotine may cause erectile failure, presumably due to a local vasoconstriction.[17]

Hormones Androgens, estrogens, corticosteroids, and cancer chemotherapeutic agents which affect gonadal function have all been shown to produce impotence. These effects are probably related to the dose of the drug as well as the duration of therapy.

H_2 antagonists Cimetidine can negatively affect erection by increasing prolactin secretion and opposing the effects of androgenic hormones; this effect is considered to be dose dependent. Higher doses of ranitidine also increase prolactin secretion but appear to have no antiandrogen activity.[15] There has been at least one report of impotence associated with nizatidine, but no significant sexual dysfunction has been associated with famotidine.

Miscellaneous drugs As stated previously, virtually any drug which affects the autonomic nervous system could potentially lead to impotence. The drugs most commonly implicated are listed in Table 12-1.

Table 12-1 Drugs known to cause sexual dysfunction

ANTIHYPERTENSIVE AGENTS

- Diuretics
  - Amiloride
  - Chlorthalidone
  - Spironolactone
  - Thiazides
- Beta-adrenergic blocking agents
  - Atenolol
  - Labetalol
  - Metoprolol
  - Pindolol
  - Propranolol
  - Timolol
- Direct vasodilators
  - Hydralazine
  - Minoxidil
- Centrally acting antiadrenergics
  - Clonidine
  - Guanabenz
  - Guanfacine
  - Methyldopa
- Peripherally acting antiadrenergics
  - Doxazosin
  - Guanadrel
  - Guanethidine
  - Prazosin
  - Reserpine
  - Terazosin

ANTIHYPERTENSIVE AGENTS (*Cont.*)

- Calcium channel blockers
  - Verapamil

DRUGS AFFECTING CNS

- Antianxiety agents/hypnotics
  - Alprazolam
  - Diazepam
- Antipsychotics
  - Chlorpromazine
  - Chlorprothixene
  - Fluphenazine
  - Haloperidol
  - Mesoridazine
  - Perphenazine
  - Pimozide
  - Thioridazine
  - Thiothixene
  - Trifluoperazine
- CNS stimulants
  - Amphetamines/anorexiants
- Antidepressants
  - Amitriptyline
  - Amoxapine
  - Desipramine
  - Doxepin
  - Imipramine
  - Isocarboxazid

DRUGS AFFECTING CNS (*Cont.*)

  - Maprotiline
  - Nortriptyline
  - Pargyline
  - Phenelzine
  - Protriptyline
  - Tranylcypromine
  - Trazodone
- Narcotic analgesics

CARDIOVASCULAR DRUGS

- Antiarrhythmics
  - Amiodarone
  - Digoxin
  - Disopyramide
  - Mexiletine

GASTROINTESTINAL AGENTS

- H_2 antagonists
  - Cimetidine
  - Nizatidine
  - Ranitidine
- Others
  - Anticholinergics
  - Metoclopramide
  - Propantheline

ANTICONVULSANTS

  - Barbiturates
  - Carbamazepine
  - Ethosuximide
  - Phenytoin
  - Primidone

ANTI-INFECTIVE AGENTS

- Ethionamide
- Ketoconazole

MISCELLANEOUS DRUGS

- Acetazolamide
- Baclofen
- Clofibrate
- Danazol
- Disulfiram
- Estrogens
- Interferon
- Levodopa
- Lithium
- Naproxen
- Progesterone

DIAGNOSTIC TECHNIQUES

History

This is the clinician's single most important diagnostic tool. Often, simply listening to the patient will reveal why he is impotent. If the patient has a good idea of what he wants to do about his dysfunction, further evaluation is often unnecessary before proceeding to treatment. The importance of a detailed past medical history, surgical history, and drug history is obvious from the foregoing discussion regarding etiology. Men who awaken regularly at night or in the morning with a rigid penis rarely have organic erectile problems. Short-lived, occasional, or absent nocturnal erections by history, on the other hand, may simply mean that the patient is a poor historian, wakes up at the wrong time, or has a sleep disorder. Listening to details of timing regarding the sexual history often directs further evaluation and management. Organic impotence is generally of gradual onset or, if sudden, is temporarily related to a new medicine, trauma, or surgical insult. Psychologically based impotence is frequently of sudden onset and related to a life event, a new partner, or other stress. Most men do not volunteer such data, and solicitation of such historical detail from an often embarrassed, anxious male takes a great deal of time and patience. It is almost always time well spent.

Physical Examination

Surprisingly, this is not generally very helpful in most evaluations. It is important to perform a simple neurologic examination, including an attempt to elicit a bulbocavernosus reflex, as this may provide evidence of neurologic impairment. Generally, however, other historic or physical evidence of such disease is present. Diminished lower extremity pulses are very common in the elderly and generally not correlated well with penile vascular status. Eunuchoid proportions and small testes may suggest Klinefelter's syndrome and impotence which is secondary to mid-life Leydig cell failure. Gynecomastia is rare but may result from the increased estrogen production seen in individuals impotent from hyperthyroidism or from drug therapy.[5]

Serum Hormone Determinations

Serum testosterone levels should be measured in all impotent men and serum prolactin levels measured in those with subnormal testosterone. Hyperprolactinemia rarely occurs in the absence of a low testosterone.[22] Other hormone levels should be measured only when clinically indicated on the basis of history or physical. Patients may need referrals for appropriate endocrine evaluations.

Nocturnal Penile Tumescence Monitoring

Nocturnal penile tumescence (NPT) monitoring is the best noninvasive means of differentiating psychogenic from organically based impotence. A variety of devices are available to monitor the three to five erections that occur during REM sleep at night in healthy men. The simplest is probably a ring of postage stamps wrapped around the penis before bedtime and simple patient observation as to whether or not the band has broken during sleep.[23] While inexpensive, reliability is questionable; most prefer the RigiScan (Dacomed), a portable computerized unit which the patient uses in his own bed at home. Penile circumference and rigidity changes are monitored at the penile tip and base and recorded on a memory chip within a tamperproof box. The patient returns the box after two to three nights of monitoring and the data are downloaded into a computer and printed out for reading. Clearly, the presence of the usual number of erections of adequate size and rigidity during a night's sleep "prove" a physically normal erectile response. Absence of such response, however, does not necessarily indicate organic impotence. A variable small number of men do respond to external erotic stimuli but do not have normal nocturnal erections for reasons not well understood. Because of this, absence of erections on NPT is not absolute proof of inability to get erections in an erotically stimulating situation. NPT monitoring is generally not necessary for most impotent patients since history often suggests probable causative factors. However, when history is confusing or the patient is manipulative, NPT monitoring is invaluable in guiding further evaluation and therapy.

Arterial Evaluation

In the past decade, *penile brachial index* (PBI) has frequently been used as a measure of adequate penile blood flow. A small blood pressure cuff placed about the flaccid penis was inflated and a Doppler stethoscope used to measure penile systolic blood pressure, which was then compared with systolic brachial pressure. A penile-brachial ratio of 0.7 or higher is considered normal. This is an inaccurate test and of little value, since many impotent men with cavernosal arterial insufficiency have normal PBIs. The dorsal and urethral arteries make up most of the blood flow measured by the PBI; their flow is irrelevant to erectile hemodynamics, which largely depend on cavernosal artery blood flow. Additionally, the test indirectly measures penile blood flow in the flaccid state, which has little or nothing to do with capacity to increase blood flow in response to sexual stimuli.[24]

The arterial side of the erectile mechanism can, however, be evaluated accurately and functionally using intracorporal injection of vasoactive agents in conjunction with duplex ultrasonography of the penis. In the early 1980s, Virag[25] and Brindley[26] demonstrated that vasodilators (papaverine and phenoxybenzamine) induced erections in normal and in some impotent men when injected into the corpora. Subsequent workers have refined and expanded on the initial observations to demonstrate that when injected into the corpus, such agents relax arteriolar and lacunar smooth muscle directly to produce erections lasting minutes to hours in normal men and in men with psychologic or neurologically caused impotence.[27] Erection also results when vascular disease is mild. In effect, these drugs act directly on intracorporal erectile smooth muscle, bypassing dysfunctional nerves and minimizing effects of psychologic inhibition, and dilate moderately narrowed arteries to achieve an increase in blood flow sufficient for erection. When atherosclerosis is severe, arteries cannot respond and erection does not result. When venous leakage is severe, erection does not occur despite increased arterial dilation and increased blood flow, as sufficient blood cannot be sequestered in the lacunae to pressurize the corpora.

Today most workers use a papaverine-phentolamine combination, prostaglandin E_1 (PGE_1), or a combination of the above for such testing. When men do not respond to intracorporal vasodilators with an erection, one can determine whether this is due to severe arterial disease or venous leakage by monitoring arterial response over a 30-min period using duplex ultrasonography as described by Lue.[24] After an injection of 20 μg of PGE_1, an adequate arterial response 5 to 10 min after injection consists of >60 percent increase in cavernosal arterial diameter and a peak systolic velocity in these arteries in excess of 25 cm/s. If arterial response to injection approximates these parameters yet no erection results, then the cause must be a venous leak since arterial inflow is normal. Conversely, lack of erection in response to the injected vasodilator associated with a lesser arterial response indicates an arterial etiology of the impotence.

Not all patients require intracorporal injection of vasoactive agents or duplex ultrasonography as part of their evaluation. However, when patients would realistically consider a home self-injection program as a therapeutic measure, office test injections are certainly worth trying. Frequently, individuals with neurogenic or mild arterial disease as the cause of their impotence experience the drug-induced erection as part of their evaluation and are then anxious to use it therapeutically. Similarly, when injections produce suboptimal erections in typical doses in the office, it makes it clear to patients that a home injection program is not practical in their particular instance.

Duplex ultrasound is often valuable in differentiating arterial from venous causes of impotence in candidates for vascular reconstructive surgery. However, it is an expensive test not generally available in all medical centers and is certainly not necessary in most patients. Arteriography is another specialized diagnostic tool that is useful in providing a preoperative final road map in individuals with arterial insufficiency documented on duplex ultrasound who wish to pursue revascularization as an option. This is not the case in most impotent elderly men presenting in the primary practitioner's office.

Venous Evaluation

When a man does not get an erection and has good arterial flow parameters on duplex ultrasound, a venous leak exists. When penile venous ligation surgery is a realistic option for the patient, one should evaluate the extent and site of leakage with pharmacologic cavernosometry and cavernosography. After the corpus is injected with PGE_1, it is infused with saline via a scalp vein needle in one corpus at progressively faster rates until intracorporal pressure, monitored by a pressure transducer connected to a second needle in the opposite corpus, approaches 90 mmHg (systolic pressure) and an erection occurs. The flow rate required to achieve erection estimates the magnitude of the venous leak. The corpus is then continuously infused with contrast, while digital subtraction films are taken to localize venous leakage sites from the corpora. Such studies are indicated in the small minority of men who are realistic candidates for venous surgery.

Neurologic Assessment

Multiple sophisticated diagnostic studies including measurement of sacral-evoked response can be used to assess the erectile reflex arc. These are rarely indicated clinically, and in practice one depends upon basic history, neurologic examination, and response to intracorporal vasoactive agents to evaluate therapy of neurologically caused impotence.

TREATMENT

Psychologic Treatment/Sex Therapy

When evaluation indicates that psychologic or relationship disorders are partly or totally the cause of impotence, referral to a qualified "sex therapist" or other mental health professional is indicated. Patients are often reluctant to accept such advice and may be embarrassed concerning the prospect of sharing intimate details with yet "another third party." The RigiScan printout is helpful in such instances to demonstrate quite clearly that physical components of the erectile mechanism are in "working order." Faced with such evidence, many men are more likely to accept an appropriate referral for counseling. The likelihood of success depends on many factors. Masters and Johnson reported a 5-year 70 percent success rate for secondary impotence, but other studies report rates ranging from 33 to 80 percent.[28] In most cases therapy takes weeks to months, is costly, and generally requires involvement of an interested and open-minded patient and partner. In most communities, only a small minority of mental health practitioners are interested in and/or capable of treating male sexual dysfunction effectively. Identifying these capable individuals generally requires initiative and follow-up on the part of the referring practitioner.

Drug Therapy

Yohimbine The drug is an alpha-$_2$ adrenoreceptor blocker derived from the bark of the yohimbine tree and has been considered an aphrodisiac in herbal medicine circles for years. It is administered orally and has been tested in several clinical trials over the past 10 years. Morales et al have tested the drug in double-blind trials of patients whose impotence resulted primarily from organic[29] and psychogenic[30] causes. Eighteen milligrams per day in three divided doses resulted in a positive response in 42.6 percent of patients with organic impotence versus a 27.6 percent response rate with placebo. The results were not significantly different statistically. When 48 patients with psychogenic impotence were tested, however, 62 percent reported a positive response versus 16 percent treated with placebo. These results are significantly different. There is a lag period of 2 to 4 weeks between onset of therapy and any observed efficacy.

At a recommended dose of 5.4 mg orally three times daily, the drug is inexpensive, and side effects are generally minimal. Occasionally, patients exhibit anxiety; hypotension is theoretically possible, although it is rarely seen. Cholinergic stimulation produced by the drug limits its use in patients with ulcers and gastrointestinal disorders. It may be tried in patients who want to exhaust "simple" potential remedies before embarking on a complex evaluation or more invasive therapies. Most have experienced results that are less impressive than those reported by Morales's group.

Hormones Impotent men are frequently referred to the urologist after failing prior empirically administered testosterone injections. In most series, testosterone deficiency is an unusual cause of impotence and is involved in less than 5 percent of cases treated. In the other 95+ percent whose serum testosterone is normal, supplemental testosterone is of no value. However, when serum testosterone is less than 300 ng/dL, replacement therapy is indicated, inexpensive, and effective. Alkylated oral preparations of testosterone are available, but they are poorly absorbed and may cause liver damage.[5] Long-acting parenteral esters, testosterone cypionate, or enanthate in doses of 200 mg every 2 weeks to 400 mg every 3 weeks are preferred. Patients are usually begun on 200 mg every 3 weeks. Serum testosterone levels are measured in 2 weeks, and the dose is titrated to achieve "normal range" levels 5 to 7 days prior to the next scheduled dose. Some men describe erratic mood swings at 3-week dose intervals; in such cases a 2-week interval allows for narrower fluctuations in serum drug levels and associated affect. Adult-onset acne is one minor side effect.

The prostate is examined regularly to detect any testosterone-accelerated growth of latent prostate carcinoma. Because prostate cancer is generally androgen dependent, men with this disease are not candidates for testosterone replacement. When significant hyperprolactinemia is associated with diminished serum testosterone, patients should be referred to an endocrinologist for treatment in addition to prescribing testosterone replacement therapy as described above. Additionally the pituitary fossa should be evaluated radiologically with a computed tomography (CT) scan or magnetic resonance imaging (MRI) as a screen for prolactin-secreting tumor.

Miscellaneous drugs Other drugs which have been reported to be beneficial in the treatment of impotence include trazodone,[31] topical nitroglycerin,[32] bromocriptine,[33] erythropoietin,[34] vasoactive intestinal polypeptide,[35] naltrexone,[36] and bethanechol.[37] At the present time, these have been reported as single cases or anecdotal reports. Their potential in treating impotence on a large-scale basis is uncertain.

Intracavernous self-injection In the past decade literally thousands of men have successfully treated themselves for impotence in supervised chronic self-injection programs. The drugs used are all direct or indirect vasodilators and act to relax the smooth muscle in the walls of small intracorporal arterioles and lacunae by bypassing the normal neuromuscular control mechanism. The drugs and drug combinations most often used clinically at the present time are listed in Table 12-2.[38,39]

Both papaverine and PGE_1 are direct smooth muscle relaxants, while phentolamine is an $alpha_1$ blocker. Papaverine was the first drug widely used clinically, and phentolamine was later added as a synergist to augment response. These drugs have been noted to cause intracorporal fibrosis and secondary iatrogenic Peyronie's disease (penile curvature when erect) in a small minority of patients. The fibrotic complications generally are dose and duration related, but idiosyncratic non-dose-dependent fibrotic reactions have also been observed. Some have been sufficiently severe as to make subsequent penile prosthesis placement or subsequent effective treatment with vasoactive drugs difficult or impossible. Mild liver function abnormalities have been noted in 10 percent of patients during chronic drug administration. Similar fibrotic side effects and/or liver function abnormalities have not been observed with PGE_1 use. However, intracorporal injection with this drug does cause penile pain in 15 to 30 percent of patients. This is generally mild but can be sufficiently severe to make the drug unsuitable for use in a sexual setting. The three-drug combination in Table 12-2 has very recently been introduced, and to date, painful injections or fibrosis have not been reported.

Table 12-2 Intracavernous drug therapy for impotence

Drug	Concentration	Usual dose
Papaverine	30 mg/mL	0.2-2.0 mL
Papaverine hydrochloride Phentolamine mesylate	30 mg/mL 0.5-1.0 mg/mL	0.1-1.0 mL (total)
Prostaglandin E_1	10μg-20 μg/mL	0.1-1.0 mL
Papaverine hydrochloride Phentolamine mesylate Prostaglandin E_1 Normal saline	2.5 mL of 30 mg/mL 0.55 mL of 5 mg/mL 0.05 mL of 500 μg/mL 1.2 mL	0.1-0.25 mL (total)

The major short-term complication reported with self-injection is priapism or prolonged erection. Treatment is straightforward when initiated early (<6 h) and consists of an intracorporal injection/irrigation of epinephrine (20 μg/20 mL saline) or phenylephrine (500 μg/mL saline). When the duration of erection is substantially longer than 6 h, a surgical shunt procedure is often necessary to reduce the erection, and permanent impotence and fibrosis can result from the hypoxia, acidosis, and tissue ischemia of the insult as well as from the surgery.[40]

When using any of the drugs listed in Table 12-2, duration of erection is linearly related to the amount of drug injected in a given individual. Priapism does not occur if one does not inject too much drug. Of course, self-injection programs should be limited to stable, responsible individuals who will follow directions carefully. In addition, before issuing any prescriptions, it is necessary to determine the therapeutic dose to be prescribed by using several office visits to titrate gradually increasing doses of drug with observed erectile response until a dose that results in an erection lasting 45 to 90 min is reached. During these visits, it is important to discuss potential complications with the patient, to teach injection technique to him and/or his partner, and to assess and deal with problems in technique as they are observed. Figure 12-2 is presented as a very useful teaching aid in illustrating penile anatomy and injection technique.[41] Before the patient leaves the office, he must feel confident that he can easily inject himself and must understand the danger of

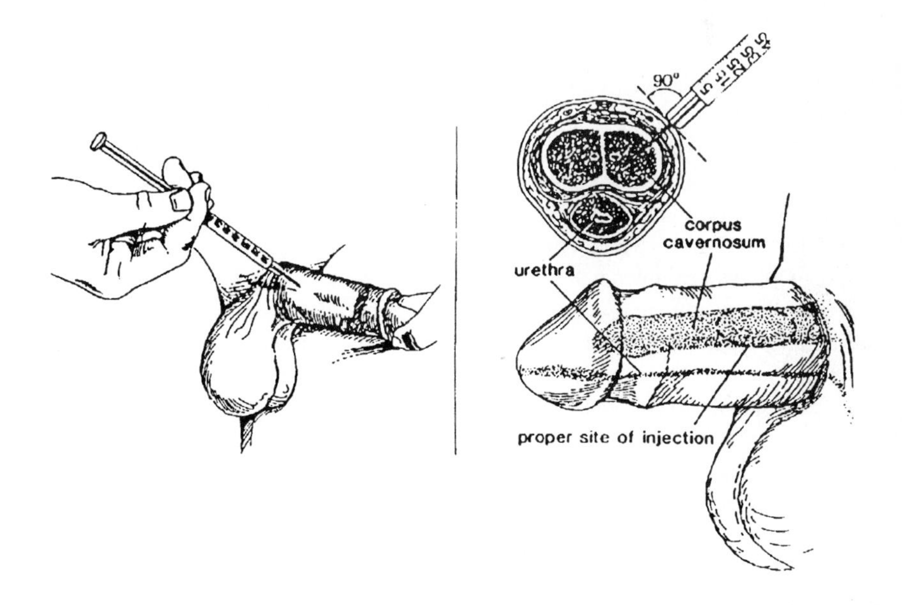

Figure 12-2 Self-injection technique. (From Duffy LM, Lange PH: Vasoactive intracavernous pharmacotherapy—the nursing role in teaching self-injection therapy. *J Urol* 138:1198, 1987. © 1987 by Williams & Wilkins. Reprinted with permission.)

injecting more than the prescribed amount of drug. Patients should be advised to inject no more than once in 24 h. PGE_1 is an excellent first choice because at a concentration of 20 μg/mL, it is convenient to mix and low in cost. Less than 10 percent experience significant pain sufficient to interfere with sexual pleasure. Those who do can use a two-drug papaverine-phentolamine combination. The three-drug combination described in Table 12-2 is becoming increasingly popular because it minimizes the chance of fibrotic complications. Most patients with modest arterial compromise require 10 to 20 μg of PGE_1 chronically as the usual therapeutic dose, while those with pure neurogenic impotence [multiple sclerosis, spinal cord trauma, post-transurethral prostatic resection (TURP) impotence] require 2 to 4 μg of the drug. Of those patients initially achieving satisfactory erections, 40 to 70 percent continue the program on an ongoing basis.[38,42] If PGE_1 is utilized as the principal agent, there is little corporal fibrosis. With careful patient selection and education, priapism is rare.

Vacuum Devices

These mechanical devices have been used safely and effectively to enhance erection for many years in this country. As can be seen in Fig. 12-3, they consist of a plastic cylinder closed at one end placed over the flaccid penis to form a tight seal at the base, a pump used to evacuate the cylinder after it is placed, and a constriction ring. After the cylinder is evacuated, the penis generally becomes engorged, presumably via enhanced arterial blood flow in the vacuum. At this time, the constriction ring, which has previously been placed over the base of the cylinder, is slipped off onto the penile base to inhibit venous return and the cylinder is removed. The constriction ring may be safely left in place for 30 min while intercourse takes place.[43,44]

Several companies market various design variations for about $400 to $600. All include a detailed instruction book as well as a VCR instruction tape and are sold by prescription only. Most men are able to master the technique of achieving an erection in four to five practice sessions, and after this point, an erection can be obtained in a few minutes with the device.[43] Many men experience minor discomfort from the vacuum and/or ring initially, but generally this is not enough to limit use or cause physical harm. It generally diminishes with time. The erection obtained with the vacuum device is rigid only distal to the applied ring, which also limits antegrade ejaculation at orgasm. In a recent survey of 100 men who chose vacuum device therapy for impotence and purchased a device, 83 were able to maintain erection sufficient to complete intercourse, and 69 expressed overall satisfaction with such therapy.[45] Minor bruising and small hematomas are common, but significant bleeding is rare even with patients on anti-platelet therapy or formal anticoagulation. Vacuum devices or constriction rings alone may also be used in conjunction with intracorporal injection as effective therapy. High satisfaction rates have been reported by most investigators, particularly in elderly patients in established intimate relationships. Satisfaction has been less in younger and/or single men.

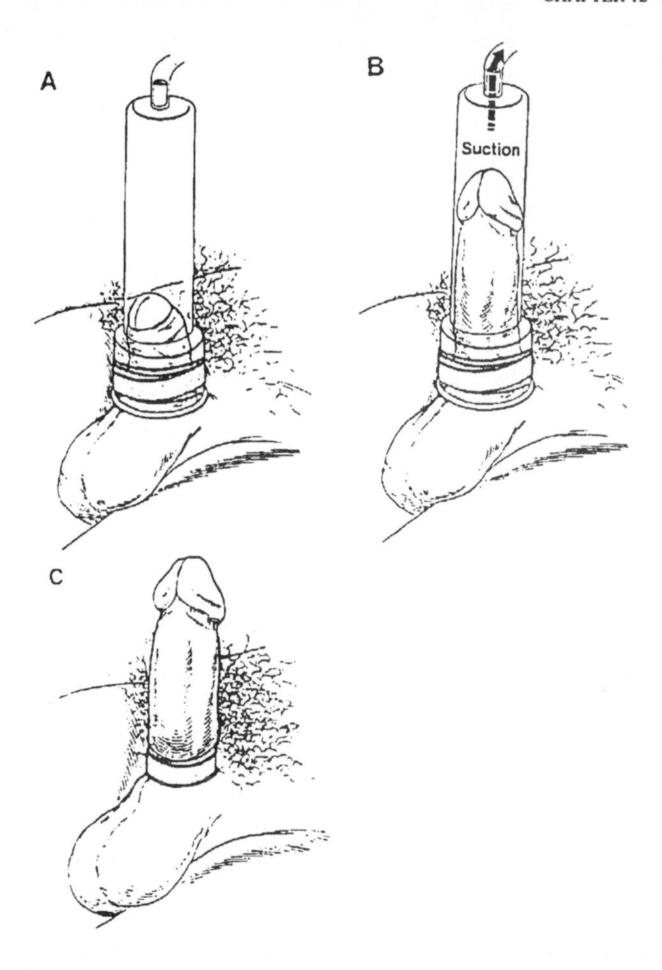

Figure 12-3 Vacuum device technique. *A*. Vacuum chamber placed over penis. *B*. Negative pressure draws blood into penis to produce erectionlike state. *C*. Tension band guided from device to base of penis. Entrapment of blood occurs, which maintains tumescence. (Reprinted with permission from Witherington R: External aids for treatment of impotence. *J Urol Nurs* 6:10, 1987.)

Penile Prostheses

All the treatment entities described above are reversible. If the patient is unhappy with one, he simply discards it and may try another. Penile prostheses, on the other hand, are not reversible; once one is inserted and corporal tissue surgically disrupted to make room for the prosthesis, the patient generally must depend on the prosthesis to achieve erections for the rest of his life. For this reason, men are generally encouraged to work with "reversible" options before committing to a prosthesis.

All penile prostheses involve surgical insertion of paired cylinders into the corpora cavernosa via a penoscrotal, infrapubic, or subcoronal incision in an operation lasting about 45 to 90 min. The "spongy tissue" within the corpora is dilated or spread apart to make room for the cylinders, and thus the physiologic erectile mechanism is further compromised by the surgery. The cylinders make the corpora cavernosa rigid enough for penetration, but the devices do not make the glans rigid. Sexual excitation, however, often produces turgidity of the glans and the corpus spongiosum in many men. Although prostheses can be inserted in outpatient procedures using a local anesthetic, generally 24 h of hospitalization is necessary and a general or regional anesthetic is employed. Postoperatively, discomfort requiring oral narcotic analgesics lasts 1 to 2 weeks and the prosthesis is not used sexually for about 6 weeks. Three general types of prostheses are employed today:

(1) *Semirigid rods.* These are the least expensive and most reliable prostheses available. They are simplest in design and easiest to implant, and since few or no moving parts are involved, malfunction within the first 5 to 10 years is quite unusual. All are sufficiently rigid to allow sexual intercourse. Various design characteristics allow the devices to bend sufficiently when not in use sexually to allow reasonably good concealment. The Small Carrion (Mentor) device has been in use for the longest period of time and consists of a silicone foam center covered by a solid silicone coating. The Flexi-rod (Surgitek) has a silicone "hinge" which bends beneath the pubis to aid concealment. The Jonas prosthesis (Bard) and the AMS 600 cover metal wires with silicone and use the malleability of the wire to vary position and assist in concealment. A related more complex device is the Duraphase (Dacomed) (Fig. 12-4), in which articulated plastic segments are manipulated by a cable and spring assembly to provide rigidity or "flaccidity." Satisfaction rates with these devices are comparable and approach 80 to 90 percent in men who know what they are getting. Their major advantage is reliability, while their principal drawback is that they are somewhat less concealable in restrooms, showers, and when wearing swim suits than their inflatable counterparts. They are always firm and can be felt through clothing by "lap sitters," dance partners, etc.

(2) *Fully inflatable prostheses.* These hydraulic devices consist of paired fluid-filled intracorporal cylinders which are connected to a scrotal pump and a fluid-filled reservoir by "kink resistant" tubing. In *two-part prostheses* (Fig. 12-5) like the Surgitek Uniflate and the similarly constructed Mentor GFS Mark II, the reservoir holds about 25 mL of fluid and is combined in the scrotum with the pump. In *three-part prostheses* like the Mentor inflatable prostheses and the AMS 700 Ultrex (Fig. 12-6), the fluid reservoir is placed separately inside the abdomen in the prevesical space, holds about 60 mL of fluid, and is connected by tubing to both cylinders and the scrotal pump. To activate these inflatable devices for sex, one pumps fluid from the reservoir to the cylinder by gently squeezing the scrotal pump and empties the cylinder during nonsexual activity by pushing an intrascrotal release valve. The Mentor devices are composed largely of polyurethane while the others are made primarily of silicone. Each has its advocates and detractors in the urologic community.

These fully inflatable prostheses mimic physiologic erection more closely than do the semirigid devices. The rigidity achieved by fluid transfer into the cylinders

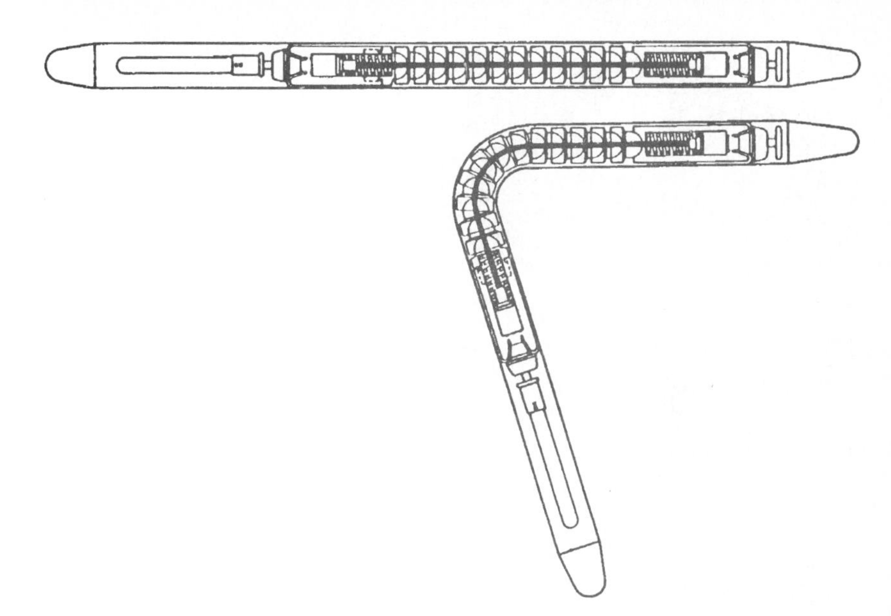

Figure 12-4 DuraPhase prosthesis. (Courtesy of Dacomed Corporation, Minneapolis, Minnesota.)

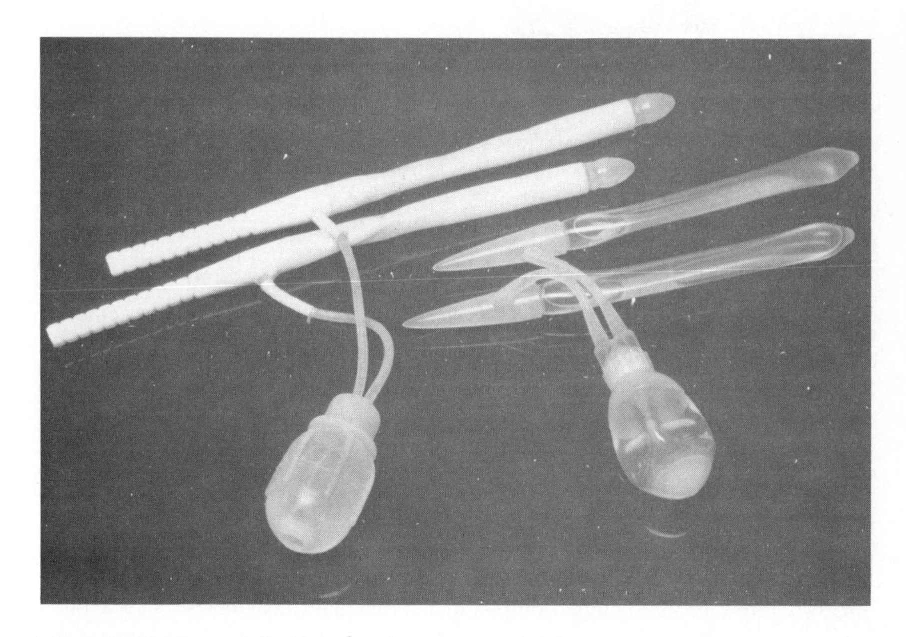

Figure 12-5 Two-part inflatable prosthesis: the Surgitek Uniflate (*left*) and the Mentor GFS Mark II (*right*).

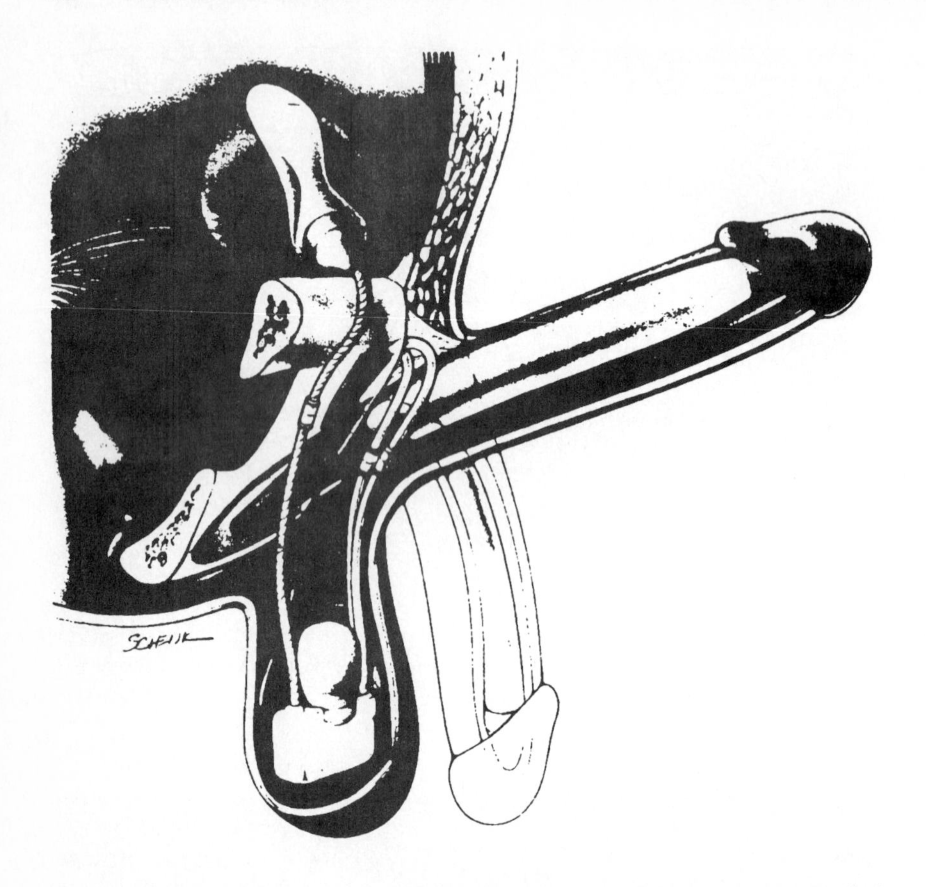

Figure 12-6 Three-part inflatable AMS-700 Ultrex prosthesis in place. (Courtesy of American Medical Systems, Inc., Minnetonka, Minnesota. Medical illustration by Michael Schenk.)

is adequate for penetration, and the "feel" of the implanted penis more closely resembles that of normal tissue, which is largely water. The size difference achieved by pumping fluid into and out of the penis with erection/flaccidity is also more physiologic. The trade-off for these advantages is a more complex design and an associated higher mechanical malfunction rate of 5 to 15 percent in the short term (2 to 5 years).[46] Most companies guarantee the devices for at least 5 years, replacing all or part of the cost of the prosthesis if malfunction occurs. Technology has advanced so rapidly in this field that long-term performance figures are simply unavailable for models currently being implanted, but common sense suggests that malfunction rates will naturally increase with time due to wear and tear. Replacement surgery is generally much simpler than initial placement, costs less, and hurts less. However, doctor and hospital bills other than the replacement costs of the device itself are not paid for by the manufacturers.

(3) *Self-contained hydraulic implants.* These devices consist of a miniaturized pump, fluid reservoir, and pressurizable chamber in each of two chambers which are totally implanted in the penile shaft. Figure 12-7 demonstrates one such device, the FlexiFlate II. With pumping they become rigid but not bigger than in the flaccid state, and when a release valve is pressed, flaccidity results but the penis does not become smaller. The cost and mechanical malfunction rates of these devices resemble those of the fully inflatable prostheses. They are somewhat easier to implant than the multicomponent devices. They are made rigid by pumping an inflate valve in the distal penis and are "deflated" either by bending the shaft or by pushing a deflate valve.

The AMS Hydroflex and the Surgitek FlexiFlate (later FlexiFlate II) were introduced in the mid-1980s, and large numbers of each have been implanted subsequently. Problems learning the inflation-deflation mechanism have been reported with the Hydroflex, and spontaneous deflation problems have been noted with FlexiFlate. In general, however, patients implanted with either device report acceptable satisfaction rates. A new *self-contained* device, the Dynaflex, has recently been introduced by AMS, but reported experience to date is minimal.

Risk of infection is common to all prostheses. When this occurs, as it does in 2 to 3 percent, the entire prosthesis must generally be removed and not replaced for at least 6 months, at which time intracorporal scarring may make replacement difficult or, rarely, impossible. To prevent late hematogenous infection, implanted patients are frequently advised to take antibiotics before oral, gastrointestinal, or urinary tract manipulation. Penile prostheses are expensive ($6000 to $10,000, with actual costs for the individual depending upon prosthesis selection, hospitalization time, and other factors). While such expenses are generally covered by Medicare and most commercial insurers, patients should check preoperatively with their own insurer when considering a prosthesis. Specific exclusions and/or requirements on the part of insurers for penile prosthetic surgery are not uncommon. Geographic differences in coverage are also common.

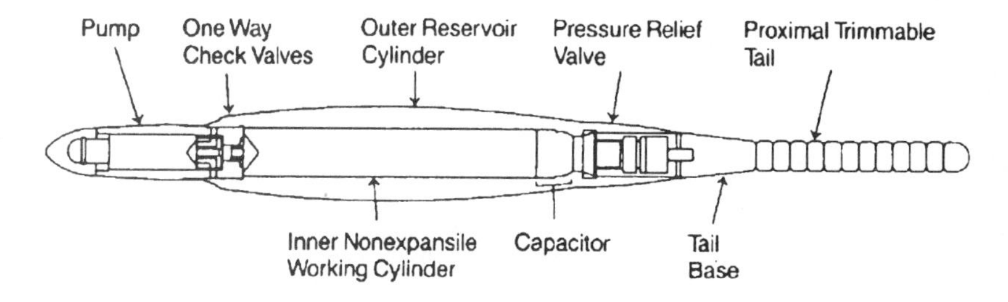

Figure 12-7 A one-part "self-contained" inflatable prosthesis, the FlexiFlate II (Surgitek).

Vascular Surgery for Impotence

Two types of vascular surgery are currently being performed to correct impotence: (1) arterial reconstruction using the inferior epigastric artery to bring new blood flow into the penis[47] and (2) penile vein ligation to correct "venous leaks" which may inhibit erection by allowing too much blood to escape from the penis during sexual excitation. Very few men in the geriatric age group are realistic candidates for such vascular surgery. While rearterialization has an 80 percent short-term success rate in young men with isolated occlusive lesions secondary to trauma, results are extremely poor (less than 25 percent short-term success)[47] when diffuse atherosclerosis is present. Such disease is, of course, ubiquitous in the elderly population. Penile venous surgery is still in its developmental stages, and surgical and diagnostic techniques are evolving. Currently, reported short-term improvement rates range from 50 to 80 percent and long-term rates are certainly far less.[48] Most agree that the procedure works best in individuals without associated atherosclerotic occlusive disease. Although neither arterial nor venous penile corrective surgery "closes the door" on subsequent treatment with prostheses or more conservative measures, most elderly men are probably best advised to limit themselves to more *time-tested* options at this time.

REFERENCES

1. Kinsey AC, Pomeroy W, Martin C: Age and sexual outlet, in Kinsey AC, Pomeroy W, Martin C (eds): *Sexual Behavior in the Adult Male*. Philadelphia, W. B. Saunders, 1948, p 218.
2. McCulloch DK, Campbell IW, Wu FC, et al: The prevalence of diabetic impotence. *Diabetologia* 18:279, 1980.
3. Lue TF, Tanagho EA: Hemodynamics of erection and functional anatomy and mechanism of penile erection, in Tanagho E. Lue TF, McClure RD (eds): *Contemporary Management of Impotence and Infertility*. Baltimore, Williams & Wilkins, 1988, pp 28–55.
4. Krane RJ, Goldstein I, Saenz de Tejada I: Impotence. *N Engl J Med* 321:1648, 1989.
5. McClure RD: Endocrine evaluation and therapy of erectile dysfunction. *Urol Clin North Am* 15:53, 1988.
6. Torrens MJ: Neurologic and neurosurgical disorders associated with impotence, in Krane RJ, Siroky MB, Goldstein I (eds): *Male Sexual Dysfunction*. Boston, Little Brown, 1983, p 55.
7. Moss HB, Procci WR: Sexual dysfunction associated with oral antihypertensive medication. *Gen Hosp Psychiatry* 4:121, 1982.
8. Rajfer J, Rosciszewskik A, Mehringer M: Prevalence of corporal venous leakage in impotent men. *J Urol* 140:69, 1988.
9. Metz P, Ebbehaj J, Uhrenholdt A, et al: Peyronie's disease and erectile failure. *J Urol* 130:1103, 1983.
10. Ellis WJ, Grayhack JT: Sexual function in aging males after orchiectomy and estrogen therapy. *J Urol* 89:895, 1963.
11. Melman A: Iatrogenic causes of erectile dysfunction. *Urol Clin North Am* 15:33, 1988.
12. Brendler CB, Steinberg GD, Marshall FF, et al: Local recurrent and survival following nerve-sparing radical cystoprostatectomy. *J Urol* 144:1137, 1990.
13. Dhabuwala CB, Hamid S, Katsikas DM, Pierce JM: Impotence following delayed repair of prostatomembranous urethral disruption. *J Urol* 144:677, 1990.

14. Hogan MJ, Wallin JD, Baer RM: Antihypertensive therapy and male sexual dysfunction. *Psychomatics* 21:234, 1980.
15. Abramowicz M (ed): Drugs that cause sexual dysfunction. *Med Lett* 29:65, 1987.
16. Buffam J: Pharmacosexology update: prescription drugs and sexual function. *J Psychoact Drugs* 18:97, 1986.
17. Wein AJ, Van Arsdalen KN: Drug-induced male sexual dysfunction. *Urol Clin North Am* 15:23, 1988.
18. Van Arsdalen KN, Wein AJ: Drug-induced sexual dysfunction in older men. *Geriatrics* 39:63, 1984.
19. Moss HB, Procci WR: Sexual dysfunction associated with oral antihypertensive medication: a critical survey of the literature. *Gen Hosp Psychiatry* 4:121, 1982.
20. Croog SH, Levine S, Sudilovsky A, et al: Sexual symptoms in hypertensive patients: a clinical trial of antihypertensive medications. *Arch Intern Med* 148:788, 1988.
21. King BD, Pitchon R, Stern EH, et al: Impotence during therapy with verapamil. *Arch Intern Med* 143:1248, 1983.
22. Benson GS: The clinical evaluation of the patient presenting with erectile dysfunction: What is reasonable? *Semin Urol* 8:94, 1990.
23. Barry JM, Blank B, Boileau M: Nocturnal penile tumescence monitoring with stamps. *Urology* 15:171, 1980.
24. Lue T: Functional evaluation of penile arteries with papaverine, in Tanagho E, Lue TF, McClure RD (eds): *Contemporary Management of Impotence and Infertility.* Baltimore, Williams & Wilkins, 1988, pp 57-64.
25. Virag R: Intracavernous injection of papaverine for erectile failure. *Lancet* 2:938, 1982 (Letter to Editor).
26. Brindley GS: Cavernosal alpha-blockade: a new technique for investigating and treating erectile impotence. *Br J Psychiatry* 143:332, 1983.
27. Abber JC, Lue TF, Orvis BR, et al: Diagnostic tests for impotence: a comparison of papaverine injection with the penile-brachial index and nocturnal tumescence monitoring. *J Urol* 135:923, 1986.
28. Smith AD: Psychologic factors in the multi-disciplinary evaluation and treatment of erectile dysfunction. *Urol Clin North Am* 15:41, 1988.
29. Morales A, Condia M, Owen JA, et al: Is yohimbine effective in the treatment of organic impotence? Results of a controlled trial. *J Urol* 137:1168, 1987.
30. Reid K, Morales A, Harris C, et al: Double blind trial of yohimbine in treatment of psychogenic impotence. *Lancet* 2:421, 1987.
31. Lal S, Rios O, Thavundayil J: Treatment of impotence with trazodone: a case report. *J Urol* 143:819, 1990.
32. Owen JA, Saunders F, Harris C, et al: Topical nitroglycerin: a potential treatment for impotence. *J Urol* 143:546, 1989.
33. Baum N: Treatment of impotence: nonsurgical methods. *Postgrad Med* 81:133, 1987.
34. Imagawa A, Kawanishi Y, Numata A: Is erythropoietin effective for impotence in dialysis patients? *Nephron* 54:95, 1990.
35. Roy JB, Petrone RL, Said SI: A clinical trial of intracavernous vasoactive intestinal peptide to induce penile erection. *J Urol* 143:302, 1990.
36. Franzese A, Lazzari R, Fraioli F, et al: Endorphins in male impotence: evidence for naltrexone stimulation of erectile activity in patient therapy. *Psychoneuroendocrinology* 14:103, 1989.
37. Yager J: Bethanechol chloride can reverse erectile and ejaculatory dysfunction induced by tricyclic antidepressants and mazindol: case report. *J Clin Psychiatry* 47:210, 1986.
38. Nelson RP: Non-operative management of impotence. *J Urol* 139:2, 1988.
39. Bennet AH, Carpenter AJ: An improved vasoactive drug combination for a pharmacological erection program. *J Urol* 143:317A, 1990 (abstract).
40. Lue TF, Hellstrom WJG, McAninch JW, et al: Priapism, a refined approach to diagnosis and treatment. *J Urol* 136:104, 1986.

41. Duffy LM, Sidi AA, Lange PH: Vasoactive intracavernous pharmacotherapy—the nursing role in teaching self injection therapy. *J Urol* 138:1198, 1987.
42. Lakin MM, Monague DK, Medendorp SV, et al: Intracavernous injection therapy: analysis of results and complications. *J Urol* 143:1138, 1990.
43. Witherington R: Mechanical aids for treatment of impotence. *Clin Diabet* 7:1, 1989.
44. Leslie SW: *Impotence: Current Diagnosis and Treatment: Patient Education Guide.* Augusta, Georgia, Charter, 1989.
45. Sidi AA, Becher EF, Zhang G, Lewis JH: Patient acceptance of and satisfaction with an external negative pressure device for impotence. *J Urol* 144:1154, 1990.
46. Stanisic TH, Dean JC: The Flexi-Flate and Flexi-Flate II penile prostheses. *Urol Clin North Am* 16:39, 1989.
47. Goldstein I: Penile revascularization. *Urol Clin North Am* 14:805, 1987.
48. Lewis RW: Diagnosis and management of corporal venoocclusive dysfunction. *Semin Urol* 8:113, 1990.

CHAPTER

13

EPILEPSY

Edward P. Armstrong

Epilepsy is a common disease in the elderly and has unique characteristics from epilepsy in a younger population.[1] A seizure is defined as a temporary and reversible behavioral alteration resulting from excessive electrical activity of the brain. Recurrent seizures are termed *epilepsy*. The physical signs of the seizure depend upon the site of electrical stimulus origin and the path of electrical discharge within the brain.

The incidence of patients who develop chronic seizures is difficult to define. Some seizures may occur from isolated events, such as alcohol withdrawal, and others may occur from acute diseases, such as hyponatremia or meningitis, or other complications including theophylline toxicity or uremia. Seizures from these isolated events do not represent epilepsy.

Overall, approximately 2 percent of the general population is estimated to have a chronic seizure disorder, and approximately 10 percent of the general population will have at least one seizure in their lifetime. These estimates may be low, since all patients may not contact a health care facility after their seizure. It is difficult to determine the prevalence of seizures in the elderly, since there are limited age-specific studies and because of the varied ages of patients examined. The largest epidemiologic study on epilepsy which collected data between 1935 and 1968 noted that the incidence of seizures was highest in the population less than 1 year of age, gradually decreased in each successive decade of life, and then increased dramatically again after 60 years of age.[2] Their data specifically noted that there was a significant rise in focal seizures in patients older than 60 years of age. Similar results were reported in another study which identified an annual incidence of seizures of 77 per 100,000 population per year in patients 60 years of age or older.[3]

SEIZURE CLASSIFICATION

Seizures are classified as *generalized* when there is abnormal electrical involvement throughout the entire brain. They are classified as *partial* when abnormal electrical impulses are limited to one segment of the brain. However, a partial seizure may spread throughout the brain to become *secondarily generalized.* The classification of epileptic seizures is based on the International Classification of Epileptic Seizures and is summarized in Table 13-1.[4] A primary characteristic of this classification is that it stresses the clinical seizure type and the electroencephalographic pattern of the seizure rather than the etiology of the seizure. A major category in the seizure classification is that some seizures, such as partial or focal, begin in one portion of the brain and either remain localized or generalize throughout the brain. The location of the seizure focus determines the clinical presentation of the seizure.[6] In contrast, another seizure category is those seizures that appear to be general from their earliest symptom by involving both cerebral hemispheres in their clinical and electroencephalographic changes.

ETIOLOGY OF EPILEPSY

A majority of seizures in the elderly are partial in onset and have secondary generalization of the seizure activity. In addition, approximately 30 to 40 percent of seizures in the elderly are simple partial seizures.[7]

The rise in the incidence of seizures in patients over age 60 appears to be

Table 13-1 Classification of epileptic seizures

I. Partial, or focal, seizures (seizures begin in one brain segment)
- A. Simple partial seizures (without impairment of consciousness, but with motor, sensory, autonomic, or psychic signs)
- B. Complex partial seizures (with impairment of consciousness; also called *psychomotor*, or *temporal lobe*, seizures)
- C. Secondary generalized partial seizures (partial onset progressing to generalized tonic-clonic seizures)

II. Primary generalized seizures (bilaterally symmetrical and without local onset)
- A. Tonic-clonic (grand mal)
- B. Tonic
- C. Absence (petit mal)
- D. Atypical absence
- E. Myoclonic
- F. Atonic
- G. Clonic

III. Unclassified seizures (e.g., neonatal)

Source: Adapted from Ref. 5.

attributed to their increased vulnerability to disorders that produce seizures. The elderly's reduced homeostatic mechanisms and increased risk of brain tumors, cerebrovascular accidents, and infections make them more likely to develop seizures. In addition, the elderly are exposed to a larger number of medications and often have altered medication pharmacokinetics. Many drugs have altered absorption, distribution, metabolism, and excretion in the elderly, which may contribute to additional adverse drug reactions. In addition, if an elderly patient has any additional diseases which contribute to cerebral hypoxia or ischemia, this may increase the chances of seizures from other conditions.

Cerebrovascular disease is a major contributor to seizures in the elderly. Cerebral infarction, from either thrombosis or embolus, intracranial bleeding, or vasculitis may result in 30 percent of all seizures in the elderly.[8] Brain tumors, either primary or metastatic, are a much more frequent cause of seizures in the elderly than in the younger population. These seizures are usually focal in nature. The tumors most commonly associated with seizures are glioblastomas and meningiomas; however, tumors from metastatic lesions in the lung, breast, and gastrointestinal tract can also produce seizures.

Systemic disorders linked to seizures include metabolic abnormalities such as hyponatremia, uremia, nonketotic hyperosmolar coma, hypoglycemia, hepatic failure, hypocalcemia, hypoxic encephalopathy, and central nervous system (CNS) infections. Seizures from CNS infections usually occur during the acute stage of the disease. These disorders may cause either focal or generalized seizures.[9] In addition, a number of medications are known to produce seizures. Some examples are theophylline, lidocaine, penicillin, and withdrawal from barbiturates and alcohol. Table 13-2 summarizes medications associated with generalized seizures at a large tertiary care institution, excluding withdrawal from alcohol or sedative drugs.[10]

A large study of 342 patients whose seizure activity started after 60 years of age noted that cerebrovascular disease was the most common cause (39 percent),

Table 13-2 Medications associated with generalized seizures

Isoniazid
Psychotropic agents
Bronchodilators
Insulin
Stimulants
Lidocaine
Narcotic analgesics
Anticholinergics
Cefazolin
Loxapine/benztropine
Thioridazine/pentazocine

Source: Adapted from Ref. 10.

followed by head injury (21 percent), brain tumors (11 percent), metabolic disorders (7 percent), multifactorial etiology (6 percent), CNS infection (4 percent), and undetermined (11 percent).[11] In the 132 patients whose seizures were due to cerebrovascular disease, 43 percent had cerebral infarctions, 19 percent had cerebral hemorrhage, 17 percent had subarachnoid hemorrhage, and 20 percent had recurrent stroke. The majority of patients with recurrent stroke had cerebral infarcts. Simple partial seizures, with or without secondary generalization, were the most common type and accounted for 71 percent of all seizures; simple partial seizures alone accounted for 35 percent, and partial seizures with secondary generalization accounted for 36 percent. In addition, simple partial seizures were also the most common seizure type with metabolic disorder etiologies, although approximately half of the patients had secondary generalization. In comparison, complex partial seizures and generalized tonic-clonic seizures without focal onset were uncommon in the elderly patients. The onset of seizures was within 1 month of insult in 95 percent of subarachnoid hemorrhage patients, 86 percent of head injury patients, 80 percent of CNS infection patients, and 76 percent of intracerebral hemorrhage patients. In cerebral infarction, seizures occurred either in the acute stage (32 percent) or within 6 months to 3 years after the stroke (44 percent).

TREATMENT OF EPILEPSY

Treatment of a patient with epilepsy is primarily focused on eliminating the cause of the seizures, suppressing the manifestations of the seizures, and minimizing the psychosocial consequences which may occur. If the seizure is a result of a metabolic abnormality such as uremia or hypoglycemia, correction of metabolic function usually results in elimination of seizure activity. If a structural abnormality such as a brain tumor is the etiology for the seizures, removal of the tumor may abolish the seizure activity.

The primary therapy in the management of epilepsy is the use of pharmacologic therapy. The proper treatment of epilepsy is primarily based on the classification of the seizure type and the administration of the most effective antiepileptic drug. Monotherapy is preferred and is effective in the majority of epilepsy patients. Since some agents may cause significant adverse effects, such as sedation, the proper selection of an antiepileptic agent must address the avoidance of adverse drug effects as equally important as suppression of the seizure activity.[12] These factors emphasize that antiepileptic drug regimens must be individualized for each patient. In addition, effective antiepileptic therapy is based upon the pharmacokinetic and pharmacodynamic characteristics of the drug, optimal titration of dosage, potential adverse drug reactions experienced by the patient, patient compliance with the medication regimen, and chronic therapy monitoring.

The primary treatment goals are to minimize the frequency of seizures and to allow the patient to maintain an otherwise normal lifestyle. It is optimal for the seizure activity to be eliminated; however, in some cases, this must be balanced by some of the adverse drug reactions experienced by the patient. For example, if oversedation is severe, some seizure control may have to be reduced in order to improve cognitive function.

If the patient experiences seizures from correctable causes, for example hyponatremia, the antiepileptic drugs may be used acutely, but they are not needed for chronic administration if the seizure cause is correctly identified and remedied. The classification of epileptic seizures (Table 13-1) has proven very useful in the selection of the most effective antiepileptic drugs. For example, generalized tonic-clonic seizures do not respond well to ethosuximide, which is frequently a drug of choice in absence seizures.

As previously discussed, partial seizures are the most common seizure disorder in the elderly population. Carbamazepine is currently regarded as the agent of first choice in the management of partial seizures. Useful alternatives include phenytoin, phenobarbital, and valproic acid. The management of tonic-clonic seizures is undergoing reevaluation. Historically, the drugs of choice have been phenytoin and phenobarbital; however, since carbamazepine and valproic acid have been shown to have equal efficacy and a lower incidence of adverse effects, many clinicians are now recommending these drugs as agents of first choice.[13] Table 13-3 summarizes the drugs of choice and alternative agents in the treatment of different seizure types.

The first agent chosen should be adjusted until either the maximum reduction in seizure activity has occurred or intolerable adverse effects are seen. It is important to stress to patients regarding the need for proper compliance with the antiepileptic regimen in order to evaluate its effectiveness. If the initially selected agent has been administered in appropriate doses and proven to be ineffective in controlling the seizure activity, an alternative monotherapy antiepileptic agent should be selected.[14] If a patient will fail a specific therapy from either lack of seizure control or the development of adverse effect, the failure usually occurs within the first 6 months of therapy.[15] If an alternative agent is needed, the second agent should be adjusted to the proper dose before the initial antiepileptic agent is tapered off. If this therapy proves unsuccessful, a combination of antiepileptic agents may be effective in achieving seizure control.

Some evidence is available which indicates that there may be different thera-

Table 13-3 Anticonvulsant therapy for seizure type

	Simple partial	Complex partial	Generalized tonic-clonic
Primary agents	Carbamazepine	Carbamazepine	Carbamazepine
	Phenytoin	Phenytoin	Phenytoin
	Phenobarbital	Phenobarbital	Valproic acid
Alternative agents	Valproic acid	Valproic acid	Phenobarbital
	Primidone	Primidone	Primidone

peutic ranges for the antiepileptic drugs, depending upon the seizure classification. Simple or complex partial seizures may require higher concentrations of phenytoin, phenobarbital, or carbamazepine than those needed in patients with tonic-clonic seizures.[16]

Adjustment of the antiepileptic dose to achieve optimum therapeutic benefit and minimization of adverse drug effects is important. Many antiepileptic drugs are known to produce CNS depression during the first several days of therapy. Other common complaints with the initiation of therapy include tiredness, drowsiness, and lack of energy. Often these effects are seen for the first week or two of therapy and then diminish in significance. Since tolerance to these effects often develops, the agents are often initiated in low doses, unless there is an urgent condition, and the dose is gradually raised until seizure control is reached or the patient develops significant adverse effects. Elderly patients, particularly, are often started on one-fourth to one-third of the estimated final dose with the dose gradually raised over several weeks in order to lower the incidence of adverse effects.

A major advance in the utilization of antiepileptic drugs is the application of therapeutic drug monitoring. Since there are large differences in milligram-per-kilogram doses and pharmacokinetic characteristics for given antiepileptic drugs between patients, blood level monitoring of these agents considerably improves the likelihood of identifying the proper dose for these drugs. The desired plasma concentration is a range that is correlated with minimizing seizure activity and reducing risk of toxicity. However, these are guidelines and not absolute values; some patients may achieve control of their seizures below the general minimum therapeutic level, and some patients may experience toxic effects at concentrations below the upper limit of the therapeutic range.[17] On the other hand, some patients may require concentrations above the therapeutic range to achieve acceptable seizure control and not suffer significant adverse drug reactions. Despite these limitations, therapeutic drug monitoring has proven extremely useful in managing the antiepileptic drug regimens of most patients with epilepsy.

The determination of "free" concentrations of antiepileptic agents has been shown in research settings to be helpful for monitoring some antiepileptic drug therapy. Many antiepileptic drugs are highly bound to plasma proteins, such as albumin. The unbound, or free, drug concentration is the amount of drug which is able to penetrate the blood-brain barrier and produce therapeutic effects. Newer assay techniques may enable this technology to be useful on a clinical basis to monitor patients. Due to its expense and lack of correlation with improved outcomes, free level monitoring is not indicated for routine use in all patients on antiepileptic drugs.[18] However, monitoring free concentrations may be particularly useful in patients who are not responding or who are having side effects at "therapeutic" concentrations of total drug. In addition, in patient populations who are known to have altered plasma protein binding, such as hypoalbuminemia, renal failure, or concurrent therapy with some interacting drugs, free concentration monitoring may be especially useful rather than relying on total drug concentration alone.

Carbamazepine

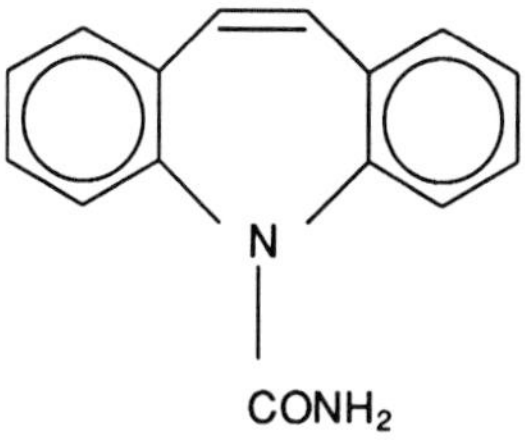

Carbamazepine

Carbamazepine's relative lack of adverse effects as compared with phenytoin and phenobarbital has contributed to its increased use in a variety of seizure disorders. Carbamazepine is considered the antiepileptic of first choice in the treatment of partial seizures.[19] It is also very effective for generalized seizures other than absence.

Carbamazepine acts on sodium channels in the brain to produce an inhibition of high-frequency discharges in and around epileptic foci with minimal disruption of normal neuronal impulses. In addition to its seizure inhibition properties, carbamazepine is also known to have efficacy in trigeminal neuralgia and bipolar disorders.

Carbamazepine's absorption is delayed and inconsistent because it has low water solubility. Table 13-4 summarizes the pharmacokinetic characteristics of the anticonvulsants. Overall, the absorption of carbamazepine exceeds 75 percent, although its variable absorption leads to considerable fluctuation in time to reach peak concentration. Following oral administration, the peak concentration is usually reached in 2 to 8 h; however, this may be delayed until 24 h, particularly following the administration of larger doses. Food may raise its bioavailability.

Table 13-4 Pharmacokinetic characteristics of the anticonvulsants

Drug	Bioavailability, %	Volume of distribution, L/kg	Elimination half-life, h	Elimination type	Therapeutic range, μg/mL
Carbamazepine	>75	0.8–1.4	15–26 with chronic monotherapy	Linear	6–12
Phenytoin	>90	0.75	24, varies	Linear→ nonlinear	10–20
Phenobarbital	>90	0.7	96	Linear	15–40
Valproic acid	>95	0.15–0.4	15 with monotherapy	Linear	50–100
Primidone	>90	0.6	5–19	Linear	5–12

Carbamazepine distributes well into tissues and is approximately 74 percent bound to plasma proteins, and its free drug concentration in the plasma is similar to the drug concentration within the cerebrospinal fluid (CSF). Carbamazepine is eliminated from the body primarily by metabolism; 2 percent of the parent drug is recovered in the urine.[20] The primary path of metabolism is conversion to the 10,11-epoxide, which is an active metabolite. This metabolite is then further broken down to other inactive compounds.

Carbamazepine is unique in that it induces its own metabolism. Carbamazepine's half-life is much longer in a patient who has only received a single dose than during chronic therapy. The enzyme induction begins to occur within the first few days of therapy and is usually complete at the end of 1 month. Because of this induction of metabolism, it is possible to start a patient on carbamazepine, achieve therapeutic blood levels, and then observe the carbamazepine blood levels to become subtherapeutic despite proper compliance with their drug regimen. During chronic administration, carbamazepine's plasma half-life is usually between 15 and 26 h. In a patient receiving concurrent phenytoin or phenobarbital, which may further enhance the liver's metabolic rate, carbamazepine's half-life will decrease to approximately 9 to 10 h.

The most common adverse effects with chronic administration of carbamazepine are dizziness, drowsiness, vertigo, fatigue, unsteadiness, ataxia, diplopia, nystagmus, and blurred vision. These adverse effects occur in one-third to one-half of patients. As expected, they are more frequent when therapy is initiated and may become less significant with chronic therapy. Some of these side effects may be minimized by giving a larger dose at bedtime. Other adverse effects which may be seen are nausea, vomiting, significant hematologic side effects such as aplastic anemia and agranulocytosis, and allergic reactions including dermatitis, eosinophilia, and lymphadenopathy. Carbamazepine is also known to sometimes produce a retention of free water with resultant decrease in serum osmolality and sodium concentration. This adverse effect, similar to the syndrome of inappropriate antidiuretic hormone secretion, may be more common in elderly patients. Of the adverse effects known to occur, aplastic anemia is probably most feared by clinicians. However, this appears to occur infrequently; the prevalence rate of aplastic anemia appears to be about 1 in 200,000 patients who are treated with the drug.[21] Leukopenia is the most frequent hematologic side effect; however, in most patients this is transient despite continued administration. The mild and transient depression of the leukocyte count should not be confused with significant bone marrow depression.[22] A primary reason many clinicians select carbamazepine is that it appears to have minimal effects on cognitive functioning.[23]

Since medications that alter the liver's metabolic rate will change the pharmacokinetics of carbamazepine, there are several important drug interactions. Table 13-5 summarizes important drug interactions with the anticonvulsants. Concurrent medications such as phenytoin, phenobarbital, or primidone, which can increase drug metabolism, may produce clinically significant decreases in carbamazepine plasma concentrations if its dosage is not properly adjusted. Similarly, other

Table 13-5 Important drug interactions with the anticonvulsants

Anticonvulsant	Interacting drug(s)	Effect
Carbamazepine	Phenytoin Phenobarbital Primidone	Induce carbamazepine metabolism and lower its plasma concentration
	Cimetidine Erythromycin Propoxyphene Isoniazid	Decrease carbamazepine metabolism and raise its plasma concentration
	Theophylline Valproic acid Warfarin	Carbamazepine will increase the metabolism of these drugs and lower their plasma concentration
Phenytoin	Cimetidine Valproic acid Isoniazid	Decrease phenytoin metabolism and produce a rise in plasma concentration
	Carbamazepine	Increases phenytoin metabolism and lowers its plasma concentration
	Phenobarbital	Effect unpredictable
	Enteral feedings Calcium	Reduce gastrointestinal absorption of phenytoin
	Vitamin D Folic acid	Decrease concentration of vitamin D and folic acid
Phenobarbital	Valproic acid Cimetidine Phenytoin	Reduce phenobarbital metabolism and increase its plasma concentration
	Warfarin Quinidine Others	Increase metabolism of other drugs, producing a decrease in their effect
Valproic acid	Phenobarbital Phenytoin Carbamazepine Primidone	Increase elimination of valproic acid, reducing its plasma concentration
	Aspirin	Increases free concentration of valproic acid
Primidone	Phenytoin Carbamazepine	Enzyme induction to increase plasma concentration of phenobarbital
	Phenobarbital metabolite	Interactions as above with parent drug

medications which are known to decrease the enzyme activity are known to decrease the elimination of carbamazepine and potentially lead to toxicity. Agents in this class include cimetidine, erythromycin, propoxyphene, and isoniazid.[24] Since a number of the drugs which can alter carbamazepine are other anticonvulsants, it is especially important to monitor their effects on carbamazepine when single therapy is not effective. In addition to the drugs that can affect carbamazepine, carbamazepine's enhancement of metabolism can increase the clearance of theophylline, valproic acid, and warfarin.

When carbamazepine therapy is initiated, it is usually started at 25 to 33 percent of the anticipated final total dose. For most adults, 200 mg orally twice daily is selected as initial therapy. Larger doses are generally not used since the CNS and gastrointestinal adverse effects are more prominent. The dose is then gradually increased at 2- to 3-week intervals to achieve adequate therapeutic concentrations and to adjust for autoinduction of its own metabolism. The most common dosage range for the ultimate chronic dose for adults is 7 to 15 mg/kg/day. Since carbamazepine induces its own metabolism, the drug must usually be given at least twice daily.

The therapeutic range of carbamazepine is generally defined as 6 to 12 μg/mL. Some patients require a concentration of 8 μg/mL to attain therapeutic effects. Concentrations exceeding 11 to 12 μg/mL are more likely to produce significant CNS adverse effects. In providing therapeutic drug monitoring of carbamazepine, it must be kept in mind that autoinduction of its metabolism occurs and that this will impact the length of time required to reach steady-state concentrations within the blood following dosage adjustments. Typically, trough blood samples are obtained and the dosing regimen is adjusted using first-order kinetics to achieve a trough level above 4μg/mL if seizures are inadequately controlled.

Phenytoin

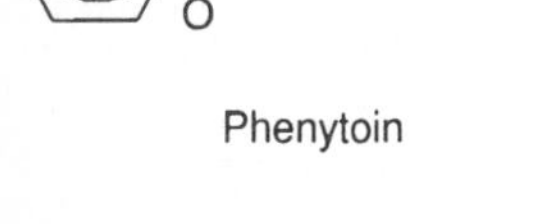

Phenytoin

Phenytoin is a primary drug for all seizure types except absence seizures. Phenytoin is effective in limiting the development of maximal seizure activity and minimizing the spread of seizure activity from an active focus. It has minimal action to raise the threshold for seizures. These actions are probably due to phenytoin's inhibition of sodium channels and action on calcium channels.

Phenytoin has markedly unique pharmacokinetic properties since it has limited water solubility and dose-dependent elimination. Oral absorption of phenytoin is slow and its bioavailability exceeds 90 percent. Limited data indicate there may also be a decreased or delayed absorption of phenytoin in the elderly.[25] Significant differences in bioavailability of oral phenytoin by different manufacturers have been detected. It is therefore recommended that patients be chronically maintained on one specific manufacturer's product and very carefully monitored if the brand is changed. The time to peak for an oral dose is between 3 and 12 h.[26] The absorption time for oral phenytoin is especially dependent on particle size of the product, and this causes some brands to be absorbed faster than others. Products designed for single daily dosing are described as extended-release preparations. In addition, the amount of phenytoin available for absorption varies depending on the product selected. Sodium phenytoin capsules contain 92% phenytoin (e.g., 30- and 100-mg capsules and the 50-mg/mL product for injection). Products which contain phenytoin acid contain 100% phenytoin (e.g., 50-mg chewable tablets and suspension). Formulations which contain phenytoin acid will produce a higher plasma concentration than phenytoin sodium products because of the 8 percent increase in phenytoin content.[27]

Following absorption, phenytoin is distributed throughout the body tissues. Phenytoin is also extensively (95 percent) bound to plasma proteins, primarily albumin. However, it is extremely important to note that the amount of unbound, or free, phenytoin is increased in patients with hypoalbuminemia or uremia. These patients may, therefore, become toxic on phenytoin at "therapeutic" phenytoin total drug concentrations. The phenytoin concentration in the CSF is equal to the unbound amount in the plasma.

Phenytoin is extensively metabolized to inactive metabolites, with only a small portion excreted unchanged in the urine. The rate of phenytoin metabolism (V_{max}) has been shown to be significantly lower in patients older than 60 years of age compared to patients 20 to 39 years of age.[28] A unique feature of phenytoin is that at concentrations below approximately 10 μg/mL, the elimination of phenytoin is first order, or exponential. However, when the phenytoin concentration exceeds this concentration, the elimination becomes dose-dependent and the plasma half-life increases with higher concentrations of phenytoin. This appears to be due to saturable metabolism, and no additional drug can be eliminated once this concentration is reached. This can lead to large increases in plasma concentration with small increases in phenytoin dose.[29] This unique characteristic describes why it is very difficult to predict the resultant plasma concentration following dosage adjustment of phenytoin. Similarly, serum concentrations do not decline by a constant percentage after the drug has been discontinued. The time required for 50 percent of the dose to be eliminated typically averages approximately 24 h, but there is a very large range. Since higher plasma concentrations lead to a longer time for the drug to be eliminated, higher plasma concentrations also lead to a longer time to reach steady-state plasma concentrations.

The most frequent adverse effects with the initiation of phenytoin include

CNS-depressant effects including drowsiness, incoordination, blurred vision, and lethargy and gastrointestinal effects such as nausea, vomiting, anorexia, and epigastric pain. When serum concentrations exceed 20 μg/mL, nystagmus, ataxia, and impaired coordination become more frequent. Coma may occur at concentrations exceeding 40 μg/mL. Gingival hyperplasia is also well known to occur with chronic therapy. The gum changes appear to be due to altered collagen metabolism and can be minimized by good oral hygiene including gum massage. This adverse effect is reversible when the drug is discontinued. Phenytoin is also known to possibly impair cognitive abilities related to memory and mental and motor speed.[30] Intestinal malabsorption of vitamins and minerals and enhanced metabolism of vitamin D and folic acid may also occur. This may lead to hypocalcemia and osteomalacia in some patients on chronic therapy. Megaloblastic anemia is uncommon, but macrocytosis may be seen in many phenytoin patients. Hypersensitivity reactions, serious skin reactions, including Stevens-Johnson syndrome, and hematologic reactions such as leukopenia, neutropenia, agranulocytosis, aplastic anemia, and thrombocytopenia have also been reported. Lymphadenopathy resembling lymphoma, hepatotoxicity, and fever are other known adverse effects of phenytoin.

Some adverse effects may be related to the route of administration. When phenytoin is administered intravenously, the maximum rate should be 25 to 50 mg/min. Elderly patients should generally receive the lower rate of administration. Hypotension, arrhythmias, and other cardiovascular complications are known to occur with rapid intravenous administration from the propylene glycol diluent in the intravenous product.[31] In addition, caution should be exercised due to the risk of extravasation. Small hand veins should be avoided, particularly in elderly patients.

There are many important drug interactions with phenytoin. Since phenytoin is highly bound to plasma proteins, it may be displaced by other agents and increase the percentage of phenytoin that is free, or unbound. However, the rise in free concentration allows the clearance rate to increase and the total phenytoin concentration to decrease, and this allows the new steady-state free concentration to approximately equal the previous free concentration but at a lower total concentration. Although the widespread use of free phenytoin plasma concentration monitoring is criticized, it may be useful when evaluating the clinical effects in a patient when another medication known to compete for binding sites is added to or subtracted from the regimen. In addition, agents such as cimetidine, valproic acid, and isoniazid can decrease the clearance of phenytoin and produce a rise in the plasma concentration. Carbamazepine, through its enzyme induction ability, can lead to an increased clearance of phenytoin and a subsequent decrease in plasma concentrations. Phenobarbital may also alter phenytoin's clearance, but its effects are less predictable. The gastrointestinal absorption of phenytoin is known to be reduced by concomitant enteral feedings and calcium.

The dosing of phenytoin has several unique characteristics. For most patients there is a good correlation between the total concentration of phenytoin in the plasma and its resultant clinical effect. The therapeutic range is defined as 10 to 20 μg/mL. Most patients have control of seizures with plasma concentrations above 10 μg/mL, and toxic effects such as nystagmus often occur at approximately 20 μg/mL. Ataxia typically occurs at 30 μg/mL, and lethargy may be seen as levels reach 40 μg/mL. However, these numbers serve as guidelines; some patients may not achieve seizure control with 11 μg/mL but may achieve control with 17 μg/mL. For most patients, the free fraction of phenytoin is 10% of the total drug concentration. Therefore, the therapeutic range for free phenytoin is 1 to 2 μg/mL.

Since phenytoin undergoes nonlinear elimination, therapeutic drug monitoring is very important. Monitoring the plasma phenytoin concentration is much more accurate than monitoring the total daily dose a patient receives. Although 300 mg/day is the most common dosage in clinical practice, some patients may be subtherapeutic and others may be toxic on this dose. Monitoring of plasma levels to be sure the levels are within the therapeutic range is preferred since phenytoin doses must be individualized.

When a loading dose of phenytoin is required, phenytoin doses are based on the patient's total body weight. A loading dose may be given either orally or intravenously. When a full loading dose is needed, the intravenous dose is 15 to 20 mg/kg. The loading dose may be administered by direct intravenous injection or via intravenous infusion diluted in a volume of 50 to 100 mL of sodium chloride or lactated Ringer's just prior to use.[32] Intravenous phenytoin should not be added to dextrose solutions since it may precipitate. Some clinicians recommend starting the infusion immediately after mixing and using an in-line filter. As previously stated, the administration rate should not exceed 25 to 50 mg/min.

If the patient is alert and can swallow, the phenytoin loading dose could alternatively be administered orally. A 20-mg/kg loading dose may be administered in three to four divided doses at 1- to 2-h intervals. The total oral loading dose is not given in one dose in order to minimize the risk of significant gastrointestinal adverse effects.

In nonurgent situations, phenytoin can generally be started at a dose of 200 to 300 mg/day (3 to 6 mg/kg) and the dose can be titrated as needed. Due to the unique saturable metabolism of phenytoin, predictions of steady-state serum concentrations on specific dosing regimens are extremely difficult. Nomograms and sophisticated computer software systems have been developed to try and improve the selection of proper phenytoin doses. As previously stated, small increases in dose may result in disproportionately large increases in phenytoin plasma concentrations. Because of this characteristic, chronic daily dose changes are usually modified in increments of only 30 to 100 mg. For therapeutic drug monitoring, plasma concentrations are often obtained approximately 7 days after each dosage adjustment; however, full steady-state levels in some patients often require 10 to 14 days or longer. As the daily dose is raised, the time to reach steady state is prolonged because of the dose-dependent metabolism.

Many patients are acceptable candidates to receive phenytoin (extended-release phenytoin sodium) as a single daily dose, given at bedtime. Developing a drug regimen which is simple to follow is important in the chronic management of epilepsy. Patients who have had difficulty achieving seizure control on a divided-dose regimen may be poor candidates for single daily dose administration.

If a patient on phenytoin has inadequate seizure control, therapeutic drug monitoring may separate failure to respond to adequate phenytoin plasma concentrations from a problem with phenytoin absorption or noncompliance. As with other drugs, the therapeutic phenytoin plasma concentration of 10 to 20 μg/mL is a guideline for monitoring. The most important monitoring parameter for antiepileptic efficacy is the clinical status of the patient regarding his or her frequency of seizure activity. It may also be useful to document the results of dosage adjustments or the subsequent effects of adding or subtracting other medications to the patient's drug regimen. Usually a trough blood sample is obtained for blood level monitoring.

Patients who have a significant impairment in renal function, jaundice, increased bilirubin, and concurrent therapy with other highly protein bound drugs may have a reduced binding of phenytoin to plasma protein. In addition, disease states such as malnutrition, burns, nephrotic syndrome, pregnancy, and hepatic cirrhosis may produce significant changes in phenytoin protein binding due to a decrease in albumin concentration. For example, renal failure results in the retention of metabolic products which may compete for plasma protein binding sites with phenytoin. This produces an increase in free phenytoin; however, since the free phenytoin available for metabolism is also increased, the total phenytoin plasma concentration will actually decrease. Although the total phenytoin concentration may be below the therapeutic range, the patient may still have a therapeutic free phenytoin concentration from the increased percentage of free phenytoin. If free phenytoin concentrations are unable to be measured, the following formula may be used to estimate a correction for the phenytoin concentration in renal failure[33]:

$$C_{corrected} = \frac{C_{observed}}{0.1 \times \text{Albumin} + 0.1}$$

In addition, alterations in the patient's serum albumin must be considered when evaluating plasma phenytoin concentrations. If a patient is hypoalbuminemic, this will also lower the total phenytoin concentration but produce a higher percentage of phenytoin in the free form. In this setting, monitoring free phenytoin may prove helpful; if unavailable, the phenytoin concentration may be corrected with the following equation:

$$C_{corrected} = \frac{C_{observed}}{0.2 \times \text{Albumin} + 0.1}$$

Phenobarbital

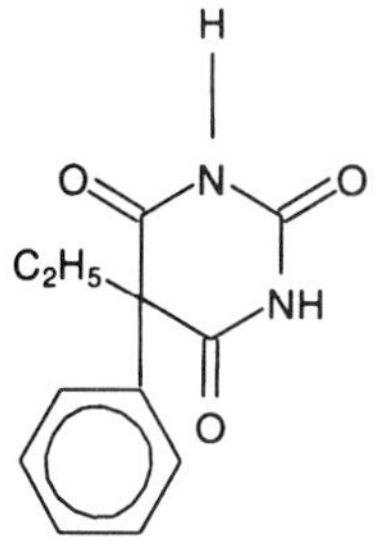

Phenobarbital

Phenobarbital has proven to be a useful antiepileptic agent through its ability to limit the spread of seizure activity and elevate the seizure threshold. It is useful in the treatment of generalized seizures, except absence, and may be an alternative agent in partial seizures.

Following oral administration, phenobarbital is extensively absorbed, and peak concentrations occur in 8 to 12 h. Phenobarbital is known to rapidly cross the blood-brain barrier and eventually distributes to all body tissues. The half-life of phenobarbital is approximately 4 days and follows first-order pharmacokinetics.[34] Approximately 25 percent of a dose is eliminated unchanged in the urine. The remaining drug is inactivated by hepatic microsomal enzymes.

Phenobarbital is well known to produce numerous adverse effects. Primarily CNS adverse effects are of greatest concern. Drowsiness, sedation, and fatigue are the primary limitations, although tolerance often develops to these effects with chronic dosing. It is also important to note that phenobarbital may produce confusion, agitation, or depression in the elderly. Impairment of cortical function is also known to occur with phenobarbital. Less commonly, rashes, megaloblastic anemia, and osteomalacia may be seen.

Since phenobarbital is known to induce hepatic microsomal enzymes, it may enhance the elimination of many drugs. Other medications may also alter the elimination of phenobarbital. Cimetidine, valproic acid, and phenytoin may all reduce the metabolism of phenobarbital, thus requiring a reduction in dose.

In nonemergent indications, phenobarbital therapy may be started orally. Often the initial starting dose is 60 to 100 mg/day in adults. Because phenobarbital has such a long half-life, it usually takes 3 to 4 weeks for a patient to reach steady-state plasma concentrations. Its prolonged elimination rate also enables patients to take their phenobarbital as a single daily dose, usually at bedtime. The dose can gradually be titrated to obtain the desired clinical effects and/or attainment of therapeutic plasma concentrations.

In emergent indications, phenobarbital can be administered intravenously. Careful monitoring of blood pressure, heart rate, and respiratory rate is important during this route of administration. In addition, preparations for endotracheal intubation and a ventilator should be available when phenobarbital is being administered intravenously. Often the dose is given slowly in increments of 60 to 120 mg until the clinical or therapeutic goals are achieved, until significant adverse effects occur, or until a maximum of 20 mg/kg total dose has been given.

Therapeutic drug monitoring may be very useful with phenobarbital. The therapeutic range is defined as 15 to 40 μg/mL. As with other anticonvulsants, this range is a guideline for clinical monitoring, not an absolute value. In addition, since phenobarbital is not extensively bound to plasma proteins, free concentration monitoring is rarely useful. Phenobarbital plasma concentrations are linear in relation to the patient's dose. However, it must be kept in mind that doses should not be changed too quickly because of the prolonged time to reach steady-state plasma concentrations. When obtaining blood samples, trough levels are usually preferred; however, there is often minor peak-trough variation since phenobarbital has a prolonged half-life.

Valproic Acid

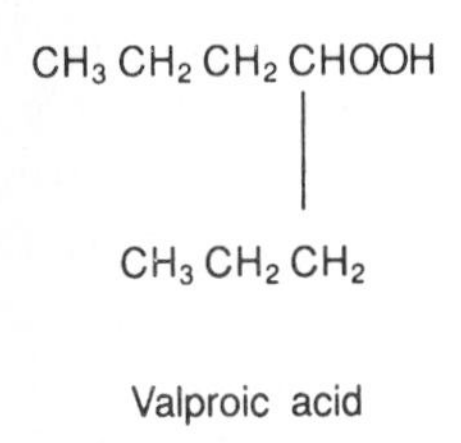

Valproic acid

The use of valproic acid is increasing because it is effective against a number of seizure disorders and usually does not cause significant CNS adverse effects.[35] Some clinicians recommend that valproic acid be the drug of first choice in the treatment of clonic-tonic-clonic or tonic-clonic seizures.[36] Its mechanism of action appears to be enhancing the accumulation of gamma-aminobutyric acid (GABA), potentiating the effects of GABA, and the action on sodium channels to stabilize neuronal membranes. Valproic acid is rapidly and completely absorbed following oral administration. Peak concentrations are often reached within 1 to 4 h. Enteric-coated products may delay the absorption by several hours. Following absorption, valproic acid is well distributed throughout the body. It is highly bound to plasma proteins (90 percent), and this binding may be saturable as the plasma concentration increases. Only a small amount of valproic acid is eliminated unchanged into the urine. Valproic acid is extensively metabolized by the liver. Numerous metabolites have been identified, some with some anticonvulsant activity. The half-life of valproic acid is approximately 15 h but may decrease to 8 to 9 h in patients concurrently receiving other enzyme-inducing anticonvulsants.[37]

The most frequent adverse effects produced by valproic acid often involve the gastrointestinal tract.[38] These include anorexia, vomiting, and nausea. Taking the dose with meals or changing to an enteric-coated product may reduce these complaints.[39] The primary CNS adverse effects with valproic acid are sedation, ataxia, and tremor. Valproic acid usually causes minimal effects on cognitive function. The adverse effect of greatest concern to clinicians is often the risk of hepatotoxicity. Elevation of hepatic enzymes or hyperammonemia is common, and it frequently occurs asymptomatically during the initial few months of therapy. The asymptomatic changes usually resolve despite continuation of valproic acid therapy. Most patients who have died from fulminant valproic acid–induced hepatitis are young (less than 2 years of age), received multiple antiepileptic agents, and had other medical conditions. There is some evidence that one metabolite of valproic acid may be responsible for the liver toxicity. Patients receiving other enzyme-inducing antiepileptic drugs may increase the formation of this toxic metabolite and increase the risk of hepatotoxicity. This may explain the association with hepatotoxicity and multiple epileptic agents. Other less common adverse effects include thrombocytopenia and alopecia.

There are numerous drug interactions known to occur with valproic acid. Many of these interactions involve other antiepileptic agents. Through their ability to increase liver metabolism, phenobarbital, phenytoin, and primidone have all been shown to increase the elimination of valproic acid. Some medications such as aspirin may compete with protein binding sites and increase the free concentration of valproic acid. Another well-known interaction is the effect of valproic acid on phenobarbital. Valproic acid inhibits the metabolism of phenobarbital and may lead to a considerable increase in phenobarbital plasma concentrations if the phenobarbital dose is not reduced. The effect of valproic acid on phenytoin is more complicated; phenytoin's metabolism may be decreased, but its displacement from binding sites by valproic acid may minimize the effects of reduced metabolism.

Valproic acid is usually initiated with a dose of approximately 15 mg/kg/day, given in divided doses. The dose is then increased in several days by approximately 5 to 10 mg/kg/day. Many patients experience significant gastrointestinal and/or CNS adverse effects if the dose is initiated too high. Most patients receiving valproic acid must take the drug more often than once a day. Some patients may have long half-lives enabling single daily dosing, but this is less common. Twice daily dosing is most frequent; however, patients receiving other enzyme-inducing drugs may require receiving the drug more frequently. If the patient experiences significant gastrointestinal distress with the valproic acid capsule, the enteric-coated tablet may be tried as an alternative.

Therapeutic drug monitoring of valproic acid may be very useful. The lowest effective anticonvulsant concentration appears to be approximately 50 μg/mL. The upper level of the therapeutic range is less clear. The most commonly noted upper limit is 100 μg/mL; however, some patients may attain better seizure control with concentrations above 100 μg/mL.

Primidone

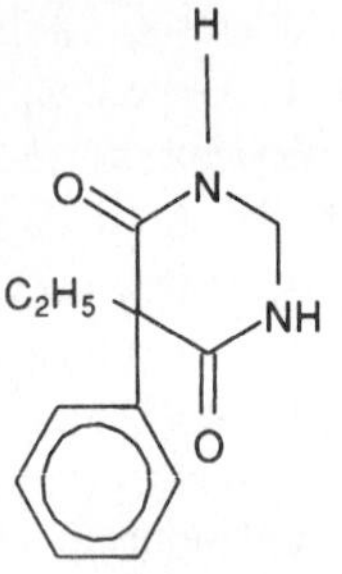

Primidone

Primidone is an alternative antiepileptic agent that may be used in generalized tonic-clonic and partial seizures. Since other agents have fewer adverse effects, it is not considered a first-line antiepileptic agent. The anticonvulsant actions of primidone are due to both the effects of the parent drug and its active metabolite, phenobarbital. Primidone also has a second metabolite, phenylethylmalonamide (PEMA), which may also be active. As with phenobarbital, primidone is a CNS depressant.

Primidone is well absorbed orally and peaks in the plasma 3 h after ingestion. The half-life of primidone varies but is often 5 to 19 h; the half-life of PEMA is 16 h. During chronic therapy, approximately 15 to 25 percent of a dose is eliminated unchanged in the urine, 50 to 70 percent is metabolized to PEMA, and 15 to 25 percent is metabolized to phenobarbital. The ratio of primidone to phenobarbital plasma concentrations is not consistent between patients. The accumulation of phenobarbital metabolite over time may induce the metabolism of primidone and gradually increase its clearance.

The side effects of primidone and phenobarbital are very similar. Since phenobarbital accumulates with chronic primidone therapy, the relative side effects between primidone and phenobarbital are often difficult to distinguish. The most frequent adverse effects are sedation, dizziness, ataxia, diplopia, nystagmus, and nausea. Rashes, leukopenia, and thrombocytopenia have also been reported. Megaloblastic anemia and osteomalacia may occur as discussed with phenobarbital.

Several primidone drug interactions are known. Phenytoin and carbamazepine are both known to increase the concentration of phenobarbital through enzyme induction. In addition, the accumulation of phenobarbital with chronic primidone therapy would also be expected to interact as discussed with phenobarbital.

Primidone therapy is usually initiated in doses of 50 to 125 mg and increased every few days. The usual adult daily dose is 750 to 1500 mg, given in divided doses. Although less clearly established between the concentration of primidone in the plasma and the antiepileptic effect, the therapeutic range is listed as 5 to 12 μg/mL.[40] Primidone concentrations exceeding 10 to 12 μg/mL are associated with a significant increase in adverse effects.

CONCLUSION

Epilepsy within the elderly population has several important characteristics in comparison to other age groups. There is a significant rise in focal seizures in patients older than 60 years of age, and many of these patients will have secondary generalization of the seizure activity. Many of these seizures are caused by cerebrovascular diseases, head injury, and brain tumors.

Treatment of epilepsy in the elderly is focused on eliminating the precipitating cause, if possible, and suppressing the manifestations of the seizures. Monotherapy with an appropriate antiepileptic drug is the foundation of pharmacologic therapy. The proper selection of an antiepileptic agent must address the avoidance of adverse effects as equally as important as suppression of the seizure activity. Carbamazepine is currently regarded as the agent of first choice in the management of partial seizures. If a properly administered and monitored initial therapy proves unsuccessful, an alternative monotherapy agent or a combination of antiepileptic agents may be effective in achieving seizure control.

REFERENCES

1. Theodore WH: Clinical pharmacology of antiepileptic drugs: selected topics. *Neurol Clin* 8:177-91, 1990.
2. Hauser WA, Kurland LT: The epidemiology of epilepsy in Rochester, Minnesota, 1935 through 1967. *Epilepsia* 16:1-66, 1975.
3. Luhdorf K, Jensen P, Plesner AM: Epilepsy in the elderly: incidence, social function, and disability. *Epilepsia* 27:135-141, 1986.
4. Commission on Classification and Terminology of the International League Against Epilepsy: Proposal for classification of epilepsies and epileptic syndromes. *Epilepsia* 26:268-278, 1985.
5. Dreifuss FE: Classification of epileptic seizures and the epilepsies. *Pediatr Clin North Am* 36:265-279, 1989.
6. Delgado-Escueta AV, Treiman DM, Walsh GO: The treatable epilepsies: Part 1. *N Engl J Med* 308:1508-1514, 1983.
7. Roberts MA, Godfrey JW, Caird FI: Epileptic seizures in the elderly: I. Aetiology and type of seizure. *Age Ageing* 11:24-28, 1982.
8. Schold C, Yarnell PR, Earnest MP: Origin of seizures in elderly patients. *JAMA* 238:1177-1178, 1979.
9. Dickinson ES: Seizure disorders in the elderly. *Prim Care* 9:135-142, 1982.
10. Messing RO, Closson RG, Simon RP: Drug-induced seizures: A 10-year experience. *Neurology* 34:1582-1586, 1984.
11. Sung CY, Chu NS: Epileptic seizures in elderly people: Aetiology and seizure type. *Age Ageing* 19:25-30, 1990.
12. Treiman DM: Efficacy and safety of antiepileptic drugs: A review of controlled trials. *Epilepsia* 28(suppl 3) :S1-8, 1987.
13. Wilder BJ: Treatment considerations in anticonvulsant monotherapy. *Epilepsia* 28(suppl 2):S1-7, 1987.
14. Beghi E, DiMascio R, Tognoni G: Drug treatment of epilepsy: outlines, criticism and perspectives. *Drugs* 31:249-265, 1986.
15. Homan RW, Miller B, Veterans Administration Epilepsy Cooperative Study Group: Causes of treatment failure with antiepileptic drugs vary over time. *Neurology* 37:1620-1623, 1987.

16. Schmidt D, Einicke I, Haenel F: The influence of seizure type on the efficacy of plasma concentrations of phenytoin, phenobarbital, and carbamazepine. *Arch Neurol* 43:263-265, 1986.
17. Troupin AS: The measurement of anticonvulsant agent levels. *Ann Intern Med* 100:854-885, 1984.
18. Levy RH, Schmidt D: Utility of free level monitoring of antiepileptic drugs. *Epilepsia* 26:199-205, 1985.
19. Mattson RH, Cramer JA, Collins JF, et al: Comparison of carbamazepine, phenobarbital, phenytoin, and primidone in partial and secondarily generalized tonic-clonic seizures. *N Engl J Med.* 313: 145-151, 1985.
20. Bertilsson L: Clinical pharmacokinetics of carbamazepine. *Clin Pharmacokinet* 3:128-143, 1978.
21. Rall TW, Schleifer LS: Drugs effective in the therapy of the epilepsies, in Gilman AG, Rall TW, Nies AS, Taylor P (eds): *The Pharmacological Basis of Therapeutics.* New York, Pergamon, 1990, pp 436-462.
22. Engel J, Troupin AS, Crandall PH, et al: Recent developments in the diagnosis and therapy of epilepsy. *Ann Intern Med* 97:584-598, 1982.
23. Vining EPG: Cognitive dysfunction associated with antiepileptic drug therapy. *Epilepsia* 28(suppl 2):S18-22, 1987.
24. Pippenger CE: Clinically significant carbamazepine drug interactions; an overview. *Epilepsia* 28(suppl 3):S71-76, 1987.
25. Ensom RJ, Nakagawa RS: Phenytoin absorption in adults: effect of aging. *N Engl J Med* 313:697, 1985.
26. Richens A: Clinical pharmacokinetics of phenytoin. *Clin Pharmacokinet* 4:153-169, 1979.
27. Raebel MA: Nonequivalence of phenytoin capsules and tablets. *N Engl J Med* 309:925, 1983.
28. Bauer LA, Blouin RA: Age and phenytoin kinetics in adult epileptics. *Clin Pharmacol Ther* 31:301-304, 1982.
29. Richens A, Dunlop A: Serum-phenytoin levels in management of epilepsy. *Lancet* 1:247-248, 1975.
30. Trimble MR: Anticonvulsant drugs and cognitive function: A review of the literature. *Epilepsia* 28(suppl 3):S37-45, 1987.
31. Dela Cruz FG, Kanter MZ, Fischer JH, Leikin JB: Efficacy of individualized phenytoin sodium loading doses administered by intravenous infusion. *Clin Pharm* 7:219-124, 1988.
32. Boike SC, Rybak MJ, Tintinalli JE, et al: Evaluation of a method for intravenous phenytoin infusion. *Clin Pharm* 2:444-446, 1983.
33. Winter ME, Tozer TN: Phenytoin, in Evans WE, Schentag JJ, Jusko WJ (eds): *Applied Pharmacokinetics: Principles of Therapeutic Drug Monitoring*, 2d ed. Spokane, Applied Therapeutics, 1986, pp 493-539.
34. Eadie MJ: Anticonvulsant drugs: An update. *Drugs* 27:328-363, 1984.
35. Penry JK, Dean JC: Valproate monotherapy in partial seizures. *Am J Med* 84(suppl 1A):14-16, 1988.
36. Delgado-Escueta AV, Treiman DM, Walsh GO: The treatable epilepsies: part 2. *N Engl J Med* 308:1576-1584, 1983.
37. Gugler R, Von Unruh GE: Clinical pharmacokinetics of valproic acid. *Clin Pharmacokinet* 5:67-83, 1980.
38. Browne TR: Valproic acid. *N Engl J Med* 302: 661-666, 1980.
39. Pugh CB, Garnett WR: Current issues in the treatment of epilepsy. *Clin Pharm* 10:335-358, 1991.
40. Mahler ME: Seizures: Common causes and treatment in the elderly. *Geriatrics* 42:73-78, 1987.

CHAPTER

14

TREATMENT OF PARKINSON'S DISEASE

Erwin B. Montgomery
Robert J. Lipsy

CLINICOPATHOLOGIC CONSIDERATIONS

Parkinson's syndrome is characterized by tremor, rigidity, bradykinesia, akinesia, and postural abnormalities. Diagnosis usually requires the presence of at least two of these symptoms. However, any of these symptoms can be variable within and between individuals. This variability can cause diagnostic confusion.

The tremor occurs primarily at rest, although not exclusively. The tremor most often affects the distal upper extremity, but it can affect any part of the body. The tremor is usually at 4 to 5 cycles per second. Stress of any origin may exacerbate or bring out tremor. As many as 30 percent of patients may not have tremor.

Akinesia refers to the absence of movement. For example, the normal arm swing associated with walking is often lost. Facial expression may be lost, resulting in a "masklike" facies. Bradykinesia refers to slowness of movement. Patients may take much more time to dress or eat. Any movement may be affected, such as speech, writing, eating, and walking. The patient may walk with a short shuffling gait of small step length. Patients may find that they have difficultly starting to walk or suddenly freeze. Some patients may start to fall forward at an increasing pace until they fall or encounter an obstacle. This is called a *festinating gait*. Handwriting may be affected, with the writing becoming smaller as the patient continues to write. This symptom is called *micrographia*.

Rigidity is identified by resistance to passive movement of the limb or head. The increased resistance associated with parkinsonism may be of the cogwheel or intermittent type or of the lead pipe or plastic type, which is continuous. Many parkinsonian patients may not have rigidity.

Postural abnormalities include a flexed or stooped posture. Postural reflexes are also slowed, leading to frequent falls. Other symptoms which may be present include autonomic dysfunction such as orthostatic hypotension and bladder dysfunction. Some patients may have dysphagia causing increased risk of aspiration.

A distinction between Parkinson's disease and Parkinson's syndrome must be maintained. Idiopathic Parkinson's disease is associated with characteristic pathologic changes such as depigmentation of the substantia nigra, loss of dopamine neurons in the substantia nigra, and the presence of eosinophilic cytoplasmic inclusions called Lewy bodies. Idiopathic Parkinson's disease accounts for approximately 80 percent of patients with Parkinson's syndrome.

Approximately 10 percent of parkinsonism is caused by drugs which deplete the brain of dopamine or block dopamine receptors. These drugs include some antihypertension medications such as alpha-methyldopa and reserpine, antipsychotics such as haloperidol, chlorpromazine, and other medications such as metoclopramide and amoxapine.

A variety of rare neurodegenerative disorders produce parkinsonism. The presence of severe autonomic dysfunction suggests Shy-Drager disease or multisystem atrophy. Loss of vertical eye movements, particularly in the upward direction, suggests progressive supranuclear palsy. Some patients with Alzheimer's disease may also appear parkinsonian.

Parkinson's disease will become an increasingly important health care problem. The incidence of Parkinson's disease is approximately 200 per 100,000 general population. However, the prevalence is 2 percent in the population over age 80, and it is this segment of the population which is growing at the greatest rate. While the onset of Parkinson's disease is greatest in the sixth and seventh decades, the disease can affect the young. It is not uncommon to see Parkinson's disease in patients in their twenties and thirties.

The primary cause is related to degeneration of the substantia nigra pars compacta. Loss of nigral dopamine-containing neurons results in a deficiency of dopamine in the caudate nucleus and putamen of the basal ganglia. Rarely lesions of the globus pallidus may be associated with parkinsonism. The neuronal basis of these pathogenic mechanisms is unknown. Therapy is usually symptomatic, primarily designed to replace dopaminergic activity, although anticholinergic medications and stereotactic surgery probably utilize different mechanisms. Recently, protective therapy has been introduced aimed at slowing the rate of progression of the disease.

SYMPTOMATIC TREATMENT

The clinician has a wide array of therapeutic agents for the treatment of Parkinson's disease. The individual agents are reviewed below followed by a discussion of treatment strategy. Recommended dosing regimens for initiation and maintenance of therapy of the various agents are provided in Table 14-1.

Levodopa

Levodopa is a precursor of dopamine, and its decarboxylation in the brain restores dopamine. Dopamine will not cross the blood-brain barrier whereas levodopa will. Dopamine replacement therapy with levodopa has dramatically improved the quality of life and has normalized the life expectancy of Parkinson's disease patients.

However, replacement of dopamine is complicated by the pharmacokinetics and pharmacodynamics of levodopa and dopamine. Levodopa must be transported across multiple compartments including the gastrointestinal tract, blood plasma, and brain (Fig. 14-1). There are multiple factors influencing transport across these compartments as well as metabolism within each of these compartments. Furthermore, progression of the disease and possibly continued exposure to medications may have adverse effects on dopamine receptor function, thereby influencing the physiologic effect of medications.

Initial management of the early or mildly affected patient is relatively straightforward. For many patients there may be a "honeymoon" period of gratifying response to levodopa only to be followed by frustrating side effects. A few years after the introduction of levodopa, numerous complications emerged.[1] These included involuntary movements called *dyskinesias* and involuntary postures termed *dystonias*. Another complication is the appearance of marked fluctuations in the clinical control of the parkinsonian symptoms.[2] These fluctuations have been referred to as *on-off effects*, *wearing-off effects*, *end-of-dose deterioration*, and *yo-yoing*. Any of these complications can be more disabling than the parkinsonian symptoms, and they may occur in half of patients who have been on levodopa for 4 years or more.

Pathophysiology of dyskinesias, dystonias, and clinical fluctuations Most dyskinesias and dystonias are dose related and are most severe at the time of peak levodopa effect. These dyskinesias are termed *peak-dose dyskinesias*. Reduction in the levodopa dose reduces or eliminates the dyskinesias. However, the reduction of levodopa necessary to eliminate dyskinesias often results in worse parkinsonian features. For some patients, a decision has to be made as to whether the parkinsonian symptoms or the peak-dose dyskinesias are more disabling and dosing decisions made accordingly. Another rare form of dyskinesias is called *biphasic* and is associated with the rapid raise and fall of plasma levodopa levels.

Recent evidence suggests that most fluctuations in clinical response are secondary to failure to maintain constant brain levels of dopamine. This failure is most often due to the inability to provide a constant supply of levodopa to the brain. Alternative means of providing a more continuous supply of levodopa by intravenous[3] or intraduodenal[4] infusions, by augmentation with dopamine agonists such as bromocriptine and pergolide or the monoamine oxidase type B (MAO-B) antagonist selegiline, or by controlled-release levodopa preparation (Sinemet CR)[5] may reduce the frequency and severity of motor fluctuations. Usually the failure

Table 14-1 Suggested doses of commonly used agents in Parkinson's disease

Drug name	Dosage form	Starting dose	Maximum dose
Dopaminergics			
Levodopa (Larodopa, Dopar, various)	100-, 250-, 500-mg tablets and capsules	250–500 mg daily	2 to 8 g daily in 3–4 divided doses
Levodopa-carbidopa (Sinemet, Sinemet Cr)	10/100, 25/100, 25/250-mg tablets; 50/200-mg sustained-release tablet	75/300-mg daily in 3–4 divided doses	200/2000 mg daily in 3–4 divided doses
Amantadine (Symmetrel)	100-mg capsule; 50 mg/5 mL syrup	100 mg daily for 1 week	100 mg twice daily[a]
Pergolide (Permax)	0.05-, 0.025-, 1-mg tablets	0.05 mg daily for 2 days increased by 0.1 or 0.15 mg every 3 days, after 12 days can increase by 0.25 mg daily	2.5–6 mg daily
Bromocriptine (Parlodel)	2.5-mg tablet; 5-mg capsule	1.25 mg twice a day, increase every 14–21 days by 2.5 mg/day	100 mg in divided doses
Anticholinergics			
Benztropine (Cogentin)	0.5-, 1-, 2-mg tablets; 1 mg/mL 2-mL ampules	0.5–1 mg daily, increase by 1–2 mg daily	0.5–6 mg daily
Trihexyphenidyl (Artane)	2, 5-mg tablets; 5-mg sustained-release capsule; 2 mg/5 mL	1–2 mg daily, increase by 1–2 mg every 3 days	6–10 mg daily

Diphenhydramine (Benadryl, various)	25, 50-mg tablets and capsules; 12.5 mg/5 mL elixir; 10- and 50 mg/mL injection	25–50 mg daily	5–100 mg daily in divided doses
Biperiden (Akineton)	2-mg tablet; 5-mg/mL ampule	2 mg twice a day	2 mg 3–4 times a day
Procyclidine (Kenadrin)	2-, 5-mg tablets	2.5 mg 2–3 times a day	10–20 mg daily in divided doses
Ethopropazine (Parsidol)	10-, 50-mg tablets	50 mg once or twice daily	100–600 mg daily
Monoamine oxidase type "B" inhibitors			
Selegiline (Eldepryl)	5-mg tablets	10 mg daily in divided doses	10 mg

[a]Amantadine is excreted solely by the kidneys. The drug's elimination closely parallels creatinine clearance. Dosage should be adjusted for patients with decreased renal function (see below):

Creatinine clearance, mL/min/1.73 m^2	Estimated half-life, h	Suggested daily dosage
>80	11	100 mg twice a day
60–80	17	100 mg alternated with 200 mg daily
40–60	25	100 mg daily
30	40	200 mg twice weekly
20	66	100 mg 3 times a week
<20	200	200 mg, alternate with 100 mg every 7 days or hemodialysis 3 times a week

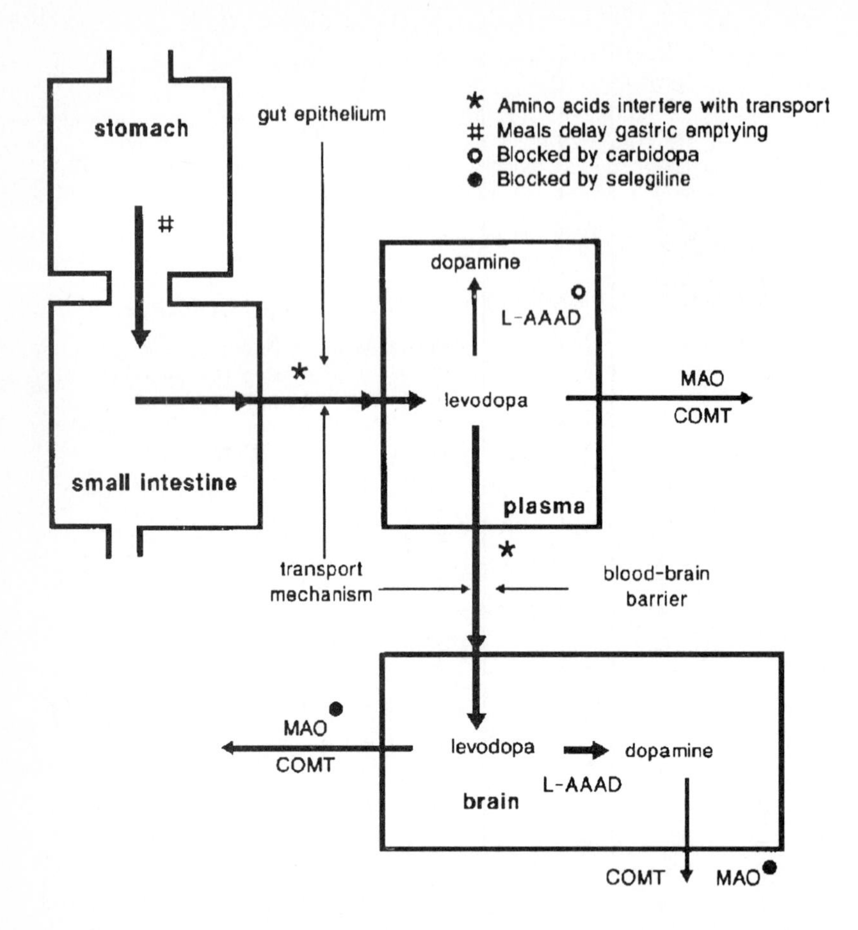

Figure 14-1 The different compartments levodopa must cross in order to reach the brain and be converted to dopamine to exert its clinical effect. There are numerous factors that influence transport across compartments and metabolism within an effected compartment. Many of these factors can be influenced so as to improve treatment.

to provide constant dopamine replacement is due to failure to maintain constant plasma levels (wearing-off effects).

Distinction between plasma levodopa and physiologic response Parkinson's disease patients vary in the duration of their clinical response to levodopa. While the variation represents a continuum, the extremes are identified as long- and short-duration responders.[6] For the long-duration responder there is continued improvement despite declining plasma levodopa levels after a dose of levodopa. The improvement and decline in the disability for the short-duration responder

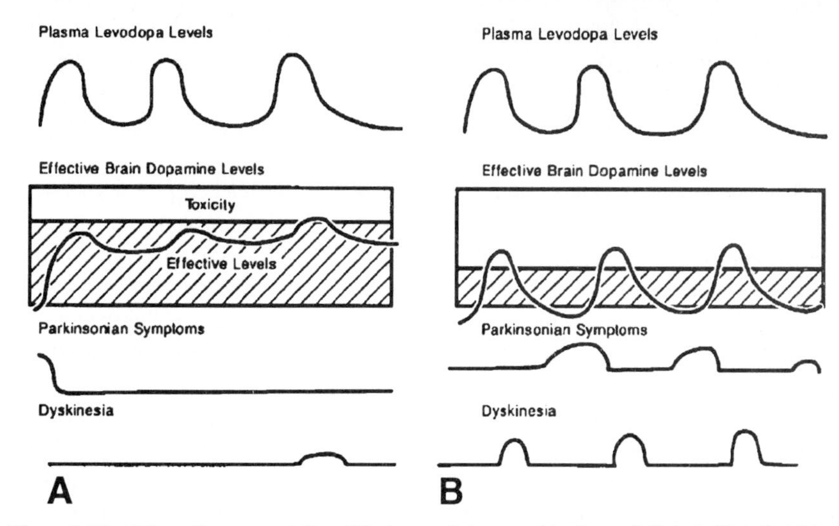

Figure 14-2 Schematic representation of the issues of pharmacokinetics and clinical effects in (*A*) long- and (*B*) short-duration responders. The plasma kinetics are similar in the two types of responders, resulting in the same plasma level profiles, but the net effective brain levels as interpreted from the clinical response differ. As a consequence, short-duration responders are more likely to have dyskinesia and wearing-off effects with a reappearance of parkinsonian symptoms.

parallels the plasma levodopa levels. Furthermore, short-duration responders have a lower plasma levodopa level threshold for dyskinesias (Fig. 14-2).

It is probable that the short-duration responders are the ones who have motor fluctuations. This is particularly true if the dosing interval is longer than the duration of response. As the patient's plasma levels of levodopa rise, there is an improvement in the bradykinesia. However, dyskinesias may appear. As the plasma levels fall, there is worsening of the patient's bradykinesia and a lessening of the dyskinesias. If the same patient is given a constant infusion of levodopa, there results more consistent plasma levodopa levels and more consistent control of the parkinsonian symptoms.[3]

Since the plasma clearance of dopamine is approximately 1 to 2 h and is the same in long- and short-duration responders, the difference in response between the groups must be related to central nervous system mechanisms. These mechanisms include the conversion of levodopa to dopamine; the response of postsynaptic and, possibly, presynaptic receptors; the reuptake of dopamine into presynaptic terminals; and the metabolic breakdown of levodopa and dopamine. With progression of the disease or continued exposure to levodopa, there may be changes in any of these mechanisms such that the duration of beneficial response decreases with time and the severity and incidence of adverse effects increase.

Another central mechanism may be the significant reduction of aromatic L-amino-acid decarboxylase (L-AAAD) in the basal ganglia necessary to convert levodopa to dopamine. There is no significant reduction of MAO and only a 25 percent decrease in catechol-*O*-methyltransferase (COMT).[7] Thus, there may be a reduction in the conversion of levodopa to dopamine but continued conversion of levodopa to metabolites such as 3-*O*-methyldopa. These metabolites may interfere with conversion of levodopa to dopamine or binding of dopamine to its receptor. With progression of the disease there may be further decreases in substantia nigra neurons with secondary decreases in L-AAAD.

There also may be changes in the postsynaptic dopamine receptor associated with continued loss of presynaptic elements and/or continued exposure to dopamine. Motor fluctuators (short-duration responders by inference) have a lower plasma levodopa threshold to dyskinesia compared to long-duration responders. These observations suggest changes in the physiologic response of the receptors. This may be caused by intermittent administration of levodopa compared to continuous administration of the same dose.[8]

Another central mechanism mediating the duration of levodopa response may be the degree of preservation of substantia nigra neurons. Patients must lose approximately 80 percent of their substantia nigra neurons before becoming symptomatic.[9] Furthermore, dopamine released from the synaptic terminal is inactivated by reuptake. It has been hypothesized that new onset Parkinson's disease patients may have some substantia nigra neurons remaining which can take up dopamine derived from exogenously administered levodopa. These neurons are then able to release dopamine as the brain levodopa levels are decreasing. In this way, the remaining substantia nigra neurons are able to buffer the effects of changing plasma levodopa levels such that the clinical effects outlast the plasma levodopa levels. As the disease progresses, there are fewer remaining substantia nigra neurons left to buffer the dopamine levels and the patient becomes dependent on the plasma to supply the levodopa to be converted to dopamine.[1,10] There may be differences in the number of presynaptic nigrostriatal terminals in the long- versus the short-duration responders.

As the duration of beneficial clinical response lessens with decreased ability of the brain to buffer dopamine levels, the brain levels of dopamine become more dependent on brain levodopa levels, which in turn are dependent on plasma levodopa levels. Since the plasma half-life of levodopa is between 1 and 2 h, the duration of clinical response becomes 1 to 2 h. Less frequent oral dosing of levodopa will result in fluctuating plasma levels and, therefore, fluctuating clinical control of symptoms.

Multicompartment distribution and metabolism of levodopa The aim of levodopa replacement therapy is the constant delivery of dopamine to the postsynaptic receptors in the basal ganglia. For the short-duration responders (i.e., motor fluctuators) this requires the constant delivery of levodopa to the brain and constant levodopa conversion to dopamine. Since oral administration is currently the only practical approach, levodopa has to be transported across multiple compartments (e.g., gastrointestinal tract, blood plasma, and brain) before it reaches the striatal dopamine receptors. Within each compartment there are many factors which influence the fate of levodopa and, thus, the patient's clinical response.

Gastrointestinal compartment Absorption of levodopa from the gastrointestinal tract into the blood occurs in the small intestine with approximately 80 percent of an oral dose reaching the plasma (Fig. 14-1).[11] Factors which influence delivery of levodopa to the small intestine will affect delivery of levodopa to the plasma compartment and subsequently to the brain. Meals delay gastric emptying. If levodopa is taken with meals, it may be held up in the stomach and delayed in reaching the small intestine. In the study of Nutt et al,[3] meals caused an average delay of 34 min in reaching peak plasma levels and 27 percent reduction in peak plasma levels. Most patients should be instructed to take levodopa at least 1 h before meals or 2 h after meals. However, as long as the drug is taken at the same time in relation to meals, intake of some food with each dose may help reduce nausea and the dose can be titrated to patient response. When administered with levodopa, iron may cause up to a 50 percent reduction in adsorption[12] (Table 14-2). Therefore, patients should be instructed to separate their levodopa dose by 1 or 2 h from foods rich in iron, iron supplements, or multivitamins with iron.

Transport of levodopa across the gut endothelium is also enzyme mediated. The enzyme also transports neutral amino acids.[3] Ingestion of a large amount of protein could increase the concentration of neutral amino acids within the gut, which would compete with transport of levodopa into the plasma. Decreases in plasma concentrations can be as great as 20 percent and are most severe when daily protein exceeds 2 g/kg. Dietary intake of 0.5 g/kg/day or less appears to be safe[13] (Table 14-2).

Plasma compartment Once levodopa is absorbed into the plasma, numerous enzymes act to metabolize and eliminate levodopa (Fig. 14-1). Less than 1 percent of levodopa is excreted unchanged in the urine. A major enzyme is L-AAAD. This enzyme converts levodopa to dopamine. Dopamine itself cannot be transported across the blood-brain barrier. Therefore, plasma dopamine is of no clinical use. Carbidopa inhibits L-AAAD in the periphery but not in the brain, where decarboxylation to dopamine is necessary. Coadministration of carbidopa prolongs the serum half-life of levodopa from 1 to 2 h and increases the amount of unmetabolized levodopa excreted in the urine to 6 percent. With carbidopa, five times the blood level of levodopa on half the oral dose of L-dopa can be achieved. Peripheral dopamine levels remain the same.[14] As a consequence, smaller amounts of levodopa can be administered, thereby reducing the incidence and severity of peripheral side effects such as anorexia, nausea, vomiting, and cardiac irritability.

The optimal dose of carbidopa in an adult is 75 to 100 mg/day. However, many patients require larger doses.[15] Carbidopa is generally well tolerated. The carbidopa dose becomes a factor in deciding which form of Sinemet (levodopa-carbidopa combination) to use. There are three forms used, 10/100, 25/100, and 25/250. The first number refers to the carbidopa dose and the second to the levodopa dose. For most patients, the 25/100 form is most appropriate because the 10/100 form does not provide sufficient carbidopa and the 25/250 form often gives excessive amounts of levodopa, resulting in dyskinesias.

Table 14-2 Drug and food interactions with levodopa

Drug or food	Interaction	Severity	Probable mechanism
Benzodiazepines	Decreased anti-Parkinson effect in some patients	Moderate	Unknown
Clonidine	Decreased anti-Parkinson effect in some patients	Moderate	Stimulation of central alpha-adrenergic receptors
Dietary protein	Decreased anti-Parkinson effect; diets containing over 2 g/kg of body weight per day cause greatest effect; diets with 0.5 g/kg appear safe	Severe	Competition between large amino acids and levodopa for intestinal absorption or with dopamine for passage across blood-brain barrier
Iron	Decreased anti-Parkinson effect	Moderate	Iron binds with levodopa, reducing absorption by 50%
Methyldopa	May increase or decrease anti-Parkinson effect; may also either attenuate or potentiate orthostatic hypotension	Mild	May increase effect by acting as decarboxylase inhibitor; mechanism for decreasing effect unknown
MAO inhibitors, e.g., pargyline, isocarboxazid, phenelzine, tranylcypromine	Hypertensive crisis	Severe	Increase in storage and release of dopamine, norepinephrine, or both
Neuroleptics, e.g., haloperidol, chlorpromazine	Decreased anti-Parkinson effect	Moderate	Inhibition of dopamine reuptake and blockade of dopamine receptors
Pyridoxine	Decreased anti-Parkinson effect; does not occur in patients receiving carbidopa	Severe	Increased decarboxylation of levodopa in periphery
Phenytoin	Decreased anti-Parkinson effect in an occasional patient	Mild	Unknown
Papaverine	Decreased anti-Parkinson effect in an occasional patient	Mild	Unknown

It may be difficult in some cases to provide patients with sufficient carbidopa without giving excessive amounts of levodopa, due to the fixed ratios of carbidopa to levodopa in commercially available preparations. It is possible to obtain plain carbidopa directly from the manufacturer as Lodosyn 25 mg. Note that regular Sinemet went off patent in 1991. The types of possible generic levodopa-carbidopa preparations and their formulations are unknown at present.

Brain compartment Levodopa must be transported across the blood-brain barrier via an enzyme-mediated system. This system also transports neutral amino acids. High plasma concentrations of these neutral amino acids following a high-protein meal may compete with levodopa. Consequently, there may be a fall in the brain levodopa levels and, subsequently, a fall in brain dopamine levels despite maintained plasma levodopa levels. As with transportation across gut endothelium, the interaction appears to be dose related with daily intake of 2 g/kg of protein being associated with the most severe effects and intake of 0.5 g/kg being relatively safe[13] (Table 14-2).

Levodopa must be converted to dopamine in the brain. Reduced basal ganglia levels of L-AAAD may cause a reduction in brain dopamine levels. Relatively intact MAO and COMT systems may further reduce brain dopamine levels by catabolizing both levodopa and dopamine. There may be accumulations of catabolic products such as 3-*O*-methyldopa which can interfere with levodopa and dopamine.

Dopamine receptor Ultimately, the dopamine must interact with the postsynaptic dopamine receptor in order to exert its physiologic and clinical effect. Changes in receptor function may complicate the clinical response. This is suggested by the change in the levodopa plasma threshold to produce dyskinesias.[2,16] These thresholds are lower in the short-duration responders compared to the long-duration responders, thereby narrowing the therapeutic window. In some patients, the therapeutic window can "invert," and the patients experience dyskinesias while bradykinesia persists. It is possible that these changes in threshold to dyskinesias are related not just to exposure to levodopa but rather to pulsatile administration. Continuous infusions may widen the therapeutic window.[17]

Sinemet CR Sinemet CR is a controlled-release form of carbidopa-levodopa. Fifty milligrams of carbidopa and 200 mg of levodopa are embedded in a slowly dissolving matrix which releases drug, slowly producing a longer plasma presence of approximately 4 h following an oral dose. The plasma half-life of levodopa is not affected. The prolonged plasma presence may be an advantage for short-duration responders but does not appear to be helpful in patients experiencing the on-off phenomenon.[18] Sinemet CR does not produce as high peak plasma levels of levodopa as does regular levodopa-carbidopa levels. This may lessen the maximum severity of dyskinesias in those patients with peak-dose dyskinesia. However, more patients appear to have a longer duration of dyskinesias during the on period with the sustained-release product.[19] Some patients with rare biphasic dyskinesias may have worsened dyskinesias with Sinemet CR. This preparation takes longer to reach peak plasma levels (1 to 2 h), so some patients may not "turn on" suddenly as with regular levodopa-carbidopa compounds. This can produce dissatisfaction and compliance problems. At this time, the benefits of the sustained-release preparation appear to be short-lived in many patients. At 1 year following initiation of therapy solely with Sinemet CR, 50 to 75 percent of patients have required addition of regular Sinemet as a supplement, or "booster," for early morning and other predictible off periods.[20,21] In one study, the mean number of tablets taken daily (regular plus CR) at the end of 1 year was 11.9 and the mean number of doses was 8.0.[20]

Beneficial response to regular levodopa-carbidopa compounds depends critically on plasma and brain pharmacokinetics. Response to Sinemet CR may be dependent on gastrointestinal kinetics, which may be abnormal in the elderly. Abnormally slow gastrointestinal motility may result in increased time in the small intestine causing greater than usual absorption. This could produce increased dyskinesias. Abnormally fast gastrointestinal motility may result in a shortened presence of Sinemet CR in the small intestine and less than usual absorption. This would reduce the effectiveness of Sinemet CR. Day-to-day variations in gastrointestinal motility may account for the day-to-day variations in response to Sinemet CR, which is more variable than regular levodopa-carbidopa compounds.

The bioavailability of levodopa in Sinemet CR is less than in regular Sinemet.[22] Therefore, in the conversion from regular Sinemet to Sinemet CR, the total daily dose of levodopa from regular Sinemet is multiplied by 125 percent. Generally, when converting from Sinemet to Sinemet CR, the dosing interval is doubled to a maximum of 4 h. Patients not previously on levodopa compounds can be initiated on a once or twice a day regimen. In clinical trials, dosing frequency was usually reduced from an average of six to eight times a day with the non-sustained-release product to four to five times a day with CR. However, conversion is inexact and careful titration is required.

Toxicity of levodopa compounds Levodopa is associated with a number of peripheral and central adverse effects (Table 14-3). The most common side effects of levodopa are nausea and emesis. These are caused by local irritation of the gastric mucosa and stimulation of the chemoreceptive areas in the brain. Local irritation of the gastrointestinal tract can be reduced by taking levodopa with meals. Adequate use of carbidopa can reduce or eliminate gastrointestinal irritation by levodopa.

Dyskinesias and dystonias also suggest excessive levodopa and can be relieved by reduction of dose. Levodopa can also cause nocturnal myoclonus characterized by jerklike movement during sleep. Levodopa may also produce vivid dreams which can be disturbing to the patient or family members. These problems may also be reduced or eliminated by decreasing the last dose of levodopa prior to bedtime.

Hallucinations, delusions, confusion, or paranoia can be produced by levodopa. Reduction of the levodopa dose can reduce or eliminate this problem but possibly at the cost of control of the parkinsonian symptoms. Use of traditional

Table 14-3 Adverse effects of anti-Parkinson agents

Drug name	Adverse effects
	Dopaminergics
Levodopa	*Frequent:* Nausea, vomiting, anorexia, choreiform or dystonic movements, ataxia, increased hand tremor, headache, dizziness, numbness, confusion, insomnia, nightmares, hallucinations *Less frequent:* Orthostatic hypotension, behavioral changes, cardiac arrhythmias, "on-off" phenomenon
Levodopa-carbidopa	Same as levodopa with less frequent systemic effects of nausea, vomiting, cardiac arrhythmias
Amantadine	*Frequent:* Slurred speech, tremor, ataxia, hyperexcitability *Less frequent:* Insomnia, depression, hallucination, livedo reticularis In overdose increased CNS adverse reactions including choreiform or dystonic movements and seizures.
Pergolide	Same as levodopa with the addition of rhinitis, somnolence, and peripheral edema; possibly a higher incidence of CNS reactions
Bromocriptine	Same as levodopa with a higher incidence of hallucinations, confusion, nausea and possibly orthostatic hypotension
	Anticholinergics
Benztropine, biperiden, trihexyphenidyl, procyclidine, diphenhydramine	*Frequent:* Blurred vision, dry mouth, drowsiness, muscle weakness, mild confusion, constipation, urinary retention *Less frequent:* In higher or toxic doses tachycardia, hallucinations, agitation, elevation of body temperature, seizures
	MAO-B inhibitors
Selegiline	*Frequent:* Nausea, confusion, depression, ataxia, insomnia, agitation, involuntary movements *Less frequent:* Hallucinations, orthostatic hypotension, chorea, bradykinesia, hypertension

antipsychotic medications can control psychosis but often exacerbate the parkinsonism. A new antipsychotic called *clozapine* (Clozaril) may control psychotic symptoms without exacerbating the parkinsonian symptoms. In some patients in which psychosis limits the use of levodopa compounds, adjunctive use of clozapine may allow increases in levodopa dose necessary to control symptoms.[23] However, there is a 2 percent incidence of agranulocytosis, and therefore careful weekly monitoring of white blood cell counts is necessary. The agranulocytosis improves with discontinuation of clozapine. Some patients may be successfully restarted on clozapine once the white cell counts return to normal.

The side effects of Sinemet CR are the same as regular Sinemet; however, they occur over a longer time course. For example, dyskinesias which last 15 to 30 min on regular Sinemet may last hours on Sinemet CR. Another disadvantage to Sinemet CR is that response may be more erratic than with regular Sinemet. Sinemet CR cannot be ground up to be administered. This defeats the slow-release design. The incidence of hallucinations appears increased on Sinemet CR, compared to regular Sinemet.[7]

Adverse drug interactions with levodopa A number of drug interactions have been reported with levodopa (Table 14-2). The most severe have been reported to occur with nonspecific monoamine oxidase inhibitors (MAOIs) such as pargyline, tranylcypromine, and phenelzine and with pyridoxine.[24] MAOIs increase the storage and release of dopamine, norepinephrine, or both. Concomitant use of levodopa with these agents or use within 1 to 2 weeks after their discontinuation may lead to severe hypertensive crisis. Pyridoxine increases the decarboxylation of levodopa in the periphery, which can lead to a decreased anti-Parkinson effect. This interaction does not take place in patients receiving carbidopa.[25] Other drugs reported to diminish the anti-Parkinson effects of levodopa include clonidine, methyldopa, neuroleptics such as haloperidol and chlorpromazine, phenytoin, and papaverine. Often the nature of the interactions has not been determined and the effects in individual patients are variable.[25]

Adjunctive use of monoamine oxidase type B inhibitors Selegiline (Eldepryl), which selectively blocks MAO-B, may be useful in increasing the response to levodopa by decreasing brain metabolism of levodopa and dopamine. Selegiline can prolong the response to regular levodopa-carbidopa compounds. Well absorbed following oral administration, selegiline is rapidly metabolized. The three major metabolites, desmethyldeprenyl, amphetamine, and methamphetamine, have much longer half-lives of 2, 17.5, and 20.5 h, respectively.[26] Maximum inhibition of MAO-B by selegiline may not occur for 2 to 3 days. Some patients must reduce their levodopa dose by as much as 10 to 30 percent when selegiline is added.[27] Selegiline prolongation of levodopa response will probably not be clinically significant when Sinemet CR is used.

Toxicity Selegiline is relatively selective for MAO-B and spares MAO type A in the periphery. As such, there is little risk of hypertensive crises associated with general MAOIs. However, a few patients may have increased blood pressure on recommended doses. At doses higher than 10 mg/day significant inhibition of MAO-A occurs, and the risk of hypertensive crises and other sympathomimetic-mediated adverse drug reactions increases. Selegiline also causes a number of adverse effects associated with increased amounts of dopamine (Table 14-3). In addition, selegiline is metabolized to amphetamine. This may cause feelings of anxiety and sleep disturbance. For this reason it is recommended that selegiline be given as 5 mg in the morning and 5 mg in the afternoon. Generally, selegiline is started at half this dose and gradually increased to the recommended dose as tolerated.[28]

Direct Dopaminergic Agonists

Direct dopaminergic agonists, such as bromocriptine (Parlodel) and pergolide (Permax), act as dopamine but do not require activation or conversion as does levodopa. Additionally, the plasma half-life of bromocriptine is 3 h and that of pergolide is 27 h, although the duration of clinical benefit is approximately 5 h in most patients.[29] The longer half-lives of these compounds result in less fluctuations in clinical response. Thus, these compounds are effective adjuncts to levodopa-carbidopa compounds in short-duration responders.[30,31]

These compounds are generally not as effective as monotherapy. However, if research confirms that exposure to levodopa contributes to the development of dyskinesias and motor fluctuations, then direct dopaminergic agonists may be indicated initially as monotherapy in newly diagnosed or mildly affected patients.

Pergolide is generally more potent than bromocriptine in terms of binding affinities to the dopamine receptor. However, this does not immediately translate to increased clinical effectiveness. Patients who fail with bromocriptine may respond to pergolide, yet patients who fail to respond to pergolide usually do not respond to bromocriptine. Generally, pergolide may be less expensive compared to bromocriptine.[29]

Bromocriptine is supplied as 2.5-mg tablets and as 5-mg capsules. The usual starting dose is 1.25 mg twice a day slowly titrated upward until satisfactory response or the appearance of limiting side effects. Most patients require 12.5 mg or more for symptomatic relief when used as monotherapy. Doses in excess of 40 mg/day are unlikely to provide additional benefit although doses up to 100 mg daily have been effective in some patients.

Pergolide comes as 0.05-mg, 0.25-mg, and 1.0-mg scored tablets. The initial dose is 0.05 mg twice a day slowly titrated upward until satisfactory response or the appearance of limiting side effects. Most patients require 2.5 mg or more for symptomatic relief when used as monotherapy. Doses in excess of 6 mg per day are unlikely to provide additional benefit.

Toxicity Bromocriptine and pergolide are ergot alkaloid compounds and are generally associated with more limiting side effects than levodopa compounds, particularly in the elderly. Twenty-seven percent of patients may stop pergolide because of side effects which include nausea, vomiting, confusion, hallucinations, hypotension, and lightheadedness[29] (Table 14-3). Their use is problematic in patients with coronary artery disease. They can exacerbate angina and congestive heart failure. Direct dopaminergic agonists may exacerbate dyskinesias associated with simultaneous use of levodopa compounds.

Amantidine

The exact mechanisms of action of amantidine (Symmetrel) are not known. The drug does possess both anti-Parkinson and anticholinergic properties. Amantidine works principally by augmenting the presynaptic synthesis and release of dopamine and by diminishing dopamine uptake into storage terminals.[25] Amantidine, when used as monotherapy, has a short duration of effective use. Positive effects have usually diminished or are absent by 4 to 6 weeks.[32] Amantadine has been compared to placebo, levodopa, and anticholinergic agents. It is more effective than placebo but less effective than levodopa. Amantidine may be equally effective as anticholinergic agents.[25]

Toxicity Amantidine shares many of the same side effects as the anticholinergics (Table 14-3). Additional side effects include livedo reticularis, a purplish blotchy discoloration of the lower extremities. This side effect does not necessitate discontinuation of amantadine. This drug can also cause pedal edema and exacerbation of congestive heart failure.[25,31] The usual starting dose is 100 mg daily for 1 week followed by a maintenance dose of 100 mg twice a day. Amantadine is excreted virtually unchanged in the urine. Doses should be reduced in elderly patients and others with reduced renal function when dosing amantidine[25] (Table 14-1). Generally, amantadine side effects are better tolerated in the elderly compared to the anticholinergic agents.

Anticholinergic Agents

Anticholinergic compounds have been used since the 1890s when Charcot used the extract of the belladonna plant. Modern anticholinergics include trihexyphenidyl (Artane), benztropine mesylate (Cogentin), ethopropazine (Parsidol), diphenhydramine (Benadryl), biperiden (Akineton), and procyclidine (Kemadrin). Doses should begin small and be gradually titrated until satisfactory response or the appearance of rate-limiting side effects (Table 14-1).

The exact mechanisms of action in improving parkinsonian symptoms are unknown. However, the proposed mechanism involves the suppression of cholinergic overactivity in the brain. Anticholinergics improve tremor and rigidity by only 25 percent and are ineffective for bradykinesia and postural imbalances. They have a longer plasma half-life and may be useful as adjunctive therapy particularly in short-duration responders. These medications are not as potent as levodopa and, therefore, are usually not effective as long-term monotherapy.[25,30]

Toxicity The high incidence of significant side effects, particularly in the elderly, make the use of these compounds highly problematic.[32] These medications frequently cause confusion, disorientation, memory disturbances, and hallucinations. Other side effects include dry mouth and eyes, cycloplegia, constipation, and urinary retention (Table 14-3). Anticholinergics may delay gastric emptying, thereby complicating levodopa delivery to the small intestine when used as adjunctive therapy. Anticholinergic agents should not be abruptly stopped. Doing so can greatly exacerbate the parkinsonian symptoms.

PROTECTIVE THERAPY

Parkinson's disease is a progressive disorder. There must be an 80 percent reduction in substantia nigra neurons before a patient becomes symptomatic. There is also a normal age-related decline in these neurons. It is possible that the progression of the disease as well as the transition from the long-duration responder to the short-duration responder may be related to the continued decline in substantia nigra neurons. Treatments which slow or stop the continued decline may then slow the progression of the disease and the transition to the short-duration response, which makes symptomatic treatment problematic.

Selegiline may slow the progression of parkinsonian symptoms. The development of this drug was a result of research on a "designer drug" called *MPTP* (*n*-methyl-4-phenyl-1,2,3,6-tetrahydropyridine), which causes selective degeneration of the substantia nigra and parkinsonism in experimental animals and in humans. However, MPTP must first be converted to 1-methyl-4-phenyl-pyridinium ion $(MPP)^+$ by MAO in order to produce toxicity. Blockage of MAO blocks the toxicity of MPTP in experimental animals. This leads to the testing of selegiline in slowing progression of Parkinson's disease.

Two studies of de novo patients demonstrated increased time to development of symptoms severe enough to require medical treatment in patients on selegiline compared to those on placebo.[33,34] This endpoint of the studies could have been complicated by any symptomatic benefit of selegiline. However, both studies included a wash-in and a wash-out period which would identify any symptomatic benefit of the selegiline. In one study there was no difference as a result of the wash-in or wash-out, suggesting little or no symptomatic benefit.[33] In the second study a significant wash-in effect was noted, suggesting a symptomatic effect.[34] However, when the population was subdivided into those with and those without a wash-in effect, selegiline still showed a prolonged time to the end point even in patients without a wash-in effect.

The data support MAO-B inhibition as slowing the progression of the symptoms. It is problematic whether slowing of symptom progression translates to decreased destruction of substantia nigra neurons. However, slowing of only the symptoms can have significant health, psychologic, and economic advantages.

TREATMENT STRATEGIES

The specific approach utilized in any given patient depends on age, risks of adverse effects, and to a lesser extent, the stage of disease. Potency is not generally a consideration because it is not predictive of response. Specific approaches differ among different experts.

Assuming the protective effect of selegiline, most patients should be started on selegiline. If it were possible to identify those patients with insignificant remaining substantia nigra pars compacta neurons, selegiline would not be indicated in those patients. Currently, it is not possible to identify those patients. Short-duration responders may be shown to have insignificant nigra neurons and would not warrant selegiline. Selegiline may provide sufficient symptomatic benefit so that other medications are not needed. Some patients whose symptoms are not disabling or embarrassing may not require any further treatment.

The choice of agent for symptomatic treatment is predicated on assessing the risk of side effects. Generally, carbidopa-levodopa compounds are better tolerated than the anticholinergics and direct dopaminergic agents, especially in the elderly. However, if the development of dyskinesias and motor fluctuations is consequent to levodopa exposure, then a reasonable argument can be made for using other agents first. This issue is further complicated by the possibility that it is the pulsatile administration of levodopa associated with regular Sinemet which is responsible. Sinemet CR may not carry that risk. However, this issue remains unresolved.

Generally, younger patients tolerate the anticholinergics and direct dopaminergic agents better than the elderly. Younger patients face a longer illness duration and, therefore, a longer duration of exposure to levodopa if instituted early. Younger patients could be started on anticholinergic medications or direct dopamine agonists first. Generally, if these agents help but are insufficient, the next drug can be added. If the original drug was of no help, it is gradually discontinued as the second drug is started. When levodopa-carbidopa therapy is needed, indirect evidence favors use of Sinemet CR.

Elderly patients are less likely to tolerate anticholinergic and direct dopaminergic agonist agents. Most specialists use levodopa-carbidopa compounds as first choice for symptomatic relief. These compounds are titrated by considering peak-dose effects and duration of response. Many parkinsonologists will introduce direct dopaminergic agents when the duration of levodopa effect becomes impractically short or some arbitrary level of daily levodopa is reached, such as 5000 mg in 1 day.

Selegiline may be used as adjunctive therapy to increase the effectiveness and duration of response to regular levodopa-carbidopa compounds. Selegiline is unlikely to provide significant benefit as adjunctive to Sinemet CR. Similarly, the direct dopaminergic agonists may be useful adjuncts to regular levodopa-carbidopa treatment in patients whose dosage interval becomes impractically short. However, direct dopaminergic agonists are unlikely to be useful as adjuncts to Sinemet CR.

REFERENCES

1. Wooten GF: Progress in understanding the pathophysiology of treatment-related fluctuations in Parkinson's disease. *Ann Neurol* 23:363–365, 1988.
2. Fabbrini G, Mouradin MM, Juncos JL, et al: Motor fluctuations in Parkinson's disease: central pathophysiological mechanisms. *Ann Neurol* 23(Part I): 366–371, 1988.
3. Nutt JG, Woodward WR, Hammerstad JP, et al: The "on-off" phenomenon in Parkinson's disease. *N Engl J Med* 310: 483–488, 1984.

4. Kurlan R, Rubin AJ, Miller C, et al: Duodenal delivery of levodopa for on-off fluctuations in parkinsonism: preliminary observations. *Ann Neurol* 20: 262-265, 1986.
5. Cedarbaum JM, Hoey M, McDowell FH: A double-blind crossover comparison of Sinemet CR4 and Sinemet 25/100 in patients with Parkinson's disease and fluctuating motor performance. *J Neurol Neurosurg Psychiatr* 52: 207-212, 1989.
6. Muenter MD, Tyce GM: L-Dopa therapy of Parkinson's disease: plasma L-dopa concentration, therapeutic response, and side effects. *Mayo Clin Proc* 46: 231-239, 1971.
7. Goetz LG, Tanner CM, Shannon KM, et al: Controlled-release carbidopa, levodopa (CR-4 Sinemet) in Parkinson's disease patients with and without motor fluctuations. *Neurology* 38: 1143-1146, 1988.
8. Juncos JL, Engber TM, Raisman R, et al: Continuous and intermittent levodopa differentially affect basal ganglia function. *Ann Neurol* 25: 473-478, 1989.
9. Bernheimer H, Birkmayer W, Hornykiewicz O: Brain dopamine and the syndrome of Parkinson and Huntington: Clinical, morphological and neurochemical correlations. *J Neurol Sci* 20: 415-455, 1973.
10. Marsden CD, Parkes JD, Quinn N: Fluctuations of disability in Parkinson's disease—clinical aspects, in Marsden CD, Fahn S: (eds): *Movement Disorders*. Butterworth Scientific, London, 1982, pp 96-122.
11. Lloyd KG, Davidson L, Hornykiewicz O: The neurochemistry of Parkinson's disease: effect of L-dopa therapy. *J Pharm Exp Ther* 196: 453-464, 1975.
12. Campbell NRC, Hasinoff B: Ferrous sulfate reduces levodopa bioavailability: chelation as a possible mechanism. *Clin Pharmacol Ther* 45: 220-223, 1989.
13. Gillespie NG et al: Diets affecting treatment of parkinsonism with levodopa. *J Am Diet Assoc* 62: 525-530, 1973.
14. Boomsma F, Meerwaldt JD, Man in't Veld AJ, et al: Treatment of idiopathic parkinsonism with L-dopa in the absence and presence of decarboxylase inhibitors: effects on plasma levels of L-dopa, dopa decarboxylase, catecholamines and 3-O-methyldopa. *J Neurol* 236: 223-230, 1989.
15. Cedarbaum JM, Kutt H, Dhar AK, et al: Effect of supplemental carbidopa on bioavailability of L-dopa. *Clin Neuropharm* 9: 153-159, 1986.
16. Mouradin MM, Juncos JL, Fabbrini G, et al: Motor fluctuations in Parkinson's disease: central pathophysiological mechanisms. *Ann Neurol* 23(Part II): 366-371, 1988.
17. Mourdian MM, Heuser IJE, Baronti F, Chase TN: Modification of central dopaminergic mechanisms by continuous levodopa therapy for advanced Parkinson's disease. *Neurology* 39: 888-891, 1989.
18. Ahlskog JE, Muenter MD, McManis PG, et al: Controlled-release sinemet (CR-4): a double-blind crossover study in patients with fluctuating Parkinson's disease. *Mayo Clin Proc* 63: 876-886, 1988.
19. Cedarbaum JM, Hoey M, McDowell FH: A double-blind crossover comparison of sinemet CR4 and standard sinemet 25/100 in patients with Parkinson's disease and fluctuating motor performance. *J Neurol Neurosurg Psychiatr* 52: 207-212, 1989.
20. Mark MH, Sage JI: Long-term efficacy of controlled-release carbidopa/levodopa in patients with advanced Parkinson's disease. *Ann Clin Lab Sci* 19(6): 415-421, 1989.
21. Mark MH, Sage JI: Controlled-release carbidopa-levodopa (sinemet) in combination with standard sinemet in advanced Parkinson's disease. *Ann Clin Lab Sci* 19(2): 101-106, 1989.
22. Yeh KC, August TF, Bush OF, et al: Pharmacokinetics and bioavailability of Sinemet CR: a summary of human studies. *Neurology* 39(suppl 2): 25-38, 1989.
23. Pfeiffer RF, Kang J, Graber B, et al: Clozapine for psychosis in Parkinson's disease. *Movement Disorders* 5: 239-242, 1990.
24. Teychenne PF et al: Interactions of levodopa with inhibitors of monoamine oxidase and L-aromatic amino acid decarboxylase. *Clin Pharmacol Ther* 18: 273-276, 1975.
25. Berg MJ et al: Parkinsonism—drug treatment: Part I. *DICP Ann Pharmacother* 21: 10-21, 1987.
26. Golbe LI: Deprenyl as symptomatic therapy in Parkinson's disease. *Clin Neuropharmacol* 11: 387-400, 1988.

27. Giovannini P, Martiignoni E, Piccolo I, et al: Deprenyl in Parkinson's disease: a two year study in the different evolutive stages. *J Neural Transm* 22(suppl): 235–246, 1986.
28. Eldepryl package information, Somerset Pharmaceuticals, Denville, New Jersey, 1989.
29. Langtry HD, Clissold SP: Pergolide: a review of its pharmacological properties and therapeutic potential in Parkinson's disease. *Drugs* 39: 491–506, 1990.
30. Tanner CM, Goetz CG, Glantz RH, et al: Pergolide mesylate: four years experience in Parkinson's disease. *Adv Neurol* 45: 547–549, 1986.
31. Erwin WG: Current concepts in clinical therapeutics: Parkinson's disease. *Ther Rev* 5: 742–745, 1986.
32. Aminof MJ: Parkinson's disease in the elderly: current management strategies. *Geriatrics* 42(7): 31–37, 1987.
33. The Parkinson Study Group: Effect of deprenyl on the progression of disability in early Parkinson's disease. *N Engl J Med* 321: 1364–1371, 1989.
34. Tetrud JW, Langston JW: The effect of deprenyl (selegiline) on the natural history of Parkinson's disease. *Science* 245: 519–522, 1989.

CHAPTER

15

DEPRESSION

Rubin Bressler

Depression is probably the most common psychiatric problem in the elderly population. The prevalence of major depression ranges from 2 to 14 percent, and an additional 15 percent experience milder forms of depression.[1-3] Depression is the most frequent psychiatric diagnosis in hospitalized elderly patients.[4]

Depression in the elderly has been characterized as early or late onset using the criterion of onset before or after age 60.[5,6] Depression onset in later life is more often associated with medical illness, whereas genetic and familial factors are more common in early onset depression.[5,6]

The signs and symptoms of depression in elderly people may represent an appropriate response to adverse life events such as loss of friends, health, and mobility, and financial difficulties. Such reverses cause a sadness that is of brief duration and appropriate intensity. Major depressions are disorders from which elderly patients usually recover and which are amenable to successful treatment.[7,8] Many depressed patients seek help from primary care physicians rather than psychiatrists. There are ample data attesting to the underrecognition and misdiagnosis of depression by primary care physicians.[9-11] The failure of primary care physicians to diagnose and treat depression is unfortunate, since only around 20 percent of depressed patients are treated by psychiatrists.[9-11]

The signs and symptoms of major depression should allow the alert physician to readily make the diagnosis. The diagnostic criteria of major depression are shown in Table 15-1.

Table 15-1 DSM-III-R Diagnostic criteria of major depression

For the diagnosis of major depression, at least five of the following (which must include 1 and 2) have been present during the same 2-week period:

1. Depressed mood
2. Diminished interest or pleasure in all or almost all activities
3. Weight loss or weight gain or decreased or increased appetite
4. Insomnia or hypersomnia
5. Psychomotor agitation or retardation
6. Fatigue or loss of energy
7. Feelings of worthlessness or excessive or inappropriate guilt
8. Diminished ability to think or concentrate or indecisiveness
9. Recurrent thoughts of death or suicidal ideation

DEPRESSED PATIENTS

Depressed patients generally lose interest in and fail to find enjoyment in usually pleasurable work, social, and sexual activity. They usually describe themselves as feeling sad and blue and not caring about anything and sometimes experience delusional or paranoid thinking. Frequently they become preoccupied with somatic symptoms (i.e., headache, constipation) and/or are overly sensitive to criticism, particularly in atypical depression, wherein mood may fluctuate dramatically upward in response to positive experiences or plummet in response to negative events.

Depression in the elderly is more often associated with medical illness and is characterized by early morning insomnia, somatization (*hypochondriasis*), agitation, and delusions.[8,12] Atypical presentations (*masked depressions*) are more common in the elderly. Masked depressions present more somatic and cognitive symptoms and lesser degrees of emotional manifestations of depression. These patients may deny sadness and anxiety and attribute their discomfort to medical illness.[3,8,13,14] This is often a difficult diagnosis, since many elderly people have organic illnesses and are taking drugs. The neurovegetative symptoms of depression are shown in Table 15-2. Some medical diseases associated with depression are shown in Table 15-3, and drugs which may cause depression are shown in Table 15-4.

Mania appearing for the first time in elderly patients is unusual.[15] Most patients have documented episodes of bipolar illness at an earlier age. Characteristically elderly manic patients have experienced recurrent cycles of mania and depression which have increased in frequency and intensity with aging.[15] The diagnosis of mania in the elderly is based on the usual criteria used in younger patients. However, certain features are more prominent in the elderly patient. These include confusion, paranoia, and some of the following:

1. Lability of affect, irritability
2. Flight of ideas with morbid or depressive content

3. Dysphoria with augmented psychomotor output (like *agitated depression*)
4. Long latency period between initial depressive episode and the onset of mania
5. Distractibility, diminished attention span, decreased concentration, and disorientation resembling dementia or delirium

The neurovegetative symptoms of mania are shown in Table 15-5.

Table 15-2 Neurovegetative symptoms of major affective disorders

Type of symptom	Depression
Physical	Anhedonia (decreased interest in things previously enjoyed; loss of sex drive)
	Fatigability, loss of energy
	Social withdrawal
	Psychomotor retardation or agitation
	Insomnia with fatigue
	Somatic complaints
	Loss of appetite, loss of weight
	Decreased hygiene
	Crying spells for no significant reason
Cognitive	Decreased ability to concentrate
	Indecisiveness
Emotional	Dysphoric mood, sad thoughts of or attempts at suicide
	Hopelessness, helplessness
	Worthlessness, guilt, shame

Source: From Lake CR, Moriarty KM, Alagna SW: Neurovegetative symptoms of major affective disorders—depression. *Psychiatr Clin North Am* 7:662, 1984. Reproduced with permission.

Table 15-3 Medical diseases that may produce depression

Endocrine system
Hypothyroidism, hyperthyroidism (apathetic), diabetes mellitus, hyperparathyroidism, Cushing's disease, Addison's disease

Central nervous system
Brain tumors, Parkinson's disease, multiple sclerosis, Alzheimer's disease, Huntington's disease

Cardiovascular system
Myocardial infarction, congestive heart failure, cerebrovascular accident

Miscellaneous
Rheumatoid arthritis, pancreatic disease, carcinoma, systemic lupus erythematosus, infectious disease, metabolic abnormalities, pernicious anemia, malnutrition

Table 15-4 Drugs that may produce depression

Antihypertensive and cardiovascular drugs
Guanethidine, methyldopa, reserpine, hydralazine, propranolol, metorolol, prazosin, clonidine, digitalis, procainamide
Sedative-hypnotic agent
Alcohol, chloral hydrate, benzodiazepines, barbiturates, meprobamate
Anti-inflammatory agents and analgesics
Indomethacin, phenylbutazone, opiates, pentazocine
Steroids
Corticosteroids, oral contraceptives, estrogen withdrawal
Miscellaneous
Antiparkinson drugs, antineoplastic agents, ethambutol, neuroleptic, stimulant withdrawal

PATHOPHYSIOLOGY OF DEPRESSION

Theories of the pathophysiology of depression involve two central nervous system (CNS) classes of neurons, the noradrenergic and the serotonergic. These neurons are separate and distinct, utilizing norepinephrine (NE) and 5-hydroxytryptamine (5-HT, or serotonin), respectively, as neurotransmitters. These neurotransmitters are stored in neuronal vesicles and released into the synaptic cleft following nerve stimulation.

Table 15-5 Neurovegetative symptoms of mania

Type of symptom	Mania
Physical	Increased activities and energy (inappropriate buying, phoning, driving, and sexual behavior)
	Increased gregariousness
	Increased talkativeness, pressured speech
	Decreased need for sleep without fatigue
	Increased intake of alcohol, drunkenness
	Physically threatening, combative, dangerous behavior
Cognitive	Distractibility
	Flight of ideas, speeded thinking, racing thoughts
	Poor judgment, impulsive actions and decisions
Emotional	Elevated mood, increased self-confidence, elation, euphoria, grandiosity
	Irritability, hostility
	Easily angered

Source: From Lake CR, Moriarty KM, Alagna SW: Neurovegetative symptoms

Two pools of NE are discernible: the vesicle pool and a protected cytoplasmic nonvesicle pool. The nonvesicle pool is not released by nerve action potentials but can be secreted by the action of some indirectly acting sympathomimetic drugs, such as tyramine. The released NE is cleared from the synapse primarily by neuronal reuptake (85 percent) and inactivated to a lesser extent by catechol-*0*-methyltransferase (COMT) (15 percent). The intraneuronal NE stores are actively turning over because of neuronal NE synthesis and catabolism catalyzed by mitochondrial monoamine oxidase (MAO) (Fig. 15-1).

The physiology of the serotonergic neurons and 5-HT, their neurotransmitter, is similar to the physiology of the noradrenergic system, although the serotonergic neurons affect different postsynaptic actions.

The physiology of neurotransmitters in the CNS is shown in Fig. 15-1. Some postsynaptic receptors are shown.

A number of hypotheses on the biologic nature of affective disorders (unipolar and bipolar depressions) have postulated a relationship between depression and CNS monoamine transmission.[3,8,16] These theories include the following:

1. *Permissive hypothesis.* Depression and mania are viewed as a continuum: decreases of both NE and 5-HT characterizing depression and decreases of 5-HT and increases of NE characterizing mania.
2. *Receptor sensitivity hypothesis.* Depression is considered to be due to abnormalities in the amine receptors. Antidepressant drug effects on amine receptors are slow and are consonant with clinical antidepressant drug efficacy. Postsynaptic receptor sensitivity changes are consistently produced by antidepressant drugs and electroconvulsive therapy (ECT). Following antidepressant therapy β-receptor sensitivity is decreased, α_2-receptor sensitivity is decreased, whereas α_1- and 5-HT-receptor sensitivities are increased.[17-19]

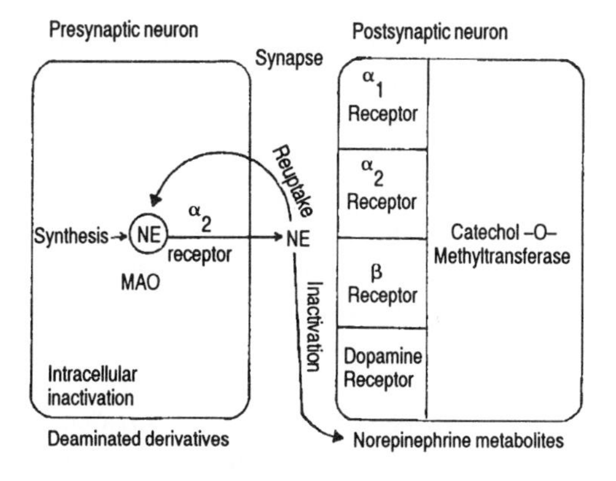

Figure 15-1 Physiology of neurotransmitters in the central nervous system. NE=norepinephrine; MAO=monoamine oxidase.

3. *Dysregulation hypothesis* postulates that in depression neuronal discharge is both erratic and increased. However, there is less NE released per stimulus. Changes are thought to be presynaptic and to involve the α_2 receptor. Tricyclic antidepressants (TCAs) desensitize the α_2 receptor and decrease the neuronal firing rate. This increases the NE released per nerve impulse.

Studies of blood, urine, and cerebrospinal fluid (CSF) monoamines and monoamine metabolites have been inconsistent in both unipolar and bipolar depressions.[19,20] The several theories on the pathophysiology of depression are as yet unproven.

The rates of major depression in the elderly are not increased.[8,12] However, much of the depression in the elderly occurs in a setting of bereavement, isolation, chronic illness, disability, and financial stress. The elderly depressed patient has a good prognosis for recovery with antidepressant therapy. The prognosis is better if the patient is under 70 years of age and the depression is less than 2 years in duration.[3,8] Although initial drug-induced recovery rates are around 90 percent, 75 percent later relapse if antidepressant maintenance therapy is not employed.[3,8] The overall prognosis for elderly depressed patients who receive antidepressant therapy is as follows: one-third stay well following therapy, one-third recover but later relapse, and one-third remain depressed. The relapse is often successfully treated with the drug to which the patient initially responded but which was later discontinued.

Depression is the emotional disorder of the elderly that is perhaps most amenable to successful therapy. As with other diseases of the elderly, depression is confounded by a variety of special factors, including chronic cardiovascular disease, renal disease, and organic brain syndromes. The use of cyclic antidepressants (CAs) and monoamine oxidase inhibitors (MAOIs) by the elderly is attended by the risk of cardiovascular toxicities and anticholinergic effects. These adverse effects are more frequent and more severe in a population with a higher incidence of cardiovascular disease, renal disease, and cerebrovascular disease.[7]

Depression in the elderly is not a direct cause of mortality in that no characteristic morbid target organ pathology has been ascertained. However, suicide deriving from depression is a distinct threat. Elderly people with spouse loss due to divorce or death who are living alone with decreased capacity for self-care due to physical illnesses are more prone to experience depression and have thoughts of wishing to die. There are a greater number of suicides among elderly men. The prospect of suicide in the elderly depressed patient who is moderately to markedly afflicted with characteristic signs and symptoms should lead the primary care physician both to seek psychiatric help and to hospitalize the patient.

When the diagnosis of depression has been considered in elderly patients, the medical and psychiatric history must be carefully assessed. A number of organic illnesses have been associated with depression (Table 15-3), and a variety of pharmacologic agents used in the therapy of some diseases found in elderly patients, such as hypertension, pain syndromes, insomnia, and allergies, may be associated with onset of depression (Table 15-4). A complete drug history, including over-the-counter drug use, is important in treatment consideration of the elderly depressed patient. This is essential to rule out both drug and disease contributions to the depression but also to avoid drug-drug interactions with the CAs or MAOIs, which may be used for therapy of the depression. Some of these antidepressant drugs, other drug interactions, and their consequences are shown in Tables 15-6 and 15-7.

The primary care physician often has the initial contact with the patient. The presentation made usually encompasses the criteria for depression (Table 15-1). The history must ascertain precipitating events such as loss of a loved one, loss of close friends, retirement, isolation, moving to a new setting, and financial stresses. Onset of depression is usually a rapid syndrome of signs and symptoms. These may appear in a few days to weeks, unlike senile dementia, which is a more gradual course of mental and physical deterioration extending over years in an unrelenting progressive manner.

CYCLIC ANTIDEPRESSANT DRUGS

The CAs are chemically similar to the phenothiazines and share a number of their properties. The 6-6-6 ring structure of the phenothiazines is replaced by an ethylene bridge in the middle ring of the TCAs, converting it to a 6-7-6 structure. This change converts the relatively two-dimensional planar structure of the phenothiazines to a skewed three-dimensional structure. The TCAs contain tertiary or secondary propylamino side chains. The drugs available in the United States are shown in Fig. 15-2.

Pharmacology The pharmacology of the TCAs and CAs has been extensively studied, but the mechanisms responsible for their antidepressant efficacy are not known. This is understandable in light of the uncertain nature of the pathophysiology of depression and the absence of animal models in which to study the disease and its response to therapy. In animal studies, the CAs have been found to alter a number of neuronal adrenergic receptors.[7,17-19] Changes in adrenergic receptors due to chronic TCA treatment have been proposed as being consistent with the clinical efficacy of the antidepressant drugs. The presynaptic α_2 receptors become less sensitive with chronic antidepressant therapy, resulting in an increased neuronal release of NE per nerve impulse. Increased sensitivity of the postsynaptic α_1-adrenergic receptors occurs with TCA therapy, whereas postsynaptic β-adrenergic receptor sensitivity decreases.[17,19] The relationship of TCA action and receptor responses may not be important indices of drug potency or efficacy.

The CA compounds marketed in the United States are classified as tertiary amines, secondary amines, and atypical antidepressants. These are shown in Fig. 15-2.

Table 15-6 Drug interactions with psychotropic drugs: cyclic antidepressants

Drug	Clinically significant	Mechanism of action	Clinical effect
Anticholinergics Antihistamines Neuroleptics	Yes	Additive effect, Trihexyphenidyl increases metabolism of antidepressant	Increased anticholinergic toxicity, decreased blood levels of antidepressant
Epinephrine	Yes	Unopposed beta-mediated vasodilation	Augmentation of hypotension, increased bleeding during nasal surgery
Cimetidine	Yes	Interference with hepatic metabolism of antidepressant	Increased toxicity secondary to increased blood level of antidepressant
Methylphenidate Acetaminophen Oral contraceptives Chloramphenicol Disulfiram Isoniazid	?	Interference with hepatic metabolism	Increased toxicity secondary to increased TCA blood level
MAOI Guanethidine Bethanidine Debrisoquine	Yes	Blockade of reuptake of neurotransmitter	Decreased antidepressant effect, decreased antihypertensive effect
Propoxyphene	?	Decreased hepatic metabolism, displacement of antidepressants from plasma protein-binding sites	Increased doxepin toxicity, theoretic increase in free fraction of antidepressant
Clonidine	Yes	Probably stimulates CNS α_2 NE secretion	Decreased antidepressant effect
Quinidine Procaine amide Disopyramide	Yes	Additive effects on cardiac conduction	Prolongation of cardiac conduction, heart block
Coumarin anticoagulants	?	Increased metabolism of anticoagulant	Instability of anticoagulation
Neuroleptics	?	Inhibition of anti-depressant metabolism	Higher plasma concentration
Thiazide diuretics	Yes	Decreased intravascular volume	Decreased blood pressure

Table 15-6 (*continued*) Drug interactions with psychotropic drugs: cyclic antidepressants

Drug	Clinically significant	Mechanism of action	Clinical effect
Barbiturates Nonbarbiturate hypnotics (e.g., glutethimide, methaqualone) Dichlorphenazone Rifampin Doxycycline Griseofulvin Phenylbutazone Carbamazepine Phenytoin Chloral hydrate	?	Increased metabolism of antidepressant	Decreased plasma concentration
Activated charcoal Kaolin	?	Decreased absorption of antidepressant	Helpful in antidepressant overdoses
Triiodothyronine (T_3)	?	Not established	Conflicting reports about potentiation of antidepressant effect

Source: From Salzman C: Psychotropic drug dosages and drug interactions, in Salzman C (ed): *Clinical Geriatric Psychopharmacology*. McGraw-Hill, New York, 1984, pp 206–207. Reproduced with permission.

Table 15-7 Antidepressant interactions

Unwanted effect	Interacting drug	Mechanism	Onset	Significance
Anticholinergic	Antihistamines Antiparkinson drugs Antipsychotics Meperidine	Additive effects	Fast	Minor
Sedation	Narcotics Sedative hypnotics Antipsychotics Alcohol	Additive effects	Fast	Minor
Sympathetic stimulation	Norepinephrine Epinephrine Phenylephrine	Additive effects	Fast Fast Fast	Major Major Moderate
Cardiotoxicity	Quinidine Procainamide Disopyramide	Additive cardiac conduction effects	Fast	Minor

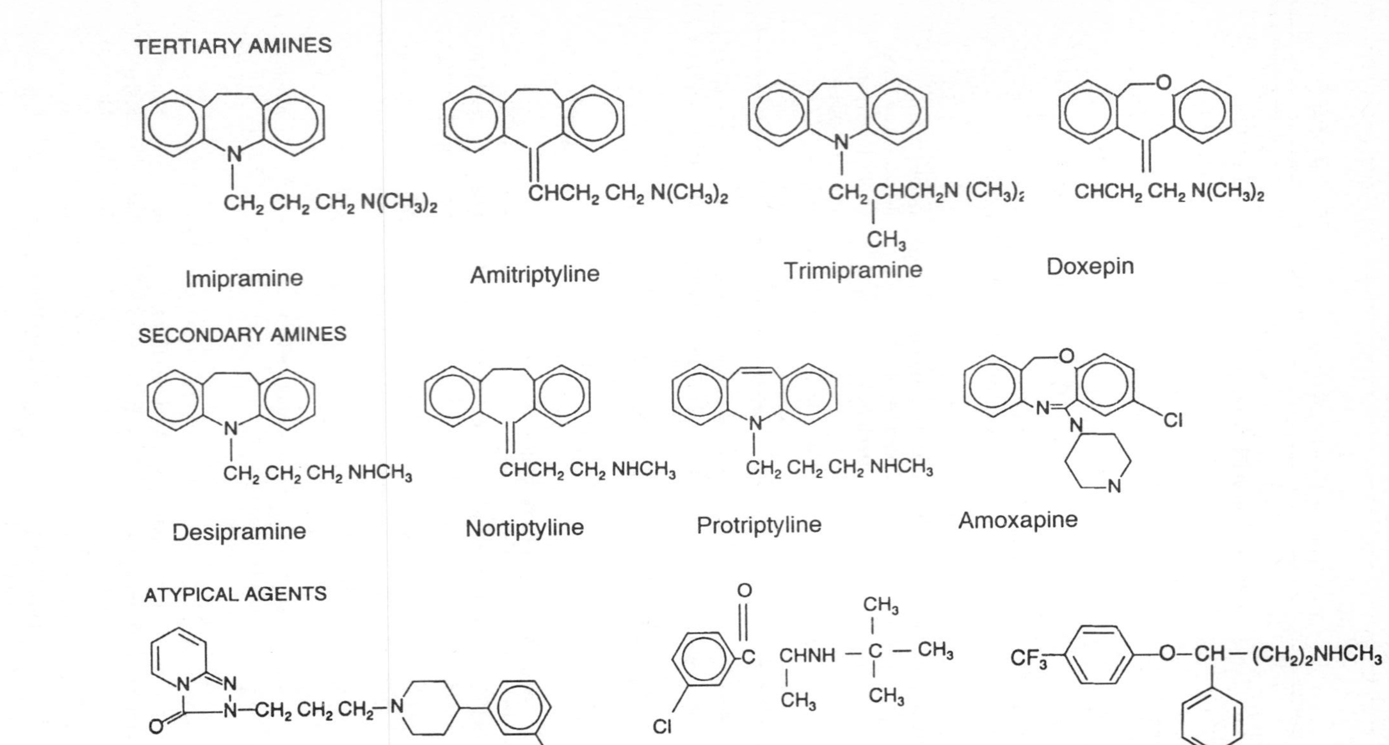

Figure 15-2 Chemical structures of antidepressants.

Table 15-8 Pharmacokinetics of cyclic antidepressants

Antidepressants	Availability (oral), %	Bound in plasma %	V_d, L/kg	Half-life, h	Dosage range, mg	Plasma level, ng/mL
Secondary amines						
Protriptyline	77–93	92	21–23	67–89	15–60	100–200
Nortriptyline	46–56	92	14–22	18–44	50–200	50–150
Desipramine	51	90	26–42	12–24	75–300	40–160
Tertiary amines						
Amitriptyline	37–59	95	12–16	10–22	75–300	60–220[a]
Doxepin	17–37	ND	12–28	11–23	75–300	30–150[a]
Imipramine	19–35	95	15–31	11–25	75–300	100–300
Newer agents						
Amoxapine	ND	90	ND	8–30	100–600	180[a]
Bupropion	10	80	1.4–3.2	8–24	200–300	ND
Fluoxetine	100	94	12–97	24–72	20–80	ND
Maprotiline	37	88	23	27–57	150–300	200–300
Trazodone	ND	92	ND	10–12	50–600	ND

ND = Not done.
[a]Parent compound plus active metabolite.

Pharmacokinetics of Cyclic Antidepressants

The antidepressants are rapidly absorbed from the gastrointestinal tract. They undergo extensive first-pass extraction by the liver, where they are metabolized.[21,22] There is a low-to-moderate order of bioavailability of these drugs, as shown in Table 15-8. The antidepressants are highly bound to plasma proteins and have a large apparent volume of distribution because of their lipid solubility.[21,22] These drugs are widely distributed in tissues, leaving only a small fraction of the body's content of the drug in the blood. This property precludes significant drug removal in overdose cases by either hemoperfusion or dialysis.[21]

The value of plasma concentrations of the CAs is unsettled. Blood levels vary widely following standard oral doses.[21,22] An unusual situation has been ascertained in the case of nortriptyline: There appears to be a blood level below which therapeutic efficacy is not obtained and above which clinical effects are minimal. Antidepressant doses are generally determined by patient responses in regard to efficacy and/or unacceptable toxicity. Amitriptyline and imipramine are among the more commonly used antidepressant drugs. Studies with these agents have shown a linear dose-response relationship.[23]

Mechanism of Action of the Cyclic Antidepressants

The CAs have a number of well-characterized neuronal effects. These include inhibition of neurotransmitter reuptake, stimulation of neurotransmitter release via inhibition of the α_2-adrenergic receptor, and inhibition of a number of other receptors.[17,19] The correlation of the antidepressant drug effects on neurotransmitters and/or receptors is not known, but the drug effects on receptors correlate with adverse drug reactions. The effects of the several classes of CA drugs on neurotransmitter reuptake inhibition are shown in Tables 15-9 and 15-10.

The three types of antidepressants shown in Tables 15-9 and 15-10 have differential effects on the inhibition of neuronal reuptake of NE and 5-HT. The tertiary amine antidepressants are the more potent blockers of 5-HT reuptake, whereas the secondary amine antidepressants more potently inhibit NE reuptake.[7,21,24,25] The atypical antidepressants have predominant effects on either NE reuptake (amoxapine, maprotiline) or 5-HT reuptake (trazodone, fluoxetine).

A number of unwanted effects of the antidepressant drugs are to varying degrees inseparable from the drugs' efficacy. This is because of the binding of these drugs to the several receptors shown in Table 15-11. The adverse effect is a function of the potency of antidepressant binding. The several prominent adverse effects follow below.

Sedation The CAs are sedative drugs. The quality of the sedative effect is similar to that of the phenothiazines. The onset of the sedative effect is immediate, unlike that of the antidepressant effect.[21,24,26] The sedative effect decreases over time, further distinguishing it from the drugs' antidepressant effects. Tertiary amines (Fig. 15-2) such as amitriptyline, doxepin, and imipramine are more sedative than

Table 15-9 Neurotransmitter actions

Antidepressants	Reuptake inhibition[a,b] NE	5-HT	DA	Anticholinergic potency[b]	Neurologic[b] Sedation	Seizures	Cardiac[b] Orthostasis	Arrhythmias
Secondary amines								
Protriptyline	+++	++	-	+++	+	++	++	++++
Nortriptyline	+++	++	-	+++	+++	++	+	+++
Desipramine	++++	+	-	++	++	++	+++	+++
Tertiary amines								
Doxepin	+	++	-	+++	++++	+++	++	++
Amitriptyline	++	++++	-	++++	++++	+++	+++	++++
Imipramine	+++	+++	-	+++	+++	+++	++++	++++
Trimipramine	+	+	-	++++	++++	+++	+++	++++
Newer agents								
Amoxapine	+++	++	-	+++	++	+++	+	++
Bupropion	-	-	+	-	+	+++	-	-
Fluoxetine	-	+++	-	-	+	+	+	+
Maprotiline	+++	+	-	+++	+++	++++	++	+++
Trazodone	-	++	-	-	+++	++	+++	+

[a]NE = norepinephrine; 5-HT = serotonin; DA = dopamine.
[b]High = ++++; moderate = +++; low = ++; very low = +; none = -.

Table 15-10 In vitro inhibition by antidepressants and other agents of uptake of amines in brain tissue

Agent	Potency (IC_{50}, nmol/L)			Potency ratio
	NE	5-HT	DA	(NE : 5-HT)
Typical tricyclic type				
Desipramine	1.2	1,100	9,000	916
Protriptyline	1.4	1,000	5,200	714
Amoxapine	14	570	46	40
Maprotiline	14	13,500	9,300	960
Nortriptyline	20	1,000	5,300	50
Imipramine	30	260	16,000	9
Amitriptyline	50	170	5,800	3
Doxepin	100	1,850	7,700	18
Atypical tricyclic type				
Fluoxetine	740	6.9	12,000	0.009
Bupropion	3,000	19,000	1,800	6
Trazodone	10,000	760	60,000	13

Source: From Baldessarini RJ: Chemotherapy in Psychiatry: Principles and Practice, 1985, Chap. 4, p.154. Reprinted by permission of the publishers from *Chemotherapy in Psychiatry: Principles and Practice, Revised and Enlarged Edition*, by Ross J. Baldessarini, M.D., Cambridge, Massachusetts: Harvard University Press. Copyright © 1985, 1977 by the President and Fellows of Harvard College.

are secondary amines such as desipramine and nortriptyline. Protriptyline is without sedative action.[21] Drug choice is sometimes made on the basis of the sedative action. Elderly patients who have hypersomnia and are depressed are not good candidates for treatment with tertiary amine TCA. Hyperkinetic, depressed elderly patients might benefit from the more sedative TCAs because they may correct sleep disturbances quickly.[7,25,27]

Anticholinergic activity The TCAs have both peripheral and central anticholinergic activity.[21,24] This activity is not considered to play a significant role in the drugs' antidepressant activity. The available agents have different anticholinergic potency: Amitriptyline is the strongest and desipramine is the weakest of the TCAs but not the weakest of all the CAs.[21,27-29] These data are summarized in Tables 15-9 and 15-12. Because the anticholinergic effects are usually undesirable for elderly patients, drug choice may be based on this adverse effect. The problems of precipitating glaucoma, urinary retention, and excessive sedation must be considered. Moreover, the effects of anticholinergic drugs on drying of the mouth and visual accommodation may be disturbing to elderly patients who are anxious and depressed. The TCAs are more potent anticholinergic agents than the phenothiazines. The newer antidepressant drugs, which will be discussed later, have minimal anticholinergic activity.

Antihistamine activity The TCAs have been shown to be blockers of the histamine H_1 and H_2 receptors.[21,24] Other than sedation, however, the clinical signifi-

Table 15-11 Potency of antidepressants and other agents for amine receptors (IC_{50}, nmol/L)

Agent	Cholinergic	Adrenergic			Dopaminergic	Serotonin		Histamine	
	ACh_m	α_1	α_2	β	(D-2)	$5\text{-}HT_1$	$5\text{-}HT_2$	H_1	H_2
Typical tricyclic type									
Amitriptyline	34	26	765	6,800	290	1,480	13	0.1	54
Protriptyline	70	200	6,700	3,100	360	—	640	48	420
Doxepin	138	24	1,000	7,100	380	720	250	0.03	160
Imipramine	186	74	3,200	38,000	610	5,000	245	16	153
Nortriptyline	550	66	2,100	15,000	800	920	40	17	400
Maprotiline	590	90	9,100	—	—	—	—	—	—
Amoxapine	1,000	50	2,600	—	100	—	—	—	—
Desipramine	1,200	136	7,000	4,200	980	9,500	540	250	320
Atypical tricyclic type									
Fluoxetine	8,000	8,000	13,000	10,000	6,600	>10,000	1,300	—	—
Bupropion	47,600	50,000	>100,000	—		—	—	—	—
Trazodone	320,000	70	1,000	>10,000	3,000	1,700	111	460	50,000
Others									
Atropine	2	—	—	—	—	—	—	—	—
Chlorpromazine	5,700	4	>10,000	25	3,500	15	28	41	300

Source: From Baldessarini RJ: Chemotherapy in Psychiatry: Principles and Practice, 1985, Chap. 4, pp 156–157. Reprinted by permission of the publishers from *Chemotherapy in Psychiatry: Principles and Practice, Revised and Enlarged Edition*, by Ross J. Baldessarini, M.D., Cambridge, Massachusetts: Harvard University Press.

Table 15-12 Potency of antidepressants in blocking receptors

Drug	Muscarinic receptor blockade	Histaminergic-H_1-receptor blockade	α_1-Adrenergic receptor blockade
Amitriptyline	++++	+++	++++
Amoxapine	±	++	+++
Desipramine	+	+	++
Doxepin	+++	++++	++++
Fluoxetine	±	±	±
Imipramine	+++	++	+++
Maprotiline	±	+++	+++
Nortriptyline	++	++	+++
Protriptyline	++++	++	++
Trazodone	0	+	++++
Trimipramine	+++	++++	++++

cance of the antihistaminic effects are unknown. It has been suggested that the H_1-receptor blockade plays a role in the appetite-stimulating effects of the TCAs.[24] A serious adverse effect of TCA therapy is weight gain, which might result from blockade of the H_1 receptor in the brain. This could be a consideration for the use of TCAs by obese elderly patients. The H_1-receptor blocking activity of these agents does not parallel their anticholinergic activity (Table 15-12). Trazodone, fluoxetine, and bupropion have minimal to no H_1-receptor blocking activity, and their use is not associated with weight gain.

α-Adrenergic blockade Tricyclic antidepressants cause both central and peripheral α-adrenergic receptor blockade.[24,27] This results in orthostatic hypotension in a significant number of patients being treated with TCAs.[28,29] Animal studies have demonstrated that the drugs bind to α_1-adrenergic receptors in the brain. The tertiary amine TCAs (amitriptyline, doxepin) have a greater affinity for the α-adrenergic receptor than do the secondary amine TCAs (desipramine, nortriptyline). The tertiary amine agents are very effective for patients with psychomotor agitation (Tables 15-11 and 15-12), but they have more pronounced sedative and hypotensive effects (Table 15-9). The secondary amine TCAs are less sedative and hypotensive (Table 15-9). The newer antidepressants bupropion and fluoxetine have no α-adrenergic blocking activity, whereas trazodone has moderate α-adrenergic blocking activity.

The sedative and hypotensive effects may be important for the treatment of elderly patients, for whom decreases in blood pressure can precipitate cardiac arrhythmias and ischemia and in whom sedation predisposes to falls and other accidents.[21,30,31]

Receptor blockade by antidepressants and associated adverse affects are shown in Tables 15-13 and 15-13a.

Table 15-13 Receptor blockade of antidepressants

	Receptor				
Drugs	Cholinergic	Histaminergic	α_1	α_2	DA
Imipramine (Tofranil)	+2	+2	+3	+1	+1
Desipramine (Norpramin)	+1	+1	+2	+/0	+1
Amitriptyline (Elavil)	+3	+3	+4	+2	+1
Nortriptyline (Pamelor)	+1	+1	+3	+1	+1
Doxepin (Sinequan)	+2	+4	+4	+2	+1
Amoxapine (Asendin)	+/0	+2	+3	+1	+2
Maprotiline (Ludiomil)	+/0	+3	+3	+/0	+1
Trazodone (Desyrel)	0	+1	+4	+2	+1
Fluoxetine (Prozac)	+/0	+/0	+/0	+/0	+1
Bupropion (Wellbutrin)	0	+/0	+/0	0	0
Reference drug	Atropine (belladonna alkaloid) +4	Diphenhydramine (Benadryl) +2	Phentolamine (Regitine) +4	Phentolamine (Regitine) +3	Haloperidol (Haldol) +4

Source: From Richelson E: Antidepressant: pharmacology and clinical use, in Karasu TB (ed): *Treatments of Psychiatric Disorders*, Chap. 164, pp 1773–1787, 1989. Copyright 1989, the American Psychiatric Association. Reprinted by permission.

Table 15-13a Potential adverse effects of antidepressant drugs' blockade of receptors

Cholinergic	Histaminergic	α_1	α_2	DA
Blurred vision	Sedation, drowsiness	Postural hypotension	Block antihypertensive effects of clonidine, guanabenz, and methyldopa	Extrapyramidal movement disorders
Dry mouth	Weight gain	Dizziness		Endocrine changes (prolactin elevation)
Sinus tachycardia	Hypotension	Reflex tachycardia		
Constipation	Potentiation of CNS depressants	Additive with antihypertensive prazosin		
Urinary retention				
Memory dysfunction				
Decreased sweating				

Drug Commentary

Maprotiline has a longer half-life than most antidepressants (around 2 days).[32,33] This could promote drug accumulation in elderly patients. Maprotiline has two adverse effects which are relatively unique to antidepressant therapy. Around 5 percent of maprotiline users develop an erythematous skin rash within the first 2 weeks of drug use, and drug use may result in seizures at both elevated and therapeutic serum drug concentrations in normal patients and perhaps more so in those with preexisting neurologic diseases. It has been suggested that an active maprotiline metabolite may be responsible for the seizures.[34] The drug does not have therapeutic advantages for elderly patients. Its cardiotoxicity and seizure potential in association with its delayed excretion makes it unsuitable for elderly patients.

Amoxapine Pharmacologic tolerance within 6 to 12 weeks has been reported.[32,35] The drug has neuroleptic adverse effects including tardive dyskinesia, and overdoses have resulted in renal failure, seizures, and high lethality.[32] The claims of earlier onset of antidepressant have not been substantiated.[32]

Trazodone An inhibitor of 5-HT reuptake, trazodone has been found to be inactive in some preclinical animal behavioral screening tests for antidepressant activity, whereas it has demonstrated antianxiety and sedative effects. The efficacy of trazodone as an antidepressant has been questioned, whereas it has been successfully used in anxiety disorders and agitated states.[32,36] Trazodone has been considered to be safe in regard to cardiotoxicity. However, arrhythmias have occurred with trazodone use in patients with and without preexisting heart disease.[36,37] Trazodone is regarded as a safe drug even in overdose.[32,36,38] A unique and rare side effect is priapism (protracted, painful penile erection).[39] Trazodone has a very low anticholinergic potency and a moderate sedative action. This could make it a useful drug in treating the elderly anxious patient.

Fluoxetine A selective 5-HT reuptake inhibitor, fluoxetine has a long half-life ranging from 1 to 4 days. Its demethylated active metabolite has an even longer half-life of 7 to 15 days. The time to plasma steady state with daily dosing is around 12 to 42 days. The long half-lives of fluoxetine and norfluoxetine promote insidious drug accumulation, which takes considerable time to correct.[40,41] Excess drug effects resemble those of the amphetamines. They include jitteriness, anxiety, anorexia, headache, and insomnia. Additional adverse effects include gradual sedation, fatigue, and emotional blunting after relief by a decrease in dose. Like other CAs, fluoxetine is metabolized in the liver, resulting in its interference with the metabolism of other drugs.[40-42] Concurrent use of fluoxetine and TCAs has been associated with increased plasma levels and toxicity of the TCAs.[40,41,43] This probably represents an inhibition of TCA metabolism.

Fluoxetine has been successfully used in obsessive compulsive disorder,[40,44]

Table 15-14 Summary of pharmacokinetics of fluoxetine

Active metabolite	Norfluoxetine
Serum protein binding	94.5%
Peak plasma concentration (initial dose)	6–8 h
Serum half-life	
Fluoxetine	2–3 days
Norfluoxetine	7–9 days
Steady-state plasma concentration	2–4 weeks
Volume of distribution	20–45 L/kg
Plasma clearance	
Fluoxetine	20 L/h
Norfluoxetine	9 L/h

panic, and anxiety disorders.[44] Fluoxetine is structurally different from the CAs and does not have inhibitory effects on the cholinergic, histaminic, or adrenergic neuronal receptors. The drug is devoid of sedative, hypotensive, anticholinergic, and cardiac side effects.[40,41]

The antidepressant efficacy is equal to other CAs. Amphetamine-like adverse effects are dose-related.[40,41,45] Several studies comparing fluoxetine with CAs or placebo showed antidepressant efficacy comparable to the cyclics and superior to placebo. Fluoxetine has been shown to have efficacy in unipolar depression in the elderly.[46] Doses as low as 2.5 to 5 mg/day have been used in elderly patients.

Weight gain is a common adverse effect of TCA therapy and is not an uncommon cause of discontinuing therapy. Fluoxetine has only rarely been associated with weight gain during the course of antidepressant therapy but has caused nausea, vomiting, and some anorexia. The unique absence of characteristic TCA adverse effects makes fluoxetine a drug to be considered in the therapy of unipolar depression in the elderly. A number of cases of extrapyramidal symptoms (EPSs) have been reported in patients on fluoxetine.[40,47] Akathisia due to fluoxetine has responded to reduction in dose.[48] These data suggest an indirect inhibitory effect of fluoxetine on dopaminergic neurons.[40]

A serious fluoxetine-MAOI interaction[49] has been reported. The resultant syndrome of hyperthermia, neuromuscular irritability, and altered mental state is thought to be due to excessive central nervous system 5-HT. The interaction may occur because of an MAOI being given to a patient before fluoxetine is completely cleared from the body. The long half-life of fluoxetine makes it a possible interacting drug for several weeks after it has been stopped. A 5-week washout period has been recommended between stopping fluoxetine and starting on MAOI. The pharmacokinetics of fluoxetine are shown in Table 15-14.

Bupropion Chemically related to the central stimulant unicyclic aminoketone diethylpropion hydrochloride (Fig. 15-3), bupropion is a nonpotent inhibitor of

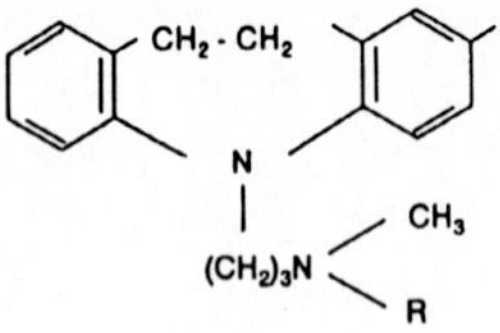

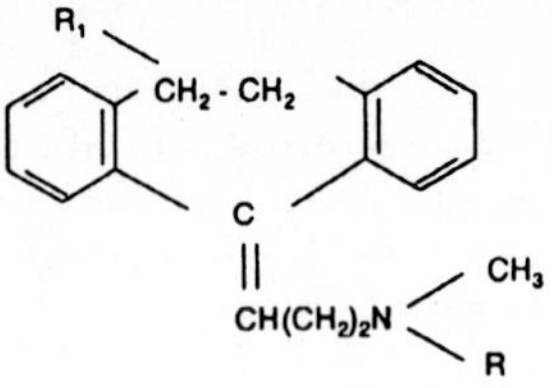

R = CH_3-R_1 = H   Imipramine
R = R_1 = H   Desipramine
(R_1 = OH Hydroxylated derivatives)

R = $CH_3$$R_1$ = H   Amitriptyline
R = R_1 = H   Nortriptyline
(R_1 = OH Hydroxylated derivatives)

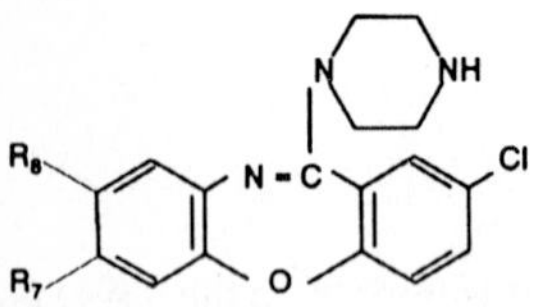

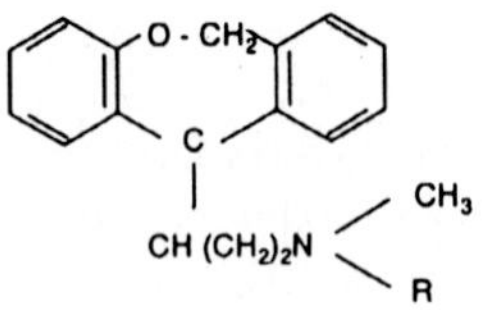

R_7, R_8 = H   Amoxapine
R_7 = H, R_8 = OH   8-Hydroxyamoxapine
R_7 = OH, R_8 = H   7-Hydroxyamoxapine

R = CH_3 Doxepin
R = H   Nordoxepin

Figure 15-3 Structures of TCAs and their main metabolites.

Table 15-15 Pharmacokinetics of antidepressants

Drug	Elimination half-life, h	Average daily dose, mg	Therapeutic range, µg/L	Time to steady state, days
Amitriptyline	21-40	150-300	80-250	4-10
Nortriptyline	15-93	50-100	50-150	4-19
Imipramine	6-25	150-300	150-250	2-5
Desipramine	12-76	150-300	125-300	2-11
Doxepin (desmethyldoxepin)	8-36(33-80)	200-400	150-250	2-8
Trimipramine	9	100-200	150-250	2
Protriptyline	54-198	30-60	70-260	10+
Maprotiline	27-58	100-200	200-600	5-10
Amoxapine	8(30)	200-300	200-600	2(5)
Trazodone	13	200-300	800-1600	3
Fluoxetine (norfluoxetine)	24-96 (7-15 days)	20-40	—	12-42
Alprazolam	12	4-10	20-55	3
Bupropion	14	225-450	—	4-8

Source: From Husseini K, Potter MZ: The new generation antidepressants. *Hosp Ther* 15:696,1990. Reproduced with permission.

neuronal reuptake of NE, 5-HT, and dopamine (DA). Multiple controlled studies have shown bupropion to be as efficacious in the treatment of depression as other CA drugs.[50,51] As with fluoxetine, patients do not gain weight and may lose weight with bupropion use.[50,52] Bupropion has no anticholinergic, sedative, or cardiovascular effects. Common adverse effects include anxiety, restlessness, insomnia, agitation, and tremor. Activation of the dopaminergic system may be responsible for the induction of psychosis in some depressed patients.[50,53] Seizures have occurred at both therapeutic and toxic blood levels of drug.[54] The manufacturer has reported a higher incidence of adverse effects when bupropion is used with levodopa.[50]

The drug has been shown to be an effective antidepressant without causing sedation, weight gain, sexual dysfunction, or orthostatic hypotension. As such, it is a good choice for therapy of the elderly in spite of the need to avoid its use in patients with seizure history and those with a history of psychosis. Pharmacologic data are shown in Table 15-15.

Alprazolam This agent is a triazolobenzodiazepine with antianxiety and putative antidepressant activity.[55] The pharmacokinetics are shown in Table 15-15. Its short duration of action necessitates its use three times a day. Like the benzodiazepine class, in general, alprazolam use has been associated with tolerance and dependence. The antidepressant efficacy of alprazolam has been found to be equal to that of TCAs with fewer and less severe side effects.[36,56] These studies have been criticized on the basis of the populations studied, the TCA dose used, and the indices used to assess antidepressive efficacy.[56,57] The compound lacks anticholinergic and cardiovascular adverse effects and has a good margin of safety. Obviously sedation is a prominent feature of its actions. Its use in the depressed elderly patient is complicated by the need to take the drug several times a day and the rapid development of dependence.[32,36] Moreover, the sedative effects may result in decreased cognitive function and falls in the elderly patient. A severe alprazolam withdrawal syndrome consists of severe anxiety, autonomic arousal, perceptual distortions, delirium, and seizures.[36] The drug has no special virtues in the therapy of depression in the elderly.

Metabolism The cyclic and atypical antidepressants are generally lipophilic compounds which are metabolized in the liver. The metabolism involves several phases. These include oxidative demethylation of tertiary amines to secondary amines in the hepatic microsomal enzyme systems, further oxidative hydroxylations of ring structures at the 2 and 10 positions, and conjugation of the metabolized compounds to facilitate renal elimination.[58,59] The demethylation of tertiary to secondary amines produces biologically active compounds which are long-acting and have large volume of distribution. Microsomal oxidative metabolism in the liver is the rate-limiting step, which is influenced by age, sex, diseases, and inducing and inhibiting agents.[58-60] The metabolic products of metabolism of the marketed antidepressants are shown in Figs. 15-3 and 15-4.

Patients treated with tertiary amine TCA, like imipramine, amitriptyline, and doxepin, are also exposed to their secondary amine metabolites desipramine,

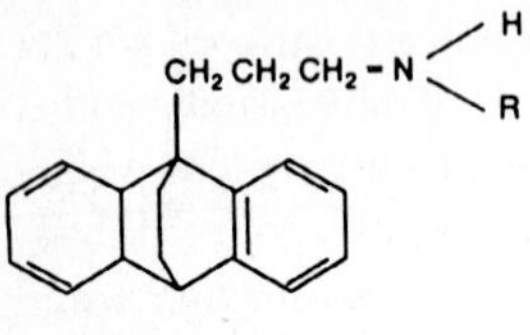

$R = CH_3$ Maprotiline

$R = H$ Desmethyl-maprotiline

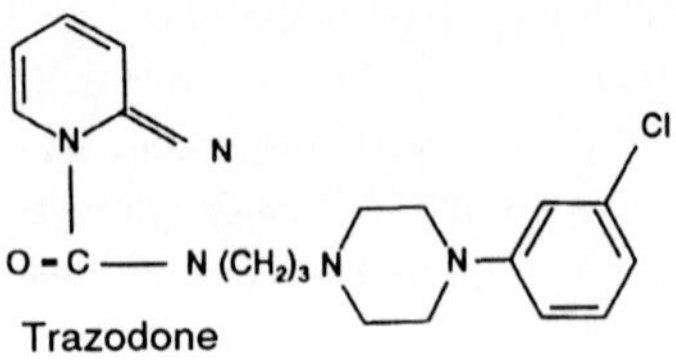

Trazodone

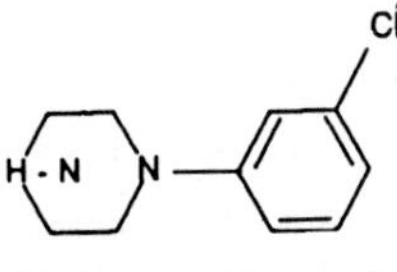

m-Chlorophenylpiperazine

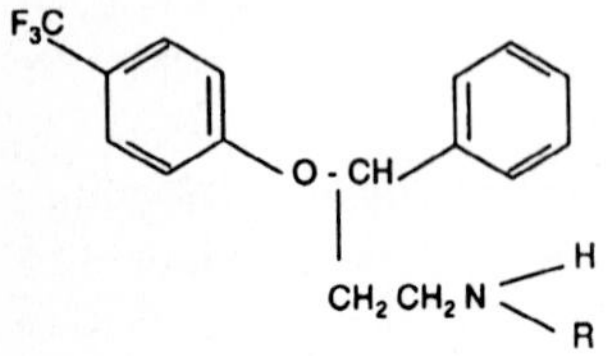

$R = CH_3$ Fluoxetine

$R = H$ Norfluoxetine

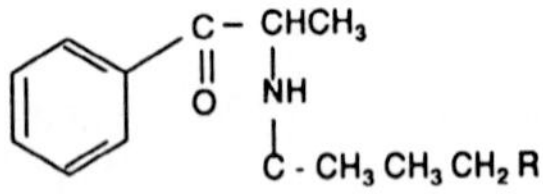

$R = H$ Bupropion

$R = OH$ Hydroxy-bupropion

Figure 15-4 Structures of cyclic antidepressants and their main metabolites.

nortriptyline, and nordoxepin, which are biologically active but affect NE more than 5-HT. Therefore, the metabolites are less sedative and less anticholinergic and cause less orthostatic hypotension via α_1-adrenergic blockade.

The metabolism of amoxapine, the *N*-desmethyl derivative of the neuroleptic loxapine, involves aromatic ring hydroxylation (at positions 7 and 8) followed by conjugation. Like the parent drug, both the 7- and 8-hydroxy metabolites inhibit reuptake of NE. The potent antidopaminergic activity in vitro of the 7-hydroxy derivative is of pharmacologic importance in that in overdose it engenders extrapyramidal adverse effects. Maprotiline, tetracyclic compound, is demethylated, but the pharmacologic activity of the metabolite has not yet been elucidated.[60] Fluoxetine is extensively demethylated. The metabolite norfluoxetine is eliminated more slowly (half-life 7 to 9 days) than the parent drug ($t_{1/2}$ of 2 to 3 days) and is a blocker of 5-HT reuptake. At steady state, the plasma concentrations of the two compounds are about equal. Trazodone undergoes cleavage of the phenylpiperazine to form *m*-chlorphenylpiperazine (*m* CPP), a potent 5-HT agonist. Bupropion undergoes reduction of the amino ketone to amino alcohol derivatives, which are less potent antidepressants but at steady state are at higher plasma concentration than bupropion.

The metabolism of antidepressant drugs has been extensively reviewed in recent years.[60-63]

Elderly patients treated with amitriptyline and imipramine attained higher plasma concentrations of imipramine, desipramine, and amitriptyline (but not nortriptyline) than did younger patients.[64] The $t_{1/2}$ of desipramine was also prolonged in the elderly. In another study, the plasma clearance of nortriptyline was lower in elderly patients than in younger ones. This study suggested that if nortriptyline (75 mg/day) were given to elderly patients, more than half of them would attain plasma levels higher than the suggested upper limit.[65]

Metabolism and elimination of TCAs decrease in the elderly. This is shown in Table 15-16.[66,67]

Cyclic Antidepressant Therapy

Depression is generally a self-limited disease with a natural history of spontaneous recovery in 6 to 9 months.[7,8,27,29] However, the risk of suicide, the social disruptions caused by depression, and the lessened life expectancy of elderly patients are adequate reasons to prescribe drug therapy.

The efficacy of antidepressant drugs in the treatment of geriatric depression is well established.[8,25,62] Although ECT has been found to be as effective as antidepressant drugs, it is possible that some patients who did not respond to antidepressant drug therapy did not receive adequate doses.[7,8]

Elderly patients in whom antidepressant drug therapy is likely to be successful tend to have the following characteristics: (1) onset of depressive symptoms before age 70; (2) positive family history of affective disorders; (3) predepression outgo-

Table 15-16 Effect of aging on metabolism and elimination of antidepressants[a]

Measurement	Under 65 years	Over 65 years	Change in elderly, %
Imipramine dose, mg/day	150	92	61
Total plasma [TCA], ng/mL	52	141	271
[TCA]/dose, ng/mL/mg	0.35	1.52	434
[DMI]-[IMI] ratio	0.66	0.68	103
Half-life, h			
Imipramine	19	24	126
Desipramine	34	76	224

[a]Depressed adults were tested in a steady state of drug metabolism after at least a week of treatment; data are means for group of about six patients. Similar results were obtained with amitriptyline. There was a significant correlation of total tricyclic antidepressant (TCA) plasma level [imipramine (IMI) + desipramine (DMI)] versus age (r = 0.54).

Source: Adapted from Nies AS et al: Relationship between age and tricyclic antidepressant plasma levels. *Am J Psychiatry* 134:790, 1977. Copyright 1977, the American Psychiatric Association. Reprinted by permission.

ing personality and multiple interests; (4) severe symptoms, including confusion and agitation; (5) preservation of emotional responsibility; and (6) good recovery from previous depression. Features associated with a poorer response to TCA therapy include serious physical illness, dependency, obsessiveness, and schizoaffective states.[3,7,27,28]

The pharmacologic doses and effects of the marketed antidepressant drugs are shown in Tables 15-17 and 15-18. The tertiary amines are more sedative, anticholinergic, and hypotensive. However, since they are in good part metabolically demethylated to secondary amines, the theoretical differences in the two drug classes may not be clinically significant.

In clinical practice drug choice is empirical. The more sedating drugs are usually used by persons with high degrees of anxiety, agitation, and sleep disturbances. Tertiary amine TCAs such as amitriptyline, doxepin, and imipramine are often used for such patients.[24,27,62] Dosage schedules for TCAs are given in Table 15-17. These are guidelines, and therapy must be individualized based on therapeutic efficacy and adverse effects. Elderly patients are treated with a lower dose of drug because of the higher incidence of adverse effects at standard adult doses.[7,64-67] Since these adverse effects can be life threatening, doses are approximately one-third to one-half of the usual adult dose.

It is worthwhile to start medications at a low dosage and to increase the dosage gradually over a period of days. This permits assessment of the adverse effects such as sedation and hypotension and the several anticholinergic effects. Drug dose may be limited by these adverse effects. Divided doses may be of value for some elderly patients because the twice daily or three times daily schedule may dampen the drug's anticholinergic, hypotensive, and sedative effects. Patience and a gradual buildup of drug dose are helpful, since some degree of tolerance develops to the sedative, hypotensive, and anticholinergic effects with continued use.[21,27,29] Unwanted effects of TCA are avoided by giving the entire dose at bedtime.

The TCAs have relatively long half-lives and a large volume distribution. At

Table 15-17 Daily dosage ranges of tricyclic antidepressants

	Initial dose, mg/day		Maintenance dose, mg/day	
Drug	Average adult	Elderly	Average adult	Elderly
Imipramine (Tofranil)	75–300	20–100	75–150	20–75
Amitriptyline (Elavil)	150–300	20–100	75–150	20–75
Desipramine (Norpramin)	150–300	20–100	75–150	20–75
Notriptyline (Aventyl)	50–150	10–75	50–100	10–50
Doxepin (Sinequan)	200–400	30–200	150–250	30–150
Protriptyline (Vivactil)	30–60	10–30	20–40	20–30

Source: From Rosenbaum AH, Maruta T, Richelson E: Drugs that alter mood. I. Tricyclic agents and monoamine oxidase inhibitors. *Mayo Clin Proc* 54:338, 1979. Reproduced with permission.

Table 15-18 Comparison of antidepressant treatments with placebo

Agent	Trials, n	Agent superior to placebo, %[a]
Tricyclic		
Imipramine	38	68
Amitriptyline	20	70
Maprotiline	12	75
Nortriptyline	8	62
Desipramine	6	66
Amitriptyline+perphenazine	5	80
Protriptyline	3	100
Doxepin	1	100
Atypical		
Trazodone	12	75
Other treatments		
Electroconvulsive therapy	9	89

[a]Summarizes controlled trials with a variety of depressive disorders in inpatient and outpatient settings where a test agent produced results better than a placebo, with statistical significance at least 5 percent. The mean placebo response rate, by patients, averaged 34 percent.

Sources: Morris JB, Beck AT: The efficacy of antidepressant drugs. *Arch Gen Psychiatry* 30:667–674, 1974. Copyright © 1974 American Medical Association. Reproduced with permission. Appleton WS, Davis JM: *Practical Clinical Psychopharmacology*, 3d ed. Baltimore, Williams & Wilkins, 1988, pp 133–134. Reproduced with permission.

any fixed drug dose, it takes at least 5 to 7 days to reach a steady-state plasma level. Therefore, it is probably a safe practice to use the lower usual doses for approximately 5 to 10 days before increasing the dose. It is important to treat for a sufficient period of time. The TCAs have a characteristic latent period of approximately 3 weeks.[3,19,29] The initial response to the drugs takes this period of time even at an effective dose level. The drugs have some degree of efficacy prior to this time because of their effects on sleep disturbances.

Response to therapy The patients should be made aware of the expected response to treatment. Because of the rapid effects of the TCAs on sleep disturbances, the patients may have unrealistic expectations of a rapid dissipation of the symptoms of depression. The physician must emphasize that a number of weeks of treatment may be necessary before definite results are noted. The usual sequence of events in response to adequate doses of TCAs is as follows:

1. The patient's sleep disturbance is improved in the first week of therapy.
2. By 2 to 3 weeks, the patient becomes more aware of and interested in his or her surroundings and responds more appropriately to people and activities.

3. The physician, nurses, family, and friends note this improvement, but the patient may not yet feel much better.
4. The patient feels better. The symptoms are markedly improved or gone.

The selection of a CA can be made on the basis of the degree of anxiety and agitation or retardation. If there is retardation, nortriptyline, bupropion, fluoxetine, maprotiline, or desipramine may be used, whereas amitriptyline or doxepin is useful when anxiety and agitation are prominent.

The efficacy of TCAs has been well established.[25,27-29]

The effectiveness of some CAs versus placebo therapy or other drugs is shown in Tables 15-18 and 15-19.

Maintenance therapy The characteristic course of depression is to recur following successful treatment if maintenance therapy is not used.[8,28,29] This is true of depressions in any age group. Table 15-20 shows the high relapse rate in a number of studies in which depression was successfully treated and maintenance was with either a placebo or antidepressant drugs. The placebo relapse rate was over twice that of the antidepressant drugs.

Table 15-19 Efficacy of antidepressant treatment compared with a standard tricyclic

Agent	Trials, *n*	Similar, %	Inferior, %	Superior, %
Tricyclic				
Amitriptyline (vs. imipramine)	11	71	0	29
Amitriptyline+perphenazine (vs. imipramine)	7	57	14	29
Desipramine (vs. imipramine)	11	82	18	0
Doxepin	11	64	9	27
Imipramine (vs. amitriptyline)	11	36	45	19
Maprotiline	22	100	0	0
Nortriptyline	9	100	0	0
Protriptyline	8	75	25	0
Atypical				
Trazodone	21	100	0	0
Other treatments				
Electroconvulsive therapy	7	57	0	43

Sources: From Morris JB, Beck AT: The efficacy of antidepressant drugs. *Arch Gen Psychiatry* 30:667, 1974. Copyright © 1974 American Medical Association. Reproduced with permission. Appleton WS, Davis: *Practical Clinical Pharmacology*, 3d ed. Baltimore, Williams & Wilkins, 1988, pp 133–134. Reproduced with permission.

Table 15-20 Antidepressant treatment and early relapse in nonbipolar major affective illness[a]

Study	Year	Total, *n*	Relapse rate, % Placebo	Relapse rate, % Antidepressant	Protection ratio
Seager and Bird	1962	28	69	17	4.1
Mindham et al	1973	92	50	22	2.3
Prien et al	1973	77	67	37	1.8
Klerman et al	1974	99	29	12	2.4
Coppen et al	1978	29	31	0	>30
Stein et al	1980	55	69	28	2.5
Prien et al	1984	73	52	28	1.9
Total or mean (7 studies)		453	52.4	20.7	2.5

[a]Studies involved the use of a placebo and imipramine or amitriptyline and followed patients for 3 to 8 months after recovery of an index episode of major depression. Means are weighted by the number of patients per study.

Sources: Review and references therein from Prien RF, in Rifkin A (ed): *Schizophrenia and Affective Disorders: Biology and Drug Treatment.* Wright-PSG, Boston, 1983, pp 95–115; six-month data from Prien RF, Kupfer DJ, Mansky PA, et al: Drug therapy in the prevention of recurrences in unipolar and bipolar affective disorders. *Arch Gen Psychiatry* 41:1096, 1984. Copyright © 1984 American Medical Association. Reproduced with permission.

A number of maintenance therapies have been employed to prevent relapse of depression for a year. These treatments are shown in Tables 15-21 and 15-21a. The same high relapse rate has been found following therapy of the elderly depressed patient.

A patient who has undergone TCA therapy for previous episodes of depression should probably be maintained on the TCA even with amelioration of the depressive state. Maintenance therapy is especially indicated, since successive depressive episodes are usually more severe and more resistant to therapy.[8,29] In studies of adults treated with TCAs for depression, 22 percent of those receiving maintenance therapy for 6 months relapsed, whereas 50 percent of those receiving no therapy relapsed.[8,29] Maintenance therapy has generally been prescribed at a lower dose (50 to 66 percent of the usual therapeutic dose) because of the lower incidence of adverse effects. More recent studies have suggested that better maintenance therapy is effected by full-strength antidepressant therapy.[31] This strategy may be limited by the patient's response to the drug's adverse effects. Over 50 percent of patients who experience a depressive episode suffer a recurrence. Following two episodes of depression, the probability of a recurrence is even higher and the period between episodes is shorter.[29] Studies have shown that maintenance therapy with CAs is a partially effective prophylaxis against recurrent episodes of depression. The relatively long half-life and extensive tissue distribu-

Table 15-21 Treatment to prevent relapse or recurrence of nonbipolar depression for one year

Treatment	Patients, *n*	Relapse rate, %	Protection ratio
Placebo	321	67.2	1.0
Antidepressant[a]	281	40.6	1.7
Lithium salt	226	37.3	1.8
Antidepressant plus lithium	105	25.9	2.6

[a]Most studies used imipramine or amitriptyline (without systematic evaluation of the effect of dose); a few used maprotiline or mianserin.

Source: Prien RF, Kupfer DJ, Mansky PA, et al: Drug therapy in the prevention of recurrences in unipolar and bipolar affective disorders. *Arch Gen Psychiatry* 41:1096, 1984. Copyright © 1984 American Medical Association. Reproduced by permission.

Table 15-21a Antidepressant treatment and late recurrence in nonbipolar major depression

Study	Year	Total, *n*	Relapse rate, %		Protection ratio
			Placebo	Antidepressant	
Peselow et al	1981	83	84	69	1.2
Quitkin et al	1981	12	100	83	1.2
Kane et al	1982	24	77	55	1.4
Prien et al	1984	73	65	33	2.0
Total or mean (4 studies)		192	76.9	54.4	1.4
Annual relapse	—	—	39.8	28.6	1.4

Source: From Baldessarini RJ: *Chemotherapy in Psychiatry: Principles and Practice*, 1985, p 177. Reprinted by permission of the publishers from *Chemotherapy in Psychiatry: Principles and Practice, Revised and Enlarged Edition*, by Ross J. Baldessarini, M.D., Cambridge, Massachusetts: Harvard University Press. Copyright © 1985, 1977 by the President and Fellows of Harvard College.

tion of these drugs allow for once daily administration. When taken once per day at bedtime, the drugs can be used for their sedative effects, and the anticholinergic effects are less apparent.

Adverse Effects of Antidepressants

Common adverse effects of TCAs in the elderly are orthostatic hypotension, sedation, anticholinergic toxicity, cardiac toxicity, and memory loss.[7] These effects are shown in Table 15-22.

Table 15-22 Adverse effects of antidepressants

Effects	Frequent	Infrequent
Anticholinergic	Blurred vision Constipation Urinary hesitancy Memory loss	Aggravation of glaucoma Paralytic ileus Urinary retention Delirium
Cardiovascular/ sympathomimetic	Tachycardia Tremor Sweating Orthostatic hypotension Electrocardiogram abnormalities Cardiomyopathy Sudden death	Agitation Insomnia Aggravation of psychosis Delayed cardiac conduction Arrhythmias
Neurologic	Paresthesia Electroencephalogram alteration	Seizure
Allergic/toxic	—	Cholestatic jaundice Agranulocytosis
Metabolic/endocrine	Weight gain Sexual disturbance	Gynecomastia Amenorrhea

Although the drugs are fairly safe when used in a reduced dose range appropriate for elderly patients (25 to 50 percent of usual therapeutic dose),[7,21,27,29] adverse effects are more frequent and severe in the elderly. The higher incidence of adverse effects (Table 15-22) is in part due to the higher incidence of cardiovascular, renal, and cerebrovascular disease in the elderly, which causes impaired compensatory responses to TCA overdoses, and because of age-related decreases in TCA clearance.

Table 15-23 lists some marketed antidepressants and their potential for engendering adverse effects at usual therapeutic doses.

The sedative effect of antidepressant drugs is beneficial in relieving insomnia of depression. However, the long action of these agents may result in daytime hangover and drowsiness, which are unwanted. Some degree of tolerance to the sedative effect develops with drug use.[21,25,27,29]

Orthostatic hypotension is potentially dangerous in elderly patients, who are subject to serious injuries when they fall. Postural hypotension is not predictable by type of antidepressant used or its dose. It occurs more in elderly, cardiac patients and those with preexisting postural hypotension (Table 15-24). This adverse effect can be more frequent and serious in the elderly because of an impaired baroreceptor and/or insensitive sinus node.[21] Anticholinergic excess can be manifest as peripheral or central effects (Table 15-23). Urinary retention occurs more frequently in elderly men with benign prostatic hypertrophy. Constipation occurs commonly on TCAs. Narrow-angle glaucoma can be precipitated or worsened by TCAs.

Table 15-23 Relative side effects of cyclic antidepressants in the elderly patient

Drug	Sedation	Hypotension	Anticholinergic side effects	Altered cardiac rate and rhythm
Tertiary amines				
Imipramine	Mild	Moderate	Moderate to strong	Moderate
Doxepin	Moderate to strong	Moderate	Strong	Moderate
Amitriptyline	Strong	Moderate	Very strong	Strong
Trimipramine	Strong	Moderate	Strong	Strong
Secondary amines				
Desipramine	Mild	Mild to moderate	Mild	Mild
Nortriptyline	Mild	Mild	Moderate	Mild
Amoxapine	Mild	Moderate	Moderate	Moderate
Protriptyline	Mild	Moderate	Strong	Moderate
Maprotiline	Moderate to strong	Moderate	Moderate	Mild
Atypical antidepressants				
Trazodone	Moderate	Moderate	Mild (except dry mouth)	Mild to moderate
Fluoxetine	None	None	None	Low
Bupropion	None	None	None	Low

Blockade of the histamine H_1 receptor by TCAs may be the cause of weight gain.[21,24,29] Cardiovascular side effects are potentially the most dangerous. A number of electrocardiographic changes have been noted with use of TCAs. These changes include frequent T-wave changes, QRS widening related to plasma levels of drug, and intraventricular conduction delays.[68-72] Tricyclic antidepressants should be prescribed with care of patients with cardiac disease.[69,72] Elderly patients with heart disease should be carefully monitored. Imipramine and desipramine

Table 15-24 Incidence of postural hypotension with tricyclic antidepressants

	Incidence of hypotension, %		
Patient group	Mild	Moderate	Severe
Cardiac	37	14	24
Medically well	28	7	0

Source: From Muller OF et al: The hypotensive effect of imipramine hydrochloride in patients with cardiovascular disease. *Clin Pharmacol Ther* 2:300, 1961.

have been used successfully at therapeutic doses to treat arrhythmias in young adults.[68,69,71]

A decrement in recent memory with intact remote memory has been noted in patients on CAs.[7,29] This has been attributed to the anticholinergic activity of the drugs. Elderly patients are more susceptible to the anticholinergic effects of the antidepressant drugs, which include confusion, delirium, and coma. The effect of CAs on cerebral function in the elderly is shown in Fig. 15-5.

Cyclic Antidepressant Overdose

Increased use of TCAs by the elderly has led to a rise in the number of overdose cases. However, death from these overdoses is unusual.[73-76] In a study of 40 TCA overdose cases with plasma levels ranging tenfold or more over therapeutic levels, only two deaths occurred.[73]

The serious clinical signs of overdose encompass anticholinergic and cardiovascular effects.[73,74,76] The cardiovascular effects include sinus tachycardia (more than 70 percent), hypotension (more than 40 percent),[67,73,74] prolongation of the QRS complex (more than 40 percent), and prolongation of the Q-T interval (20 percent to 45 percent). The width of the QRS complex may be followed as an index of TCA drug clearance.[68,74]

Less frequent but more serious findings include other supraventricular tachycardias, intraventricular conduction defects, atrioventricular blocks, bradycardia, nodal rhythms, ventricular ectopy with recurrent ventricular tachycardia, and occasional ventricular fibrillation.

The tachycardia derives from the anticholinergic effect of TCAs, hypotension from α-adrenergic blockade, and the widened Q-T interval and QRS complex from

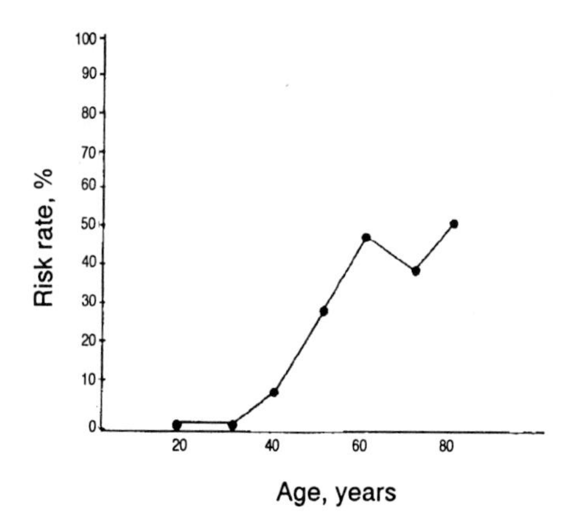

Figure 15-5 Effect of increasing age on risk of confusional states with tricyclic antidepressants. (From Davis et al: Confusional episodes and antidepressant medication. *Am J Psychiatry* 128:95, 1971. Used by permission of the American Psychiatric Association.)

the membrane effects (quinidine-like). Respiratory depression, which occurs in severe overdoses, is probably the result of cardiac arrhythmias, acidosis, and the direct CNS effects of TCAs.

Treatment of cardiovascular toxicity is supportive, although alkalinization by means of hyperventilation or intravenous sodium bicarbonate has been beneficial.[68,76]

MONOAMINE OXIDASE INHIBITORS

If CA drugs do not successfully treat depression in elderly subjects, MAOIs or ECT are alternatives. MAOIs are thought to be especially beneficial in the treatment of atypical depressions.[77-79] This designation characterizes patients with marked anxiety, hypochondriasis, and phobic features.[7,8,16] However, there are no controlled studies on MAOI use in elderly depressed patients.[79]

MAO is an enzyme found in neuronal tissue and elsewhere, predominantly in the mitochondrial fraction of cells. It exists in two forms. These two MAOs have different substrate specificities and are subject to differential inhibitions.[80,81] Type A MAO metabolizes 5-HT and NE and is inhibited by clorgyline, a nonmarketed MAOI. Type B MAO has a relative substrate specificity for benzylamine and phenylethylamine, both nonendogenous substrates. Dopamine, tryptamine, and tyramine are metabolized by both A and B forms of MAO. Type B is inhibited by selegiline.[80-82]

MAO activity has been found to be increased in the plasma, platelets, and brain of elderly humans. However, this elevation in tissue levels of the elderly does not identify depression.

The currently available MAOIs for the treatment of depression (Fig. 15-6) are all nonspecific in that they inhibit the activities of types A and B MAO. The ideal MAOI would be specific for type A and would be rapidly transported into the CNS so that it could be used in a small dose to avoid peripheral toxicity.

Table 15-25 lists the available MAOIs used in antidepressant therapy and their average daily dose.

The MAOIs are of two chemical types: hydrazides and nonhydrazides (Fig. 15-6). The nonhydrazide drug tranylcypromine resembles dextroamphetamine in that it has a cyclopropyl chain rather than an isopropyl chain. It is the only clinically useful antidepressant of the nonhydrazide series. Its ability to inhibit MAO is greater than that of dextroamphetamine. Tranylcypromine has some of the same sympathomimetic actions as dextroamphetamine, which would made it suitable for use in withdrawn, apathetic patients.[79,81,83]

Clinically available MAOIs produce an irreversible inactivation of MAO by forming stable complexes with the enzyme. MAO normally limits intracellular levels of biologically active amines. Consequently, MAOIs increase the amounts of endogenous amines such as NE, epinephrine, DA and 5-HT in various tissues including brain, heart, intestine, and blood.

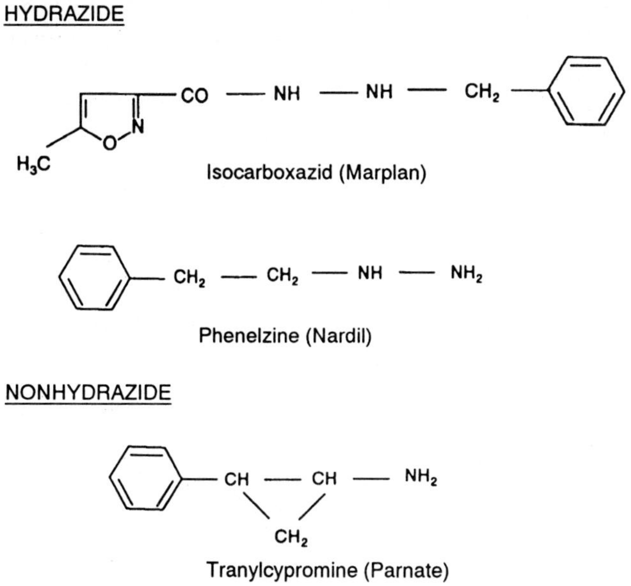

HYDRAZIDE

CO — NH — NH — CH_2

N O

H_3C

Isocarboxazid (Marplan)

CH_2 — CH_2 — NH — NH_2

Phenelzine (Nardil)

NONHYDRAZIDE

CH — CH — NH_2

CH_2

Tranylcypromine (Parnate)

Figure 15-6 Monoamine oxidase inhibitor antidepressants.

There are several amine oxidases. The clinically useful MAOIs are not entirely specific for MAO, since they also inhibit the metabolism and inactivation of certain drugs such as barbiturates and meperidine by other pathways. MAOIs also inhibit *l*-aromatic amino acid decarboxylase and choline, diamine, and methylamine oxidase.

The amine theories of depression postulate that a decreased availability of biogenic amines at central synapses is associated with depression. It is hypothesized that MAOIs raise the levels of biogenic amines (NE, 5-HT, DA) by inhibiting their intracellular destruction, which results in greater release of neurotransmitters.[21,78,81]

Clinical efficacy in the treatment of depression with MAOIs is thought to

Table 15-25 Usual daily dosages of monoamine oxidase inhibitor antidepressants

	Dosage, mg/day	
Drug	Adult	Elderly
Hydrazides		
Isocarboxazid (Marplan)	20-60	15-40
Phenelzine (Nardil)	60-90	40-60
Nonhydrazides		
Tranylcypromine (Parnate)	20-40	15-30

correlate with the degree of MAOIs. The MAO of platelets is assumed to be an index of brain MAO. MAOI efficacy is greater when over 80 percent of platelet MAO is inhibited in the course of drug therapy.[80,84]

Tranylcypromine probably possesses two modes of action. One is the result of its potent inhibition of MAO and the second is the result of an amphetamine-like action. The latter effect has been attributed to the release of NE from central neurons and also possibly to a reduction in the neuronal reuptake of NE. Tranylcypromine's rapid onset of action is a consequence of its amphetamine-like action, and its sustained antidepressant effects are related to the inhibition of MAO.[78,80,81,83]

The MAOIs are rapidly absorbed from the gastrointestinal tract. They are rapidly cleared from the plasma and are metabolized in the liver.[78,80,81] However, the inhibition of MAO continues for several days after a single dose of drug. This is thought to be caused by irreversible inhibition of MAO enzyme.[78,80,81] Termination of the drug effect results from enzyme regeneration.

The hydrazide MAOIs are metabolized in the liver to active products. Tranylcypromine is already active and combines directly with MAO.

Pharmacologic Action

The MAOIs have two distinct pharmacologic actions, antidepressant and antihypertensive, which result from the central and peripheral actions of MAOIs, respectively.

Antidepressant action Except for tranylcypromine's amphetamine-like action, the clinical effects of MAOIs do not become fully apparent for several weeks. This period approximately corresponds to the period for maximal inhibition of MAO.[85,86] Because acetylation by liver microsomal enzymes is a step in the metabolism of MAOIs, it has been thought that the genetically determined rate at which this reaction occurs in an individual may determine his or her other responses to a MAOI. Results to date, however, have been equivocal. However, patients who are elderly or have liver disease may be more sensitive to the effects of these agents.[77-79, 87]

Some studies suggest that an inadequate inhibition of MAO might be responsible for the equivocal antidepressant effects found.[19,29,84,85]

The cessation of sleep disturbances and amelioration of mood disorders by MAOI therapy are associated with a marked suppression of REM sleep.

Antihypertensive action The MAOI, especially pargyline, cause a decrease in blood pressure. The hypotensive effect is frequent, and the postural blood pressure decrease may be a serious adverse effect, especially for elderly patients.[29,79,81,85]

A body of literature exists that shows that compounds chemically similar to natural neurotransmitters could be stored in nerve terminals and could be released by nervous impulses or sympathomimetic agents. The release of these compounds, like that of normal neurotransmitters, has effects on receptor cells. However, these compounds have lesser effects on the receptor cells. They have been called substitute or false neurotransmitters. The false transmitters derive from two sources: (1) endogenous intermediates in the pathway of NE synthesis from tyrosine (octopamine) and (2) dietary tyramine, which is β-hydroxylated to octopamine. These compounds may attenuate reflex pressor impulses to the heart and blood vessels. Centrally, false transmitters may serve as α-adrenergic activators to lower blood pressure.[78,79,81,85,86]

Adverse effects Adverse effects of MAOI include the following:

1. Weight gain
2. Dry mouth
3. Aggravation of memory loss
4. Confusional reactions progressing to disorientation
5. Hyperreflexia, increased muscle tone, and generalized weakness. May progress to hyperthermia, seizures and death.
6. Conversion of retarded depressions to states of severe anxiety and agitation and occasionally hypomania
7. Hypertensive crisis ("cheese reaction")

The sympathomimetic amines in food such as tyramine are normally destroyed by gastrointestinal tract MAO. MAO inhibition permits the amines contained in cheese, certain wines, and other foods to be absorbed as active amines, which can stimulate the release of the enlarged stores of neuronal biogenic amines. This results in a series of adverse reactions including the following (in progressive order): (1) headache, tachycardia, sweating, anxiety, tension, pallor, and restlessness; (2) palpitations, hypertension, agitation, chest pains, hyperactive reflexes, and hyperthermia; and (3) involuntary movements of the jaw and face, hallucinations, intracranial bleeding, convulsions, and coma.

All stimulant drugs can detrimentally alter behavior by increasing tension, producing insomnia, aggravating psychoses, and possibly converting a retarded depression into an agitated one. Excitatory reactions are more likely with MAOIs than with TCAs, since the latter have an intrinsic sedative effect.

The occurrence of acute hypertensive crisis with fatal subarachnoid or intracranial hemorrhage led to the sharply curtailed use of tranylcypromine. Although it is a unique drug in that the direct sympathomimetic effects may ultimately be potentiated by the slower-developing inhibition of MAO, all MAOIs have been associated with such reactions.

Tremors, twitches, hyperreflexia, convulsions, and other neurologic signs have been produced by some MAOIs. The appearance of hyperreflexia may be used to signify the upper dosage level of hydrazide derivatives, and thus more disabling neuromuscular disturbances may be avoided by a reduction in dosage. Peripheral neuropathy associated with the hydrazide drugs presumably has the same basis as that associated with isoniazid; that is, it is related to pyridoxine deficiency.

Drug interactions The MAOIs account for a large number of drug interactions (Table 15-26). The drugs should be prescribed with caution and should rarely be used by elderly patients. In summary, the interaction problems are as follows:

1. MAOIs pose problems of drug-food interactions with foods rich in tyramine or other pressor amines and with various environmental chemicals.[27-29,88]
2. They primarily influence systems mediated by epinephrine, NE, DA, and 5-HT.
3. They inhibit hepatic drug-metabolizing enzymes and thus may prolong or intensify the action of other concomitantly administered drugs whose metabolism takes place primarily at hepatic sites.

Extensive experience with MAOI therapy for the elderly is lacking, and potential toxicities discourages use of the agents in preference to the CAs.

MANIA

The initial appearance of mania in the elderly patient is unusual. However, preexisting mania with exacerbations in later life is not unusual. The characteristic history of mania is that of a life-long series of manic depression episodes which increase in frequency and intensity with aging. There is a 2 : 1 ratio of females to males afflicted with later life episodes of mania.[89]

Although the diagnosis of mania is basically the same at all ages, elderly subjects have certain pronounced features. These include[89,90] (1) confusion, (2) paranoid ideation, (3) labile affect and irritability, (4) flight of ideas with morbid or depressive content, and (5) dysphoria and increased psychomotor output. Like an agitated depression, also included are (6) the long period of time between initial episode of depression and the onset of mania and (7) reduced attention span, distractibility, impaired concentration, and disorientation. The diagnosis may be more difficult if the elderly patient is suspect for dementia.

Lithium

Lithium is the major drug used for the prophylaxis and treatment of episodes of mania and depression in elderly patients with bipolar disorder.[89,90]

Patients being considered for lithium therapy should undergo a pretreatment evaluation which assesses renal function (serum creatinine and 24-h creatinine clearance), thyroid function [serum T_3, T_4, and thyroid-stimulating hormone (TSH)], and an electroencephalogram (EEG). The EEG may be decisive in the use of lithium and can serve as a baseline for ascertaining toxic lithium effects on the EEG. Assessment of memory, cognitive function, and neurologic function is made so as to be able to gauge lithium-induced changes.

Absorption of lithium is rapid and complete. Distribution is in total body water.

Table 15-26 Partial list of drugs that may interact with monoamine oxidase inhibitors

Agent	Effect
Sympathomimetics	
d- and *d, l*-amphetamine, methamphetamine, ephedrine, pseudoephedrine, norephedrine, oxymetazoline, phenylephrine, tranylcypromine, all catecholamines (including epinephrine or other vasoconstrictors added to procaine), L-dopa, foods or beverages containing pressor substances and possibly serotonin and its precursor amino acids	Potentiation, excess CNS stimulation or intoxication, hypertension with organ damage, or intracranial hemorrhage
Central depressants	
General anesthetics, alcohol, antihistamines, barbiturates, nonbarbiturates sedatives, benzodiazepines, neuroleptics, anticonvulsants, narcotics (except meperidine)	Potentiation, excessive CNS depression or intoxication; may also diminish MAO inhibition by hepatic induction
Analgesics	
Meperidine	Hyperpyrexia, seizure, coma
Aspirin	May induce hypertension(?)
Antiparkinsonism agents and anticholinergics	
All anticholinergic antiparkinsonism agents, atropine, scopolamine	Potentiate, atropinic intoxication syndrome; may decrease metabolism of MAO inhibitor(?)
L-Dopa	Potentiate; unpredictable changes in blood pressure; may induce CNS excitation or intoxication
Antihypertensive agents	
Reserpine (and congeners), α-methyldopa, guanethidine	When added to an MAO inhibitor can induce acute paradoxical hypertension and CNS excitation; unpredictable
Bethanidine, debrisoquin	Potentiate (not known to have acute press response as with guanethidine)
Clonidine	May potentiate
Hydralazine	Potentiate
Salt-losing diuretics	Hypotension
Tryptophase	When added to MAOI can induce hyperthermia and seizures
Other antidepressants and MAO inhibitors	
Imipramine and all typical tricyclic antidepressants (and possibly carbamazepine and cyclobenzaprine); all antidepressant MAO inhibitors, pargyline, nitrofuran antibiotics, and procarbazine (or other agents with MAO inhibitory activity)	Additive toxicity; unpredictable hypertension or hypotension; may induce rare but catastrophic CNS excitation, seizure hyperpyrexia of unknown cause (not due to pressor amines)

Table 15-26 (*continued*) Partial list of drugs that may interact with monoamine oxidase inhibitors

Agent	Effect
Sympathetic receptor-blocking agents	
Alpha antagonists	May potentiate.
Beta blockers	Unpredictable; may antagonize early and potentiate later
Antidiabetic agents	
Insulin, oral hypoglycemics	Potentiate
Anticoagulants	
Coumarins and indanediones	May potentiate (?)
Fluoxetine[a]	Mental status changes (confusion, hypomania), myoclonus, hypertension, tremor, diarrhea

[a]Adapted from Feighner JP, Boyer WF, Tyler DL, Neborsky RJ: Adverse consequence of fluoxetine-MAOI combination therapy. *J Clin Psychiatry* 51:222-225, 1990.

Source: From Baldessarini RJ: *Chemotherapy in Psychiatry: Principles and Practice,* 1985, Chap. 4, pp. 212–213. Reprinted by permission of the publishers from *Chemotherapy in Psychiatry: Principles and Practice, Revised and Enlarged Edition,* by Ross J. Baldessarini, M.D., Cambridge, Massachusetts: Harvard University Press.

Since total body water is decreased in the elderly, blood levels will be higher. There is no plasma protein binding of lithium. The reduced renal function of the elderly reduces lithium clearance, since this is its route of elimination. Half-lives of lithium rise from 18 to 20 in the young to 36 h in the elderly.[90,91] Lithium has a low therapeutic index and a broad range of individual tolerance differences. These features and the variable decrements in renal function found in the elderly patient make toxicity more frequent and have led to the use of dosing three times a day to minimize the excursions of plasma lithium[89-92] or the use of sustained-release lithium preparations.

Adverse reactions with lithium occur at therapeutic plasma levels of lithium in the elderly. The several adverse effects of lithium are mild in the elderly patient. However, in elderly patients who are frail, physically ill, dehydrated, on low salt diets and/or using diuretics, or with severely impaired renal function, lithium toxicity may be severe.[89-92]

Lithium is employed in both the therapy of and prophylaxis of exacerbations of bipolar illness. In the course of therapy of acute mania, lithium as a sole therapy is too slow, and drugs such as neuroleptic agents and sedatives are used.[89,90] A key feature of lithium's use is to decrease the frequency and severity of exacerbations of bipolar disease. Lithium has been demonstrated to do this, as shown by the data of Table 15-27 and Figs. 15-7 and 15-8.[27,29,90,93]

A number of studies in recent years have shown lithium to have efficacy in

Table 15-27 Prevention of bipolar relapse by lithium

			Relapse rate, %		
Study	Year	Total	Placebo	Lithium	Protection ratio
Baastrup et al	1970	50	45.5	0.0	>45
Persson	1972	24	91.7	41.7	2.2
Prien et al	1973	236	79.5	39.5	2.0
Coppen et al	1978	38	100.0	17.6	5.7
Fieve et al	1978	53	86.2	58.3	1.5
Quitkin et al	1978	6	66.7	0.0	>67
Quitkin et al	1981	11	71.4	25.0	2.9
Total or mean (7 studies)	—	78.5	34.3	2.3	

Sources: Appleton WS, Davis JM: *Practical Clinical Psychopharmacology*, 3d ed. Baltimore, Williams & Wilkins, 1988, pp. 133–134; Quitkin F, Kane JM, Rifkin A, et al: Lithium and imipramine in the prophylaxis of unipolar and bipolar depression : A prospective, placebo-controlled comparison. *Psychopharmacol Bull* 17:142, 1981. Used with permission.

preventing relapses in unipolar depression (Table 15-28). However, its efficacy as therapy of acute unipolar depression has been unimpressive.[93]

The use of lithium and the generation of a variety of adverse reactions have in recent years led to recommendations of lower serum levels of lithium for maintenance therapy.[94] Earlier lithium therapy aimed for serum levels of 0.8 to 1.2 meq/L. More recent lithium use aimed for serum levels of around 0.6 meq/L.[95] A recent study published by Gelenberg and his associates[96] demonstrated that serum lithium levels of 0.8 to 1.0 meq/L were more effective in prevention of recurrences of bipolar disease, predominantly mania, than lower serum lithium levels. The age range in the study was 18 to 74 years with average ages 37 to 40.

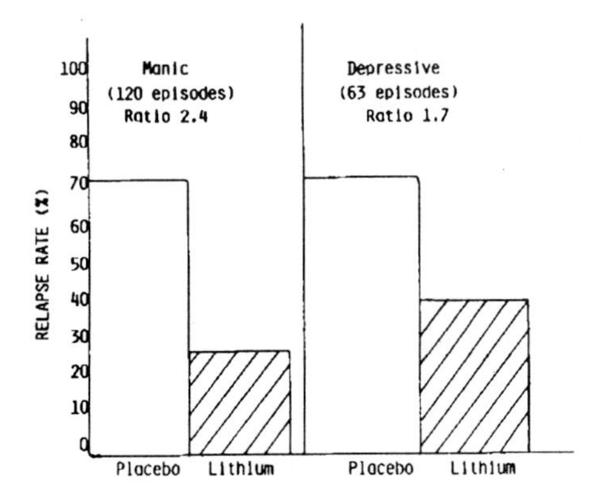

Figure 15-7 Rate of recurrence of mania or depression in bipolar manic-depressive patients with lithium or placebo. (From Davis JM: *Am J Psychiatry* 133:1, 1976. Used by permission.)

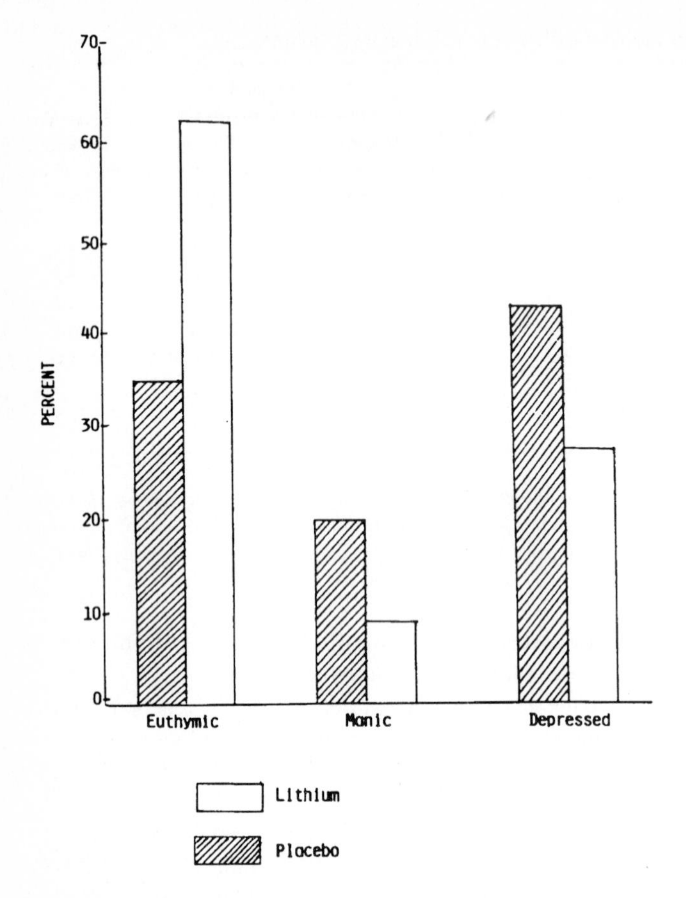

Figure 15-8 Proportion of time in mood state. (From Dunner DL et al: *Compr Psychiatry* 18:561, 1977. Used by permission.)

Age-related changes in renal blood flow, glomerular filtration, and tubular secretion reduce the clearance of drugs dependent on renal excretion. Lithium clearance is proportional to the glomerular filtration rate. In elderly subjects, renal excretion of lithium is often prolonged. Concomitant renal disease or congestive heart failure further decreases renal function and lithium excretion.[90-93]

Lithium toxicity Adverse effects of lithium may occur in elderly patients at doses and plasma levels which would be considered in the therapeutic range in younger patients. The adverse effects of lithium are often mild, but toxicity can be serious in elderly patients who are physically ill. The lithium adverse effects include (1) fine resting tremor; (2) nausea, vomiting, diarrhea, and gastric upset; (3) polyuria and polydypsia due to nephrogenic diabetes insipidus; (4) benign nontoxic goiter; (5) confusion, disorientation, and memory loss; and (6) flattening or inversion of T waves on the electrocardiogram.[91-93]

Table 15-28 Prevention of nonbipolar relapse by lithium

Study	Year	Total *n*	Relapse rate, % Placebo	Relapse rate, % Lithium	Protection ratio
Baastrup et al	1970	34	52.9	0.0	>53
Persson	1972	42	66.7	28.6	2.3
Prien et al	1973	43	87.5	48.1	1.8
Coppen et al	1978	26	80.0	9.1	8.8
Fieve et al	1978	28	64.3	57.1	1.1
Quitkin et al	1978	10	80.0	40.0	2.0
Peselow et al	1981	77	84.3	62.2	1.4
Quitkin et al	1981	13	100.0	28.6	3.5
Kane et al	1982	24	76.9	27.3	2.8
Prien et al	1984	71	65.0	57.0	1.1
Total or mean (10 studies)		445	75.5	43.5	1.7

Source: From Baldessarini RJ: *Chemotherapy in Psychiatry: Principles and Practice*, 1985, Chap. 3, p. 111. Reprinted by permission of the publishers from *Chemotherapy in Psychiatry: Principles and Practice, Revised and Enlarged Edition*, by Ross J. Baldessarini, M.D., Cambridge, Massachusetts: Harvard University Press.

The tremor is often mistaken for the senile tremor of elderly patients. It is a function of lithium dose. The gastrointestinal toxicity tends to occur early in the course of lithium therapy as the dose is being raised. Lithium causes polyuria with excretion of large quantities of dilute urine, a classic nephrogenic diabetes insipidus. This abnormality generally completely reverses within several weeks after discontinuing lithium. A variety of other renal insults have been reported including tubular damage.[90,93,97] Lithium may inhibit release of thyroxine and triiodothyronine from the thyroid gland, and lithium can cause hypothyroidism with classic signs and symptoms and elevated plasma TSH concentrations.[90,92,93,97] Elderly patients are susceptible to lithium-induced confusion and delirium. They may experience loss of memory and cognitive function and become disoriented. These CNS effects may be evident at high or even therapeutic serum lithium levels. The elderly patient may have this toxicity precipitated by diuretics, anti-inflammatory drugs, and dehydration. The confusion can progress to neuromuscular irritability, seizures and coma. Lithium's cardiac effects are rarely a manifestation of toxicity. The T-wave changes are frequent at therapeutic and toxic levels but revert with discontinuance of lithium. The elderly population with a higher incidence of heart disease may be more susceptible to cardiotoxic effects of lithium overdose. Cardiac abnormalities due to lithium are rare and are usually associated with other factors.[90,97]

The abnormalities cited are most often present during the course of therapy and disappear with discontinuance of lithium therapy.

REFERENCES

1. Blazer D, Williams CD: Epidemiology of dysphoria and depression in an elderly population. *Am J Psychiatry* 137: 439-444, 1980.
2. Blazer D: Depression in the elderly. *N Engl J Med* 320: 164-166, 1989.
3. Garland BJ, Meyers BS: Geriatric psychiatry, in Talbott JA, Hales RE, Yodofsky SC (eds): *Textbook of Psychiatry*. Washington, D.C., American Psychiatric Press, 1988, pp 1128-1133.
4. Mei-Tal V, Myers BS: Major psychiatric illness in the elderly: empirical study on an inpatient psychogeriatric unit. Part I; diagnostic complexities. *Int J Psychiatry Med* 15:91-109, 1985.
5. Cohen D, Eisdorfer C: Major psychiatric and behavioral disorders in the aged, in Andres R, Bierman EL, Hazzard WR (eds): *Principles of Geriatric Medicine*. New York, McGraw-Hill, 1985, pp 867-889.
6. Alexopoulos GS, Meyers BS, Young RC, et al: Brain changes in geriatric depression. *Int J Geriatr Psychiatry* 3:157-161, 1988.
7. Salzman C, van der Kolk B: Treatment of depression, in Salzman C (ed): *Clinical Geriatric Psychopharmacology*. New York, McGraw-Hill, 1984, pp 77-115.
8. Klerman GL: Depression and related disorders of mood, in Nicoli AM Jr (ed): *The New Harvard Guide to Psychiatry*. Cambridge, Massachusetts, Harvard University Press, 1988, pp 309-336.
9. Perez-Stable EJ, Miranda J, Munoz RF, Ying YW: Depression medical outpatients. Underrecognition and misdiagnosis. *Arch Intern Med* 150: 1083-1088, 1990.
10. Gerber PD, Barrett J, Manheimer E, et al: Recognition of depression by internists in primary care: A comparison of internists and "gold standard" psychiatric assessments. *J Gen Intern Med* 4: 7-13, 1989.
11. Keller MB: Depression. Underrecognition and undertreatment by psychiatrists and other health care professionals. *Arch Intern Med* 150: 946-948, 1990.
12. Berezin MA, Liptzin B, Salzman C: The elderly person, in Nicoli AM Jr (ed): *The New Harvard Guide to Psychiatry*. Cambridge, Massachusetts, Harvard University Press, 1988, pp 129-138.
13. Katon W, Sullivan MD: Depression and chronic medical illness. *J Clin Psychiatry* 51 (suppl):3-11, 1990.
14. Ruegg RG, Ziscook S, Swerlow NR: Depression in the aged: An overview. *Psychiatry Clin North Am* 11:83-108, 1988.
15. Liptzin B: Treatment of mania, in Salzman C (ed): *Clinical Geriatric Psychopharmacology*. New York, McGraw-Hill, 1984, pp 116-130.
16. Hirschfeld RMA, Goodwin FK: Mood disorders, in Talbott JA, Hales RE, Yodofsky SC (eds): *Textbook of Psychiatry*. Washington, D.C. American Psychiatric Press, 1988, pp 403-441.
17. Siever LJ, Uhde TW, Potter WZ, Murphy DL: Norepinephrine in the affective disorders: receptor assessment strategies, in Lake CR, Ziegler MG (eds): *The Catecholamines in Psychiatric and Neurologic Disorders*. Boston, Massachusetts, Butterworth, 1985, pp 235-268.
18. Asakura M, Tsukamoto T, Hasegawa K: Modulation of rat brain alpha-2 and beta-adrenergic reception sensitivity following long-term treatment with antidepressants. Brain Res 235: 192-197, 1982.
19. Heninger GR, Charney DS: Mechanism of action of antidepressant treatments: implications for the etiology and treatment of depressive disorders, in Meltzer H (ed): *Psychopharmacology. The Third Generation of Progress*. New York, Raven, 1987, pp 535-544.
20. Coyle JT: An introduction to the world of neurotransmitters and neuroreceptors, in Hales RE, Francis AJ (eds): *APA Annual Reviews*, vol 4, Washington, D.C. American Psychiatric Press, 1985, pp 5-94.
21. Bressler R: Antidepressant agents, in Conrad K, Bressler R (eds): *Drug Therapy for the Elderly*. St. Louis, Mosby, 1982, pp 295-315.
22. Caccia S, Garattini S: Formation of active metabolites of psychotropic drugs: An updated review of their significance. *Clin Pharmacokinet* 18: 434-459, 1990.
23. Risch SC, Janowsky DS, Huey LY: Plasma levels of tricyclic antidepressants and clinical efficacy,

in Enna SJ, Malick JB, Richelson, E (eds): *Antidepressants: Neurochemical, Behavioral and Clinical Perspectives.* New York, Raven, 1981, pp 183-217.

24. Richelson E: Antidepressants: pharmacology and clinical use, in Karasu TB (ed): *Treatment of Psychiatric Disorders*, vol 3. Washington, D.C. American Psychiatric Association, 1989, pp 1773-1787.
25. Gurland BJ, Myers BS: Antidepressant drugs, in Talbott JA, Hales RE, Yodofsky SC (eds): *Textbook of Psychiatry.* Washington, D.C. American Psychiatric Press, 1988, pp 788-805.
26. Richelson E, Nelson A: Antagonism by antidepressants of neurotransmitter receptors of normal human brain in vitro. *J Pharmacol Exp Ther* 230:94-100, 1984.
27. Hollister L, Gsernansky JG: *Clinical Pharmacology of Psychotherapeutic Drugs*, 3d ed. New York, Churchill Livingstone, 1990, pp 59-96.
28. Bernstein JG: Tricyclic and heterocyclic antidepressants. Handbook of drug therapy, in *Psychiatry*, 2d ed. Littleton, Massachusetts, PSG, 1988, pp 123-160.
29. Baldessarini RG: Antidepressant agents, in *Chemotherapy in Psychiatry.* Cambridge, Massachusetts, Harvard University Press, 1985, pp 130-234.
30. Salzman, C: Clinical guidelines for the use of antidepressant drugs in geriatric patients. *J Clin Psychiatry* 46:38-44, 1985.
31. Jackson JE: Cardiovascular effects of tricyclic antidepressants, in Ewy GA, Bressler R (eds): *Cardiovascular Drugs and the Management of Heart Disease.* New York, Raven, 1982, pp 285-310.
32. Manji HK, Rudorfer MV, Potter WZ: The new-generation antidepressants, Part I. The first wave. *Drug Ther* 15:683-700, 1990.
33. Wells BG, Gelenberg AJ: Chemistry, pharmacology, pharmacokinetics, adverse effects and efficacy of the antidepressant maprotiline hydrochloride. *Pharmacotherapy* 1:121-139, 1981.
34. Dessain EC, Schatzberg AF, Woods BT, Cole JO: Maprotiline treatment in depression: A perspective on seizures. *Arch Gen Psychiatry* 43:86-90, 1986.
35. Zetin M, Aden G, Moldawsky R: Tolerance to amoxapine antidepressant effects. *Clin Ther* 5:638-643, 1983.
36. Rudorfer MV, Potter WZ: Antidepressants—a comparative review of the clinical pharmacology and therapeutic use of the "newer" versus the "older" drugs. *Drugs* 37:713-738, 1989.
37. Aronson MD, Hafez H: A case of trazodone induced ventricular tachycardia. *J Clin Psychiatry* 47:388-389, 1986.
38. Kulig K: Management of poisoning associated with "newer" antidepressant agents. *Ann Emerg Med* 15:1039-1045, 1986.
39. Warner MD, Peabody CA, Whiteford HA, Hollister LE: Trazodone and priapism. *J Clin Psychiatry* 48:244-245, 1987.
40. Rudorfer MV, Manji HK, Potter WZ: The new-generation antidepressants, Part II. Fluoxetine and other selective reuptake inhibitors. *Drug Ther* 15:767-790, 1990.
41. Benfield P, Heel RC, Lewis SP: Fluoxetine: A review of its pharmacodynamic and pharmacokinetic properties, and therapeutic efficacy in depressive illness. *Drugs* 32:481-508, 1986.
42. Lemberger L, Rowe H, Bosomworth JC, et al: The effect of fluoxetine on the pharmacokinetics and psychomotor responses of diazepam. *Clin Pharmacol Ther* 43:412-419, 1988.
43. Ciravlo DA, Shader RI: Fluoxetine drug-drug interactions: I. Antidepressants and antipsychotics. *J Clin Psychopharmacol* 10:48-50, 1990.
44. Fountaine R, Chouinard G: Fluoxetine in the long-term maintenance treatment of obsessive-compulsive disorder. *Psychiatry Ann* 19:88-91, 1989.
45. Fabre LF, Putnam HP III: A fixed-dose clinical trial of fluoxetine in outpatients with major depression. *J Clin Psychiatry* 48:406-408, 1987.
46. Feighner JP, Cohn JB: Double blind comparative trials of fluoxetine and doxepin in geriatric patients with major depressive disorder. *J Clin Psychiatry* 46:20-25, 1985.
47. Bouchard RH, Pourcher E, Vincent P: Fluoxetine and extrapyramidal side effects. *Am J Psychiatry* 146:1352-1353, 1986.

48. Baldessarini RJ, Marsh E: Fluoxetine and side effects. *Arch Gen Psychiatry* 47:191-192, 1990.
49. Feighner JP, Boyer WF, Tyler DL, Heborsky RJ: Fluoxetine and MAOI's: Adverse interactions. *J Clin Psychiatry* 51:222-225, 1990.
50. Rudorfer MV, Manji HK, Potter WZ: The new generation antidepressants, Part III. Bupropion and medications under development. *Drug Ther* 15:911-929, 1990.
51. Golden RN, Rudorfer MV, Sherer MA, et al: Bupropion in depression. I. Biochemical effects and clinical response. *Arch Gen Psychiatry* 45:139-143, 1988.
52. Gardner EA: Effects of bupropion on weight in patients intolerant to previous antidepressants. *Curr Ther Res* 35:188-199, 1984.
53. Golden RN, James SP, Sherer MA, et al: Psychosis associated with bupropion treatment. *Am J Psychiatry* 142:1459-1482, 1985.
54. Davidson J: Seizures and bupropion: A review. *J Clin Psychiatry* 50:256-261, 1989.
55. Hicks F, Robins E, Murphy GE: Comparison of adinazolam, amitriptyline, and placebo in the treatment of melancholic depression. *Psychiatry Res* 23: 221-227, 1988.
56. O'Shea B: Alprazolam: Just another benzodiazepine? *Int Psychol Med* 6:89-94, 1989.
57. Fawcett J, Edwards JH, Kravitz HM, Jeffries H: Alprazolam: An antidepressant? Alprazolam, desipramine and an alprazolam-desipramine combination in the treatment of adult depressed outpatients. *J Clin Psychopharmacol* 7:295-310, 1987.
58. Amsterdam J, Brunswick D, Mendels J: The clinical application of tricyclic antidepressant pharmacokinetics and plasma levels. *Am J Psychiatry* 137:653-662, 1980.
59. Ereshefsky I, Tran-Johnson T, Davis CM, LeRoy A: Pharmacokinetic factors affecting antidepressant drug clearance and clinical effect: evaluation of doxepin and imipramine: new data and review. *Clin Chem* 34:863-880, 1988.
60. Caccia S, Garattini S: Formation of active metabolites of psychotropic drugs. An updated review of their significance. *Clin Pharmacokinet* 18:434-459, 1990.
61. Coccaro EF, Siever LJ: Second generation antidepressants: A comparative review. *J Clin Pharmacol* 25:241-260, 1985.
62. Hollister LE: Current antidepressants. *Ann Rev Pharmacol Toxicol* 26:23-37, 1986.
63. Rudorfer MV, Potter WZ: Pharmacokinetics of antidepressants, in Meltzer HY (ed): *Psychopharmacology: Third Generation of Progress*. New York, Raven, 1987, pp 1353-1363.
64. Crooks J, O'Malley K, Stevenson IH: Pharmacokinetics in the elderly. *Clin Pharmacokinet* 1:280-296, 1976.
65. Nies A, Robinson DS, Friedman MJ, et al: Relationship between age and tricyclic antidepressant plasma levels. *Am J Psychiatry* 134:790-793, 1977.
66. Ouslander JG: Drug therapy in the elderly. *Ann Intern Med* 95:711-722, 1981.
67. Triggs EJ, Nation RL: Pharmacokinetics in the aged: A review. *J Pharmacokinet Biopharmaceut* 3:387-418, 1975.
68. Jackson JE: Cardiovascular effects of tricyclic antidepressants, in Ewy G, Bressler R (eds): *Cardiovascular Drugs and the Management of Heart Disease*. New York, Raven, 1982, pp 285-309.
69. Glassman BH, Bigger T: Cardiovascular effects of therapeutic doses of tricyclic antidepressants. *Arch Gen Psychiatry* 38:815-820, 1981.
70. Jefferson JW: A review of the cardiovascular effects and toxicity of tricyclic antidepressants. *Psychosom Med* 37:160-179, 1975.
71. Kantor SJ, Glassman AH, Bigger JT, et al: The cardiac effects of therapeutic plasma concentrations of imipramine. *Am J Psychiatry* 135:534-538, 1978.
72. Richie JL: Cardiovascular effects of tricyclic antidepressants in depressed patients with chronic heart disease. *N Engl J Med* 306:954-959, 1982.
73. Biggs JT, Spiker DG, Petit JM, Ziegler VE: Tricyclic depressant overdose: incidence of symptoms. *JAMA* 238:135-138, 1977.
74. Callaham M: Tricyclic antidepressant overdose. *J Am Coll Emerg Phys* 8:413-425, 1979.
75. Serafimovski N, Thorball N, Asmussen I, Lunding M: Tricyclic antidepressive poisoning with special reference to cardiac complications. *Acta Anaesth Scand* 57:55-63, 1975.

76. Frommer DA, Kulig KW, Marx JA, Rumack B: Tricyclic antidepressant overdose: review. *JAMA 257:521–526, 1987.*
77. Quitkin F, Rifkin A, Klein DF: Monoamine oxidase inhibitors: A review of antidepressant effectiveness. *Arch Gen Psychiatry* 36:749–759, 1979.
78. Baldessarini RJ: Treatment of depression by altering monoamine metabolism: precursors and metabolic inhibitors. *Psychopharmacol Bull* 20:224–239, 1984.
79. Robinson DS: Monoamine oxidase inhibitors and the elderly, in Raskin A, Robinson DS, Levine J (eds): *Age and the Pharmacology of Psychoactive Drugs.* New York, Elsevier, 1981, pp 151–162.
80. Murphy DL, Lipper S, Campbell IC, et al: Comparative studies of MAO-B inhibitors, in Singer TP, Von Korff RW, Murphy DL (eds): *Man in Monoamine Oxidase Structure, Function and Altered Functions.* New York, Academic, 1979, pp 457–475.
81. Knoll J: Analysis of the pharmacologic effects of selective monoamine oxidase inhibitors, in Wolstenholme GEW, Knight J (eds): *Monoamine Oxidase and Its Inhibition.* Amsterdam, Elsevier, 1976, pp 135–161.
82. Mendelwicz J, Youdim MBH: L-Deprenil, a selective monoamine oxidase type B inhibitor in the treatment of depression: A double-blind evaluation. *Br J Psychiatry* 142:509–511, 1983.
83. Overall JE, Hollister LE, Shelton J, et al: Tranylcypromine compared with dextroamphetamine in hospitalized depressed patients. *Dis Nerv Syst* 27:653–658, 1966.
84. Pare CMB: The present status of monoamine oxidase inhibitors. *Br J Psychiatry* 146:567–584, 1985.
85. Murphey DL, Sunderland T, Cohen RM: Monoamine oxidase inhibiting antidepressants: A clinical update. *Psychiatry Clin North Am* 7:549–562, 1984.
86. Lowe MC, Horita A: Preclinical pharmacology of antidepressants. 1. Monoamine oxidase inhibitors, in Clark WG, del Giudice J (eds): *Principles of Psychopharmacology*, 2d ed, New York, Academic, 1978, pp 311–317.
87. Nies A, et al: Changes in monoamine oxidase with aging, in Eisdorfer C, Fann WF (eds): *Psychopharmacology and Aging.* New York, Plenum, 1972, pp 41–54.
88. Shulman KI, Walker SE, MacKenzie S, Knowles S: Dietary restriction, tyramine, and the use of monoamine oxidase inhibitors. *J Clin Psychopharmacol* 9:397–402, 1989.
89. Shulman KI, Post F: Bipolar affective disorder in old age. *Br J Psychiatry* 136:26–32, 1980.
90. Liptzin B: Treatment of mania, in Salzman C (ed): *Clinical Geriatric Psychopharmacology.* New York, McGraw-Hill, 1984, pp 116–131.
91. Chapron DJ, Cameron IR, White LB, et al: Observations on lithium disposition in the elderly. *J Am Geriatr Soc* 30:651–655, 1982.
92. Van der Velde CD: Toxicity of lithium carbonate in elderly patients. *Am J Psychiatry* 127:1075–1077, 1971.
93. Baldessarini RJ: Lithium salts and antimanic agents. In *Chemotherapy in Psychiatry.* Cambridge, Massachusetts, Harvard University Press, 1985, pp 93–129.
94. Report of the APA Task Force: The current status of lithium therapy. *Am J Psychiatry* 132:977–1001, 1975.
95. NIMH-NIH Consensus Development Conference Statement: Mood disorders: pharmacologic preventing of recurrences. *Am J Psychiatry* 142:469–475, 1985.
96. Gelenberg AJ, Kane JM, Keller MB, et al: Comparison of standard and low serum levels of lithium for maintenance treatment of bipolar disorder. *N Engl J Med* 321:1489–1493, 1989.
97. Simard M, Gumbiner B, Lee A, et al: Lithium carbonate intoxication. A case report and review of the literature. *Arch Intern Med* 149:36–46, 1989.

CHAPTER

16

ANTIPSYCHOTIC AGENTS

Alan J. Gelenberg
Michael D. Katz

The focus of this chapter is on antipsychotic agents—drugs also known as neuroleptics, antischizophrenic agents, and major tranquilizers (a misnomer). This pharmacologic family has become a mainstay in the treatment of schizophrenia and other psychotic disorders as well as many nonpsychotic conditions.

The most firmly grounded indication for using antipsychotic drugs is in the treatment of schizophrenia. These agents can suppress the more florid and acute symptoms of schizophrenic psychosis such as hallucinations, delusions, other aspects of thought disturbance, and excited, aggressive behavior. In addition, they may alleviate similar symptoms in patients with other syndromes, such as paranoid disorders, schizophreniform disorder, brief reactive psychosis, schizoaffective disorder, atypical psychosis, and psychosis associated with mood disorders such as melancholia and mania. Furthermore, antipsychotic drugs may alleviate psychotic symptoms or excited and assaultive behavior in patients with organic mental disorders, retardation, and childhood psychoses. At times, these agents have been effective in the treatment of patients with severe pain syndromes and difficult personality disturbances.

INDICATIONS FOR ANTIPSYCHOTICS IN THE ELDERLY

While schizophrenia is the most accepted indication for the use of antipsychotics, elderly patients may receive these drugs for a variety of indications. A disproportionately large percentage of psychotropic drugs are prescribed for the elderly. It is estimated that up to 90 percent of nursing home residents have a significant neuropsychiatric disability, and up to 75 percent of these patients receive antipsychotic medications. Common indications for antipsychotic agents include acute mania, psychotic or agitated depression, agitation associated with delirium, dementia or mental retardation, and miscellaneous medical disorders such as nausea and vomiting and hiccups.[1]

ANTIPSYCHOTIC DRUGS

Introduction

The introduction of the first antipsychotic drugs—reserpine and the phenothiazines—in the early to mid-1950s revolutionized psychiatry. For the first time, chemotherapy offered more than sedation to acutely disturbed and psychotic patients. Ultimately, antipsychotic drugs helped to diminish the previously sharp increase in the number of hospital beds in the United States occupied by schizophrenic patients. Many of these individuals could now function in their communities with periodic admission to psychiatric units, often in general hospitals. Psychiatric wards became quieter and less violent. The subspecialty of psychopharmacology was born, and many other important classes of psychopharmaceuticals have emerged. Unfortunately, the advent of antipsychotic drugs has not eliminated the problem of chronic schizophrenia. With the passage of the Community Mental Health Centers Act in 1963, President Kennedy mandated a "bold new approach" to treating the mentally ill. However, because of political and fiscal pressures, many severely ill patients were "deinstitutionalized" to nonexistent community programs. The sad result has been the re-creation of back wards in the community, with many chronic schizophrenic patients poorly medicated, hardly managed, and homeless.[2]

The rauwolfia alkaloid reserpine, especially when given in high doses, caused a number of problems, but the effects of the phenothiazine chlorpromazine were impressive. From this prototypical phenothiazine emerged a host of sister compounds with similar actions and effectiveness but with different potencies (i.e., milligram dosages) and unwanted effects. During the past three decades, various classes of antipsychotic compounds have been synthesized. They sometimes differ structurally from chlorpromazine but are pharmacologically and clinically similar.

Clinicians and researchers have labeled antipsychotic drugs with various synonyms, but the terms often have resulted in both semantic and conceptual confusion. When they were first used, these pharmaceuticals often were called *major tranquilizers*. This term developed from the observation that chlorpromazine and reserpine produce somnolence and relaxation and the consequent misbelief that their major action was sedative. However, relatively nonsedating antipsychotic compounds just as effectively combat psychotic symptoms. Moreover, patients often become tolerant to the sedating effects of antipsychotic drugs but not to the antipsychotic effects themselves. Finally, because of the implication that "major tranquilizers" are on a spectrum with but more powerful than sedative-hypnotic and antianxiety agents (sometimes called *minor tranquilizers*), this term is best avoided.

Because antipsychotic drugs frequently produce signs of neurologic dysfunction, most notably Parkinson's syndrome and other extrapyramidal reactions, the term *neuroleptic* was coined. In fact, researchers originally believed that (1) any drug effective in combating psychosis must produce extrapyramidal effects and (2) in any given patient, the induction of extrapyramidal signs indicated an optimal therapeutic dose. However, these assumptions are incorrect, based on the low incidence of extrapyramidal effects seen with thioridazine and clozaril.

Effects on Behavior and the Nervous System

In animals, antipsychotic drugs inhibit conditioned avoidance behavior, suppress electrical intracranial self-stimulation, block vomiting and aggression produced by the dopamine agonist apomorphine, and produce cataleptic immobility resembling human catatonia.[3] In early testing, researchers observed that antipsychotic drugs potentiated anesthesia and produced a state called "artificial hibernation."[4] Chlorpromazine, the prototype phenothiazine, did not by itself induce anesthesia but rather promoted sleep and diminished interest in the environment; animals required increased stimulation or motivation to perform tasks. Antipsychotic drugs have relatively little tendency to suppress vital centers in the brain stem: coma, respiratory depression, and cardiovascular collapse are rare, even at very high doses.[4]

In the electroencephalogram (EEG),[5] phenothiazines and other antipsychotic chemicals produce slowing and synchronization and a decrease in arousal-induced changes—effects that are reversed by dopamine agonists. The low-potency agents (e.g., chlorpromazine) also tend to lower the seizure threshold. Clinically, this effect is particularly important in patients predisposed to seizures, such as those with epilepsy, and in individuals undergoing withdrawal from sedative-hypnotic drugs (including alcohol).

Most antipsychotic agents (with thioridazine as an interesting exception) have antiemetic effects. They can protect against the nausea and vomiting that usually follow administration of apomorphine, presumably by blocking the latter's dopamine agonistic effects in the chemoreceptor trigger zone of the medulla.[4]

Mechanism of Action

The antipsychotic drugs block dopamine receptors in various pathways within the brain, which probably accounts for their therapeutic effectiveness as well as for some of their more prominent unwanted effects.[6-9] Table 16-1 outlines the receptor binding affinity for the antipsychotic agents.[9] According to widely held theories, antipsychotic activity depends on the blockage of postsynaptic receptors in dopamine-mediated pathways that run from the midbrain to the limbic system (septal nucleus, the olfactory tubercle, and the amygdala) and to the temporal and frontal

Table 16-1 Antipsychotic drug affinities for human brain receptors[a]

Drug	Dopamine (D_2) receptor	Muscarinic receptor	Histamine (H_1) receptor	α_1 Receptor
Chlorpromazine	5.3	1.4	11	38
Thioridazine	3.8	5.6	6.2	20
Mesoridazine	5.3	1.4	55	50
Trifluoperazine	38	0.15	1.6	4.2
Perphenazine	71	0.067	12	10
Fluphenazine	125	0.053	4.8	11
Thiothixene	222	0.034	17	9.1
Haloperidol	25	0.0042	0.053	16
Loxapine	1.4	0.22	20	3.6
Molindone	0.83	0.00026	0.00081	0.04
Clozapine	0.56	8.3	36	11
Atropine	—	42	—	—
Chlorpheniramine	—	—	6.7	—
Prazosin	—	—	—	1100

[a]Affinity = $10^{-7} \times 1/K_D$, where K_D is the equilibrium dissociation constant in molarity. Adapted from Ref. 9.

lobes of the cerebral cortex.[10] Presumably, tolerance to the dopamine-blocking action of antipsychotic drugs does not develop in these mesolimbic and mesocortical pathways, explaining the impression that tolerance does not develop to their antipsychotic efficacy.

Antipsychotic drugs also block dopamine receptors in the pathways from the substantia nigra in the midbrain to the head of the caudate nucleus in the basal ganglia.[10,11] Interruption of communication in this nigrostriatal pathway is thought to account for Parkinson's syndrome—bradykinesia, rigidity, and tremor. In this neuronal network, tolerance to the dopamine-blocking action of the drugs does seem to develop. Chemically blocked dopamine receptors are initially underactive and then become normally active to overactive, developing what is analogous to denervation supersensitivity. Underactivity of the striatal dopamine receptors presumably results in parkinsonian signs; overactivity has been postulated to cause tardive dyskinesia, a syndrome of abnormal involuntary movements.[11] Acetylcholine and gamma-aminobutyric acid (GABA) mediate transmission within adjacent connecting neuronal systems.[10] Treatment of both Parkinson's syndrome and tardive dyskinesia may involve drugs purported to act on any or all of these three neurotransmitters.

Researchers believe that a third important dopamine pathway, the tuberoinfundibular system, is affected by antipsychotic drugs. It projects from the arcuate nucleus of the hypothalamus to the median eminence, where it acts to inhibit (directly or indirectly) the release of prolactin from the anterior pituitary.[10] By blocking dopamine neurotransmission in this system, antipsychotic drugs cause increased prolactin secretion and hyperprolactinemia, producing unwanted effects and possible long-term toxicity.

A possible clue to different behavior of the various major dopamine pathways emerges from recent understanding about dopamine autoreceptors.[12,13] Autoreceptors are present on the body or axon of a nerve cell and respond to its own neurotransmitter by decreasing its synthesis and release. Thus, they serve as part of a single-cell feedback inhibition loop. Interestingly, dopamine autoreceptors do not occur in the mesocortical pathways but are present in the nigrostriatal and mesolimbic pathways. The former does not exhibit tolerance to antipsychotic drugs, but the latter two do. Similarly, it appears that tolerance does not develop to the antipsychotic actions of these drugs but does to their extrapyramidal and prolactin-raising actions. Thus, it may be the presence or absence of the dopamine autoreceptors within a system that determines whether tolerance to a clinical effect will or will not occur.

Must parkinsonian and hormonal effects accompany antipsychotic activity? The discovery of clozapine, which produced few (or perhaps no) extrapyramidal effects and had only a weak prolactin-elevating action, suggested that the answer is no. Moreover, neurophysiologic differences among the dopamine systems can mean that pharmacologic agents may act differentially at different dopamine receptors.[10] The goal, then, is to discover new drugs that are more selective dopamine blockers.

The potent effects of antipsychotic agents on the autonomic nervous system explain many of their adverse reactions.[9] They block α-adrenergic receptors,[14] which probably accounts for their hypotensive action, particularly on a postural basis. At common clinical doses, low-potency antipsychotic drugs tend to be more potent at α-adrenergic receptors and to produce a greater drop in orthostatic blood pressure. Central effects on noradrenergic systems might be involved in antipsychotic activity as well.[10]

Antipsychotic agents block muscarinic acetylcholine receptors,[9] producing other autonomic effects. As a group, antipsychotic drugs tend to be much less potent as anticholinergic agents than the tricyclic antidepressants. The most potent antimuscarinic drug among antipsychotic agents available in the United States is the phenothiazine thioridazine, which approaches the tricyclics in anticholinergic activity. High-potency antipsychotic agents act relatively weakly at cholinergic receptors.

Antipsychotic drugs produce other effects on neurotransmission,[10] including effects on GABA, histamine, serotonin, neurotensin, substance P, and endorphins. The potential significance of these effects is not clear at this time.

The hypothalamus mediates various antipsychotic drug effects. In addition to effects on prolactin, antipsychotic drugs inhibit the release of growth hormone[4,6] (which might have implications for their use in children). Some of their effects on autonomic activity may also result from actions within the hypothalamus. Furthermore, they impair the temperature-regulating mechanisms by making the normally homeothermic mammalian system poikilothermic (i.e., the body temperature drifts toward that of the environment), which has resulted in cases of hypo- and hyperthermia.[4,6] In the extreme, antipsychotic drugs have created what has been termed the *neuroleptic malignant syndrome,* also thought to involve the hypothalamus. Increase in appetite, yet another hypothalamic effect, often results in weight gain.

Classes and Chemistry

Table 16-2 presents a list of antipsychotic drugs grouped by chemical classes that are currently marketed in the United States. The first group, the phenothiazines (chlorpromazine is the prototype), are three-ring (tricyclic) molecules made up of two benzene rings linked by a sulfur and a nitrogen atom. The nitrogen atom, which is attached to a carbon side chain, determines the phenothiazine subtype. A straight chain of carbon atoms attached to the nitrogen indicates an aliphatic phenothiazine (e.g., chlorpromazine). When the amino nitrogen at the end of the chain is incorporated into a cyclic structure, the molecule is a piperidine (e.g., thioridazine). A somewhat different cyclic structure results in the piperazine phenothiazines (e.g., trifluoperazine). When a piperazine phenothiazine has a terminal hydroxyl (OH) group, esterifying it with a fatty acid results in a highly fat-soluble hybrid that diffuses into the body's adipose tissue, releasing the parent phenothiazine over a period of weeks. Examples are the enanthate and decanoate esters of the piperazine phenothiazine fluphenazine.

Replacing the nitrogen atom in the central ring with a carbon atom produces a second group of effective antipsychotic substances, the thioxanthenes. They have either aliphatic (e.g., chlorprothixene) or piperazine (e.g., thiothixene) structures and are chemically and pharmacologically similar to the phenothiazines.

The butyrophenones appear structurally quite different from the phenothiazines but are pharmacologically very similar to the piperazines. The only butyrophenone marketed for antipsychotic use in the United States is haloperidol, although the anesthetic agent droperidol also appears to have antipsychotic properties. Closely related to the butyrophenones are the diphenylbutylpiperidines, currently undergoing experimental investigation. This class includes pimozide, an extremely potent blocker of the neurotransmitter dopamine, and penfluridol (not available in the United States), which has a prolonged duration of action enabling it to be administered once weekly by mouth.

The dibenzoxazepine drugs are a fourth antipsychotic group with a three-ring structure. The only member currently labeled as an antipsychotic agent in the United States is loxapine. (The demethylation of loxapine has resulted in amoxapine, a compound with antidepressant properties.) A closely related dibenzodiazepine clozapine appears to be a nonneuroleptic antipsychotic drug.

The fifth antipsychotic group, the dihydroindolines, are solely represented by molindone.

For a tricyclic antipsychotic to be effective, three carbon atoms must lie between the amino nitrogen and the nitrogen of the center ring. The addition of an

Table 16-2 Currently available antipsychotic drugs

Nonproprietary name	Approximate potency	Available as injectable	Chemical structure (representative)
Phenothiazines			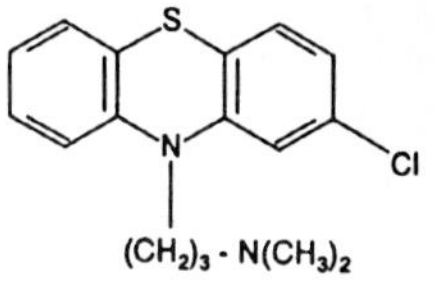
Aliphatic			
Chlorpromazine	1 : 1	Yes	Chlorpromazine
Triflupromazine	4 : 1	Yes	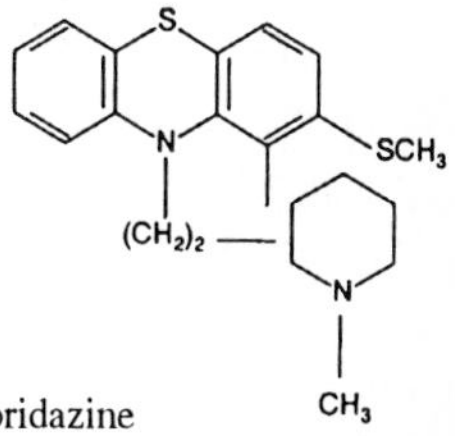
Piperidine			
Thioridazine	1 : 1	No	
Mesoridazine	2 : 1	Yes	Thioridazine
Piperazine			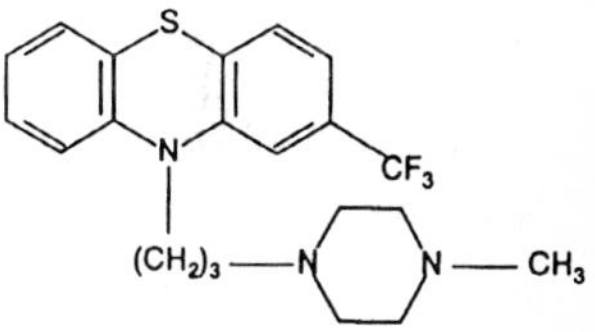
Trifluoperazine	30 : 1	Yes	
Fluphenazine	50–100 : 1	Yes	
Perphenazine	10 : 1	Yes	
Prochlorperazine	7 : 1	Yes	Trifluoperazine
Thioxanthenes			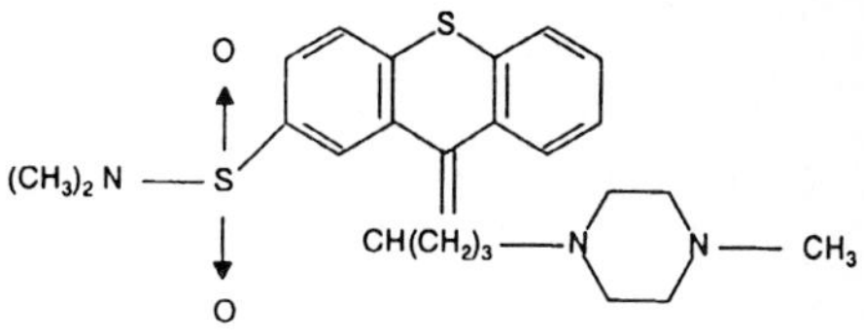
Chlorprothixene	1 : 1	Yes	
Thiothixene	25 : 1	Yes	Thiothixene
Butyrophenone			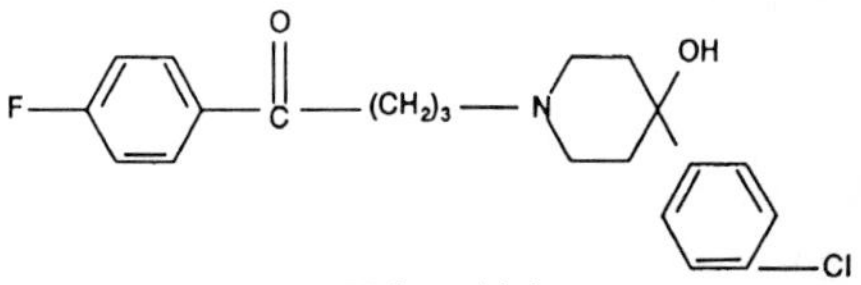
Haloperidol	50 : 1	Yes	Haloperidol

Table 16-2 (*continued*) Currently available antipsychotic drugs

Nonproprietary name	Approximate potency	Available as injectable	Chemical structure (representative)
Diphenylbutylpiperidine Pimozide	Not established	No	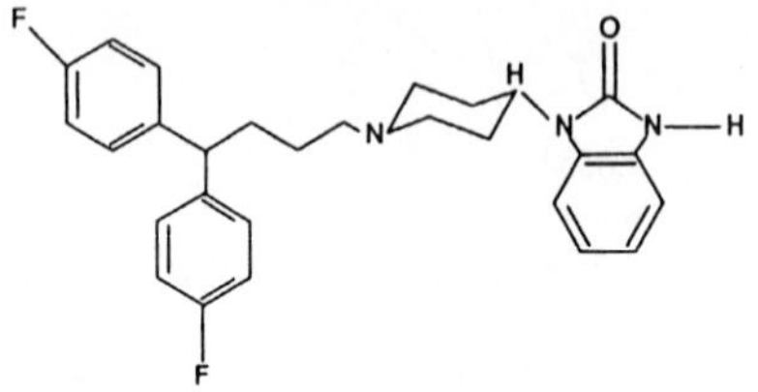 Pimozide
Dibenzodiazepine Clozapine	2 : 1	No	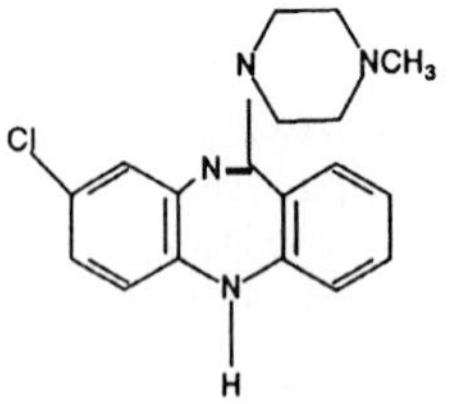 Clozapine
Dibenzoxazepine Loxapine	7 : 1	Yes	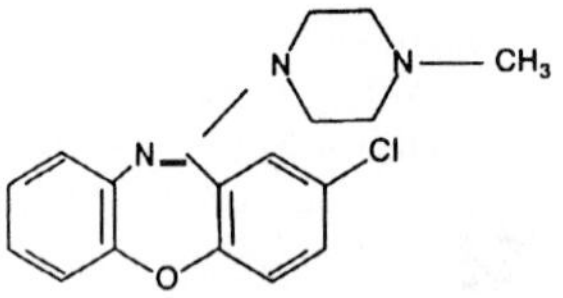 Loxapine
Dihydroindolone Molindone	10 : 1	No	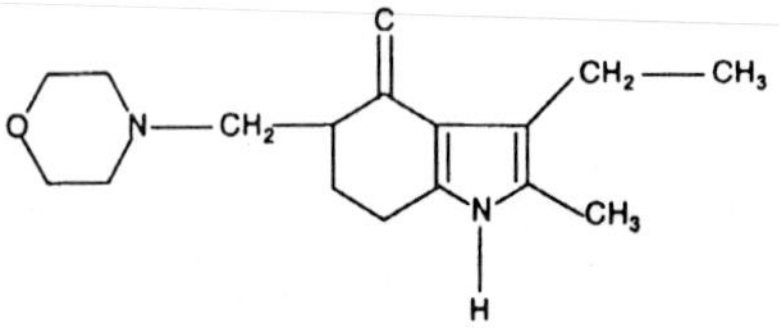 Molindone

electronegative substance to the benzene ring (e.g., Cl, SCH_3, CF_3) enhances its efficacy, whereas the piperazine group on the side chain increases its potency. As a rule, molecules with greater milligram potency produce less sedation and hypotension but more acute extrapyramidal reactions (Table 16-3).

General Principles of Use

How do clinicians choose among the various antipsychotic agents? Most importantly, they should review the patient's medication history. If the patient has previously responded favorably to a given agent, then that agent should be utilized again. In fact, if a patient has been taking a drug for maintenance therapy and an acute exacerbation occurs during a stressful period, then raising the dose of the drug may diminish the symptoms. However, if a patient has responded unfavorably to a given drug because of either lack of efficacy or unacceptable adverse effects, that agent should be avoided. Failing all of these suggestions, the clinician is free to choose among the agents on the basis of his or her own experience and the spectrum of adverse effects. In general, the high-potency antipsychotic drugs are less sedating, produce less hypotension, and have less effect on the seizure threshold, fewer anticholinergic effects, less cardiovascular toxicity, less weight gain, and very little effect on the bone marrow and liver. On the negative side, high-potency antipsychotic drugs have a greater incidence of acute extrapyramidal effects. The converse is true of low-potency agents (Table 16-3).

While the scientific evidence to support the use of antipsychotics is strongest in the treatment of schizophrenia, many elderly patients receive these agents in the managment of agitation.

Agitation in the elderly[14-16] may be a consequence of an organically impaired central nervous system (CNS), such as in dementia, or be due to a loss or a reaction to some stress or acute illness. In addition, agitation may be a manifestation of

Table 16-3 Spectrum of adverse effects caused by antipsychotic drugs

Low potency	High potency
Fewer extrapyramidal reactions (especially thioridazine)	More frequent extrapyramidal reactions
More sedation, postural hypotension	Less sedation, postural hypotension
Greater effect on the seizure threshold, electrocardiogram (especially thioridazine)	Less effect on the seizure threshold, less cardiovascular toxicity
More likely skin pigmentation and photosensitivity	Fewer anticholinergic effects
Occasional cases of cholestatic jaundice	Occasional cases of neuroleptic malignant syndrome
Rare cases of agranulocytosis	

psychosis or depression in the elderly or may result from an acute change in environment, such as admission to the hospital.

It is extremely important for the clinician to make an appropriate diagnosis and identify the underlying cause of the patient's agitation, if possible. Table 16-4 outlines the characteristics of delirium, dementia, and acute functional psychosis in the elderly.[15] A variety of drugs can cause altered mental status in the elderly. Such medications include the anticholinergics (including antidepressants, low-potency antipsychotics, antihistamines), digoxin, H-2 antagonists, benzodiazepines, nonsteroidal anti-inflammatory agents, and a variety of antiarrhythmics and antihypertensives. Drug-induced agitation or delirium should

Table 16-4 Clinical features of delirium, dementia, and acute functional psychosis

Characteristic	Delirium	Dementia	Acute functional psychosis
Onset	Sudden	Insidious	Sudden
Course over 24 h	Fluctuating, with nocturnal exacerbation	Stable	Stable
Consciousness	Reduced	Clear	Clear
Attention	Globally disordered	Normal, except in severe cases	May be disordered
Cognition	Globally disordered	Globally impaired	May be selectively impaired
Hallucinations	Usually visual or visual and auditory	Often absent	Predominantly auditory
Delusions	Fleeting, poorly systematized	Often absent	Sustained, systematized
Orientation	Usually impaired, at least for a time	Often impaired	May be impaired
Psychomotor activity	Increased, reduced, or shifting unpredictably	Often normal	Varies from psychomotor retardation to severe hyperactivity, depending on the type of psychosis
Speech	Often incoherent, slow or rapid	Patient has difficulty finding words, perseveration	Normal, slow or rapid
Involuntary movements	Often asterixis or coarse tremor	Often absent	Usually absent
Physical illness or drug toxicity	One or both are present	Often absent, especially in senile dementia of the Alzheimer's type	Usually absent

Source: Adapted from Ref. 15.

be treated primarily by removing the offending agent(s) rather than by adding additional medications. Withdrawal from alcohol, benzodiazepines, and other CNS depressants also may cause severe agitation. Other causes for agitation or a change in mental status, such as endocrine diseases (hypothyroidism, hypercalcemia, hyponatremia), renal failure, and nutritional abnormalities (vitamin B_{12} and thiamin deficiency), should be ruled out.

Drugs are frequently used to control agitation in the elderly. Antipsychotics are the third most frequently prescribed class of drugs in skilled nursing facilities.[14] Haloperidol and thioridazine are especially common agents used in the elderly. In a recent study,[17] 82 percent of 685 nursing home residents were taking one or more antipsychotic drugs.

Proper non-drug treatment is an essential component of the management of these patients.[15] A quiet and well-lighted room, a clearly visible clock and calendar, and a few familiar objects may help calm and orient the patient. The provision of reassuring, supportive nursing care that assists the patient in reestablishing orientation is vital. If the patient is very agitated and restless, drug therapy may be indicated. In general, antipsychotic agents are the most effective, while benzodiazepines appear to be less effective in many studies.

While a variety of antipsychotics have been used, haloperidol is currently the most popular. In general, a high-potency agent with little anticholinergic or cardiovascular effects should be used. Low doses of antipsychotics should be used, such as 0.5 mg haloperidol once or twice daily (Table 16-5). If nighttime agitation is most problematic, a larger percentage of the daily dose may be given at bedtime. If the initial dose is not effective, the dose should be slowly escalated. Excessive amounts of antipsychotics in these patients may cause severe extrapyramidal effects as well as CNS depression. Because the underlying cause of the patient's agitation may be reversible, short-term therapy should be

Table 16-5 Selected antipsychotics: pharmacologic factors of special relevance for the elderly

Agent	Relative potency[a]	Predominant side effects	Usual initial daily dose for the elderly
Chlorpromazine	100	Sedating, anticholinergic	10-25 mg twice or three times a day
Thioridazine	95-100	Sedating, anticholinergic	10-25 mg twice or three times a day
Thiothixene	5	Extrapyramidal	2-3 mg
Haloperidol	2	Extrapyramidal	0.5-2 mg
Fluphenazine	2	Extrapyramidal	0.5-2 mg

[a]Chlorpromazine was arbitrarily assigned a potency of 100 for the sake of comparison with other agents.

Source: Adapted from Ref. 1.

the rule. Long-term therapy with these agents in the elderly may cause debilitating tardive dyskinesia.

Pharmacokinetics[18-21]

Table 16-6 outlines the pharmacokinetic properties of the antipsychotic agents. The pharmacokinetics of chlorpromazine, the prototypical phenothiazine, has been extensively studied. Chlorpromazine is virtually completely absorbed from the

Table 16-6 Pharmacokinetics of antipsychotic agents

Antipsychotic agents	Time to peak after oral dose, h	Elimination half-life, h	Protein binding, %	Active metabolites
Phenothiazines				
Chlorpromazine	2-4	16-37 (but active metabs probably much longer)	98-99	Many, unclear which of >160 metabs active
Fluphenazine (oral)	—	12-24	—	None?
Mesoridazine	—	~6	~25	
Perphenazine	—	8-21	—	None
Thioridazine	2 (concentrate) 4 (tablets)	7-42	96-99	Mesoridazine Sulphoridazine
Trifluoperazine	3-6	17-18	Unknown	Uncertain (possibly demethylated and hydroxylated metabolites)
Butyrophenones				
Haloperidol	2-6	12-40	~90	Reduced haloperidol?
Dibenzoxepines				
Loxapine	1 IM/2 PO	3.4 (loxapine) (9 8-OH loxapine 30 8-OH amoxapine)	~90	8-OH loxapine 8-OH amoxapine
Dibenzodiazepines				
Clozapine	1-4	6-33	>90	Uncertain (demethylated metabolites may be active)
Indolones				
Molindone	0.5	1.5	None	?
Thioxanthenes				
Thiothixene	1-3	α = 3.5 β = 34	Not studied	None identified

gastrointestinal tract. The antipsychotics are highly bound to serum proteins and distributed widely into tissue, with a volume of distribution of 10 to 20 L/kg. Brain concentrations of chlorpromazine are fivefold those in serum after chronic administration. The antipsychotics are extensively metabolized by the liver. Over 100 chlorpromazine metabolites have been identified, and these metabolites are excreted renally. While the initial elimination half-life of chlorpromazine is approximately 6 h, with long-term administration the elimination half-life ranges from 16 to 30 h. The rate of clearance of the phenothiazines is highly variable, with plasma levels varying 10 - to 100-fold. It has been demonstrated that the rate of disposition of several phenothiazines depends on the debrisoquine hydroxylation phenotype.[19]

Clozapine[22,23] has an oral bioavailability of 50 to 60 percent, with extensive first-pass hepatic metabolism. The apparent volume of distribution of clozapine is 5 L/kg, lower than other antipsychotic agents but still quite large. The average elimination half-life is 12 h, but long-term pharmacokinetic studies evaluating the terminal elimination have not been done. Remoxipride, an investigational benzamide antipsychotic, has an elimination half-life of 3 to 6 h.[24]

While there are not extensive studies evaluating the pharmacokinetic differences of antipsychotics in the elderly versus the young, one study has found that the elderly have higher serum chlorpromazine and thioridazine levels than younger patients.[18] There is conflicting evidence regarding any pharmacokinetic differences of haloperidol in the elderly.[14] Elderly patients receiving clozapine have a twofold increase in serum levels versus younger patients.[22] The half-life of remoxipride in elderly patients was twice that of younger patients, and serum levels were significantly higher in the elderly as well.[24]

Because of the high degree of interpatient variability of the pharmacokinetics of the phenothiazines and butyrophenones, it is not clear whether there are consistent age-related differences in absorption, distribution, or clearance. There is good evidence to support such differences with clozaril and remoxipride. The clinician would be wise to assume such age-related differences with all antipsychotics in the elderly and use lower initial doses and slower dose titrations in this patient population (see Table 16-5).

Attempts to correlate plasma concentrations of antipsychotic drugs with their clinical efficacy have yielded contradictory results. This unsatisfying situation reflects problems in research methodology as well as in biochemical assays and questions about active drug metabolites. Although it was once thought that a radioreceptor assay measuring the level of dopamine-blocking activity in serum would replace direct chemical measurements of drug concentrations, this is less clear-cut at present.[25] Available evidence hints at the existence of a curvilinear (*therapeutic window*) relationship for the butyrophenone haloperidol, a drug with no (or possibly one) active metabolite(s), although the precise upper and lower boundaries on this "window" remain to be delineated.

Regardless of any given antipsychotic drug's specific half-life, virtually all of these agents can be administered in a once-daily dose, usually at bedtime. The clinical effectiveness of this regimen presumably reflects the drugs' prolonged brain effects and gradual elimination from the body. After chronic dosing, biologic effects of these agents persist for many weeks. After prolonged use of decanoate preparations, clinical and biologic effects can extend beyond 6 months.

Use of Clozapine

Clozapine[22,23] is a relatively new and unique antipsychotic. Encouraging evidence accumulated in the late 1980s suggests that clozapine, besides having a lower profile of extrapyramidal effects, can also alleviate chronic symptoms of psychosis in patients previously resistant to standard neuroleptics. A large collaborative study[26] showed substantial improvement in 33 percent of patients with treatment-resistant schizophrenia. Additional longitudinal data suggest that, after a year's treatment, more than two-thirds of patients in this category may become responders. Thus, although encumbered by agranulocytosis and other potentially serious side effects,[22,23] clozapine may bring relief to a substantial subset of previously treatment-resistant schizophrenics.

Because of clozapine's unique side-effect profile (Table 16-7), specific approaches to clinical management are required for patients maintained on the drug.[22,23] As mentioned earlier, patients who have recovered from clozapine-induced agranulocytosis should never again be exposed to this drug. Those with seizures can, however, be reexposed, possibly in conjunction with an anticonvulsant, and certainly at a lower initial dose. Sedation can be managed with a lower dose or a bedtime biasing of the dosage schedule and, as with other psychotropic medications, symptomatic hypotension may be treated with support stockings, increased dietary sodium, or the mineralocorticoid fludrocortisone. Hyperthermia is common with clozapine, but it is usually benign and transient.

Table 16-7 Common side effects of clozapine

Side effect	Incidence, %
Sedation and fatigue	34±24
Sialorrhea	23±23
Weight gain	34±29
Hypotension	11±12
Gastrointestinal symptoms	17±23
Tachycardia	7±7
Fever	5±4
Seizures	4±0
Electrocardiographic changes	2±2
Leukopenia or agranulocytosis	1±2

Source: Adapted from Ref. 22.

However, infection and neuroleptic malignant syndrome must be ruled out. Occasional patients who develop nausea and, less commonly, vomiting after weeks or months of clozapine therapy have been treated successfully with metoclopramide.

Adverse Effects and Toxicity

The relative side-effect profile[1,4,27,28] of the antipsychotics is outlined in Table 16-8.

Neurologic

Extrapyramidal syndromes Antipsychotic drugs may cause four types of extrapyramidal syndromes: acute dystonic reactions, akathisia, Parkinson's syndrome, and after longer-term use, tardive dyskinesia.

Acute dystonic reactions Acute dystonic reactions, including acute dyskinesias (i.e., abnormal involuntary movements of various types) and oculogyric crises, typically occur during the early hours or days following the initiation of antipsychotic drug therapy or after marked dosage increments. Involuntary muscle contractions are common, particularly about the mouth, jaw, face, and neck. The symptoms are episodic and recurrent, lasting from minutes to hours. There may be trismus ("lockjaw"), dystonia or dyskinesias of the tongue, opisthotonus (spasms of the neck that arch the head backward), or eye closure. In oculogyric crises, there is a dystonic reaction of the extraocular muscles, and gaze is fixed in one position.

Acute dystonic reactions are distressing, particularly to the patient, family member, or clinician who is unfamiliar with them. They may be uncomfortable.

Table 16-8 Relative incidence of antipsychotic drug adverse effects

	Sedation	Extra-pyramidal symptoms	Anticholinergic	Cardiovascular
Low-potency agents				
Chlorpromazine	High	Moderate	Moderate	High
Clozapine	High	Very low	High	High
Thioridazine	High	Low	High	High
High-potency agents				
Trifluoperazine	Low	High	Low	Low
Fluphenazine	Low	Very high	Low	Low
Thiothixene	Low	High	Low	Low
Haloperidol	Very low	Very high	Very low	Very low
Loxapine	Moderate	High	Low	Moderate
Molindone	Very low	High	Low	Low

They are rarely dangerous. However, in rare cases there can be respiratory compromise with the potential for a fatality.

The diagnosis of acute dystonic reaction is usually not difficult if it is clear that a patient has recently begun taking an antipsychotic drug or has had a switch in the type or dosage of medication. At times, however, eliciting this information may be difficult, especially with patients who are taking prochlorperazine suppositories (and say they are not taking any tranquilizer pills), who do not wish to acknowledge use of antipsychotic drugs, or who have sought antipsychotic drugs for illicit use (described recently). Among the many neuropsychiatric syndromes that must be considered in the differential diagnosis of acute dystonic reactions are tetanus, hypocalcemia, seizures, and conversion reactions.

The highest potency antipsychotic drugs have the greatest likelihood of producing acute dystonias, the low-potency agents much less, and thioridazine and clozapine the least. Young people are at greater risk of developing this syndrome than the elderly, and males do so more frequently than females.

The mechanism underlying acute dystonic reactions is unclear. One hypothesis is that the syndrome reflects an acute increase in dopamine neurotransmission in the basal ganglia, which transiently supervenes the blockade of dopamine receptors brought about by the same drugs. Although dystonic reactions do not occur in naturally occurring Parkinson's disease, they are observed in postencephalitic Parkinson's syndrome, which shares other features with antipsychotic drug-induced extrapyramidal reactions.

Although the mechanism may be unclear, the treatment of an acute dystonic reaction is straightforward, readily available, and usually dramatically successful. Parenteral treatment is preferred for initiating drug therapy, with intravenous therapy being more rapid than intramuscular. An injectable anticholinergic antiparkinson drug such as benztropine 1 mg may be used. Other clinicians prefer to administer an antihistamine drug such as diphenhydramine 50 mg or a benzodiazepine intravenously, such as diazepam, up to 10 mg. While diazepam is relatively safe, equipment for support of the airway should be immediately available should respiratory depression occur.

Following immediate relief of acute dystonic signs, the clinician may wish to begin oral administration of one of these drugs, using the lowest effective dose (see Table 16-9). If this successfully prevents additional reactions, the medication can usually be tapered and discontinued within several weeks. Would it be wise to coadminister an antiparkinson drug from the beginning of antipsychotic drug therapy in the hope of avoiding an acute dystonic reaction? Recent data suggest that one may offer partial protection to some patients through this "prophylactic" approach.[29] Therefore, the physician may want to consider this approach for patients at highest risk (i.e., young males receiving high-potency antipsychotic agents) and for those in whom a reaction is likely to be clinically disruptive. For other patients, it makes sense to avoid a drug that may be unnecessary, reserving treatment until signs of dystonia appear.

Table 16-9 Antiparkinson agents used in the treatment of neuroleptic-induced extrapyramidal syndrome

Generic name	Type of drug	Usual dose range, mg/day	Injectable
Amantadine	Dopamine agonist	100 to 300	No
Benztropine	Antihistamine and anticholinergic	1 to 6	Yes
Biperiden	Anticholinergic	2 to 6	Yes
Diphenhydramine	Antihistamine and anticholinergic	25 to 200	Yes
Ethopropazine	Antihistamine and anticholinergic	50 to 600	No
Orphenadrine	Antihistamine	50 to 300	Yes
Procyclidine	Anticholinergic	6 to 20	No
Trihexyphenidyl	Anticholinergic	1 to 10	No

Clinicians, family members, and anyone else who may observe a patient receiving an antipsychotic medicine should be aware of the possible occurrence of a dystonic reaction early in therapy. Treatment should be readily available. For most patients, the risk of dystonic reactions appears to wane with continued antipsychotic drug therapy.

Akathisia Akathisia is another extrapyramidal reaction associated with both antipsychotic drugs and postencephalitic Parkinson's syndrome (rarely with Parkinson's disease). Akathisia is a symptom defined as a compulsion to be in motion. Patients describe an inner restlessness, an intense desire to move about simply for the sake of moving. Patients suffering from akathisia are often observed to pace aimlessly, fidget, and be markedly restless. At times, akathisia may cause a worsening of psychosis.[30]

Akathisia can occur early in the course of drug treatment, or it may not appear for several months. It, too, appears to be more prevalent with high-potency drugs. The natural course of akathisia is less clear than that of acute dystonic reaction. At times it appears to wane; yet some patients are troubled by it for a prolonged time. Its mechanism is obscure but may involve a blockade of mesocortical dopamine receptors.

Treatment responses are variable. Nevertheless, akathisia is an important syndrome to recognize, as it may severely complicate a patient's response to antipsychotic drug therapy; perhaps most importantly, it makes patients extremely unhappy. Approaches to treatment include attempts to lower the dose of the antipsychotic drug, switch to a lower potency agent, or add a contraactive drug. The same drugs discussed for the treatment of acute dystonic reactions—anticholinergic antiparkinson agents, antihistamines, and benzodiazepines—also may be tried orally in cases of akathisia, although results are less universally successful.

Whether the dopamine agonist antiparkinson drug amantadine may play a role in the treatment of this disorder is unclear.

Recent research has shown that the beta-adrenergic blocking drug propranolol can effectively treat both subjective and objective manifestations of akathisia while producing an acceptable profile of side effects; other β-blockers may be safe and effective as well.[29] Another agent that diminishes central noradrenergic activity, the antihypertensive clonidine, also may be effective but appears to cause an unacceptable incidence of sedation and hypotension.[30]

Parkinson's syndrome Parkinson's disease is discussed extensively in Chap. 13. In neuroleptic-induced Parkinson's syndrome, tremor is typically bilateral; unilateral tremors should raise questions about the etiology. Although tremor is very common and may be one of the earlier signs in naturally occurring Parkinson's disease, it is less common than rigidity and bradykinesia and may not appear until relatively late in the drug-related syndrome.

In extreme forms of the drug-induced parkinsonism, rigidity and bradykinesia may mimic (or actually become) the waxy flexibility with sustained postures characteristic of catatonia.[31] In antipsychotic drug-induced Parkinson's syndrome, rigidity tends to be more common than tremor but less common than akinesia.

In a less severe manifestation, the slowed movements of the parkinsonian patient may appear primarily as apathy, boredom, and a "zombielike" appearance. If other signs of Parkinson's syndrome are not prominent, this social akinesia may be misdiagnosed as depression.[32]

Parkinson's syndrome usually occurs within weeks to months after the beginning of antipsychotic drug therapy. Although tolerance develops in many patients, the disorder may persist and require ongoing treatment in others. Women and the elderly are affected more commonly. Again, the high-potency agents appear more likely to promote this disturbance.

Ganzini et al [33a] have reported on the incidence of extrapyramidal reactions in 19 elderly patients treated with antipsychotics. In this report, 10 out of 19 patients had signs of Parkinson's syndrome, despite not having received antipsychotics for at least 2 weeks. Once treated with antipsychotics, none of the patients developed acute dystonia, 19 percent developed akathisia, and a dose-related Parkinson's syndrome occurred in 71 percent. The occurrence of drug-induced parkinsonism and akathisia was associated with failure to benefit clinically from antipsychotic therapy. In additon, two patients developed incontinence associated with the parkinsonian symptoms.

The treatment of Parkinson's syndrome reflects our understanding of the pathophysiology. One approach is to decrease the dose of the antipsychotic drug, presumably thereby decreasing the degree of dopamine blockade at the synaptic receptor. Alternatively, a less potent antipsychotic agent may be employed.

Among the original neuroleptics, thioridazine has the lowest incidence of parkinsonian reactions. The reason for this differential effect of antipsychotic drugs in causing Parkinson's syndrome may be related to variations in activity within the several dopamine systems or differing central anticholinergic potency. Clozapine has by far the lowest incidence of parkinsonism.

Pharmacologic contraactive therapy for parkinsonism consists of attempts to counterbalance the decreased dopamine neurotransmission either by blocking acetylcholine transmission (anticholinergic antiparkinson drugs include benzotropine and trihexyphenidyl) or by increasing dopamine neurotransmission (e.g., by the use of amantadine and others). Other dopamine agonist drugs such as L-dopa and bromocriptine may be useful in other forms of Parkinson's syndrome but are seldom employed for the drug-induced variety.

Table 16-9 lists available drugs that are useful for the treatment of drug-induced Parkinson's syndrome. With constant awareness of the pleomorphic and often subtle manifestations of extrapyramidal reactions, the clinician prescribes one of these contraactive drugs as needed for a patient's comfort and optimal functioning, always seeking the lowest effective dose. Clinicians should periodically attempt to taper and discontinue a concomitant antiparkinson drug, although many patients on maintenance neuroleptic therapy may require parallel maintenance with antiparkinson drugs.[33]

With the exception of amantadine, all of the antiparkinson drugs listed in Table 16-9 have anticholinergic and/or antihistaminic properties. Among these drugs, trihexyphenidyl has a relatively short half-life, whereas benztropine has a relatively long half-life. Amantadine is a dopamine agonist that has few anticholinergic effects. This feature may make it preferable in patients particularly sensitive to anticholinergic reactions.[33] For many patients, the strongly anticholinergic antiparkinson drugs can impair memory, time perception, and cognition: these CNS anticholinergic side effects also might prompt the use of amantadine.[34] Amantadine, 100 mg two to three times daily, may be effective in some cases of drug-induced Parkinson's syndrome, particularly the more severe variety, when anticholinergic antiparkinson drugs have been ineffectual.[35] Amantadine has a relatively long half-life (approximately 24 h). It is excreted in the urine unchanged and may lead to toxicity (including psychiatric symptoms) in elderly patients, especially those with impaired renal function.

Low-dose clozapine therapy may be an alternative management strategy, especially if the elderly psychotic patient has preexisting Parkinson's disease.[22,23]

Tardive dyskinesia Tardive dyskinesia is characterized by abnormal, involuntary, choreoathetotic movements involving the tongue, lips, jaw, face, extremities, and occasionally the trunk. Not many years after the introduction of antipsychotic agents, patients were described who displayed these movements after a period of drug treatment. For the most part, clinicians generally ignored the existence of tardive dyskinesia.

By the early 1970s, however, tardive dyskinesia was recognized as more widespread than previously appreciated, and a 1981 review even suggested that its prevalence has progressively increased over the years since the introduction of antipsychotic medication.[36]

Tardive dyskinesia typically involves orobuccolingual masticatory movements. These may include lip smacking, chewing, puckering of the lips, protrusion of the tongue, and puffing of the cheeks. A common early sign is wormlike movements of the tongue. Other movements of the face can be observed, including grimacing, blinking, and frowning. Another late-onset condition, presumably caused by antipsychotic drug exposure, is tardive dystonia, characterized by slow, sustained, involuntary twisting movements of limbs, trunk, neck, or face, including involuntary eye closure (blepharospasm).[37]

The signs of tardive dyskinesia can range in intensity from minimal to severe. Patients' awareness of the movements similarly varies. Institutionalized chronic schizophrenic patients may deny even very severe movements, whereas a highly functioning patient with a mood disorder could be extremely troubled by the most minimal symptom. The movements may embarrass the patient and interfere with important activities such as eating, talking, and dressing. In rare instances, tardive dyskinesia can impair breathing and swallowing.

Although movements identical to tardive dyskinesia occur with exposure to neuroleptics, a meta-analysis of 21 studies found that neuroleptics multiply the risk of developing dyskinesia by 2.9 times.[38] It is generally believed that for tardive dyskinesia to occur, a patient must have been exposed, more or less continuously, to an antipsychotic drug for at least 3 to 6 months, although it is probable that a rare, highly sensitive patient may develop this syndrome after an even briefer period. Presumably, increasing exposure to antipsychotic drugs increases the risk of developing tardive dyskinesia, although a patient who has not developed it after some length of time is probably less vulnerable. The only risk factor that has appeared consistently in studies of tardive dyskinesia is advanced age, although wide interindividual sensitivity to the development of this syndrome probably exists. Smith and Baldessarini[39] found that advancing age leads to a regularly increasing risk of tardive dyskinesia in terms of prevalence, severity, and remission. There is no convincing evidence that patients taking one type of antipsychotic drug, such as high or low potency, are more or less likely to develop tardive dyskinesia. It appears that "drug holidays," i.e., regular, abrupt discontinuation of antipsychotic drug therapy, do not reduce the risk of tardive dyskinesia. Although it has been suggested that drug holidays may even increase the risk,[38] this is controversial. Prospective studies suggest a link between cumulative dosage and the development of tardive dyskinesia, underscoring the wisdom of maintaining patients on the lowest effective dosage over prolonged periods of time.

Estimates of the prevalence of tardive dyskinesia have varied widely—from 1 to over 50 percent of patients currently taking these drugs.[40] However, when the most minimal cases are removed from consideration, an attempt is made at differential diagnosis, and a careful and reliable screening procedure is used, the prevalence of tardive dyskinesia in a group of patients maintained on antipsychotic drugs for a variable period of time (i.e., a typical outpatient schizophrenic population) is likely to be 20 to 30 percent.[41] In a recent prospective study of 215 elderly patients, 31 percent developed tardive dyskinesia over a 43-week period.[42] A more important question concerns the incidence of tardive dyskinesia; preliminary data suggest 3 to 4 percent per year of patient exposure.[41]

The movements of tardive dyskinesia may appear during treatment when a patient is taking a constant dose of an antipsychotic, or they may initially appear when the dosage of the drug is lowered or stopped entirely. Conversely, if movements are present, increasing the dose of an antipsychotic drug can make the movements cease. This latter phenomenon has been referred to as *masking* of the movements and gives rise to the concept of *covert dyskinesia*, in other words, dyskinesia observed only when an antipsychotic drug has been discontinued.[43] On the other hand, when an antipsychotic drug is discontinued abruptly, a patient may show transient dyskinetic movements that can disappear in a matter of days or weeks. This phenomenon has been known as withdrawal dyskinesia, and it might conceivably indicate that a patient is vulnerable to a persistent dyskinesia if the medication is reinstituted and continued. Tardive dyskinesia itself is believed to be persistent, although evidence suggests that if the movements are detected early and medication is discontinued, many patients will show gradual improvement over time.[44]

The linkage between early development of Parkinson's syndrome and later development of tardive dyskinesia, as well as possible contributing factors to the development of tardive dyskinesia from earlier use of antiparkinson drugs, is unresolved. What is clear is that anticholinergic drugs frequently exacerbate the movements of tardive dyskinesia once they are present and that administration of anticholinergic agents may even "unmask" latent movements. Conversely, discontinuing an anticholinergic drug in a patient with tardive dyskinesia may improve the movements.

The most widely held hypothesis about the mechanism of tardive dyskinesia has involved the nigrostriatal dopamine pathway. Chronic blockade of dopamine receptors within the basal ganglia leads first to receptor underactivity and then to overactivity. This state of excessive dopaminergic activity is believed to result in the abnormal movements of disorders such as tardive dyskinesia and Huntington's chorea.[45]

The "dopamine excess" hypothesis of tardive dyskinesia is not completely satisfying, however. For example, prolonged exposure to neuroleptic drugs results in dopamine receptor supersensitivity in virtually all experimental animals, but only some patients develop tardive dyskinesia. Also, such supersensitivity is *less* likely to develop in older animals, but tardive dyskinesia is *more* likely to develop in older patients. These and other objections have led many scholars to conjecture that the dopamine supersensitivity hypothesis of tardive dyskinesia is too simplistic to be universally applicable. Perhaps such a mechanism is valid in some patients, but alternative neurotransmitter systems that may contribute to the development of tardive dyskinesia include those involving GABA, acetylcholine, and norepinephrine.

Treatment approaches to tardive dyskinesia are based on our understanding and beliefs about the nature of antipsychotic drugs and tardive dyskinesia. First, of course, comes primary prevention. This means avoiding unnecessary exposure of patients to antipsychotic drugs. In particular, the use of these agents to treat relatively benign conditions or those that could respond equally well or better to other agents should be avoided whenever possible. When it is necessary to employ antipsychotic drug therapy, use the lowest dose for the shortest period of time. Of course, most schizophrenic patients will require prolonged therapy with these agents, but the clinician should find the lowest effective maintenance dose. Similarly, in the treatment of patients with other chronic disorders such as mental retardation and organic brain syndrome, the use of drugs should be minimized and constantly reevaluated.

Secondary prevention of a disorder means early detection. For tardive dyskinesia, this entails routine screening and monitoring of patients for the presence of abnormal movements. A standard neurologic examination can be employed for this purpose, or a clinician may want to use a specific examination procedure and rating scale such as the Abnormal Involuntary Movement Scale designed by the National Institute of Mental Health. It is best to perform an examination and note the results prior to the initiation of antipsychotic drug therapy (or before too long into the course) and then to repeat the examination every 6 to 12 months while the patient remains on drug therapy. If early movements are detected, the clinician will want to consider lowering the dose of the antipsychotic drug or discontinuing it altogether. In addition, the patient (or next of kin) should be fully apprised of the clinical dilemma, the options, and the clinician's recommendation for further treatment.

What does one do when the presence of abnormal involuntary movements is unequivocal? First, consider the diagnosis. Is any other diagnosis likely? Are the movements characteristic of tardive dyskinesia or might they be tremors or other movements? Are they chronic mannerisms and stereotypes characteristic of the underlying psychiatric disorder or have these movements only appeared following chronic drug treatment? Family history should be explored to rule out the presence of hereditary disorders of the CNS such as Huntington's chorea or dystonia. The patient's history also should be reexplored to establish a reasonable linkage between drug therapy and the appearance of abnormal movements. A neurologic examination should reveal only abnormal involuntary movements and specifically those characteristic of tardive dyskinesia; other neurologic systems, such as sensory or pyramidal, should not be involved. A physical examination should search for the presence of ancillary signs of other extrapyramidal disorders such as the Kayser-Fleischer rings of Wilson's disease. Finally, laboratory testing can rule out other disorders—e.g., copper and ceruloplasmin levels in Wilson's disease, radiologic evidence of caudate degeneration in Huntington's disease—if these conditions are suspected.

If the diagnosis of tardive dyskinesia appears firm, what is the course of treatment? Raising the dose of the antipsychotic drug might succeed in partially (or even completely) suppressing the movements, but the clinician should avoid this strategy if possible. Available evidence suggests that continuing neuroleptic therapy, although unlikely to exacerbate the degree of dyskinesia, may enhance the probability that the dyskinesia will become irreversible.[44,45] Of course, if continuing an antipsychotic drug is necessary to control the psychosis or prevent episodic relapses (as is often the case), then the clinician must recommend this course, and it is up to the patient (or guardian) to decide whether to consent.

If abnormal movements are detected early and it is clinically practical to taper and discontinue the antipsychotic medication, it is more likely that the dyskinesia will ultimately improve (although it may be temporarily exacerbated initially). Although this is ideal from the standpoint of the movement disorder, for most schizophrenic patients the trade-off in exacerbation of psychosis will not be worth the price. Schizophrenic psychosis usually is worse than tardive dyskinesia, and most often the clinician, patient, and family will decide to continue drug therapy, always at the lowest effective dose.

If the movements continue and are troublesome (and irrespective of whether the patient remains on antipsychotic drug therapy), the clinician will want to alleviate as much of the patient's discomfort as possible. Unfortunately, there is no standard and accepted treatment for tardive dyskinesia. Therapy with a benzodiazepine drug such as diazepam or clonazepam may help some patients, either by its sedative properties or possibly via its role in increasing GABAergic tone.

Just as Parkinson's syndrome often responds to strategies that increase dopamine neurotransmission, tardive dyskinesia may be alleviated by treatments that diminish dopaminergic tone. Thus, a dopamine-depleting agent such as reserpine or tetrabenazine may be useful. Another treatment approach focuses on the cholinergic system. Deanol was earlier employed for this purpose, but its status as a cholinergic agonist is in question, and its efficacy in tardive dyskinesia is doubtful. Choline chloride has been employed in this fashion, but initial positive results have not been sustained, and its many unwanted effects make it clinically troublesome. Phosphatidylcholine, contained in the naturally occurring lipid lecithin, also has been used for this purpose. Gelenberg et al have found lecithin to produce statistically significant but clinically minimal benefits.[46] If a patient is already taking an *anti*-cholinergic drug, the abnormal movements of tardive dyskinesia may be diminished if the anticholinergic drug is withdrawn; the "downside," however, is that parkinsonian signs may emerge or become worse.

Agents that increase GABA activity also may have some benefit in tardive dyskinesia.[47] Baclofen, a GABA agonist, and sodium valproate, a GABA transaminase inhibitor, may cause a GABA-mediated inhibition of nigrostriatal dopamine activity. Further studies are needed with these agents.

Sedation It was initially believed that sedation[1,27,28] was important for the effectiveness of antipsychotic drugs, but this no longer appears true.[4] Drugs can have a major impact on the primary symptoms of psychosis such as hallucinations and thought disorder without producing somnolence. As mentioned previously, the low-potency antipsychotic drugs such as chlorpromazine, thioridazine, and chlorprothixene tend to be more sedating. Clozapine is especially sedating. If around-the-clock sedation is desired, these drugs can be administered several times daily during initial therapy. If nighttime sedation is indicated, the drugs may be administered once daily at bedtime. Tolerance to sedation tends to develop over a matter of days or several weeks.

Administration of CNS depressant drugs in the elderly may cause global cognitive impairment. Larson et al[48] found that a variety of agents, including haloperidol and thioridazine, caused excessive morbidity, with incidence of cognitive impairment correlated with the number of CNS depressant drugs the patient was taking. Avorn et al[17] found that 16 percent of 685 nursing home residents were taking two or more antipsychotic medications. Therefore, any patient receiving these agents who develops a change in mental status should have a reassessment of the patient's medication profile.

Clozapine therapy recently has been reported to cause respiratory depression. [50a] This rare event may result in respiratory arrest and appears to be associated with concomitant clozapine and benzodiazepine therapy.

Seizures Antipsychotic drugs, particularly the low-potency agents, lower the seizure threshold.4,27,28 For most patients, this is seldom a problem. However, an occasional patient without a history of epilepsy will experience a seizure during treatment with very high doses (or a particularly rapid increase in dose) of a low-potency agent. The problem is more likely to surface in the case of a patient with marginally controlled seizures or in a state of heightened vulnerability such as withdrawal from sedative-hypnotic drugs or alcohol. Each case must be handled individually, but consideration should be given to lowering the dose of the antipsychotic drug, changing to a high-potency agent, and/or adding (or increasing) an anticonvulsant. Clozapine lowers the seizure threshold in a dose-dependent fashion.23

Neuroleptic malignant syndrome The neuroleptic malignant syndrome (NMS) is a serious disorder consisting of fever, muscular rigidity, and stupor, which develops in association with antipsychotic drug therapy.[49] Other features include autonomic dysfunction (e.g., increased pulse, respiration, sweating, and blood pressure instability) and occasionally respiratory distress. Laboratory findings commonly indicate leukocytosis and elevated serum creatine kinase (CK). This syndrome typically develops explosively over a 24- to 72-h period beginning anywhere from hours to months after initial drug exposure. A patient may have received prior treatment with antipsychotic drugs without showing this pattern.

NMS has been associated with various antipsychotic drugs but is more prevalent with high-potency agents, particularly when the dose is being raised quickly. Haloperidol has been associated with a disproportionate share of case reports. Both sexes may be affected at any age, but among reported cases, young adult males predominate. The incidence of this disorder is probably around 0.1 percent of patients exposed to neuroleptics.[50] Mortality from NMS may be 10 to 20 percent, but when the patient survives, sequelae are rare.[50,51]

The mechanism of NMS has yet to be elucidated. Most theories have focused on the basal ganglia and hypothalamus, where blockade of dopamine neurotransmission is held responsible since withdrawal of dopamine agonists, as well as institution of dopamine antagonists, has been associated with precipitation of NMS. An alternative site for the pathology of NMS could be peripheral muscles, analogous to the malignant hyperthermia of anesthesia.

Levenson and Simpson[52] have underscored the heterogeneity of cases of neuroleptic-induced extrapyramidal signs plus fever. They emphasize that many such patients have diverse and independently treatable medical or neurologic conditions, which require a careful differential diagnosis.

Since a patient may develop NMS on one exposure to a neuroleptic yet not on another, it is likely that additional factors may play a role in the pathogenesis. Dehydration may be one such factor, and clinicians would do well to attend to hydration status during antipsychotic therapy, particularly in warmer weather when patients are exerting themselves or if they have inadequate oral intake.

Appropriate management requires immediate discontinuation of antipsychotic drugs and institution of supportive measures (e.g., lowering body temperature, hydration) along with ruling out infection and other possible metabolic abnormalities. Although no contraactive treatment has been clearly proved safe and effective, most attention in recent years has focused on dantrolene and bromocriptine.

How to treat subsequent psychotic episodes in a patient with a history of NMS is capturing increasing attention among clinicians.[53] Low-potency neuroleptics may be safer than those of higher potency, although even clozapine has been associated with NMS. When a patient has a history of this syndrome, the clinician should first verify the past diagnosis. If it is validated, the clinician should consider nonneuroleptic treatments such as electroconvulsive therapy (ECT) or, in the case of a mood disorder, lithium. When a neuroleptic is thought to be required, one of lower potency should be considered, and the dose should be raised gradually. It is of particular importance that all previous signs of NMS should have ended completely at least 2 weeks before the reintroduction of an antipsychotic.

Anticholinergic

Peripheral Antipsychotic drugs block the muscarinic subtype of cholinergic receptor.[6,9] This type of receptor, which responds to interneuronal release of acetylcholine, is located on postganglionic neurons of the parasympathetic branch of the autonomic nervous system (as well as autonomic ganglion cells and certain cortical and subcortical neurons). The most strongly anticholinergic among the traditional antipsychotic drugs is thioridazine. High-potency antipsychotic drugs (e.g., fluphenazine, haloperidol) are comparatively weak in their atropine-like action.

Common anticholinergic effects include warmth and flushing of the skin, decreased sweating, mydriasis with difficulty in visual accommodation, increased intraocular pressure, xerostomia, tachycardia, decreased intestinal motility with subsequent constipation, urinary retention, and delayed or retrograde ejaculation.

In general, the elderly are more sensitive to anticholinergic effects than are younger patients. Obviously, certain illnesses are exacerbated by anticholinergic actions of drugs. An abrupt attack of narrow-angle glaucoma is a rare possibility that can occur in a predisposed individual. Fortunately, the more common open-angle glaucoma, particularly when controlled by drugs, is less likely to be made worse by drug administration. Individuals prone to dental problems may suffer from diminished salivation. Those with cardiac disorders may be compromised by tachycardia as well as by more direct cardiotoxic effects, which are discussed below. Individuals with gastrointestinal disturbances, including those who have recently had abdominal surgery, may be adversely affected by the diminished bowel motility. Similarly, a man with prostatic enlargement could find urination difficult during treatment with an anticholinergic drug.

Some degree of tolerance develops to these effects over weeks and months (and conversely, rebound can occur on drug withdrawal). When peripheral anticholinergic activity of antipsychotic drugs is a problem, the clinician may wish to lower the dose of the drug or switch to a drug with less anticholinergic activity. At times, symptomatic treatment may be offered, such as sugarless gum and lozenges for dry mouth or a stool softener or mild laxative for constipation. In occasional patients, the use of a peripherally active parasympathomimetic agent such as bethanechol may be indicated.

In its anticholinergic activity, clozapine again is something of an anomaly.[23] Its binding potency at the muscarinic receptor is higher than that of older antipsychotic drugs, even thioridazine. However, one of the common side effects of clozapine is hypersalivation.

Central Presumably through their action in blocking central muscarinic cholinergic receptors, antipsychotic drugs can at times produce memory difficulties, confusion, and in the extreme, delirium. The elderly are especially at risk of developing central anticholinergic toxicity, especially if the patient is receiving multiple agents with anticholinergic effects.

With serious intoxication, the patient suffering from an atropine-like delirium is typically confused, disoriented, and agitated. Pupils are large (although responsive), mucous membranes are dry, and skin is hot and flushed. Tachycardia and markedly diminished bowel sounds are common. The best treatment of anticholinergic intoxication is withdrawal of the offending agents. In very rare cases, the administration of the anticholinesterase physostigmine may be helpful. However, because physostigmine may cause seizures and life-threatening bradyarrhythmias, its use should be avoided.

Cardiovascular and respiratory

Hypotension Orthostatic hypotension during antipsychotic drug administration has been attributed to a combination of hypothalamic actions and peripheral alpha-adrenergic blockade. Some degree of tolerance may develop. This reaction is more common with the low-potency drugs (e.g., chlorpromazine) and may be more of a problem with the elderly or with patients with preexisting postural hypotension and vascular instability. It is likely that parenteral administration of an antipsychotic drug may provoke more severe hypotension than oral ingestion of the same drug. Clozapine produces substantial postural hypotension.

If postural hypotension does develop, it usually can be managed by keeping the patient horizontal. The next step, if necessary, is the administration of intravenous fluids to expand the vascular volume. If these two maneuvers are not effective, than a relatively pure α-adrenergic pressor agent such as phenylephrine or norepinephrine should be administered. The use of a mixed α- and β-stimulating drug such as epinephrine could lead to a paradoxical drop in blood pressure, since the α receptors are blocked, and the unopposed β stimulation can promote further hypotension. Similarly, the use of a primarily β-stimulating drug such as isoproterenol should be avoided.

Cardiac Antipsychotic drugs have both antiarrhythmic and arrhythmogenic effects. Antagonism of sympathetic activity in the hypothalamus and a local anesthetic property that stabilizes the cardiac cell membrane (similar to the effects of lidocaine) may cause the antiarrhythmic effect. In addition, antipsychotic drugs have direct quinidine-like effects on the myocardium and cardiac conduction system.

Whether antipsychotic drugs are protective or toxic to the heart probably depends on the agent, the dose, and the underlying state of a patient's cardiac physiology. Low-potency antipsychotic agents, especially thioridazine and clozapine, tend to be more cardiotoxic. On the electrocardiogram (EKG), increased heart rate, prolongation of the QT and PR intervals and T wave, and depression of the ST segment are occasionally observed, particularly with thioridazine, clozapine, and pimozide. For most patients, these effects are not clinically troublesome. Occasionally, however, a life-threatening arrhythmia, such as torsades de pointes (polymorphic ventricular tachycardia), can occur. Patients with preexisting cardiac disease should be monitored carefully (e.g., clinical examinations, vital signs, EKGs), and low-potency drugs (especially in excessive doses and particularly thioridazine, clozapine, and pimozide) should be avoided.

Overdoses of antipsychotic drugs (especially thioridazine) can cause cardiac arrhythmias. Because antipsychotic agents have quinidine-like actions, arrhythmias caused by overdoses should not be treated with quinidine or related type 1a antiarrhythmic drugs (procainamide and disopyramide). In the treatment of cardiac arrhythmias that result from overdoses with phenothiazines and related drugs, antiarrhythmics such as lidocaine, phenytoin, and propranolol may have a role. The early use of transvenous pacing also has been recommended.

Combinations of antipsychotic drugs and antidepressants can produce additive cardiotoxic effects. In particular, combinations of thioridazine, clozapine, pimozide, and tricyclic antidepressants, especially amitriptyline, are best avoided.

Occasional cases of sudden death reported in patients receiving antipsychotic drugs are difficult to interpret and probably result from various causes. However, episodes of potentially fatal ventricular arrhythmias are a possible factor.

Ocular As already noted, the anticholinergic effects of antipsychotic drugs can affect the eye. Increased mydriasis can make a patient more light sensitive. Interference with visual accommodation may result in complaints of blurred vision. Because of the rare possibility of precipitating an attack of angle-closure glaucoma, prior to treatment with any anticholinergic agent patients should be asked about history of visual symptoms—such as eye pain, blurring, and halos—that could suggest previous narrow-angle episodes. Open-angle glaucoma is less likely to be a problem, but the patient should be managed conjointly with an ophthalmologist.

Prolonged treatment with high doses of low-potency antipsychotic drugs has been associated with the deposition of pigment in the lens, cornea, conjunctiva, and retina, often together with skin pigmentation. Except in extreme cases, these are unlikely to interfere with vision. However, if it is necessary to expose a patient to high doses of a low-potency agent for long periods of time, periodic ophthalmologic examinations would be worthwhile, perhaps annually.

Of greater clinical significance is the pigmentary retinopathy that may accompany thioridazine treatment. This disorder, which can result in visual impairment, is unlikely if doses of thioridazine do not exceed 800 mg/day. Thus, thioridazine is the one antipsychotic agent that should be considered to have an absolute "ceiling dose"—800 mg daily—which must not be exceeded for even brief periods of time.

Cutaneous Virtually any drug is capable of producing an allergic rash in occasional patients, typically between 2 and 10 weeks following initial exposure. This is usually maculopapular, erythematous, and itchy, affecting the face, neck, trunk, and extremities (often the palms and soles of the feet). Allergic reactions vary in distribution and severity, the most extreme being exfoliative dermatitis, which can be life-threatening. In most cases, discontinuation of the precipitating agent is followed by prompt remission of symptoms and signs. The itching and rash can be treated symptomatically. Subsequent antipsychotic therapy should be with a drug from a different chemical group. Occasionally, contact dermatitis occurs in patients hypersensitive to antipsychotic drugs, particularly to liquid preparations.

Patients receiving low-potency antipsychotic medication sometimes become very sensitive to sunlight. The resulting reaction resembles severe sunburn. Management of the acute reaction is the same as for sunburn. Subsequent treatment should include switching to a higher potency antipsychotic drug or warning the patient to protect himself from sun, whether physically or through the use of a sunscreening preparation.

Occasional patients treated with high doses of low-potency phenothiazines for prolonged periods develop a blue-gray discoloration of the skin, specifically in skin exposed to sunlight. This usually occurs in conjunction with pigmentary changes in the eye. Aside from cosmetic concerns, it is unclear if this reaction has any clinical importance.

Hormonal, sexual, and hypothalamic reactions Antipsychotic drugs increase prolactin release from the anterior pituitary and consequently cause hyperprolactinemia, probably as a result of dopamine-blocking activity. In females, this occasionally leads to galactorrhea (also, rarely, in males), decreased frequency or flow of menstruation, and in both sexes a diminished libido. Although so far there is no convincing evidence that chronic antipsychotic drug treatment increases the risk of breast cancer, it is not inconceivable that the growth of prolactin-sensitive tumors may be enhanced by the presence of elevated circulating prolactin concentrations. Therefore, women should be asked about personal and family history of breast cancer, and women receiving long-term antipsychotic therapy should undergo periodic breast examinations. Although there is no evidence that chronic antipsychotic drug treatment can result in increased incidence of pituitary adenomas, it remains at least a theoretical possibility that lactotrophes in the pituitary will be stimulated. Therefore, in the face of chronic hyperprolactinemia, patients should be examined occasionally for possible evidence of pituitary enlargement. Persistent amenorrhea and galactorrhea suggest that the clinician should lower the antipsychotic drug dose.

Another sexual symptom, already mentioned under anticholinergic effects, is interference with ejaculation. This is most frequently observed in young males treated with thioridazine and is manifested by delayed ejaculation or retrograde ejaculation. In the latter case, the patient reports orgasm without emission, followed by urination that has a "foamy" appearance. Some males also report difficulty maintaining and sustaining erection. In these cases, change to a high-potency drug.

Both females and males taking antipsychotic drugs sometimes complain of delayed, altered, or inadequate orgasms. The mechanism is unclear but may include psychologic, hormonal, or autonomic factors. Possible therapeutic strategies can include lowering the dose of the antipsychotic agent, switching to a higher potency compound, or using a peripherally active cholinomimetic, such as bethanechol. The antiserotonin antihistaminic drug cyproheptadine has been reported helpful in reversing orgasmic dysfunction attributed to antidepressant drugs; whether it might have similar value in patients on neuroleptic therapy is untested.

In addition to effects on prolactin and the existence of the neuroleptic malignant syndrome, antipsychotic drugs seem to have many other actions at the level of the hypothalamus. These probably include cardiovascular effects as well as various hormonal and autonomic changes. Temperature regulation is also impaired by phenothiazines and their relatives, particularly the low-potency ones, making patients more vulnerable to hypo- or hyperthermia (depending on the ambient temperature).

Another unwanted effect, probably related to hypothalamic changes, is increased appetite with resultant weight gain. In some patients, this can be most marked and unpleasant. Probably, appetite increase (which may be related to antihistaminic effects) is more common with low-potency drugs. Management may include switching to a higher potency agent and dietary counseling.

Hepatic The low-potency antipsychotic drugs occasionally produce a syndrome of cholestatic jaundice, probably a combination of a direct toxic effect and an allergic reaction. Typically, within the first month of treatment, the patient develops fever, chills, nausea, malaise, pruritus, and right upper quadrant abdominal pain, followed within days by jaundice. Liver function tests reveal an obstructive pattern with increased alkaline phosphatase and conjugated (direct) bilirubin. Transaminase enzymes also may be elevated, but they do not reach the levels observed in hepatitis.

The recommended treatment for cholestatic jaundice is discontinuing the antipsychotic drug, although it is possible that patients will recover despite continued therapy. In almost all cases, recovery occurs over a matter of weeks and is complete and without sequelae. Subsequent treatment probably should be with a different antipsychotic drug, preferably a high-potency agent.

The presence of preexisting liver disease does not contraindicate the use of antipsychotic drugs. However, when the liver is impaired, metabolism of antipsychotic drugs may be slowed, and other drugs that use similar enzyme pathways could be affected by the addition of another liver-metabolized agent.

Hematologic Low-potency antipsychotic agents probably are weakly toxic to some elements of the bone marrow, particularly stem cells of the granulocyte series. Almost all patients can compensate for this and show no more than a transient leukopenia. However, a rare patient goes on to develop agranulocytosis.

Perhaps 1 in 3000 to 4000 patients treated with chlorpromazine (and possibly other low-potency drugs) will develop agranulocytosis. This occurs rarely, if at all, with high-potency drugs. For clozapine, the incidence of agranulocytosis may be much higher, perhaps as high as 2 percent.

The onset is typically within the first 2 to 3 months of drug therapy. The white blood cell count may fall below 1000, and practically all those cells will be lymphocytes.

Routine blood counts will be unlikely to detect the abrupt onset of agranulocytosis unless they are performed two to three times each week for the first several months of treatment. For this reason, they are generally not recommended (clozapine is an exception). Instead, the best approach is to maintain a high clinical index of suspicion. Thus, sore throat, fever, malaise, or other symptoms or signs of infection should prompt immediate white blood count with a differential. If the count is low, antipsychotic drugs should be discontinued immediately. If infection does not supervene, a normal blood count returns within several weeks. If infection does occur, there is substantial mortality.

Agranulocytosis associated with the new and atypical antipsychotic drug clozapine is particularly noteworthy.[22,23] First, as mentioned above, it is much more common, afflicting perhaps 1 to 2 percent of patients who take it. Second, it does not appear to show cross-tolerance with other drugs, even with the chemically similar loxapine.[54] Third, unlike the probable toxic mechanism underlying agranulocytosis induced by chlorpromazine and other phenothiazines, agranulocytosis engendered by clozapine is more likely caused by an immune mechanism.[54] This (with some empirical data) suggests that reexposure of a patient to clozapine could result in an abrupt drop in white blood cell count. Finally, there is evidence of genetic vulnerability to clozapine-induced agranulocytosis, with patients of Ashkenazi Jewish background possibly at highest risk.[54] Since at least one patient has developed agranulocytosis after more than 1 year of clozapine therapy, current requirements include indefinite, weekly white blood cell counts in patients taking this medication.

Clozapine therapy also has been associated with leukocytosis and eosinophilia.[57] Eosinphilia has been reported to occur in up to 5 to 10 percent of patients treated with clozapine.

About half of a group of patients who had been treated chronically with chlorpromazine had a positive antinuclear antibody test, and more than 75 percent showed increased serum concentrations of immunoglobulin M (IgM) associated with prolongation of partial thromboplastin time. In addition, a number of autoantibodies have been found in patients treated with chlorpromazine, often in association with splenomegaly.[55] In a recent study contrasting the immunologic effects of chlorpromazine versus those of haloperidol, 6 of 29 patients taking chlorpromazine but none of 14 taking haloperidol had progressive elevations of serum IgM at the end of 5 years.[56] By the end of 5 years, 87 percent of chlorpromazine-treated and 50 percent of haloperidol-treated patients had antinuclear antibodies, but none had developed a lupuslike syndrome.

Withdrawal reactions Habituation and addiction are not believed to occur with antipsychotic drugs. As noted earlier, tolerance does develop to some of the unwanted effects of these agents. Partial to complete tolerance may develop to sedation, and some degree of tolerance can occur for hypotension and anticholinergic actions. Conversely, when the drug is stopped, rebound reactions may occur. These can include insomnia, nightmares, and other disturbances of sleep as well as cholinergic rebound such as increased salivation, abdominal cramps, and diarrhea. To make patients more comfortable, discontinue these drugs gradually (e.g., 5 to 10 percent of dose per day) rather than abruptly.

As discussed in the section on tardive dyskinesia, discontinuation of antipsychotic drugs is occasionally followed by transient withdrawal dyskinesias. In other cases, discontinuing the drug unmasks persistent dyskinesia.

CONCLUSION

Antipsychotic medications are commonly used in the elderly for a variety of disorders. The clinician must assure that these agents are used only for appropriate indications, in the lowest effective dose, and for the shortest time possible to avoid serious and potentially permanent toxicity such as tardive dyskinesia. Elderly patients should receive lower doses and have dose titrations done more slowly than in younger patients. Patients placed on antipsychotics in the past for agitation may not require medication in the present, and efforts should be made to discontinue these agents whenever possible. However, when used appropriately, antipsychotics can be extremely effective in improving patients' mental status and quality of life.

REFERENCES

1. Thompson TL, Moran MG, Nies AS: Psychotropic drug use in the elderly (second of two parts). *N Engl J Med* 308: 194-199, 1983.
2. Gelenberg AJ: Treating the outpatient schizophrenic. *Postgrad Med* 64: 48-56, 1978.
3. Fielding S, Lal H: Behavioral actions of neuroleptics, in Iversen LL, Iversen SD, Snyder SH (eds): *Handbook of Psychopharmacology*, vol. 10. New York, Plenum, 1978, pp 91-128.
4. Baldessarini RJ: Drugs and the treatment of psychiatric disorders, in Gilman AG, Rall TW, Nies AS, Taylor P (eds): *The Pharmacological Basis of Therapeutics*, 8th ed. New York, Pergamon, 1990, pp 383-435.
5. Itil TM: Effects of psychotropic drugs on qualitatively and quantitatively analyzed human EEG, in Clark WG, del Guidice J (eds): *Principles of Psychopharmacology*, 2nd ed. New York, Academic, 1978, pp 261-277.
6. Richelson E: Pharmacology of the neuroleptics, in Palmer GC (ed): *Neuropharmacology of Central and Behavioral Disorders*. New York, Academic, 1981, pp 84-99.
7. Clark D, White FJ: Review: D1 dopamine receptor—the search for a function: a critical evaluation of D1/D2 dopamine receptor classification and its functional implications. *Synapse* 1: 347-348, 1987.
8. Borison RL, Fields JZ, Diamond BI: Site-specific blockade of dopamine receptors by neuroleptic agents in human brain. *Neuropharmacology* 20: 1321-1322, 1981.
9. Richelson E: Neuroleptic affinities for human brain receptors and their use in predicting adverse effects. *J Clin Psychiatry* 45: 331-336, 1984.
10. Ereshefsky L, Tran-Johnson TK, Watanabe MD: Pathophysiologic basis for schizophrenia and the efficacy of antipsychotics. *Clin Pharm* 9: 682-707, 1990.
11. Marsden CD, Jenner P: The pathophysiology of extrapyramidal side effects of neuroleptic drugs. *Psychol Med* 10: 55-72, 1980.
12. Roth RH: Dopamine autoreceptors: pharmacology, function and comparison with post-synaptic dopamine receptors. *Commun Psychopharmacol* 3: 429-445, 1979.
13. Kebabian JW: Dopamine-sensitive adenylate cyclase: a receptor mechanism for dopamine. *Adv Biochem Psychopharmacol* 19: 131-154, 1978.
14. Salzman C: Treatment of agitation in the elderly, in Meltzer HY (ed): *Psychopharmacology: The Third Generation of Progress*. New York, Raven, 1987, pp 1167-1176.
15. Lipowski ZJ: Delirium in the elderly patient. *N Engl J Med* 320: 578-581, 1989.
16. Watanabe M, Davis JM: Pharmacotherapeutic considerations in the elderly psychiatric patient. *Psych Ann* 20: 423-432, 1990.
17. Avorn J, Dreyer P, Connelly K, Soumerai SB: Use of psychoactive medication and the quality of care in nursing homes. *N Engl J Med* 320: 227-232, 1989.
18. Cooper TB, Robinson DS: Pharmacokinetics of neuroleptic drugs in the aged, in Raskin A, Robinson DS, Levine J (eds): *Age and the Pharmacology of Psychoactive Drugs*. Amsterdam, Elsevier North-Holland, 1981, pp 181-192.
19. Dahl SG: Pharmacokinetics of antipsychotic drugs in man. *Acta Psychiatr Scand* 82(suppl 358): 37-40, 1990.
20. Hicks R, Dysken MW, Davis JM, et al: The pharmacokinetics of psychotropic medication in the elderly: A review. *J Clin Psychiatry* 42: 374-385, 1981.

21. Rosen J, Bohon S, Gerson S: Antipsychotics in the elderly. *Acta Psychiatr Scand* 82(suppl 358): 170-175, 1990.
22. Baldessarini RJ, Frankenburg FR: Clozapine. A new antipsychotic agent. *N Engl J Med* 324: 746-754, 1991.
23. Ereshefsky L, Watanabe MD, Tran-Johnson TK: Clozapine: An atypical antipsychotic agent. *Clin Pharm* 8: 691-709, 1989.
24. Movin G, Gustafson L, Franzén G, et al: Pharmacokinetics of remoxipride in elderly psychotic patients. *Acta Psychiatr Scand* 82(suppl 358): 176-180, 1990.
25. Ko GN, Korpi ER, Linnoila M: On the clinical relevance and methods of quantification of plasma concentrations of neuroleptics. *J Clin Psychopharm* 5: 253-262, 1985.
26. Kane J, Honigfeld G, Singer J, et al: Clozapine for the treatment-resistant schizophrenic. A double-blind comparison with chlorpromazine. *Arch Gen Psychiatry* 45: 789-796, 1988.
27. Baldessarini RJ: Antipsychotic agents, in *Chemotherapy in Psychiatry*, 2nd ed. Cambridge, Massachusetts, Harvard University Press, 1985, pp 14-92.
28. Batey SR: Schizophrenic disorders, in DiPiro JT, Talbery RL, Hayes PE, et al (eds): *Pharmacotherapy. A Pathophysiologic Approach*. New York, Elsevier, 1989, pp 714-728.
29. Keepers GA, Clappison VJ, Casey DE: Initial anticholinergic prophylaxis for neuroleptic-induced extrapyramidal syndromes. *Arch Gen Psychiatry* 40: 1113-1117, 1983.
30. Van Putten T, Mutalipassi LR, Malkin MO: Phenothiazine-induced decompensation. *Arch Gen Psychiatry* 30: 102-106, 1974.
31. Gelenberg AJ, Mandel MR: Catatonic reactions to high potency neuroleptic drugs. *Arch Gen Psychiatry* 34: 947-950, 1977.
32. Rifkin A, Quitkin F, Klein DF: Akinesia: A poorly recognized drug-induced extrapyramidal behavior disorder. *Arch Gen Psychiatry* 32: 642-674, 1975.
33. Wojcik JD: Antiparkinson drug use. *Mass Gen Hosp Biol Ther Psychiatr Newslett* 2: 5-7, 1979.
33a. Ganzini L, Heintz R, Hoffman WF, et al Acute extrapyramidal syndromes in neuroleptic-treated elders: A pilot study. *J Geriatr Psychiatr Neurol* 4: 222-225, 1991.
34. Gelenberg AJ, Van Putten T, Lavori P, et al: Anticholinergic effects on memory: Benztropine versus amantadine. *J Clin Psychopharm* 9: 180-185, 1989.
35. Gelenberg AJ: Amantadine in the treatment of benztropine-refractory neuroleptic-induced movement disorders. *Curr Ther Res* 23: 375-380, 1978.
36. Jeste DV, Wyatt RJ: Changing epidemiology of tardive dyskinesia: An overview. *Am J Psychiatry* 138: 297-309, 1981.
37. Burke RE, Fahn S, Jankovic J, et al: Tardive dystonia: late onset and persistent dystonia caused by antipsychotic drugs. *Neurology* 32: 1335-1346, 1982.
38. Morgenstern H, Glazer WH, Niedzwiecki D, et al: The impact of neuroleptic medication on tardive dyskinesia: A meta-analysis of published studies. *Am J Publ Health* 77: 714-724, 1987.
39. Smith JM, Baldessarini RJ: Changes in prevalence, severity and recovery in tardive dyskinesia with age. *Arch Gen Psychiatry* 37: 1368-1373, 1980.
40. Wojcik JD, Gelenberg AJ, Labrie RA, et al: Prevalence of tardive dyskinesia in the outpatient population. *Comp Psychiatry* 21: 370-380, 1980.
41. Kane JM, Woerner M, Borenstein M, et al: Integrating incidence and prevalence of tardive dyskinesia. World Congress of Biological Psychiatry, Philadelphia, 1985.
42. Saltz BL, Woerner MG, Kane JM, et al: Prospective study of tardive dyskinesia incidence in the elderly. *JAMA* 266: 2402-2406, 1991.
43. Gardos G, Cole JO, Tarsy D: Withdrawal syndromes associated with antipsychotic drugs. *Am J Psychiatry* 135: 1321-1324, 1978.
44. Casey DE, Povien UJ, Meidahl B, et al: Neuroleptic-induced tardive dyskinesia and parkinsonism: Changes during several years of continued treatment. *Psychopharm Bull* 22: 250-253, 1986.
45. Yagi G, Itoh H: A ten year follow-up study of tardive dyskinesia with special reference to the influence of neuroleptic administration on the long-term prognosis. *Keio J Med* 34: 211-219, 1985.

46. Gelenberg AJ, Dorer D, Wojcik J, et al: A crossover study of lecithin for tardive dyskinesia. *J Clin Psychiatry* 51: 149–153, 1990.
47. Tanner CM: Treatment of tardive dyskinesia: other therapies. *Clin Neuropharmacol* 6: 159–167, 1983.
48. Larson EB, Kukull WA, Buchner D, Reifler BV: Adverse drug reactions associated with global cognitive impairment in elderly persons. *Ann Int Med* 107: 169–173, 1987.
49. Caroff SN: The neuroleptic malignant syndrome. *J Clin Psychiatry* 41: 79–83, 1980.
50. Gelenberg AJ, Bellinghausen B, Wojcik JD, et al: A prospective survey of neuroleptic malignant syndrome in a short-term psychiatric hospital. *Am J Psychiatry* 145: 517–518, 1988.
50a. Gelenberg AJ: Respiratory compromise with clozapine. *Biol Ther Psychiatr News* 14: 43–44, 1991.
51. Shalev A, Munitz H: The neuroleptic malignant syndrome: Agent and host interaction. *Acta Psychiatr Scand* 73: 3337–3347, 1986.
52. Levenson DF, Simpson GM: Neuroleptic-induced extrapyramidal symptoms with fever: heterogeneity of the "neuroleptic malignant syndrome." *Arch Gen Psychiatry* 43: 839–848, 1986.
53. Gelenberg AJ, Bellinghausen B, Wojcik JD, et al: Patients with NMS histories: What happens when they are rehospitalized? *J Clin Psychiatry* 50: 178–180, 1989.
54. Lieberman JA, Johns CA, Kane JM, et al: Clozapine-induced agranulocytosis: non-cross-reactivity with other psychotropic drugs. *J Clin Psychiatry* 49: 271–277, 1988.
55. Zarrabi MH, Zucker S, Miller F, et al: Immunologic and coagulation disorders in chlorpromazine-treated patients. *Ann Int Med* 91: 194–199, 1979.
56. Zucker S, Zarrabi MH, Schuback WH, et al: Chlorpromazine-induced immunopathy: progressive increase in serum IgM. *Medicine* 69: 92–100, 1990.
57. Stricker BC, Tielens JE: Eosinophilia with clozapine. *Lancet* 338: 1520–1521, 1991.

CHAPTER

17

DIABETES MELLITUS

Suzanne Campbell
Arshag D. Mooradian

Diabetes mellitus is a common disease in the elderly. It is estimated that approximately 18 percent of people over the age of 65 in the United States have diabetes.[1] The management of this disease in the elderly poses a unique challenge.[2,3] A host of factors commonly found in elderly people are likely to interfere with the management of diabetes (Table 17-1). Such factors include coexisting diseases, psychosocial limitations, and altered pharmacokinetics of many drugs.

Although the long-term outcome of normalizing blood glucose levels in elderly diabetic patients is still unknown, age alone should not be the sole criterion for optimization of diabetes control. It is generally accepted that chronic hyperglycemia is deleterious at all ages and overall health status of the individual is a more important determinant of the degree of blood glucose control than age of the individual.

The general principles of treating diabetes in the elderly are similar to those used in young diabetic patients. In this chapter these general principles are reviewed briefly and specific issues related to the pharmacologic management of diabetes in the elderly are addressed. Since dietary therapy and an exercise program are essential components of the management, they are also discussed briefly.

DIETARY THERAPY

Although dietary therapy has always been considered the cornerstone of the management of type II diabetes, the optimal composition of diabetic diet is not known. The long-term consequences of currently recommended high-carbohydrate

Table 17-1 Some factors that are likely to interfere with the management of diabetes in the elderly

Medical conditions	Psychosocial conditions
Coexisting diseases	Depression
Hepatic and renal insufficiency	Cognitive changes
Drugs	Social isolation
Impaired senses interfering with insulin administration or tasting of food	Poverty

diets, specifically in relation to its effect on serum lipid profile, are of concern. The uncertainty of the dietary recommendations also extends to the wisdom of total avoidance of simple sugars in the diet or the equivalency of various complex carbohydrates. The glycemic effect of poorly digestible carbohydrates, such as legumes, is certainly lower than the glycemic effect of well-cooked starch, such as mashed potatoes.[4] In addition, ingestion of simple carbohydrates in moderate quantities with a mixed meal has only modest effects on blood glucose concentrations.[5]

One dietary recommendation which has been consistently found to improve blood glucose control is total caloric restriction.[6] However, many older diabetic patients are not overweight and weight-reducing diets can be detrimental in those over the age of 70 who have borderline nutritional status.[7] It is noteworthy that up to 20 percent of diabetic nursing home patients are malnourished.[8] In these patients, weight gain and adequate nutrition is as important as the weight loss recommended for obese patients.

Elderly diabetic patients are also at particular risk for vitamin or mineral deficiencies.[9] Supplementation with micronutrients, however, should be reserved only for those with documented biochemical evidence of a deficiency state or in whom dietary history indicates marginal nutrient intake.

In general, the prescribed diet should be simple and should take into consideration the patient's preferences and food habits. Introduction of low-fat, high-fiber meals with avoidance of simple sugars and moderation in salt intake are wise dietary recommendations for most patients. For more information on dietary therapy of diabetes in the elderly, the reader is referred to the recent review of the topic by Reed and Mooradian.[9]

ROLE OF EXERCISE

Exercise induces several changes in glucose homeostasis. In poorly controlled diabetic patients, high-intensity exercise aggravates hyperglycemia. Patients on insulin therapy may experience hypoglycemia during exercise due to enhanced insulin absorption from the injection sites. In a subset of type I diabetic patients, a delayed hypoglycemia reaction can occur several hours after exercise. Patients on oral hypoglycemic agents may also be at risk of exercise-induced hypoglycemia. However, this risk is usually small. In addition to improving glucose tolerance and lipid profile, exercise in elderly diabetic patients may have other benefits such as amelioration of hypertension and hypercoagulability, increased bone density, and improved psychologic well-being.[10,11]

Exercise programs, however, are not risk free. In addition to fluctuations in blood glucose levels, there is increased risk of cardiac arrhythmias, myocardial infarction, sudden death, injury to feet, and vitreous hemorrhage or retinal detachment in those with proliferative retinopathy. These possible risks should be evaluated and the workload prescribed should be adjusted to the individual's capacity and tolerance. In general, to avoid hypoglycemia, it is easier to increase caloric intake to meet the projected fuel needs. An increase of 1 g of carbohydrates per minute of exercise is usually sufficient for most elderly diabetic patients on insulin treatment. For non-insulin-requiring patients, dietary changes are not crucial. In those patients, postprandial hyperglycemia can be improved if the exercise is scheduled after meals.

ORAL SULFONYLUREA AGENTS

In the elderly patient with insulin-dependent diabetes mellitus (IDDM), insulin is a necessary component of therapy in addition to diet and exercise. Since non-insulin-dependent diabetes mellitus (NIDDM) is seen much more commonly than IDDM in the elderly population, the practitioner has more choices in developing a treatment plan for the elderly patient with NIDDM. Diet and exercise are the initial treatments of choice for the person with NIDDM, but at least 60 percent of patients will not achieve acceptable blood glucose control with these therapies alone. In this situation, pharmacologic therapy is indicated to attain the desired therapeutic goals.

Oral hypoglycemic agents have been available for the treatment of diabetes since the 1950s. However, their popularity has waxed and waned during this time. One of the major reasons for this was the University Group Diabetes Program (UGDP), which compared patient outcome using various pharmacologic regimens in the treatment of diabetes. The results from this study indicated that there was an increase in cardiovascular mortality in the group treated with fixed-dose tolbutamide.[12] This led to a decrease in the use of these agents, and insulin was considered by some physicians as the sole modality of pharmacologic therapy. Re-analysis of these data, however, and several subsequent studies could not confirm the conclusions reached by the UGDP.[13,14] Because of these findings, the sulfonylurea drugs have regained a role in the therapy of diabetes. It is approximated that one-third of all people in the United States with diabetes are treated with sulfonylureas.[15] Seventy percent of all prescriptions for these drugs are for patients older than 60 years.

The exact mechanism of action of the sulfonylureas has not been fully elucidated. These agents appear to have both pancreatic and peripheral effects. The sulfonylureas stimulate the release of insulin from the pancreas via a sulfonylurea receptor which is found on the pancreatic beta cell.[16,17] It seems that these receptors are closely linked with adenosine triphosphate (ATP) sensitive K^+ channels on the membranes of the beta cells. Sulfonylureas block the efflux of potassium from the beta cells, causing a depolarization of the membrane followed by an influx of calcium ions. This ultimately results in activation of the pancreatic beta cell and the release of insulin. This effect was once thought to be short lived, since insulin levels returned to baseline values after a few months of therapy with the sulfonylureas. This decrease in insulin concentration, however, is an appropriate response to the lower blood glucose level, and subsequent studies have shown that chronic administration of the sulfonylureas continues to enhance insulin release. Also, hepatic glucose production, which contributes to the fasting hyperglycemia in NIDDM, is suppressed by the sulfonylureas.[17] This correlates with the increase in the basal insulin secretion. Long-term treatment with the sulfonylureas has been associated with an increased tissue sensitivity to insulin.[16] The significance of this is not known. This effect may be secondary to a reduction in hyperglycemia with a resultant increase in the tissue sensitivity to insulin rather than to a direct effect of the drugs. Evidence against the importance of extrapancreatic effects of the sulfonylureas lies in the fact that these drugs do not work without functioning pancreatic beta cells.

Currently, there are six sulfonylureas available in the United States (Table 17-2). Four are first-generation agents, and the remaining two are second-generation agents. The individual drugs are similar in efficacy but differ primarily in their pharmacokinetic profiles and in adverse effects. These properties are especially important in discerning which drug to choose for the elderly patient.

Sulfonylureas are well absorbed after oral administration.[18] Administration with food has been reported to decrease the absorption of both chlorpropamide and

Table 17-2 Oral hypoglycemic agents

Agent	Equivalent dose, mg	Maximum dose, mg/day	Initial dose in elderly	Duration of action, h
First generation				
Tolbutamide (Orinase)	1000	3000	500 mg bid	6-12
Acetohexamide (Dymelor)	500	1500	125 mg bid[a]	12-18
Tolazamide (Tolinase)	250	1000	100 mg qd	12-24
Chlorpropamide (Diabinese)	250	500	100 mg qd[a]	24-72
Second generation				
Glipizide (Glucotrol)	10	40	2.5 mg qd	10-24
Glyburide (DiaBeta, Micronase)	5	20	1.25 mg qd	18-24

[a]Use not recommended in the elderly.

glipizide.[19,20] Because of the time required for absorption, all of the sulfonylureas are more effective in diminishing the postprandial rise in glucose if administered 30 min prior to a meal.[19] For optimal effects, patients should be instructed to take their sulfonylureas 30 min in advance of eating.

All of these agents are extensively metabolized by the liver to metabolites with varying degrees of hypoglycemic activity.[16] Tolbutamide is metabolized to hydroxytolbutamide and carboxytolbutamide, which are much less potent than the parent compound. Less than 2 percent of the dose is excreted in the urine as unchanged parent drug. The primary metabolite of acetohexamide is hydroxyhexamide, and this compound is responsible for the hypoglycemic activity of acetohexamide. Approximately 65 percent of the hydroxyhexamide is excreted unchanged in the urine. Because of this, accumulation of the metabolite can be seen in the elderly with the potential for resultant hypoglycemia. Tolazamide is metabolized to several compounds which have some hypoglycemic activity although much less than tolazamide itself, and only 7 percent of the dose is excreted unchanged in the urine. Chlorpropamide is the first-generation agent with the longest duration of action. Twenty percent of the dose is renally eliminated, so like acetohexamide, accumulation can occur in the elderly. This, along with its long duration of action, places the elderly patient at great risk for hypoglycemia when taking chlorpropamide. Glipizide is metabolized to several inactive compounds, and less than 5 percent of the parent drug is found unchanged in the urine. Finally, glyburide is converted to three major metabolites. One of these metabolites, 4-hydroxyglyburide, is 15 percent as potent as glyburide. Approximately 40 percent of this compound is eliminated by the kidney, so accumulation can occur with renal dysfunction.

Few studies have investigated the pharmacokinetics of these drugs in the elderly population. The pharmacokinetics of chlorpropamide in 9 older patients with NIDDM were compared to 15 young, healthy males.[21] The average age of the study population was 56 years. These investigators found that the volume of distribution at steady state was 77 percent greater in the older patients with NIDDM. This finding probably could not be accounted for by changes in protein binding, as there were no differences in serum albumin between the two groups. Clearance was 34 percent greater in the control population and was felt to be secondary to nonrenal clearance, since creatinine clearances were similar in the control and study populations.

Single-dose glipizide pharmacokinetics were studied in 10 healthy, young volunteers and 10 healthy, elderly volunteers with an average age of 74 years.[22] These investigators found no significant differences between the groups with respect to clearance, volume of distribution at steady state, or elimination half-life. However, different results may have been found with multiple dosing.

Since limited data are available regarding dosing of the sulfonylureas in the elderly, one must look at the pharmacokinetics of the individual agent and correlate this to changes seen in drug elimination with aging. Renal function decreases as a function of aging, although this may not be reflected by the serum creatinine since lean body mass also declines. Because of this, caution must be used when choosing an agent with significant renal elimination. Less is known about the effect of aging on the ability of the liver to metabolize drugs, but liver mass does diminish with age as does hepatic blood flow. In a clinical setting, hepatic function is much more difficult to assess than renal function. Because of this, it is always best to start with a low dose of sulfonylurea in the elderly and adjust the dose based on clinical response.

All of the sulfonylureas appear to be equally efficacious hypoglycemic agents.[19] Primary failures with these drugs are seen in up to 20 percent of patients.[23] Initial success is determined in part by appropriate patient selection which is based upon the following criteria: onset of diabetes after 40 years of age, normal weight or obese, duration of diabetes less than 5 years, no history of ketoacidosis, fasting blood glucose less than 200 mg/dL, and a daily insulin dose of less than 20 to 30 units if the patient is on insulin.[18] Secondary failures with the sulfonylureas, defined as deterioration of glucose control after an initial response, are reported to be approximately 5 to 10 percent per year.[16] The exact reason for the secondary failures is not known, but dietary noncompliance, beta cell exhaustion, and poor patient selection are potential causes. Patients who have a primary or secondary failure to tolbutamide, acetohexamide, or tolazamide may respond to chlorpropamide, glyburide, or glipizide.

The sulfonylureas are generally well tolerated with the most severe adverse effect being hypoglycemia. This has been reported in up to 5 percent of patients on oral hypoglycemic therapy.[14] The incidence of hypoglycemia appears to be greatest in patients taking chlorpropamide and glyburide, but this may be attributable to their relative frequency of use.[17,24] This hypoglycemia can be quite severe and prolonged, requiring therapy with intravenous dextrose for several days until the drug is eliminated. Predisposing factors for hypoglycemia with the sulfonylureas include impaired renal function, age greater than 60 years, poor dietary intake, and drug interactions.[14] All of these risk factors are common in the elderly, who can have several disease states for which they are taking multiple medications as well as poor nutrition and declining renal function. The consequences of hypoglycemia can also be much more severe in the elderly than in a younger patient, since the precipitation of stroke, myocardial infarction, or traumatic injury secondary to syncope are associated with hypoglycemia in this population.[25] Also, elderly patients may not sense hypoglycemia as readily since beta-adrenergic function decreases with aging.[17] Education regarding the signs and symptoms and treatment of hypoglycemia is particularly important in this population as well as ongoing assessment for risk factors for developing hypoglycemia.

The syndrome of inappropriate antidiuretic hormone (SIADH) secretion can be seen with chlorpropamide with resultant hyponatremia. Chlorpropamide increases the secretion of ADH and potentiates the action of ADH on the renal tubule.[14] Risk factors for the development of hyponatremia include female gender, age greater than 60 years, and the concomitant use of thiazide diuretics.[16] This property is unique to chlorpropamide while acetohexamide, tolazamide, and glyburide actually induce a mild diuresis.

Alcohol-induced flushing similar to that seen with disulfiram can occur in 15 to 30 percent of patients taking chlorpropamide.[14] This may also occur to a lesser degree with tolbutamide. Patients should be instructed to abstain from alcohol or use it very cautiously, particularly if they are taking chlorpropamide.

Other adverse effects seen with the oral hypoglycemic agents include gastrointestinal side effects which occur in 1 to 3 percent of patients and include nausea, dyspepsia, abnormal serum liver enzymes, and abdominal discomfort.[16] Skin rashes have been noted in up to 3 percent of patients and appear to be more common with chlorpropamide.[14] Hematologic side effects are rare but can include hemolytic anemia, aplasia, and thrombocytopenia.[19] Likewise, hepatitis has been reported but is rare.

All of the sulfonylureas are highly bound to plasma proteins. The first-generation drugs are very polar and bind to albumin by ionic as well as nonionic forces.[16] Glyburide and glipizide bind to albumin through nonionic interactions.[20,26] Because of this, the second-generation agents are only weakly displaced from albumin by anionic drugs such as warfarin and salicylates. This gives the second-generation drugs a potential advantage over those that are first generation with respect to drug interactions involving protein-binding displacement. In addition to protein-binding changes, other pharmacokinetic drug interactions affecting the action of the sulfonylureas include alterations in drug metabolism and renal elimination. Pharmacodynamic interactions can also contribute to the hypoglycemic activity of these drugs as well as diminishing their efficacy. The clinically significant drug interactions reported with the sulfonylureas[27,28] are listed in Table 17-3. Because drug interactions are an important risk factor for hypoglycemia, these should be assessed any time changes are made in the patient's concomitant medications.

When choosing an oral hypoglycemic agent for the elderly patient, several factors must be considered including route of elimination, concomitant disease states, duration of action, potential drug interactions, frequency of dosing, and cost. Since renal function declines with age, it is best to avoid acetohexamide, chlorpropamide, and probably glyburide in the elderly. Chlorpropamide's long duration of action as well as its propensity to cause hyponatremia and alcohol-induced flushing also make it an undesirable choice. The second-generation agents may offer a theoretical advantage with respect to drug interactions in a patient on drugs such as salicylates or warfarin. As the elderly may be on multiple medications, ease of a dosing regimen must also be considered to assure compliance. For this reason, it is best to choose a sulfonylurea which can be administered once or twice daily. This can be accomplished with all the available agents with the exception of tolbutamide. Based on these factors, the drugs which are most suitable for the elderly are tolazamide and glipizide. When initiating sulfonylurea therapy in the elderly, it is best to start with the lowest possible dose and increase every 1 to 2 weeks based upon the clinical response.[29] If the desired clinical response is not seen at maximal dosages, the patient may need to be switched to insulin. It is important to assess compliance to diet, exercise, and medication as well as the influence of

Table 17-3 Drug interactions with sulfonylureas

Drug	Mechanism	Effect on blood glucose
	Pharmacokinetic interactions	
Phenylbutazone Sulfonamides Salicylates Clofibrate	↓Protein binding	↓
Anabolic steroids Chloramphenicol Dicumarol Phenylbutazone	↓Hepatic metabolism	↓
Chronic alcohol Phenobarbital Rifampin	↑Hepatic metabolism	↑
	Pharmacodynamic interactions	
Phenytoin Thiazide diuretics	↓Insulin secretion	↑
MAOIs	↑Insulin secretion	↓
Acute ethanol ingestion Salicylates	↓Hepatic glucose production	↓
Corticosteroids	↑Hepatic glucose production	↑

concomitant drugs or illnesses on glucose control before deeming therapy with sulfonylureas a failure.

INSULIN

The use of insulin in the elderly patient with NIDDM has been debated.[30,31] Almost everyone agrees that insulin is indicated in the symptomatic patient, but some practitioners feel that insulin is not necessary if the patient has asymptomatic hyperglycemia. They argue that the risk of hypoglycemia outweighs the benefit of maintaining euglycemia and that with advanced age, tight blood glucose control may not influence the course of long-term complications. It is important to remember, though, that with increasing longevity, the elderly are still at risk for developing the long-term complications of diabetes. Therefore, advanced age should not preclude the use of insulin, but goals for blood glucose control should be established based on the individual patient's ability and motivation.

It is not unusual to see practitioners delay the initiation of insulin therapy in the elderly patient long after the time when it is indicated. This may be due to the misperception that the elderly will not be able to adapt to daily insulin injections. However, this should not deter the initiation of insulin therapy when it is indicated. In our experience, most elderly patients readily learn the procedure for measuring and injecting their insulin in a single educational session.

Several characteristics of insulin must be considered when deciding which product to use. These include strength, onset and duration of the insulin product, purity, and species source.[32] Presently, three strengths of insulin, U-40, U-100, and U-500, are available in the United States. A vast majority of patients use U-100, and there is rarely a situation when the other strengths would be indicated. Purity refers to the presence of proinsulin or other contaminants in the insulin. This is less of an issue today than in the past, since all available insulins are quite pure, containing less than 25 ppm of proinsulin. The purified insulins, which include the human insulins, contain less than 10 ppm of proinsulin.

Insulin is available from several different sources including beef, pork, and human. Beef insulin varies from pancreatic human insulin by three amino acids while pork differs by only one amino acid. Therefore, pork insulin is less antigenic than beef. Human insulin is produced by two processes. Biosynthetic human insulin is made by Lilly and utilizes recombinant deoxyribonucleic acid (DNA) technology. Genetic material is inserted into *Escherichia coli*, which then produces insulin that is structurally identical to pancreatic human insulin. The second process involves substituting the one differing amino acid, alanine, for threonine on pork insulin to produce semisynthetic human insulin. Human insulin is produced in this manner by Novo-Nordisk. Human insulin has the lowest antigenicity of all the insulin products. Because of this, most diabetologists now feel that human insulin is the insulin of choice if cost is not an issue.[33]

The final consideration is choosing an insulin with the desired onset and duration of action (Table 17-4). After the initial clinical use of insulin, attempts were made to prolong the action of insulin to alleviate the need for multiple daily injections.[34] This has been accomplished by adding a modifying protein, protamine, in the case of NPH and protamine zinc insulin (PZI) or forming an insulin zinc suspension with the lente insulins. Presently, the most commonly used insulin is NPH.

Insulin is both hepatically and renally eliminated.[29] Approximately 50 percent of the insulin presented to the liver is eliminated by first-pass metabolism. Insulin is also filtered by the glomeruli and degraded by the renal tubules. Therefore, changes in both hepatic and renal function will affect the pharmacokinetics of insulin. When clearance of exogenously administered insulin was compared in young and old healthy subjects, the clearance was found to be 40 percent lower in the elderly population.[35]

Like the sulfonylureas, the major adverse effect of insulin is hypoglycemia. This can be of great concern in the elderly patient, especially with the use of long-acting insulin and in the context of nocturnal hypoglycemia.[36] Since hypogly-

Table 17-4 Insulin pharmacokinetics

Preparation	Onset, h	Peak, h	Duration, h
Regular	½-1	2-4	5-7
Semilente	1-2	4-6	12-16
NPH	1-1 ½	4-12	24
Lente	1-2 ½	7-15	24
PZI	4-8	14-24	36
Ultralente	4-8	10-30	>36

cemia with the sulfonylureas can also be severe, this should not limit the use of insulin. With careful blood glucose monitoring and patient education, severe hypoglycemia can be avoided.

Other adverse effects associated with insulin therapy include insulin allergies, which can be localized or systemic, and lipodystrophies. Both of these are seen much less frequently with the use of human insulin. Recently, there has been concern that insulin therapy in NIDDM may promote atherosclerosis.[37] Hyperinsulinemia has been associated with atherosclerotic disease, but a cause-and-effect relationship has not been clearly demonstrated.[36] The evidence is insufficient at this time to delete insulin from the therapeutic armamentarium of NIDDM.

One of the most important considerations in using insulin in the elderly patient is in choosing the appropriate insulin regimen. Numerous different regimens exist, but adequate glucose control can be achieved in most patients with NIDDM using a once or twice daily injection of intermediate-acting insulin. A general guideline for an initial dose is 10 to 20 units in the morning with the lower dose being more appropriate in the elderly patient. If the patient continues with fasting hyperglycemia in the morning as the insulin dose is increased, it is best to divide the insulin into two injections. This is most commonly accomplished by giving two-thirds of the total daily dose in the morning before breakfast and one-third in the evening before supper. Dividing the insulin in this manner will provide adequate coverage during the night and prevent the afternoon hypoglycemia which can be seen when larger doses of insulin are administered in the morning. Rarely, it is necessary to supplement the elderly patient's insulin regimen with short-acting regular insulin. This may be considered when the goals for blood glucose control are not met with a split dose of intermediate-acting insulin. In this situation, a few units of regular insulin are added before breakfast and possibly before supper based upon the blood glucose levels before lunch and at bedtime, respectively. Before a more complex insulin regimen such as this is implemented, however, it is important to assure that the patient will be able to administer and monitor the insulin therapy appropriately as well as eat consistent amounts of food at regular times.

There are several premixed insulin preparations available which contain 70 percent NPH and 30 percent regular (Mixtard, Novolin 70/30, Humulin 70/30).

These provide an alternative for patients who require a split-mixed insulin regimen but have difficulty mixing their insulin. The use of this premixed insulin was investigated retrospectively in 61 NIDDM patients with an average age of 65 years.[38] These patients had previously been mixing their own short- and intermediate-acting insulins. These investigators found that the glycosylated hemoglobin improved significantly and that there were fewer episodes of hypoglycemia with the premixed insulin.

Other insulin regimens which have been suggested in the treatment of NIDDM include ultralente and bedtime NPH. The use of ultralente given as a single injection in the evening has been advocated especially in the United Kingdom.[36] Theoretically, this will provide a basal level of insulin while lessening the risk for hypoglycemia since ultralente does not exhibit a significant peak effect. This regimen is not proving to be as ideal in practice as it is in theory.[39] This may be due to several factors including the shorter duration of human ultralente as compared to animal source ultralente; hypoglycemia, which does occur with this preparation despite its blunted effect; and the lack of improvement in postprandial hyperglycemia. A single dose of ultralente may not be any more effective than oral hypoglycemics in patients who have failed diet therapy.

The interest in using bedtime NPH in the treatment of NIDDM has grown.[39] This strategy attempts to time the insulin so that it peaks at approximately 8:00 A.M. to coincide with the peak of the "dawn" phenomenon. The insulin action at this time should suppress hepatic glucose output and excessive lipolysis. This also avoids the problem of nocturnal hypoglycemia which may be seen when NPH is administered before supper. If patients do not achieve adequate blood glucose control on this regimen alone, modifications can be made by adding short-acting insulin, an additional dose of intermediate-acting insulin, or sulfonylureas. It is noteworthy, however, that many elderly patients do not have the dawn phenomenon and bedtime NPH may not be an appropriate regimen.

Once an insulin regimen has been established, it is very important that the patient receives adequate education regarding the proper procedures for injecting, mixing, and storing insulin. If the patient is taking insulin before breakfast or supper, it should be injected 30 to 60 min prior to eating.[34] The site of injection can affect the absorption of insulin with the most rapid absorption from the abdomen followed by the arms, buttocks, and thighs. In the past, patients were taught to rotate their injection sites. This can lead to wide variabilities in insulin absorption profiles and a subsequent fluctuation in blood glucose control. It is now suggested that patients rotate injection sites within the same anatomic region with the abdomen being the preferred site. If it is necessary to use two different anatomic regions, they should be rotated in a systematic fashion. For example, the abdomen is always used for the morning injection and the thigh for the evening injection. In most patients, the injection can be made at a 90° angle although a 45° angle is recommended in the thin patient to prevent an intramuscular injection. Also, there is no need to aspirate prior to injecting the insulin or use alcohol on the injection site. Deleting both of these steps will simplify the procedure.

Studies have shown that errors in insulin dosage can be as great as 20 percent in the elderly patient.[40,41] Therefore, it is essential in the elderly patient that adequate instruction is given in insulin administration. This should also be assessed on an ongoing basis, since changes in visual and cognitive abilities may occur over time. In patients who have difficulty measuring their own insulin, there are aids available such as syringe magnifiers, injection devices which can be set for a specific dose, and vial holders[42] (Table 17-5). Insulin can also be prefilled in syringes and stored in the refrigerator for up to 3 weeks.[43]

Some new information has recently become available pertaining to the mixing of insulins.[43] The most common mixture of insulin is NPH and regular. This combination is stable, and contrary to past thinking, the regular insulin does retain its pharmacokinetic profile. The lente series may be mixed together in any combination and is stable for 18 months. When regular and lente are combined, the regular binds to the lente with a delay in the onset of the regular insulin. This reaction continues in a state of flux for 24 h, so it is not recommended that these two insulins be mixed. This same caveat applies for regular insulin and PZI. Insufficient data exist at this time regarding the compatibility of regular and ultralente combinations. Vials of insulin which are presently in use can be stored at room temperature for up to 1 month.[33] All other vials should be refrigerated. Insulin should not be frozen, and deterioration does occur with temperatures in excess of 86°F.

COMBINATION THERAPY

The use of combined therapy with sulfonylureas and insulin has been considered as a treatment modality for NIDDM.[44] The rationale for this approach is that sulfonylureas stimulate insulin secretion and potentiate insulin action, thereby increasing the effectiveness of both exogenous and endogenous insulin. The usefulness of this regimen has yet to be determined. Studies have shown a varying

Table 17-5 Insulin injection aids

Syringe magnifiers	Needle and vial holders
Insul-eze	Dos-Aid
Magni-Guide	Holdease
Syringe magnifier	Inject-Aid
Dose gauges	Insul-eze
Andros IDM	Load-Matic
Click-Count Syringe	Insulin Needle Guide
Count-a-dose	Magni-Guide
Dos-Aid	Vial Center Aid
Insulgauge	Insulin pens
	Autopen
	Novo Pen
	Novolin Pen

response rate, but overall, it appears that approximately 30 percent of patients will show improved glycemic control. Criteria for patient selection have not been delineated, but the role for combination therapy may be in the obese patient who has failed oral agents and is on large, escalating doses of insulin. Generally, this regimen is best avoided in the elderly patient with diabetes who may already tend toward polypharmacy.

An overview of the approach to the management of elderly patients with NIDDM is shown in Fig. 17-1. The goals of therapy should be highly individualized. Age, per se, should not be an excuse for suboptimal control of diabetes. In general, it is our policy to try to maintain the fasting serum glucose concentration between 100 and 140 mg/dL with postprandial levels not to exceed 200 mg/dL.

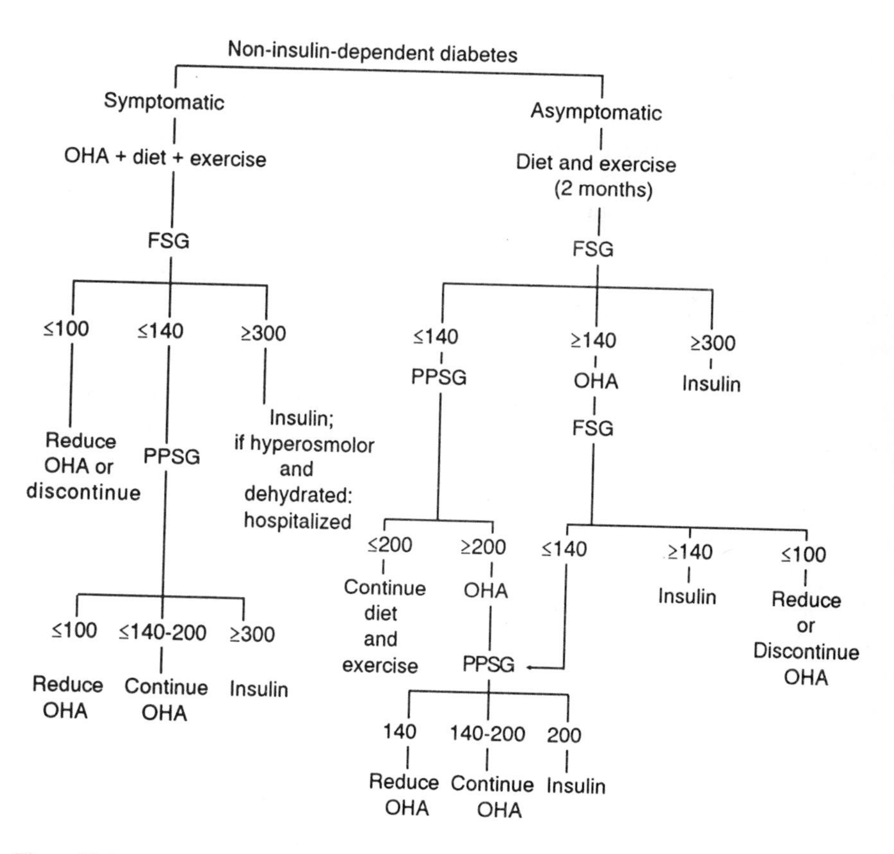

Figure 17-1 A suggested approach to the blood glucose control of elderly patients with NIDDM: OHA= oral hypoglycemic agents; FSG= fasting serum glucose concentration (mg/dL); PPSG= postprandial serum glucose concentration (mg/dL). (Adapted from Mooradian AD, Reed RL: Diabetes mellitus in the elderly, in Morley JE (ed): *Cowdry's Practice of Geriatrics*. Philadelphia, Pennsylvania, F. A. Davis, 1992.)

NEW DRUGS

Although the biguanides are not new agents in the treatment of diabetes, they have not been used in this country for many years secondary to the fatal lactic acidosis which was seen with phenformin. Metformin is currently undergoing clinical trials in patients with NIDDM.[16] The exact mechanism of action is not known, but reduced gastrointestinal absorption of glucose, inhibition of gluconeogenesis, and increased uptake of glucose by the tissues are among the proposed mechanisms. Metformin has been shown to be as efficacious as the sulfonylureas as well as being effective in up to 50 percent of patients who have failed therapy with the sulfonylureas. Metformin rarely causes hypoglycemia, which would be an advantage in the elderly population. The major side effects associated with this drug are primarily gastrointestinal. Its use is contraindicated in patients with renal insufficiency, pregnancy, liver disease, alcoholism, or cardiopulmonary disease. The incidence of lactic acidosis is very low with this drug and has been reported primarily in patients with contraindications for its use.

Acarbose is an inhibitor of the intestinal brush-border alpha-glucosidases.[45] Inhibition of the intestinal disaccharidases results in a diminished rise in postprandial blood glucose when this drug is ingested with starch-containing meals. The drug is only minimally absorbed from the gastrointestinal tract, so the side effects reported with this drug are minor and include bloating, flatulence, and diarrhea. Generally, this drug is used as an adjunct to sulfonylureas or insulin, since it only minimizes the rise in postprandial blood glucose levels. It may have a role in elderly patients with mild diabetes in whom insulin or sulfonylureas are contraindicated.[16]

Linogliride and pirogliride are two compounds which stimulate the oxidative metabolism of glucose in the peripheral tissues.[45] They may also increase insulin release in response to glucose. Both of these drugs have been shown to decrease both fasting and postprandial blood glucose levels in patients with NIDDM. Unfortunately, the toxicities may limit their clinical usefulness. Studies have been suspended with linogliride due to the occurrence of seizures during studies in dogs. Pirogliride causes an elevation in hepatic enzymes, which necessitated discontinuation of the drug in 60 percent of patients in one study. The role of these agents has yet to be determined.

MONITORING DIABETIC CONTROL

Monitoring of blood glucose control is an integral component of the management of diabetes. One of the major advances in this area is the introduction of home blood glucose monitoring. This technology should be offered to every elderly diabetic patient who has sufficient visual acuity and is capable of learning the procedure. Blood glucose monitoring is helpful not only in lowering of blood glucose levels but also in preventing hypoglycemic episodes.

The frequency of blood glucose measurements depends on individual needs and goals of therapy. This frequency ranges from an occasional use in the patient on oral agents who is concerned about hypoglycemia to six to eight times a day for the patient in intensive care settings. For most ambulatory elderly diabetic patients, a practical approach is once-a-day testing at different times during the day or four times a day for 2 days every 2 weeks. The patient's ability to accurately measure blood glucose levels should be checked periodically, since color blindness is not uncommon in the elderly patient with diabetic retinopathy.

Testing for urine glucose is unreliable and should not be used in elderly diabetic patients.

A glycosylated hemoglobin level should be checked at most every 3 months. This will allow the physician to assess the accuracy of home blood glucose measurements and will help reinforce the therapeutic recommendations. Affinity chromatography rather than anion exchange chromatography should be used in measuring glycosylated hemoglobin levels, as the latter method overestimates the level of this hemoglobin fraction in uremia, or high-dose salicylate ingestion, conditions that tend to be common in elderly patients.[2]

The use of serum fructosamine levels as an index of blood glucose control over the preceding 3 weeks is being popularized. There are no age-related changes in serum levels, and the superior precision of the test and its low cost may make it preferable to the glycosylated hemoglobin measurements.[46] However, more studies are needed to establish the usefulness of this test in elderly diabetic patients.

REFERENCES

1. Harris MI: Epidemiology of diabetes mellitus among the elderly in the United States. *Clin Geriatr Med* 6:703-719, 1990.
2. Morley JE, Mooradian AD, Rosenthal MJ, Kaiser FE: Diabetes in elderly patients: Is it different? *Am J Med* 83:533-544, 1987.
3. Lipson LG: Diabetes in the elderly: diagnosis, pathogenesis, and therapy. *Am J Med* 80(suppl 5A):10-21, 1986.
4. Jenkins DJ: Lente carbohydrate. A newer approach to the dietary management of diabetes. *Diabet Care* 5:634-641, 1982.
5. Bantle JP, Laine DC, Castle JW, et al: Postprandial glucose and insulin responses to meals containing different carbohydrates in normal and diabetic subjects. *N Engl J Med* 309:7-12, 1983.
6. Reaven GR: Dietary therapy for non-insulin dependent diabetes mellitus. *N Engl J Med* 319:862-863, 1988.
7. Mooradian AD, Kalis J, Nugent CA: The nutritional status of ambulatory elderly Type II diabetic patients. *Age* 13:87-89, 1990.
8. Mooradian AD, Osterweil D, Petrasek D, Morley JE: Diabetes mellitus in elderly nursing home patients. A survey of clinical characteristics and management. *J Am Geriatr Soc* 36: 391-396, 1988.
9. Reed RL, Mooradian AD: Nutritional status and dietary management of elderly diabetic patients. *Clin Geriatr Med* 6:883-901, 1990.
10. Rosenthal MJ, Hartnell JM, Morley JE, et al: Diabetes in the elderly. *J Am Geriatr Soc* 35:435-447, 1987.
11. Laws A, Reaven GM: Effect of physical activity on age-related glucose intolerance. *Clin Geriatr Med* 6:849-863, 1990.

12. Meinert CL, Knatterud GL, Prout TE, et al: University Group Diabetes Program: A study of the effects of hypoglycemic agents on vascular complications in patients with adult-onset diabetes. II. Mortality results. *Diabetes* 19(suppl):789-830, 1970.
13. Kilo C, Miller JP, Williamson JR: The crux of the UGDP: spurious results and biologically inappropriate data analysis. *Diabetologia* 18:179-185, 1980.
14. Lebovitz HE: Oral hypoglycemic agents. *Primary Care* 15:353-369, 1988.
15. Kennedy DL, Piper JM, Baum C: Trends in the use of oral hypoglycemic agents: 1964-1986. *Diabet Care* 11: 558-562, 1988.
16. Gerich JE: Oral hypoglycemic agents. *N Engl J Med* 321:1231-1245, 1989.
17. Halter JB, Morrow LA: Use of sulfonylurea drugs in elderly patients. *Diabet Care* 13(suppl 2):86-92, 1990.
18. Asmal AC, Marble A: Oral hypoglycemic agents: An update. *Drugs* 28:62-78, 1984.
19. Ferner RE: Oral hypoglycemic agents. *Med Clin North Am* 72:1323-1335, 1988.
20. Feldman JM: Glyburide: A second-generation sulfonylurea hypoglycemic agent. *Pharmacotherapy* 5:43-62, 1985.
21. Arrigoni L, Fundak G, Horn J, et al: Chlorpropamide pharmacokinetics in young healthy adults and older diabetic patients. *Clin Pharm* 6:162-164, 1987.
22. Kobayashi KA, Bauer LA, Horn JR, et al: Glipizide pharmacokinetics in young and elderly volunteers. *Clin Pharm* 7:224-228, 1988.
23. Washington SE, Mazzaferri EL: Type II diabetes: role of first- and second-generation drugs. *Geriatrics* 41:51-64, 1986.
24. Seltzer HS: Drug-induced hypoglycemia: A review of 1418 cases. *Endocrinol Metab Clin North Am* 18:163-183, 1989.
25. Porte D, Kahn SE: What geriatricians should know about diabetes mellitus. *Diabet Care* 13:47-54, 1990.
26. Lebovitz HE: Glipizide: A second-generation sulfonylurea hypoglycemic agent. *Pharmacotherapy* 5:63-77, 1985.
27. Jackson JE, Bressler R: Use oral hypoglycemics with caution.... *Geriatrics* 43:77-83, 1988.
28. Hansten PD, Horn JR: Antidiabetic drug interactions, in Hansten PD, Horn JR (eds): *Drug Interactions and Updates*. Vancouver, Washington, Applied Therapeutics, 1990, pp 201-217.
29. Messana I, Beizer JL: Diabetes in the elderly: practical considerations. *Practical Diabetol* 10(1):1-4, 1991.
30. Berger W: Insulin therapy in the elderly type 2 diabetic patient. *Diabet Res Clin Pract* Suppl:24-28, 1988.
31. Taylor R: Use of insulin in non-insulin-dependent diabetes. *Practical Diabetol* 8(5):1-3, 1989.
32. Francisco GE: Diabetes mellitus, in DiPiro JT, Talbert RL, Hayes PE, et al (eds): *Pharmacotherapy: A Pathophysiologic Approach*. New York, Elsevier, 1989, pp 805-821.
33. Mullen L, Hollander P: A practical guide to using insulin. *Postgrad Med* 85:227-232, 1989.
34. Skyler JS: Insulin pharmacology. *Med Clin North Am* 72:1337-1354, 1988.
35. Minaker KL, Rowe JW, Tonino R, et al: Influence of age on clearance of insulin in man. *Diabetes* 31:851-855, 1982.
36. Genuth S: Insulin use in NIDDM. *Diabet Care* 13:1240-1264, 1990.
37. Stout RW: Insulin and atheroma: 20-yr perspective. *Diabet Care* 13:631-654, 1990.
38. Bell DSH, Cutter GR, Lauritano AA: Efficacy of a premixed semisynthetic human insulin regimen. *Clin Ther* 11:795-801, 1989.
39. Riddle MC: Evening insulin strategy. *Diabet Care* 13: 676-686, 1990.
40. Kesson CM, Bailie GR: Do diabetic patients inject accurate doses of insulin? *Diabet Care* 4:333, 1981.
41. Puxty JAH, Hunter DH, Burr WA: Accuracy of insulin injection in elderly patients. *Br Med J* 287:1762, 1983.
42. Anonymous: 1991 Buyer's guide to diabetes products: insulin delivery. *Diabet Forecast*, September, 40-45, 1990.

43. Anderson JH, Campbell RK: Mixing insulins in 1990. *Diabet Educ* 16:380–387, 1990.
44. Lebovitz HE, Pasmantier R: Combination insulin-sulfonylurea therapy. *Diabet Care* 13:667–675, 1990.
45. Johnson DG, Bressler R: New pharmacologic approaches, in Rifkin H, Porte D Jr (eds): *Diabetes Mellitus: Theory and Practice*. New York, Elsevier, 1990, pp 887–895.
46. Nagoro H, Morley JE, Rosenthal MJ: Utility of serum fructosamine as a measure of glycemia in young and old diabetic and non-diabetic subjects. *Am J Med* 85:360–364, 1988.

CHAPTER

18

HORMONAL AND METABOLIC AGENTS

David G. Johnson
Suzanne Campbell

The incidence of symptoms or disease from endocrine dysfunction increases considerably with advancing age. Some of these changes, such as symptoms of estrogen withdrawal during the menopause, can be viewed as a normal part of the aging process. Nevertheless, hormonal replacement therapy may be indicated to alleviate a variety of significant diseases such as osteoporosis that are adversely affected by decreases in estrogen secretion. Other problems such as diabetes, which is more common in the elderly, obviously represent disease but may not require pharmacologic intervention. Age-related changes in other nonendocrine organs such as the heart may necessitate adjustments in the goals of therapy with hormones or other endocrinologic agents.

The effects of aging on the response of patients to hormones and drugs that affect the endocrine glands are profound and of considerable therapeutic importance. Age-related changes in the number of hormone receptors have been documented for many hormones in a wide variety of target tissues.[1] Usually the concentrations of receptors remain the same or decrease with increasing age, but examples of increases in hormone receptor concentrations have also been discovered. This chapter does not review all the effects of aging on the body's endocrine systems but concentrates on the special indications, use, and problems with the hormones and metabolic drugs most commonly prescribed for the elderly. The pharmacologic treatment of diabetes mellitus and osteoporosis is discussed in Chaps. 17 and 19, respectively. General information regarding the physiologic effects of age on the endocrine system can be found in recent reviews by Hall,[2] Hodkinson and Irvine,[3] Hall,[4] and Sanders.[5]

ESTROGENS

Estrogens are among the drugs most widely used by elderly persons. They are prescribed most frequently for the treatment of menopausal symptoms, but estrogen therapy is also used in the management of osteoporosis in women and prostatic carcinoma in men. One survey[6] indicated that almost one-half of all postmenopausal women in some communities in the United States had taken or were currently taking some kind of systemic estrogen therapy. A more recent survey found that only 17 percent of women at age 65 were using estrogen, with decreasing use down to only 4 percent for women aged 85 or older.[7]

Estrogen Use and Endometrial Carcinoma

In 1975 to 1976 three groups of investigators[8-10] reported an increased incidence of endometrial carcinoma among women receiving estrogen replacement therapy. This correlation was supported by an earlier study by Jensen and Ostergaard[11] that indicated that 33 percent of patients with endometrial carcinoma had received estrogens as compared with 21 percent of postmenopausal control patients. Previous work also indicated a close relationship between endogenous estrogen production and endometrial carcinoma. The causal relationship between estrogen therapy and endometrial cancer was challenged by several gynecologic endocrinologists, who pointed out that estrogens can cause hyperplastic changes that resemble endometrial carcinoma in situ but are reversible upon discontinuation or after a short course of progesterone therapy. The patients in Smith's study who had received estrogen therapy before development of endometrial carcinoma were much more likely to have early stages of disease than were women who had not been receiving estrogens before the development of endometrial carcinoma. Several explanations for this difference were advanced. First, women receiving estrogens under a physician's supervision were more likely to have regular checkups and to consult their physician for abnormal symptoms. Second, estrogens can make "silent" adenocarcinoma become clinically apparent by inducing bleeding. Third, without a trial discontinuation of estrogens or with addition of a progesterone agent, it is difficult to distinguish between the hyperplastic changes caused by estrogen and early carcinoma. Nevertheless, the evidence is now accepted that exogenous estrogens, like endogenous estrogens, can produce hyperplastic changes in the endometrium that can progress to carcinoma if ignored. During the past decade the addition of progestins to estrogen therapy has reversed the increased risk of endometrial carcinoma.[12,13] The use of progestin therapy may also have additional favorable effects on osteoporosis.[14] However, progestin therapy may have deleterious effects on cardiovascular disease by altering plasma lipids[15,16] or through changes in clotting mechanisms. The type of progestin used, the dosage and pattern of usage (i.e., continuous or discontinuous) may influence the effects on the cardiovascular system. Long-term studies using uniform treatment programs and collecting data on all morbid events and mortality are needed to determine the best regimen for administration of estrogen and progestins in postmenopausal women.

Contraindications

Estrogens have been associated with a number of adverse effects that limit their use. Relative and absolute contraindications to their use are outlined in Table 18-1.

Severe hypertension can develop in a small percentage of women taking estrogen. If there is a significant rise in blood pressure during therapy, the estrogen should be discontinued for at least 6 months to see if it is the cause. If the blood pressure responds to discontinuation, the estrogen should not be resumed. As stated earlier, the presence of mild hypertension before the initiation of estrogen therapy does not necessarily contraindicate its use.

Most studies have not shown any association between the use of estrogens and the development of breast cancer.[17,18] However, estrogens can have definite effects on breast cancer, causing either more rapid enlargement or regression. Therefore, most authorities believe that women who have been treated for breast cancer should not receive estrogens. A thorough breast examination must be performed before estrogen therapy is prescribed for menopausal women, and patients should be instructed in self-examination. A mammogram should also be performed. A strong family history of breast cancer suggests that caution should be used with estrogen treatment. Some authorities also advocate cyclical estrogen therapy with or without the additional use of progesterone, even for patients who have had hysterectomies, to protect the breasts from the abnormal condition of continuous estrogen stimulation.[19] It must be acknowledged that there is no convincing proof of any protective effect from this treatment.

Table 18-1 Contraindications to estrogen use

Absolute
Estrogen-caused hypertension
History of breast cancer (nonmetastatic)
Progression of fibrocystic disease of the breast
Progression of uterine leiomyomas
Relative
Obesity (increases risk of endometrial carcinoma)
Hypertension (increases risk of endometrial carcinoma)
Diabetes mellitus (increases risks of endometrial carcinoma)
Previous myocardial infarction, cerebrovascular accident, pulmonary embolism, or deep venous thrombophlebitis
Seizure disorder, migraine headaches, or multiple sclerosis
Cholelithiasis or hyperlipoproteinemia
Rheumatologic diseases

Estrogen therapy may have an adverse effect on fibrocystic disease of the breast. The presence of fibrocystic disease is not an absolute contraindication to estrogen therapy, but worsening of fibrocystic lesions is cause for discontinuation. Uterine myomas often enlarge during treatment with estrogens. The presence of small myomas before therapy is not an absolute contraindication, but if subsequent enlargement occurs during therapy, the estrogens should be stopped.

Obesity, hypertension, diabetes, and subnormal fertility from oligo-ovulation are known factors predisposing to the development of endometrial cancer.[19,20] Although the presence of one or more of these abnormalities is not a definite contraindication to the use of estrogens, close supervision is mandatory. Women taking estrogens in combination with progestins in the form of oral contraceptives have an increased risk of venous thrombosis, stroke, and myocardial infarction.[19,21] The incidence of myocardial infarction is particularly high in women who also smoke heavily.[22] The use of estrogen by postmenopausal women decreased the incidence of myocardial infarction in a recent study.[23] However, an increased incidence of myocardial infarction has been seen in other studies.[24] In view of this conflicting evidence, some physicians believe that patients with a history of myocardial infarction, cerebrovascular accident, pulmonary embolism, or thrombophlebitis should not receive estrogen therapy.

Several diseases may be adversely affected by estrogen therapy, including diabetes mellitus, seizure disorders, migraine headaches, multiple sclerosis, rheumatologic diseases, cholelithiasis, and some forms of hyperlipidemia. One must consider the presence of any of these complicating illnesses when weighing the likely risks of estrogen therapy, and significant worsening of these diseases during the course of estrogen administration may necessitate its withdrawal.

Treatment Regimens

Postmenopausal symptoms (i.e., hot flashes, mild mental depression, and emotional lability) usually respond to low or moderate doses of estrogen, such as 0.625 mg of conjugated estrogens, 20 μg of ethinyl estradiol, 0.5 mg of stilbestrol, or a 50-μg estradiol transdermal patch. Atrophic vaginitis responds, in most cases, to even lower doses, which can be given orally or as a topical cream. It is important to remember that the estrogens in the vaginal creams are well absorbed and have systemic effects. The minimal dosage required to relieve symptoms should be used and therapy should be continued only as long as necessary.

Despite the large number of studies that have been conducted using estrogen-progestin combination therapy, there is still no consensus regarding the optimal dosage or pattern of administration. In recent years, most authorities recommend that estrogen be given continuously, with progestin added either in continuous low dose or in higher dosage during only part of each cycle month.[25] The route of estrogen administration may be oral, vaginal (including intravaginal silastic rings), or via transdermal patches. Transdermal administration of 17-β-estradiol increases estradiol levels without causing an unphysiologic elevation of estrone. This prevents undesirable effects on renin substrate and the sex hormone, thyroxine, and cortisol-binding globulins.[26] Serum lipoproteins are also unchanged by transdermal estrogen therapy.[26] Estrogen patches must be replaced every 3 days. In the United States, medroxyprogesterone acetate is the most commonly employed progestin. It appears to have less adverse effects on plasma lipoprotein levels than the 19-nor progestins.[16] When medroxyprogesterone is given continuously, the usual dosage is 2.5 mg daily. When medroxyprogesterone is given intermittently, it is given according to various regimens, such as 5 mg daily for 14 days a month[27] or 10 mg daily for 10 days a month.[25] Most authorities do not advocate addition of progestin for women who have undergone hysterectomy.[28] If norethindrone is used as the progestin, 0.35 mg is comparable to 5 mg of medroxyprogesterone acetate.[27]

Follow-up Care

Opinions vary widely regarding the kind and frequency of examinations that should be given to women receiving estrogen therapy. Huppert[29] recommends routine breast, abdominal, and pelvic examinations approximately every 6 months for women taking estrogen. The indications for endometrial sampling and its frequency have not been resolved. Likewise it is not settled which of the available techniques is best for routine sampling—cytologic (Endopap, Vabra aspiration, Gravlee jet washing) or histologic (endometrial biopsy). An annual or semiannual examination that includes an endometrial aspiration and a pap smear is probably satisfactory for most patients who do not have a predisposing factor or symptoms. If abnormal bleeding occurs and endometrial hyperplasia is documented by biopsy, uterine curettage should be performed.

BREAST CANCER

The endocrine treatment of postmenopausal breast cancer has changed considerably during the past decade. Previously estrogens were used extensively to treat estrogen receptor positive breast tumors. Currently the antiestrogen, tamoxifen, is considered the first-line endocrine therapy due to its lower incidence of side effects.[30] The aromatase inhibitor, aminoglutethimide, is also used to block the peripheral conversion of androstenedione into estrone (the principal source of estrogen in postmenopausal women).[31] High-dose progestin therapy and androgen therapy are also used in advanced cases.

PROSTATIC CANCER

As mentioned previously, estrogens are effective in the treatment of prostatic cancer. Unfortunately, the use of estrogens by men is accompanied by an increased incidence of atherosclerotic vascular disease.[32] Use of estrogen to treat metastatic prostatic carcinoma is declining in the United States with the increasing use of leuprolide acetate, the nonapeptide analog of gonadotropin releasing hormone. Although leuprolide is more expensive and must be given parenterally, it does not increase the risk of atherosclerotic vascular disease. Unlike estrogens, leuprolide does not commonly cause swelling of the breasts, fluid retention, and blood-clotting problems. Both estrogens and leuprolide can cause hot flashes, a decrease in libido, and impotence as a result of the sudden decline in testosterone secretion.

When estrogens are used to treat men with metastatic prostatic carcinoma, the dosage employed is usually 3 to 5 mg of diethylstilbestrol (DES) daily. Given in this dosage, DES decreases both plasma luteinizing hormone (LH) and testosterone levels, leading to an inhibition of the growth of prostatic carcinoma. Before beginning estrogen therapy, men should receive radiation to the breasts to minimize subsequent development of gynecomastia.

Leuprolide may be given either as a daily subcutaneous injection of 1 mg or as a depot suspension of 7.5 mg given intramuscularly once a month. In a recent study the addition of flutamide, an antiandrogen, to leuprolide therapy of patients with advanced prostatic carcinoma increased the median actuarial survival time to 34.9 months versus 27.9 months for patients treated with leuprolide alone.[33] Flutamide is usually administered as two 125-mg capsules three times a day. The main side effect that occurs in patients treated with flutamide in addition to leuprolide is diarrhea. Occasionally patients develop liver function test abnormalities.

MALE HYPOGONADISM

Testosterone production diminishes with age, although the serum testosterone concentration decreases only slightly. Development of testosterone deficiency with serum testosterone values below the normal adult range (3 to 10 mg/mL) may be the result of either primary testicular failure or secondary hypogonadism from pituitary or hypothalamic disease. Elevation of the serum LH levels suggests primary hypogonadism. Secondary hypogonadism is often due to a prolactinoma. The treatment of pituitary tumors is discussed later in this chapter. Testosterone replacement therapy should be administered using intramuscular injections of esterified testosterone derivatives, usually 150 to 200 mg every 2 to 4 weeks. Oral testosterone preparations should be avoided because of the risks of hepatotoxicity. Before and periodically during testosterone therapy all elderly men should be screened for prostatic carcinoma by a careful physical examination and a serum prostatic specific antigen determination.

THYROID HORMONAL THERAPY

The circulating concentration of thyroxine does not change in elderly patients. However, plasma tri-iodothyronine concentrations are depressed 25 to 40 percent in older persons.[5] This suggests that peripheral conversion of thyroxine to tri-iodothyronine may be decreased in the elderly, since most of the circulating tri-iodothyronine appears to originate from circulating thyroxine. Physiologically, the decrease in tri-iodothyronine concentration does not elicit a compensatory rise in thyrotropin, so the lower tri-iodothyronine concentrations are not appreciated as deficient by at least one target tissue, the pituitary.[34] These physiologic alterations of thyroid hormone metabolism with aging indicate that slightly lower than normal dosages of thyroid hormone are usually sufficient for replacement therapy for older patients. When replacement therapy is begun by elderly patients, initial dosage should be small (e.g., 0.05 mg of *l*-thyroxine/day) to avoid sudden and excessive demands on sensitive body organs such as the heart. Patients should be alerted to the increased risk of angina from the augmented myocardial consumption of oxygen produced by thyroid hormone. Desiccated thyroid, which contains variable amounts of tri-iodothyronine, and other tri-iodothyronine-containing compounds are more apt to produce cardiac symptoms such as palpitations because of their potency and fluctuating plasma concentrations. For this reason they should probably be avoided as long-term replacement therapy for the elderly.

Study of hypothyroid patients taking replacement therapy with thyroxine has indicated that the sensitive thyroid-stimulating hormone (TSH) assay is the most reliable guide for ensuring correct dosage.[35,36] However, the TSH is often elevated in the first months of replacement even when the patient is clinically euthyroid.[36] Insufficient replacement therapy may lead to signs and symptoms of hypothyroidism including hypercholesterolemia. Chronic hypothyroidism predisposes to coronary artery disease.[37,38]

In recent years there has been increased concern for the excessive loss of bone mineral in patients overtreated with *l*-thyroxine.[39,40] The most reliable guide to detect overreplacement with *l*-thyroxine is a suppressed TSH.[39,40] Unfortunately, many of the commercially available "sensitive TSH" assays lack the sensitivity to differentiate reliably between low to normal and suppressed levels of TSH.[41] Nevertheless, it seems prudent to decrease the dosage of *l*-thyroxine in hypothyroid patients with nondetectable or consistently very low TSH levels.

ANTITHYROID AGENTS

Radioiodine is a particularly useful agent for the treatment of hyperthyroidism in the elderly. Although the thioamides appear to be as effective in elderly persons as they are in the young,[42] the expense and inconvenience of long-term treatment with these compounds makes them less suitable for older patients. Obviously surgery poses greater hazards for elderly patients. The ease of administering radioiodine and the freedom from concern regarding long-term effects of radiation or effects of radiation on offspring make it an especially appropriate agent for older patients. As discussed in Chap. 5, there are several changes in both the pharmacokinetics and dose-response curves to β-adrenergic receptor blocking agents in older patients. Since the appropriate dosage of β-adrenergic receptor blockers to use in the treatment of hyperthyroidism varies considerably from patient to patient, the adjustments that might be made for a patient's age are of relatively minor importance.

CORTICOSTEROIDS

Basal plasma levels of adrenocorticotropin and glucocorticoids are unchanged with age, although secretion and disposal of glucocorticoids are reduced.[2,4,5] This indicates that replacement doses of glucocorticosteroids for adrenal insufficiency should be in the low to normal range for older patients.

The indications for pharmacologic use of glucocorticoids by elderly patients are similar to those for younger patients. However, the prevalence of certain diseases that often require steroid therapy is increased in the elderly. Among these are temporal arteritis, polymyalgia rheumatica, and rheumatoid arthritis. The same principles that apply to the use of steroids by younger patients should be followed with older patients. Glucocorticoids should be reserved for persons who do not respond to less harmful drugs such as aspirin in the treatment of arthritis. Dosage should be as low as possible to achieve the necessary clinical response, and the need for continued therapy should be evaluated periodically. Whenever possible alternate-day dosage with prednisone should be used instead of daily dosage to minimize the adverse side effects of steroids, including pituitary-adrenal suppression.[43,44] Unfortunately, alternate-day therapy cannot be used to treat autoimmune hemolytic anemia, idiopathic thrombocytopenic purpura, temporal arteritis, and most cases of rheumatoid arthritis.

When the need for continued glucocorticoid therapy is judged to have passed, the dosage should usually be tapered gradually to avoid reexacerbation of the underlying disease. Patients who have received daily steroid therapy for longer than 2 weeks should be instructed to contact their physician immediately in the event of any intercurrent illness or injury that might require coverage with exogenous glucocorticoids for up to 1 year after discontinuing steroid therapy. During this time they should also carry a card or identification tag that states that they may require glucocorticoid therapy in case of illness or injury. Pharmacologic use of glucocorticoids by older patients can cause adverse effects such as the following:

1. Predisposition to infection
2. Poor wound healing
3. Sodium and water retention
4. Hypertension
5. Diabetes
6. Obesity
7. Psychotic reaction
8. Osteoporosis

9. Myopathy
10. Premature atherosclerosis
11. Cataracts
12. Change in facial appearance
13. Easy bruisability

Sodium and water retention may not be tolerated as well by patients with limited cardiovascular reserve or renal disease. The mental changes produced by high doses of glucocorticoids may exacerbate underlying dysfunction such as Alzheimer's disease or depression. Long-term use can accelerate the loss of bone that normally occurs with aging, leading to osteoporosis. The higher incidence of previous exposure to tuberculosis or systemic fungal infections increases the likelihood of reactivation during steroid therapy. Diabetes and hypertension, two highly prevalent diseases in the elderly, can be adversely affected by steroids. The catabolic effects of steroids can accelerate the loss of lean body mass that normally occurs with age, leading to extreme muscular weakness, poor wound healing, and easy bruisability. Prolonged use of high-dose steroids can cause cataracts. Although the mechanism is poorly understood, excessive corticosteroids cause premature atherosclerosis, which accounts for much of the eventual morbidity and mortality of patients undergoing long-term treatment.[45] In view of the many problems associated with corticosteroid use by older patients, the indications for employing them must be strong, and every attempt should be made to use the lowest dosage for the shortest possible time.

PITUITARY DISEASE

With advancing age growth hormone secretion decreases, leading to a similar reduction in somatomedin-C.[5] This physiologic decline may contribute to the loss of lean body mass and bone density. However, the cost, inconvenience, and uncertainty regarding adverse side effects have precluded efforts at "replacement" therapy in clinical practice. Acromegaly in the elderly is treated primarily by surgery or radiation as in younger patients. Poor operative candidates or patients not cured by surgery or radiation may be treated with bromocriptine mesylate. Patients with prolactinomas usually respond to bromocriptine with a decrease in both circulating prolactin levels and the size of the tumor. Unfortunately, the side effects of nausea and postural hypotension produced by this medication often limit the dosages that can be achieved. Initial dosage is usually 1.25 to 2.5 mg at bedtime with gradually increasing dosage to 2.5 to 5.0 mg three times daily. Octreotide acetate is more potent and better tolerated but must be given as a subcutaneous injection two to three times daily. Total daily dosage is usually 200 to 400 μg.

Diabetes insipidus in elderly patients is treated as in younger patients using oral agents or desmopressin acetate intranasally 10 to 40 μg given once or twice daily. The combination of chlorpropamide 100–250 mg plus hydrochlorothiazide

25–50 mg, both given once daily, is well tolerated by most patients. This therapy is also useful for patients with nephrogenic diabetes insipidus. Older patients have increased osmoreceptor sensitivity in the hypothalamus.[5] This causes a predisposition to the syndrome of inappropriate antidiuretic hormone secretion (SIADH). Furthermore, elderly patients are more likely to have underlying disease of the brain, heart, lung, or liver leading to SIADH. Treatment of the underlying disease and water restriction should be attempted, if possible. Alert patients who can ingest oral medications usually respond to demeclocycline 300 mg given two to four times daily.

HYPERLIPIDEMIAS

The interest in treating hyperlipidemias, especially hypercholesterolemia, has grown recently. This is due in part to data published in the past 10 years which have shown that lowering cholesterol with drug therapy can diminish cardiovascular morbidity and mortality. Because of this, guidelines for the treatment of hypercholesterolemia in adults were developed by the National Cholesterol Education Program (NCEP).[46] These guidelines state that all adults over the age of 20 years should have a plasma cholesterol level measured every 5 years. Treatment decisions are then based on the total and low-density lipoprotein (LDL) cholesterol values (Fig. 18-1). Although the NCEP did not address elderly patients specifically, this population has the highest prevalence of hypercholesterolemia and coronary heart disease (CHD).[47] Because of this, the treatment of hyperlipidemia must be considered in the elderly patient.

Dietary modification is the first line of therapy for both hypercholesterolemia and hypertriglyceridemia. In the elderly patient, it is important that a nutritionally adequate diet is maintained. Because eating habits and cost are considerations, the diet must be acceptable, affordable, and easily implemented by the patient.[47] It is also important to assure adequate vitamin and mineral intake, especially calcium, since this population is at risk for osteoporosis.

The NCEP recommends that the initial diet contain 30 percent of calories from fat, with no more than 10 percent of calories from saturated fats, and a cholesterol intake of less than 300 mg daily.[46] An additional goal of the diet is to achieve a desirable body weight in the obese patient. If there is an inadequate response to the Step-One Diet, a Step-Two Diet should be considered with a further reduction in saturated fats to less than 7 percent of total calories and cholesterol to less than 200 mg/day. At this point, patients should be referred to a dietitian for nutritional counseling. Dietary therapy should be continued for at least 6 months before drug therapy is implemented. If the LDL cholesterol remains above 160 mg/dL after an adequate trial of diet, pharmacologic therapy should be considered.

In addition to nutritional therapy, it is important to control exacerbating factors in the patient with hypertriglyceridemia.[46] Secondary causes include diabetes mellitus, obesity, excessive alcohol ingestion, hypothyroidism, renal disease, and

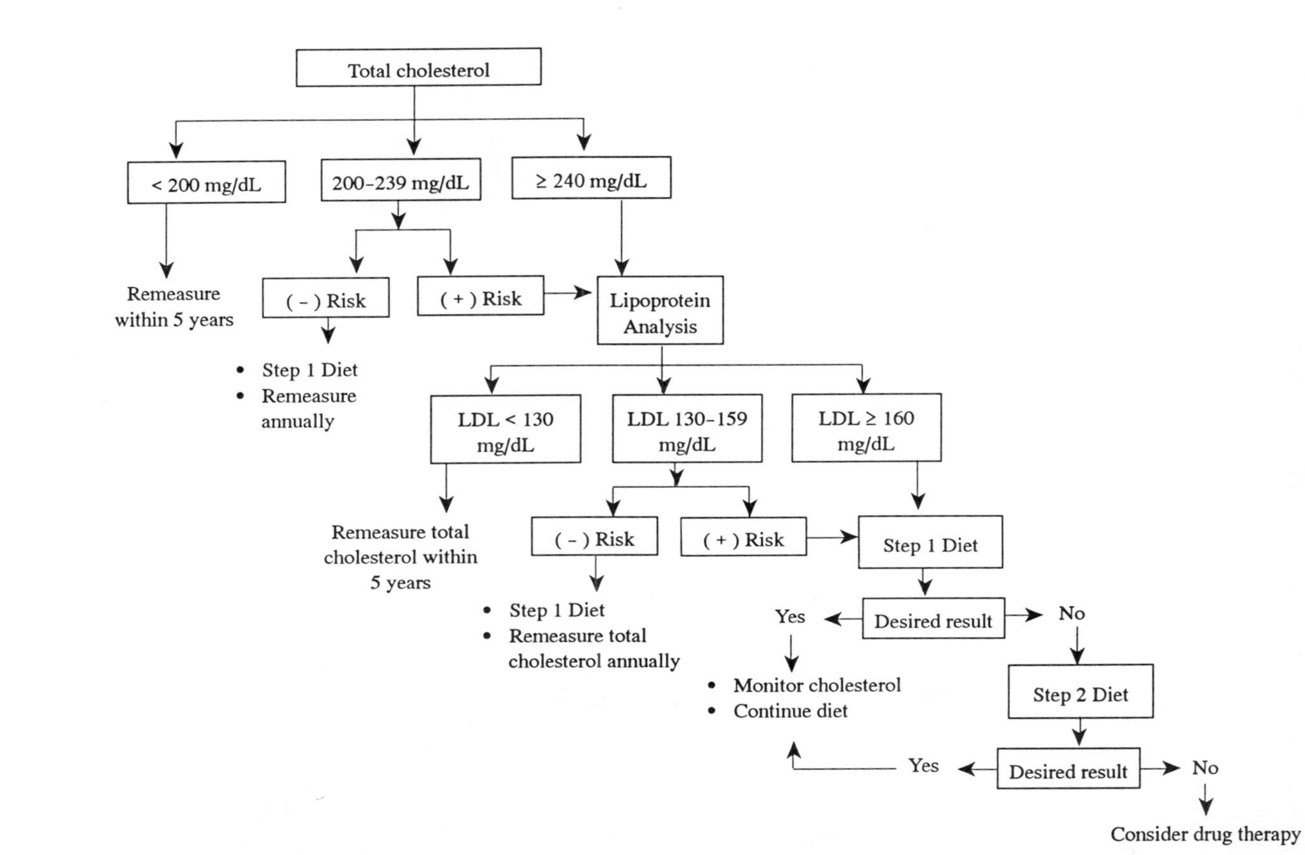

Figure 18-1 Treatment of hypercholesterolemia.

hepatic disease. In these situations, treating the underlying disorder will lower the plasma triglyceride level. If diet and minimization of secondary causes does not produce the desired effect in the plasma lipid profile, drug therapy should be considered.

Currently, there are five classes of drugs indicated for the treatment of hyperlipidemias (Table 18-2). When choosing any of these agents, the risk of drug therapy must be weighted against the potential benefit. This is especially true in

Table 18-2 Pharmacologic agents for the treatment of hyperlipidemias

Drug	Daily dose	Efficacy	Adverse effects
Bile acid sequestrants Cholestyramine Colestipol	 8–24 g 10–30 g	↓ Cholesterol 20% ↓ LDL 10–30% -/↑ Triglycerides ↓ HDL 2–8%	Constipation Nausea Abdominal pain Aggravation of hemorrhoids Indigestion ↑ Liver enzymes Interference with drug absorption
Nicotinic acid	3–6 g	↓ LDL 15–40% ↓ HDL 10–20% ↓ VLDL 15–40%	Cutaneous flushing Nausea Abdominal discomfort Diarrhea ↑ Liver enzymes ↑ Uric acid ↓ Glucose tolerance Itching
HMG CoA Reductase Inhibitors Lovastatin Pravastatin Simvastatin	 20–80 mg 10–20 mg 10–40 mg	↓ LDL 20–40% ↑ HDL 5–10% ↓ Triglyceride 15–35%	GI disturbances Nausea Headache ↑ Liver enzymes Myositis
Gemfibrozil	1200 mg	↓ LDL 0–15% ↑ HDL 10–15% ↓ VLDL 50–75%	GI disturbances Cholelithiasis ↑ Liver enzymes
Probucol	1000 mg	↓ LDL 8–15% ↓ HDL 25%	Diarrhea Flatulence Abdominal pain Nausea ECG changes

Note: GI = gastrointestinal.

the elderly, since data showing a decreased morbidity and mortality with therapy do not exist for this population. Also, the older person is generally at greater risk for adverse effects from drug therapy because of age-related alterations in drug elimination, coexisting disease states, and concomitant medications.

The bile acid sequestrants (BAS) cholestyramine and colestipol are first-line agents in the treatment of hypercholesterolemia.[46] These drugs work by binding the bile acids in the intestines with subsequent excretion in the feces.[48] Because the bile acids are synthesized from cholesterol in the liver, this reduction in bile acids causes an increase in the activity of cholesterol 7-alpha hydroxylase, which is the rate-limiting enzyme in bile acid synthesis, and a shunting of cholesterol into the bile acid synthesis pathway. The diminished hepatic cholesterol results in an increase either in the quantity of LDL receptors or in the affinity of the receptors. Through these mechanisms, the plasma LDL cholesterol concentration is decreased.

The BAS are very effective in lowering LDL cholesterol, with decreases in plasma concentrations of 10 to 30 percent. Total cholesterol is also reduced by approximately 20 percent. This effect is seen within 1 week of initiating therapy, and 90 percent of the maximal effect is reached in 2 weeks.[48] An increase in triglyceride levels can occur with the BAS especially in patients with preexisting hypertriglyceridemia. This is caused by an activation of phosphatidic acid phosphatase, which promotes hepatic triglyceride synthesis, increases the triglyceride content of the very low density lipoprotein (VLDL) particles, and subsequently increases the plasma triglyceride concentration.[48,49] For this reason, the BAS are contraindicated as single-drug therapy in patients with significant hypertriglyceridemia. The effect of these agents on high-density lipoprotein (HDL) cholesterol is minimal.

Dosing of the BAS must be individualized based on the patient's therapeutic response and tolerance of adverse effects. Four grams of cholestyramine is equivalent to 5 g of colestipol with respect to cholesterol lowering.[50] There appears to be a flat dose-response curve above 30 g/day so it is not useful to exceed this dose.[48] The usual dosage range is 8 to 24 g/day for cholestyramine and 10 to 30 g/day for colestipol. Although these drugs are commonly prescribed three to four times daily, they are just as effective when administered twice daily, which should increase compliance especially in the elderly person who may be on multiple medications.[51] The BAS should be administered within 1 hr of a meal, and one of the doses should be taken around the evening meal as this increases their cholesterol-lowering effect. It is important to initiate therapy at a low dose, such as 4 g twice daily of cholestyramine, and increase the dose gradually until the therapeutic endpoint is reached or the patient cannot tolerate the dose. Starting low and gradually titrating the dose will help to alleviate some of the adverse gastrointestinal effects seen with the BAS.

Both cholestyramine and colestipol are available as dry powders in bulk or individual packets. In addition to the original formulation of cholestyramine (Questran), a newer product is made with aspartame (Questran Light) which contains fewer calories and is sugar free. Cholestyramine is also available in a bar similar to a coated cereal bar, with each bar containing 4 g of cholestyramine and 50 to 60 calories. The dry powder should be mixed with at least 3 oz of fluid such as water, carbonated beverages, fruit, or vegetable juices. The powder may also be added to soups, liquid cereals, and applesauce. Since palatability is a major barrier to adherence to therapy, the patient should be encouraged to experiment with various diluents.

The acceptability of cholestyramine versus colestipol when combined with orange juice, water, orange drink, apple juice, grape juice, and applesauce was compared in 40 young, healthy volunteers.[52] These investigators found that cholestyramine was preferred to colestipol in all vehicles and that orange drink was the preferred vehicle for cholestyramine. A similar study also found cholestyramine superior to colestipol with respect to acceptability and that apple juice was the preferred diluent when compared to orange juice or water.[53] A third study compared cholestyramine with sucrose to cholestyramine containing aspartame in 100 volunteers with an average age of 42 years.[54] Both formulations were diluted in either orange juice or water. The cholestyramine with aspartame was preferred over the original formulation of cholestyramine in both instances. From these studies, it appears that cholestyramine is more palatable than colestipol. Since these data were from a younger population, different results may be expected in the elderly.

BAS are not absorbed systemically so they are relatively safe agents. The major adverse effects are gastrointestinal in origin, with constipation being the most commonly reported. This can be seen in up to 30 percent of patients on BAS.[48] Since the elderly are already more prone to constipation, it is important to instruct them to increase fluids and dietary fiber when BAS are prescribed.[51] If these measures do not relieve the constipation, a stool softener may be added. Abdominal distension, bloating, nausea, and vomiting can also be seen. Generally, patients will develop a tolerance to these adverse effects, and they can be minimized by starting with a low dose of BAS and titrating slowly. Other reported adverse effects include a transient rise in liver enzymes (aminotransferases and alkaline phosphatase), intestinal obstruction, and hyperchloremic acidosis.[48,50]

The BAS can interfere with the absorption of certain drugs, most importantly warfarin, thiazide diuretics, digoxin, gemfibrozil, and propranolol.[51,55] Because of this interaction, patients should be instructed to take other medications at least 1 h before or 4 h after taking the BAS. Prolonged high doses of the BAS may inhibit the absorption of the fat-soluble vitamins, and hypoprothrombinemia secondary to vitamin K malabsorption has been reported. Supplementation with vitamin K will correct the prothrombin time and alleviate any bleeding.

Since the BAS have been shown to be safe and efficacious, they should be considered as initial drug therapy for hypercholesterolemia. Their poor palatability and acceptability among patients make many practitioners reticent to prescribe these agents. However, with proper dosing and patient education, compliance with BAS therapy can be improved appreciably.

Nicotinic acid is another drug which is considered as first-line therapy for hypercholesterolemia by the NCEP.[46] As well as lowering cholesterol, it also has significant effects on plasma triglycerides that make it a good initial choice for the treatment of combined hyperlipidemias. Although the precise mechanism of action is not known, nicotinic acid appears to directly inhibit the hepatic synthesis of VLDL with a subsequent reduction in LDL production.[50] Levels of HDL cholesterol are also increased secondary to a reduction in catabolism of this particle. Overall, nicotinic acid has an ideal effect on the lipoprotein profile. It decreases LDL cholesterol by 15 to 40 percent, decreases VLDL cholesterol up to 40 percent, and increases HDL cholesterol by 20 percent.

Although nicotinic acid has a desirable effect on the serum lipoproteins, patient acceptability is a problem with the drug. Like the BAS, nicotinic acid should be initiated at a low dose and titrated based on the clinical response and tolerance of adverse effects. The recommended starting dose is 100 mg taken with the evening meal. This may be increased every 1 to 2 weeks based upon the response. Generally, 3 to 6 g/day is considered the maximal dose, and patients may have difficulty tolerating nicotinic acid at the higher doses.[51]

Nicotinic acid has a high frequency of adverse effects which makes the drug intolerable in up to 30 percent of patients for whom it is prescribed.[47] These side effects can be especially bothersome in the elderly. Flushing of the skin is the most common adverse effect about which patients complain. This effect is prostaglandin mediated and can be alleviated by pretreatment with aspirin or a nonsteroidal anti-inflammatory agent.[50] The flushing can also be minimized by starting at a low dose and titrating slowly as well as taking the drug with meals. Gastrointestinal side effects are common and include abdominal discomfort, nausea, and diarrhea. Nicotinic acid can exacerbate peptic ulcer disease and cause a dose-related elevation in liver function tests. Hyperglycemia has been noted and diabetes may result in elderly patients with preexisting glucose intolerance.[47] Nicotinic acid competes with uric acid for excretion so hyperuricemia and precipitation of acute gouty arthritis may occur. Because of these effects, nicotinic acid is contraindicated in patients with liver disease, peptic ulcer disease, and gout.[46] Liver enzymes, blood glucose, and uric acid should be monitored prior to initiating therapy and once the therapeutic dose is attained. Sustained-release nicotinic acid has been shown to diminish the flushing associated with this drug, but a higher incidence of elevated liver function tests is seen with the sustained-release product.[56] This drug is also more expensive than the immediate-release product. For these reasons, many practitioners feel that the sustained-release nicotinic acid should not be prescribed.

Although nicotinic acid can be difficult to tolerate in some patients, it is still a worthwhile drug in the treatment of hyperlipidemia. It has an optimum effect on the lipoproteins, it has been shown to be effective in decreasing CHD risk, and it is inexpensive, which is important for the elderly who may have limited financial resources. Proper titration and patient education, especially with respect to adverse effects, can improve patient compliance.

Lovastatin belongs to a class of drugs known as the 3-hydroxy-3-methylglutaryl-coenzyme A (HMG CoA) reductase inhibitors. The NCEP considers this agent a second-line drug in the treatment of hypercholesterolemia because of the lack of data showing a reduction in cardiovascular morbidity and mortality and long-term safety.[46] Lovastatin decreases plasma cholesterol levels by inhibiting the enzyme HMG CoA reductase.[57] This enzyme inhibits the conversion of HMG CoA to mevalonic acid, a rate-limiting step in the synthesis of cholesterol (Fig. 18-2). Because of the reduction in cellular cholesterol, the synthesis of hepatic LDL receptors is increased. This further contributes to the reduction in LDL cholesterol as well as VLDL cholesterol, which is also removed by the LDL receptor. Therefore, lovastatin reduces the synthesis of cholesterol as well as increases its clearance. HDL cholesterol levels are also increased by an unknown mechanism.

Lovastatin is very effective in reducing LDL with reductions of 20 to 40 percent. The drug also decreases triglycerides by 15 to 35 percent and increases HDL cholesterol by 5 to 10 percent. Lovastatin's effect on triglycerides and HDL cholesterol appears to be less consistent than that on LDL cholesterol.[58]

The recommended dose of lovastatin is 20 to 80 mg daily. Since food enhances the bioavailability of the drug, it is best to administer it with meals.[58] Therapy

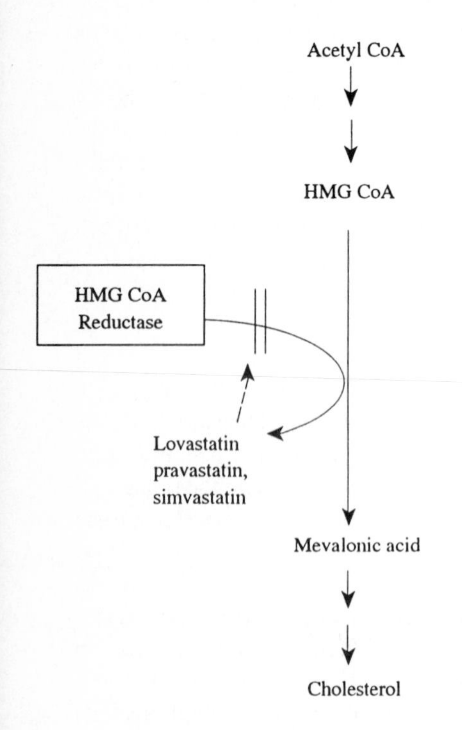

Figure 18-2 Mechanism of action of lovastatin, pravastatin, and simvastatin.

should be instituted at 20 mg with the evening meal and increased in increments of 20 mg every 4 to 6 weeks until the desired cholesterol lowering effect is obtained or maximal doses are reached. Once daily dosing in the evening appears to result in a greater lowering of cholesterol than administration in the morning but is less effective than twice daily dosing.[59] Therefore, if the patient does not respond to 20 mg in the evening, it is best to divide the dosing into a twice daily regimen.

Lovastatin is generally well tolerated with few subjective complaints by patients. The most common adverse effects are headache, diarrhea, constipation, gas, and abdominal pain.[60] Because increases in serum aminotransferases can be seen, it is recommended that these liver enzyme tests be monitored every 4 to 6 weeks for the first 15 months of therapy and periodically thereafter.[58] If the levels rise to greater than three times the baseline, the drug should be discontinued. The development of cataracts with lovastatin has been of concern since this was reported in dogs administered high doses of the drug. This has not been shown in clinical studies, but it is recommended that slit-lamp exams be performed as a baseline and annually during lovastatin therapy.[46] Increases in creatine kinase may occur, and cases of rhabdomyolysis have been reported in patients on concurrent gemfibrozil, nicotinic acid, and cyclosporine.[57] Concomitant use of lovastatin with these drugs should be avoided.

Pravastatin is a more recently approved HMG CoA reductase inhibitor and differs from lovastatin in several respects.[61] While lovastatin is lipophilic, pravastatin is a hydrophilic drug, and this property prevents the drug from readily crossing cell membranes. It appears to be taken up by the hepatocytes via an active transport mechanism and thus inhibits cholesterol synthesis selectively in the liver. In addition, pravastatin is administered as the active drug while lovastatin is administered in its inactive lactone form.

Pravastatin is similar to lovastatin with respect to efficacy and adverse effect profile. Two studies have investigated the use of pravastatin in the elderly and have found that there is a slight increase in the area under the curve and a diminished urine excretion.[62,63] Because of this, the recommended dose of pravastatin in the elderly is 10 to 20 mg daily.

Simvastatin is a third HMG CoA reductase inhibitor which has been used extensively outside the United States and has been released recently in this country.[64] It is a congener of lovastatin and is similar since it is also administered as an inactive prodrug and is lipophilic. Simvastatin appears to be approximately twice as potent as lovastatin. Studies have shown that this HMG CoA reductase inhibitor is effective and well tolerated in elderly patients.[65,66]

Overall, the HMG CoA reductase inhibitors are very effective in the treatment of hypercholesterolemia and have an acceptable adverse effect profile. If long-term safety and reduction in CHD risk can be shown, this class of drugs represents a significant advance in the treatment of hyperlipidemias.[46]

The fibric acid derivatives are the fourth class of drugs which can be used in the management of hyperlipidemias and include clofibrate and gemfibrozil. The use of clofibrate has diminished because of the results of the World Health

Organization (WHO) study which showed that there was a higher incidence of noncardiac deaths secondary to gastrointestinal neoplasms in the clofibrate group.[67] Deaths also occurred due to complications resulting from cholecystectomies necessitated by the high incidence of gallstones with clofibrate therapy. Gemfibrozil is the agent most commonly used in this country.

Gemfibrozil has a much greater effect on triglycerides than cholesterol. It inhibits the synthesis of VLDL and increases the activity of lipoprotein lipase which enhances the removal of triglyceride-rich particles from the plasma.[50] Gemfibrozil lowers VLDL cholesterol by up to 50 to 75 percent and increases HDL cholesterol by 10 to 15 percent. The effect on LDL cholesterol is more variable, but reductions of up to 15 percent can be seen.[46] Because of these effects on the lipoproteins, gemfibrozil is indicated in the treatment of type III, IV, and V hyperlipidemia and may be used in combination with other drugs such as BAS for type IIB hyperlipoproteinemia.[50] The recommended dose of gemfibrozil is 600 mg twice daily.

Gemfibrozil is usually well tolerated. The most frequent adverse effects include nausea, abdominal pain, and diarrhea in 3 to 5 percent of patients.[50] Less common side effects are rashes, eosinophilia, muscle tenderness, and increases in liver enzymes. Gemfibrozil may also increase the incidence of cholelithiasis, although this appears to be less than that seen with clofibrate. Lastly, gemfibrozil may potentiate the effects of warfarin, so it is important to monitor the prothrombin time in patients on concomitant warfarin.

Probucol is the final drug which may be considered in the management of hyperlipidemias. This drug appears to increase LDL clearance via the nonreceptor elimination pathway as well as to increase the biliary excretion of LDL.[50] It has also been proposed that probucol inhibits oxidation of LDL, which diminishes foam cell formation resulting in a decrease in atherogenesis.[68] Levels of HDL are also lowered secondary to a decrease in the synthesis of apoprotein A-I, the major apoprotein of HDL, and a reduction in lipoprotein lipase activity.[50] Probucol causes a modest reduction in LDL cholesterol of 8 to 15 percent but can also lower HDL cholesterol by as much as 25 percent. The usual dose of probucol is 500 mg twice daily.

The incidence of adverse effects with probucol is low with complaints from less than 5 percent of patients.[46] The most common side effects include diarrhea, flatulence, nausea, and abdominal pain. Probucol also prolongs the QT interval on the electrocardiogram, and although it has not been reported in humans, ventricular tachycardia has been reported in monkeys receiving the drug. For these reasons, probucol is contraindicated in patients with preexisting QT prolongation or ventricular irritability or those on other medications such as procainamide and quinidine, which also prolong the QT interval.[50] Probucol is lipid soluble and stored in adipose tissue, so it is recommended that the drug be discontinued in women 6 months prior to becoming pregnant. Because of the effect on HDL, the role of probucol has yet to be delineated, and at this time, it should be reserved as a second-line agent in the management of hyperlipidemias.

If patients do not respond adequately to a single agent, combination drug therapy can be utilized. Choosing agents with different mechanisms of action will enhance their lipid-lowering capabilities. The most effective regimens are the BAS combined with either nicotinic acid or lovastatin.[69] The BAS have also been used in combination with gemfibrozil. These regimens would be an alternative in a patient with hypercholesterolemia who does not have an optimum response to a single drug or in combined hyperlipidemia. Also, by using a lower dose of two different drugs, patient tolerance may be improved. This strategy can be especially helpful in the elderly patient.[47]

Once drug therapy has been instituted, it is appropriate to monitor both the clinical response and any adverse effects which may be occurring. The NCEP recommends measuring a LDL cholesterol 4 to 6 weeks after initiating drug therapy and again at 3 months.[46] If the therapeutic effect is not achieved at this time, compliance with diet and medication should be assessed. If it appears that the patient has been compliant, the dosage of the drug should be increased or, if a maximal dose has already been reached, changing drugs or adding a second drug should be considered. Once the LDL cholesterol goal is achieved, the total cholesterol should be measured every 4 months and the LDL cholesterol monitored on a yearly basis.

While it is clear that these drugs lower plasma lipoprotein levels, it is also important that this pharmacologic effect results in a decrease in morbidity and mortality from atherosclerotic disease. Several studies have investigated this issue. The Coronary Drug Project was designed to assess the long-term safety and efficacy of five hypolipidemic agents in 8341 males aged 30 to 64 years with evidence of a previous myocardial infarction.[70] Subjects were observed over a 6-year time period. Three of the regimens including conjugated estrogen 5 mg, conjugated estrogen 2.5 mg, and dextrothyroxine were discontinued prior to termination of the study due to excessive mortality as compared to placebo. The fourth drug, clofibrate, was not found to be effective in lowering cardiovascular or total mortality. The only drug found to be effective was nicotinic acid, which decreased the incidence of nonfatal myocardial infarction by 8.9 percent versus 12.2 percent for placebo, a statistically significant difference. However, nicotinic acid was ineffective in reducing total or cause-specific mortality during this study period. After 15 years of follow-up, mortality in the nicotinic acid group was 11 percent lower than the placebo group.[71] It is interesting that this effect was noted a minimum of 6 years after discontinuing the drug. These data suggest that nicotinic acid is effective in reducing mortality in patients with previous nonfatal myocardial infarctions.

The Lipid Research Clinics Coronary Primary Prevention Trial (LRC-CPPT) was one of the largest studies to demonstrate that lowering LDL cholesterol had a statistically significant effect on the incidence of coronary heart disease (CHD).[71,73] This study enrolled 3806 asymptomatic men aged 35 to 59 years with a total plasma cholesterol level of 265 mg/dL or greater and a LDL cholesterol of 190 mg/dL or greater. The subjects were randomized to cholestyramine 24 g daily or placebo. All subjects were placed on a low-cholesterol diet. The endpoints of the study were definite CHD death and/or a nonfatal myocardial infarction. Subjects were followed for an average of 7.4 years.

Total cholesterol was lowered 13.4 percent while LDL cholesterol was reduced 20.3 percent in the cholestyramine group. These reductions were 8.5 percent and 12.6 percent greater, respectively, than that seen in the placebo group. There were 155 definite CHD deaths and/or nonfatal myocardial infarctions in the cholestyramine group and 187 events in the placebo group. This resulted in a 24 percent reduction in definite death due to CHD and a 19 percent reduction in nonfatal myocardial infarctions in the cholestyramine group. There was no difference in overall mortality between the two groups.

A second primary prevention study was the Helsinki Heart Study, which studied 4081 asymptomatic men aged 40 to 55 years with a non-HDL cholesterol of 200 mg/dL or greater.[74] All subjects were instructed on a low-cholesterol diet and randomized to gemfibrozil 600 mg twice daily or placebo. Subjects were followed for a mean of 60.4 months with the primary endpoints being nonfatal or fatal myocardial infarction and cardiac death.

In this study, gemfibrozil decreased total cholesterol by 11 percent, LDL cholesterol by 10 percent, non-HDL cholesterol by 14 percent, and triglycerides by 43 percent and raised HDL cholesterol greater than 10 percent. There were 56 cardiac endpoints in the gemfibrozil group (27.3 per 1000) and 84 in the placebo group (41.4 per 1000). Overall, there was a 34 percent reduction in cardiac endpoints in subjects treated with gemfibrozil. Similar to the LRC-CPPT, there was no difference in overall mortality between the gemfibrozil and placebo groups.

Finally, two additional studies examined the effect of hypolipidemic drug therapy on the progression of coronary atherosclerosis. The NHLBI Type II Coronary Intervention Study compared cholestyramine 24 g/day to placebo in 116 males who had evidence of CHD on angiography and an LDL cholesterol in the upper 10th percentile.[75,76] The mean age of the subjects was 46.1 years. Coronary angiography was performed at the beginning of the study and again after 5 years of therapy.

The results showed a reduction in LDL cholesterol of 26 percent and total cholesterol of 17 percent in the subjects treated with cholestyramine. In the placebo group, LDL cholesterol was lowered 5 percent and total cholesterol 1 percent. Coronary artery disease progressed in 49 percent of the subjects on placebo and in 32 percent of the cholestyramine group.

The second study was the Cholesterol-Lowering Atherosclerosis Study (CLAS), which involved 162 males ages 40 to 59 years who had undergone previous coronary artery bypass surgery.[77] Subjects also had a total cholesterol of 185 to 350 mg/dL on admission into the study. All subjects received dietary intervention and were randomized to placebo or cholestyramine 30 g daily plus nicotinic acid 3 to 12 g daily. Doses were titrated based on the cholesterol response. Angiography was performed at baseline and after 2 years of treatment.

In the treatment group, total cholesterol decreased by 26 percent, triglycerides by 22 percent, and LDL cholesterol by 43 percent, and HDL cholesterol was increased by 37 percent. Regression of atherosclerosis was seen in 16.2 percent of subjects receiving treatment with colestipol and nicotinic acid and in 2.4 percent of subjects on placebo. A subgroup of 103 patients treated for 4 years (CLAS-II) showed regression of coronary artery lesions in 18 percent of the subjects receiving drug therapy compared with 6 percent of placebo-treated patients.[78]

Although these investigations have shown that drug therapy of hypercholesterolemia can decrease cardiovascular morbidity and mortality, the populations studied consisted primarily of middle-aged men. Therefore, it is not known if these data can be extrapolated to the elderly population. In deciding to treat the elderly person with hyperlipidemia, it is best to assess each patient individually. If the person is otherwise healthy, he or she may be a good candidate for treatment, while it may be hard to justify in the person with multiple chronic diseases and a limited life expectancy.[47] Age alone should not preclude the treatment of hyperlipidemias.

REFERENCES

1. Roth GS: Hormone receptor changes during adulthood and senescence: significance for aging research. *Fed Proc* 38:1910-1914, 1979.
2. Hall MRP: The endocrine system—the hypophysioadrenal axis, in Brocklehurst JC (ed): *Textbook of Geriatric Medicine and Gerontology*, 3rd ed. New York, Churchill Livingstone, 1985, pp 671-685.
3. Hodkinson HM, Irvine RE: The endocrine system—thyroid disease in the elderly, in Brocklehurst JC (ed): *Textbook of Geriatric Medicine and Gerontology*, 3rd ed. New York, Churchill Livingstone, 1985, pp 686-714.
4. Hall DA: The endocrine system and ageing, in *Biomedical Basis of Gerontology*. Boston, Wright PSG, 1984, pp 142-164.
5. Sanders LR: Pituitary, thyroid, adrenal, and parathyroid diseases in the elderly, in Shrier RW (ed): *Geriatric Medicine*. Philadelphia, WB Saunders, 1990, pp 475-487.
6. Stadel BV, Weiss NS: Characteristics of menopausal women: A survey of King and Pierce counties in Washington, 1973-1974. *Am J Epidemiol* 102: 209-216, 1975.
7. Canley JA, Cummings SR, Black DM: Prevalence and determinants of estrogen replacement therapy in elderly women. *Am J Obstet Gynecol* 163: 1438-1444, 1990.
8. Mack TM, Pike MC, Henderson BE, et al: Estrogens and endometrial cancer in a retirement community. *N Engl J Med* 294: 1261-1267, 1976.
9. Smith DG, Prentice R, Thompson DJ: Association of exogenous estrogen and endometrial carcinoma. *N Engl J Med* 293: 1164-1167, 1975.
10. Ziel HK, Finkle WD: Increased risk of endometrial carcinoma among users of conjugated estrogens. *N Engl J Med* 293: 1167-1170, 1975.
11. Jensen EI, Ostergaard E: Clinical studies concerning the relationship of estrogens to the development of cancer of the corpus uteri. *Am J Obstet Gynecol* 67: 1094-1102, 1954.
12. Gambrell RD Jr, Massey FW, Castaneda TA: Use of the progesterone challenge test to reduce the risk of endometrial cancer. *Obstet Gynecol* 55: 732-738, 1980.
13. Nachtigall LE, Nachtigall RH, Nachtigall RD, Beckman EM: Estrogen replacement therapy II: A prospective study in the relationship to carcinoma and cardiovascular and metabolic problems. *Obstet Gynecol* 54: 74-79, 1979.

14. Mandel FP, Davidson BJ, Erlik Y, et al: Effects of progestins on bone metabolism in postmenopausal women. *J Reprod Med* 27 (Suppl): 511-514, 1980.
15. Upton, GV: Goals and methods of hormone replacement after the menopause. *Contemporary Ob/Gyn* 25: 71-83, 1985.
16. Hirvonen E, Malkonen M, Manninen V: Effects of different progestogens on lipoproteins during postmenopausal replacement therapy. *N Engl J Med* 304: 560-563, 1981.
17. Arthes FG, Sartwell PE, Levison EF: The pill, estrogens, and the breast: epidemiologic aspects. *Cancer* 28: 1391-1403, 1971.
18. Hoover R, Gray LA, Cole P, MacMahon B: Menopausal estrogens and breast cancer. *N Engl J Med* 295: 401-405, 1976.
19. Seiler JC: Estrogens for the menopause. *Postgrad Med* 62(3): 73-79, 1977.
20. Kistner RW: Estrogen controversy updated. *Female Patient* 1(1): 25-27, 1976.
21. Dugdale M, Masi AT: Hormonal contraception and thromboembolic disease: effects of the oral contraceptions on hemostatic mechanisms. *J Chronic Dis* 23: 775-790, 1971.
22. Shapiro S, Sloan D, Rosenberg L, Kaufman DW: Oral contraceptive use in relation to myocardial infarction. *Lancet* 1: 743-747, 1979.
23. Stampfer MJ, Colditz GA, Willett WC, et al: Postmenopausal estrogen therapy and cardiovascular disease. *N Engl J Med* 325: 756-762, 1991.
24. Wilson PWF, Garrison RJ, Castelli WP: Postmenopausal estrogen use, cigarette smoking and cardiovascular morbidity in women over 50. *N Engl J Med* 313: 1038-1043, 1985.
25. Notelovitz M: Estrogen replacement therapy: indications, contraindications, and agent selection. *Am J Obstet Gynecol* 161(Suppl): 1832-1841, 1989.
26. Lignieres B, Basdevant A, Thomas G, et al: Biological effects of estradiol-17β in postmenopausal women: oral versus percutaneous administration. *J Clin Endocrinol Metab* 62: 536-541, 1986.
27. Hammond CB: Estrogen replacement therapy: What the future holds. *Am J Obstet Gynecol* 161(Suppl): 1864-1868, 1989.
28. Henderson BE, Ross RK, Lobo RA, et al: Re-evaluating the role of progestin therapy after the menopause. *Fert Steril* 49(Suppl): 9S-15S, 1988.
29. Huppert LC: Hormonal replacement therapy: Benefits, risks, doses, in Barbo DM (ed): *Medical Clinics of North America*, vol 71, number 1. Philadelphia, WB Saunders, 1987, pp 23-39.
30. Furr BJA, Jordan VC: The pharmacology and clinical uses of tamoxifen. *Pharmacol Ther* 25: 127-205, 1984.
31. Lonning PE: New endocrine drugs for treatment of advanced breast cancer. *Acta Oncol* 29: 379-386, 1990.
32. Catalona WJ, Scott W: Carcinoma of the prostate: A review. *J Urol* 119: 1-8, 1978.
33. Crawford ED, Eisenberger MA, McLeod DG, et al: A controlled trial of leuprolide with and without flutamide in prostatic carcinoma. *N Engl J Med* 321: 419-424, 1989.
34. Snyder PJ, Utiger RD: Response to thyrotropin releasing hormone (TRH) in normal man. *J Clin Endocrinol Metab* 34: 380-385, 1972.
35. Savin CT, Geller A, Hershman JM, et al: The aging thyroid. The use of thyroid hormone in older persons. *JAMA* 216: 2653-2655, 1989.
36. Helfand M, Crapo LM: Monitoring therapy in patients taking levothyroxine. *Ann Intern Med* 113: 450-454, 1990.
37. Vanhaelst L, Neve P, Chailly P, Bastenie PA: Coronary artery disease in hypothyroidism. *Lancet* 2: 800-802, 1967.
38. Steinberg AD: Myxedema and coronary artery disease—a comparative autopsy study. *Ann Intern Med* 68: 338-344, 1968.
39. Stall GM, Harris S, Sokoll LJ, Dawson-Hughes B: Accelerated bone loss in hypothyroid patients overtreated with *l*-thyroxine. *Ann Intern Med* 113: 265-269, 1990.
40. Ross DS, Neer RM, Ridgway EC, Daniels GH: Subclinical hyperthyroidism and reduced bone density as a possible result of prolonged suppression of the pituitary thyroid axis with *l*-thyroxine. *Am J Med* 82: 1167-1170, 1987.

41. Nicoloff JT, Spencer CA: Clinical review 12: the use and misuse of the sensitive thyrotropin assays. *J Clin Endocrinol Metab* 71: 553-558, 1990.
42. McGavick TM, Chevalley J, Pearson S: Variations in the response of individuals of different ages due to an antithyroid compound (methimazole). *J Am Geriatr Soc* 3: 96-105, 1955.
43. Ackerman GL, Nolan CM. Adrenocortical responsiveness after alternate-day corticosteroid therapy. *N Engl J Med* 278: 405-409, 1968.
44. McGregor RR, Sheagren JN, Lipsett MB, Wolff SM: Alternate-day prednisone therapy: evaluation of delayed hypersensitivity responses, control of disease, and steroid side effects. *N Engl J Med* 280: 1427-1431, 1969.
45. Plotz CM, Knowlton AI, Ragan C: The natural history of Cushing's syndrome. *Am J Med* 13: 597-614, 1952.
46. The Expert Panel: Report of the national cholesterol education program expert panel on detection, evaluation, and treatment of high blood cholesterol in adults. *Arch Intern Med* 148: 36-69, 1988.
47. Denke MA, Grundy SM: Hypercholesterolemia in elderly persons: resolving the treatment dilemma. *Ann Intern Med* 112: 780-792, 1990.
48. Ast M, Frishman WH: Bile acid sequestrants. *J Clin Pharmacol* 30: 99-106, 1990.
49. Shepherd J: Mechanism of action of bile acid sequestrants and other lipid-lowering drugs. *Cardiology* 76(Suppl 1): 65-74, 1989.
50. Illingworth DR: Lipid-lowering drugs: An overview of indications and optimum therapeutic use. *Drugs* 33: 259-279, 1987.
51. Hunninghake DB: The pharmacology and therapeutics of lipid lowering drugs. *Am Pharmacy* NS27: 818-825, 1987.
52. Shaefer MS, Jungnickel PW, Jacobs EW, et al: Acceptability of cholestyramine or colestipol combinations with six vehicles. *Clin Pharm* 6: 51-54, 1987.
53. Ito MK, Morreale AP: Acceptability of cholestyramine and colestipol formulations in three common vehicles. *Clin Pharm* 10: 138-140, 1991.
54. Shaefer MS, Jungnickel PW, Miwa LJ, et al: Sensory/mixability preference evaluation of cholestyramine powder formulations. *DICP* 24: 472-474, 1990.
55. Forland SC, Feng Y, Cutler RE: Apparent reduced absorption of gemfibrozil when given with colestipol. *J Clin Pharmacol* 30: 29-32, 1990.
56. Knopp RH, Ginsberg J, Albers JJ, et al: Contrasting effects of unmodified and time-release forms of niacin on lipoproteins in hyperlipidemic subjects: Clues to mechanism of action of niacin. *Metabolism* 34: 642-650, 1985.
57. Grundy SM: HMG-CoA reductase inhibitors for treatment of hypercholesterolemia. *N Engl J Med* 319: 24-32, 1988.
58. McKenney JM: Lovastatin: A new cholesterol-lowering agent. *Clin Pharm* 7: 21-36, 1988.
59. Illingworth DR: Comparative efficacy of once versus twice daily mevinolin in the therapy of familial hypercholesterolemia. *Clin Pharmacol Ther* 40: 338-343, 1986.
60. Henwood JM, Heel RC: Lovastatin: A preliminary review of its pharmacodynamic properties and therapeutic use in hyperlipidemia. *Drugs* 36: 429-454, 1988.
61. Pan HY: Clinical pharmacology of pravastatin, a selective inhibitor of HMG-CoA reductase. *Eur J Clin Pharmacol* 40(Suppl 1): S15-18, 1991.
62. Pan H, Funke P, Waclawski A, et al: Comparative pharmacokinetics of pravastatin, an HMG CoA reductase inhibitor, in healthy elderly and young male subjects. *J Clin Pharmacol* 29: 848, 1989 (abstr).
63. Pan H, Gourzis J, Kassalow L, et al: Pharmacokinetics of pravastatin, an HMG CoA reductase inhibitor, in healthy female subjects *J Clin Pharmacol* 28: 942, 1988 (abstr).
64. Mauro VF, MacDonald JL: Simvastatin: A review of its pharmacology and clinical use. *DICP Ann Pharmacother* 25: 257-264, 1991.
65. Bach LA, Cooper ME, O'Brien RC, et al: The use of simvastatin, an HMG CoA reductase inhibitor, in older patients with hypercholesterolemia and atherosclerosis. *J Am Geriatr Soc* 38: 10-14, 1990.

66. Kuhn P, Darioli R, Bovet P, et al: Dose-dependent lipid-lowering effects of simvastatin (MK-733) in the elderly. *Curr Ther Res* 46: 381-389, 1989.
67. Committee of Principal Investigators: A cooperative trial in the primary prevention of ischemic heart disease using clofibrate. *Br Heart J* 40: 1069-1118, 1978.
68. Parthasarathy S, Young SG, Witztum JL, et al: Probucol inhibits oxidative modification of low density lipoprotein. *J Clin Invest* 77: 641-644, 1986.
69. Illingworth DR: New horizons in combination drug therapy for hypercholesterolemia. *Cardiology* 76(Suppl 1): 83-100, 1989.
70. The Coronary Drug Project Research Group: Clofibrate and niacin in coronary heart disease. *JAMA* 231: 360-381, 1975.
71. Canner PL, Berge KG, Wenger NK, et al: Fifteen year mortality in coronary drug project patients: long-term benefit with niacin. *J Am Coll Cardiol* 8: 1245-1255, 1986.
72. The Lipid Research Clinics Coronary Primary Prevention Trial Results: I. Reduction in incidence of coronary heart disease. *JAMA* 251: 351-364, 1984.
73. The Lipid Research Clinics Coronary Primary Prevention Trial Results: II. The relationship of reduction in incidence of coronary heart disease to cholesterol lowering. *JAMA* 251: 365-374, 1984.
74. Frick MH, Elo O, Haapa K, et al: Helsinki heart study: primary prevention trial with gemfibrozil in middle-aged men with dyslipidemia. *N Engl J Med* 317: 1237-1245, 1987.
75. Brensike JF, Levy RI, Kelsey SF, et al: Effects of therapy with cholestyramine on progression of coronary arteriosclerosis: results of the NHLBI type II coronary intervention study. *Circulation* 69: 313-324, 1984.
76. Levy RI, Brensike JF, Epstein SE, et al: The influence of changes in lipid values induced by cholestyramine and diet on progression of coronary artery disease: results of the NHLBI type II coronary intervention study. *Circulation* 69: 325-337, 1984.
77. Blankenhorn DH, Nessim SA, Johnson RL, et al: Beneficial effects of combined colestipol-niacin therapy on coronary atherosclerosis and coronary venous bypass grafts. *JAMA* 257: 3233-3240, 1987.
78. Cashin-Hemphill L, Mack WJ, Pogoda JM, et al: Beneficial effects of colestipol-niacin on coronary atherosclerosis: A 4-year follow-up. *JAMA* 264: 3013-3017, 1990.

CHAPTER

19

THERAPY OF OSTEOPOROSIS

Michael J. Maricic

EPIDEMIOLOGY

Osteoporosis is a metabolic disorder of bone characterized by decreased total bone mass and increased susceptibility to fracture, especially of the wrist, spine, and hip. Osteoporosis is a major medical, economic, and social health problem in the United States. It is estimated that 1.2 million fractures attributable to osteoporosis occur each year in persons over age 45 years and older.[1,2] This includes 600,000 vertebral crush fractures and 250,000 fractures of the hip. The risk of hip fracture begins to rise after age 45, then rises exponentially, doubling for every 5 years of age. One-third of women over 65 will have vertebral fractures. Among those living to age 90, 32 percent of women and 17 percent of men will suffer a hip fracture.[1] For unexplained reasons, the age-adjusted incidence of hip fractures in the United States has risen over the past 30 years.[3,4] This statistic, combined with the increasing age of the population as a whole, suggests that this will become an increasingly important problem in the next few decades.

After hip fracture in the elderly, there is a 12 to 20 percent excess mortality rate in the next year[5] due to complications of immobilization (pneumonia, pulmonary embolus). Approximately 50 percent of elderly patients with hip fractures never regain the same level of functional independence, and 25 percent require long-term institutional care. The total direct and indirect annual costs for osteoporosis approach $6 billion.[6] Approximately 40 percent of these costs represents hospital care and surgery for those who have sustained hip fractures, and another 40 percent represents long-term nursing home costs.

PHYSIOLOGY OF BONE FORMATION

The three major functions of bone are to provide support for the musculoskeletal system, housing for the bone marrow, and a metabolic reservoir for calcium, phosphorus, and other ions. Bone formation and resorption occur continuously throughout life and are closely coupled. Bone matrix (osteoid) synthesized by osteoblasts is composed of collagen and noncollagenous proteins such as osteocalcin (bone Gla protein), osteonectin, and bone morphogenic protein. Mineralization of matrix starts with the laying down of amorphous calcium phosphate or octacalcium phosphate, substances which, by hydration and other changes, later convert to hydroxyapatite. Traces of fluoride are also normally found and are essential to the normal mineralization of bone. The mineral phase gives compressive strength and rigidity, but it is the fibrous organic matrix that gives bone its resistance to tractional and torsional forces. Osteoclasts are multinucleated cells, presumably derived from monocyte/phagocyte cell lines which resorb bone. It appears that most factors which activate osteoclasts act indirectly through osteoblasts. Receptors for parathyroid hormone (PTH) and 1,25-dihydroxyvitamin D, both potent stimulators of bone resorption, are not found on osteoclasts but are found on osteoblasts. Calcitonin, an inhibitor of bone resorption, has been shown to have receptors on osteoclasts. Osteocytes, which are relatively inactive osteoblasts, may also resorb bone through a process called osteocytic osteolysis and play a key role in maintaining constant levels of calcium in the body fluids.

The three major calciotropic hormones are calcitonin, PTH, and 1,25-dihydroxyvitamin D. Calcitonin levels may decrease slightly with age. However, calcitonin deficiency has not been shown to be an important etiologic cause of osteoporosis in the elderly. In fact, patients who have a total deficiency of calcitonin due to thyroidectomy have been shown to have normal bone densities.[7] PTH levels have been shown to increase slightly with age.[8] Whether this is due to decreased calcium absorption in the elderly[9] or other factors is not clear. However, this may be a contributory factor in increased bone resorption. 1,25-Dihydroxyvitamin D, obtained by 25 hydroxylation of vitamin D in the liver followed by 1-alpha hydroxylation by the kidney, has been found in most studies to be decreased in the elderly.[10] This is probably related to overall decrease in renal function in this age group. A number of other systemic hormones such as thyroid hormone, corticosteroids, growth hormones, and sex hormones also play important roles in regulating bone resorption and formation, especially in states of deficiency or excess.

The role of local regulators of bone formation and resorption is an area of intense current investigation and may provide important therapeutic options in the future. Prostaglandin E_2 and interleukin 1 stimulate bone resorption and play important roles in the osteoporosis of inflammatory disorders such as rheumatoid arthritis. Osteoclast activating factor and lymphotoxin have been shown to be mediators of resorption in myeloma. Circulating growth factors such as epidermal-, fibroblast-, and platelet-derived growth factors have direct effects on both bone formation and resorption. Thorough descriptions of these local factors of regulation have recently been reviewed.[11]

CLASSIFICATION OF OSTEOPOROSIS

Although there are over 100 disorders which can lead to osteoporosis, they may be simply separated into *involutional* and *secondary* causes. Important and treatable causes for the physician to recognize are *endocrinopathies* (hyperparathyroidism, hyperthyroidism, hypercortisolism, and premature sex hormone deficiencies), *neoplastic* disorders such as multiple myeloma and lymphoma, and *drug induced* (corticosteroids, heparin). *Involutional osteoporosis* has been further subdivided (Table 19-1) by Riggs[2] into type I (postmenopausal) and type II (senile). Postmenopausal osteoporosis is seen in women age 51 to 75, is caused by factors related to menopause, affects mainly trabecular bone, and therefore is manifest mainly by vertebral fractures. Senile osteoporosis is seen mainly after age 70 in both men and women, affects both trabecular and cortical bone, and results in both vertebral and hip fractures. Factors related more to aging [decreased 1,25-$(OH)_2D$ and decreased osteoblast function] are thought to be operative.

Osteomalacia enters into the differential diagnosis of osteopenia and must be recognized because it is potentially treatable. Common causes of osteomalacia include alimentary (postgastrectomy,[12] small intestinal,[13] and hepatobiliary diseases), renal (renal tubular acidosis[14]) and drug-induced[15] (anticonvulsants, fluoride) diseases. Vitamin D deficiency is rare, but it should be thought of in the elderly shut-ins.[16]

DIAGNOSIS AND BONE DENSITY MEASUREMENT

Most common causes of secondary osteopenia may be excluded by the history and physical and simple laboratory screening with a chemistry screen, complete blood

Table 19-1 Classification of osteoporosis

	Type I	Type II
Age	51-75	>70
Female-to-male ratio	6 : 1	2 : 1
Fracture site	Vertebrae, distal radius	Hip, vertebrae
Bone loss	Trabecular	Cortical and trabecular
Etiology	Estrogen deficiency	Factors related to aging

Source: Adapted from Riggs BL, Melton LJ: Involutional osteoporosis. *N Engl J Med* 314: 1681, 1986.

count, thyroid function tests, and urinalysis. Calcium, phosphorus, and alkaline phosphatase levels may show the following pattern:

	Calcium	Phosphorus	Alkaline phosphatase
Osteoporosis	NL	NL	NL
Osteomalacia	NL	Decreased	Increased
Hyperparathyroid	NL/increased	Decreased	Increased

Note: NL = normal

An assessment of probability of the patient being osteoporotic may be made from reviewing the patient's risk factors. They are estrogen deficiency, poor lifelong calcium intake, sedentary lifestyle, excessive alcohol and nicotine consumption, white race, small body frame, family history, and the secondary causes of osteoporosis named above.

The major means of assessing bone density are as follows:

1. Spine radiographs
2. Single-photon absorptiometry
3. Dual-photon absorptiometry (DPA)
4. Quantitative computerized axial tomography (CAT) scan
5. Dual-energy radiograph absorptiometry
6. Bone biopsy

Spine radiographs are insensitive, and one must lose 30 percent bone density before osteopenia can be detected. Single-photon absorptiometry utilizes an ^{125}Io source and is a sensitive (1 to 2 percent) tool for measuring density in the distal forearm.[17] Since the forearm is predominantly cortical in composition, however, these measurements do not accurately reflect changes occurring in more trabecular bone (spine, hip) and do not help to predict bone loss in these areas.

Dual-photon absorptiometry utilized a ^{153}G source and is useful to measure the hip and spine. It is both highly precise and reproducible (both 2 to 3 percent). The amount of radiation to the patient is about 10 mrad (one-third that of a radiograph).[18] Quantitative CAT scans have an advantage over DPA in that they can separate out trabecular (which is more metabolically active) from cortical bone.[19] The disadvantages are higher cost and radiation (300 mrad). Dual-energy x-ray absorptiometry (DEXA) replaces gadolinium in the DPA with a radiograph source and is considered the state of the art for measuring bone density because of its improved precision and accuracy (both 1 percent) and low radiation (<2 mrad).[20]

Bone biopsies are not helpful for determining bone density because of their sampling error, cost, and invasive nature. They may detect whether there is a preponderance of bone formation or resorption. However, these changes are frequently available biochemically (increased urinary calcium and hydroxyproline). Double-labeled tetracycline bone biopsies are indicated for distinguishing osteoporosis from osteomalacia.

PREVENTION AND TREATMENT

Osteoporosis is much more a preventable than a treatable disease. Prevention involves changing the changeable risk factors such as calcium deficiency, sedentary lifestyle, alcohol and nicotine abuse, and estrogen deficiency.

CALCIUM

Pharmacokinetics

Calcium is actively absorbed in the duodenum and proximal jejunum and must be in an ionized, soluble form for absorption to occur. An acidic intestinal pH is necessary for absorption of calcium. Thus absorption may be compromised in geriatric and other achlorhydric patients. Other conditions which may impair calcium absorption include uremia, steatorrhea, and the excessive consumption of certain anions (oxalates, phytates). Bone contains 99 percent of the body's calcium. The remaining 1 percent is equally distributed between the intracellular and extracellular fluids. Calcium is excreted mainly in the feces and consists of unabsorbed calcium. Most of the calcium filtered by the glomerulus is reabsorbed with only small amounts (<4 mg/kg/day) being excreted in the urine.

Use

There is a great deal of controversy in the lay and scientific literature as to the role of calcium in the prevention and treatment of osteoporosis. Most of the controversy stems from the fact that because studies have shown that calcium without estrogen replacement therapy (ERT) does nothing to retard the progress of osteoporosis, it is incorrectly stated that calcium is of no benefit. This is probably not true. Metabolic balance studies[21] have shown that premenopausal women and postmenopausal women on ERT need 1000 mg/day while postmenopausal women not on ERT need 1500 mg/day of calcium to stay in zero balance. If this is not obtained from the diet, it would probably have to be derived from bone, since a steady-state level of calcium is necessary at all times for vital body functions. Retrospective studies have correlated lifelong calcium intake to increased bone density and decreased risk of hip fracture in later life.[22] A recent double-blind, placebo-controlled study demonstrated significantly reduced bone loss in healthy older (mean age 59.9 years) postmenopausal women who had a daily calcium intake of less than 400 mg/day by increasing their calcium intake to 800 mg/day.[23]

Calcium supplementation to meet the above guidelines should be considered prudent therapy. In the elderly, calcium should be given with meals to ensure proper absorption since hypoacidity impairs calcium absorption.[24] The only relative contraindication to calcium supplementation is a history of kidney stones,[25] and the only real danger in recommending calcium is failure to recognize and treat estrogen deficiency.

ESTROGEN REPLACEMENT THERAPY

Pharmacokinetics

Oral conjugated estrogens are rapidly absorbed and undergo hepatic first-pass metabolism in the liver. They are 50 to 80 percent bound to plasma proteins and are distributed throughout most body tissues. Estrogens and their metabolites are mainly excreted in the urine, although small amounts are also present in the feces. Transdermal estradiol is rapidly absorbed through the skin and does not undergo hepatic first-pass metabolism. Distribution and elimination are similar to oral conjugated estrogens.

Use

Estrogen replacement therapy has been shown to prevent bone loss and osteoporotic fractures in postmenopausal females.[26,27] Best results are obtained when started within 5 years of the menopause. However, a recent study revealed significant benefit on bone density of the hip and lumbar spine in women an average of 14.6 years from the menopause.[28]

How long estrogen should be given for is not clear. In one study,[29] the estimated risk ratio for hip fracture in users of oral estrogens for more than 60 months was 0.42 compared to nonusers. The risk significantly decreased with increased duration of use. It is known that after stopping ERT, rapid trabecular bone loss of 4 to 5 percent per year ensues just as it would have had ERT not been started.[30] The decision to continue ERT must be based upon the risk-benefit ratio for the individual patient just as it would have been when starting it.

Most studies on bone density loss have been done with 0.625 mg conjugated equine estrogen.[31] Although 0.3 mg has also been shown to be protective,[32] it appears not to be as protective as 0.625 mg. If a woman has had a hysterectomy, she may take unopposed daily estrogen. If the uterus is intact, ERT should either be cycled with medroxyprogesterone or given in daily combination with small daily doses of progesterone,[33,34] such as medroxyprogesterone 2.5 mg/day, to protect the uterus from endometrial hyperplasia and carcinoma. The latter method is preferred by some women since withdrawal bleeding tends not to occur.

Women should have yearly mammograms while on ERT, and all breakthrough bleeding should be thoroughly investigated. The only absolute contraindication to

ERT is prior breast or uterine carcinoma. In such a patient, calcitonin should be considered if the patient is felt to be at high risk for osteoporosis.[35] Relative contraindications such as migraines, hypertension, cholelithiasis, and phlebitis may be more safely managed with the use of the estrogen patch, which does not entail first-pass hepatic metabolism. Studies have demonstrated that oral estradiol administration leads to substantial increases in renin substrate and very low density lipoprotein (VLDL) levels and significant decreases in antithrombin activity, whereas percutaneous estradiol did not induce any change in hepatic protein production.[36] Transdermal estrogen has been shown to prevent postmenopausal bone loss.[37,38] However, prevention of osteoporotic fractures has not yet been demonstrated as with oral estrogen.

CALCITONIN

Pharmacokinetics

Due to its polypeptide structure, calcitonin must be administered parentally. The duration of its osteoclastic inhibiting action following subcutaneous injection is 8 to 24 h with peak effect occurring after 4 h. The elimination half-life of salmon calcitonin is slightly longer than the human form ($t_{1/2}$= 1 h). Calcitonin is rapidly metabolized mainly by the kidney with less than 1 percent of unchanged calcitonin being excreted in the urine.

Use

Calcitonin is approved by the Federal Drug Administration (FDA) for the treatment of osteoporosis and is currently available in salmon and human preparations for subcutaneous injection.[39] The usual dose of salmon calcitonin is 50 to 100 IU every other day and for human calcitonin it is 0.5 mg three times a week. A salmon calcitonin nasal spray is currently being tested. Calcitonin has been shown to increase total body calcium by 2 to 3 percent in early short-term studies[40] and to similarly increase bone density.[41] Calcitonin has not yet been shown to decrease the incidence of osteoporotic-related fractures. However, such a study is underway.

A recent study of postmenopausal women separated into high- and low-turnover groups on the basis of serum osteocalcin levels, urinary hydroxyproline-creatine ratios, and whole-body retention of ^{99m}Tc-methylene diphosphonate demonstrated significant differences at 1 year in vertebral and hip bone densities, especially in the spine where there was a 22 percent *increase* in the high-turnover group.[35] This would indicate that measuring such parameters of bone resorption might be helpful in preselecting candidates for calcitonin therapy.

Calcitonin also appears to have an analgesic effect by enhancing beta-endorphin secretion and thus may be useful for the patient with acute vertebral crush fracture. Common adverse side effects limiting patient compliance are nausea and facial flushing.

VITAMIN D

Pharmacokinetics

Commercially available analogs of vitamin C include ergocalciferol (vitamin D_2), cholecalciferol (vitamin D_3), dihydrotachysterol, calcifediol (25-hydroxycholecalciferol), and calcitriol (1,25-dihydroxycholecalciferol). Activity of ergocalciferol and cholecalciferol is usually expressed in terms of international units.

Vitamin D analogs are readily absorbed from the intestine in the presence of normal fat absorption and bile. Absorption may thus be impaired in the presence of hepatobiliary disease. Following oral administration of ergocalciferol, the onset of hypercalcemic action is 10 to 24 h. Since it is stored in fat, the duration of action may be 2 months or more. Maximal hypercalcemic action of calcitriol is 10 h, and the duration of action is 3 to 5 days. Ergocalciferol and cholecalciferol are first hydroxylated in the liver at the 25 position and in the kidney at the 1 position to 1,25-dihydroxyergocalciferol and 1,25-cholecalciferol, respectively. When present in adequate concentration, the 25-hydroxylated compounds may be preferentially hydroxylated in the kidneys at the 24 position. These 24,25-dihydroxymetabolites may have less biologic activity. The metabolites of vitamin D analogs are excreted mainly in the bile with lesser amounts being excreted in the urine.

Use

The recommended daily allowance for vitamin D is 400 IU/day, which is usually readily achievable through the diet or exposure to sunlight. There is no currently established indication for large doses of vitamin D, including in corticosteroid-induced osteoporosis. Since high levels of vitamin D may stimulate bone resorption in addition to causing hypercalcemia and hypercalciuria, therapy with large doses is potentially harmful.[42]

1,25-Dihydroxyvitamin D levels have been shown to decline in the elderly.[10] Hence there is some rationale for examining the role of supplementation in this age group. One study using doses of up to 0.5 μg twice daily has recently been shown to be beneficial in postmenopausal osteoporosis;[43] however, other studies have not been encouraging.[44] The use of this metabolite should still be considered experimental.

SODIUM FLUORIDE

Pharmacokinetics

Sodium fluoride is rapidly absorbed in the stomach. Solubility may be decreased in the presence of calcium, magnesium, and aluminum hydroxide. Following absorption, fluoride is stored in bone and developing teeth. Fluoride is mainly eliminated in the urine, with small amounts being excreted in the feces.

Use

Since the discovery of fluorosis and increased skeletal density in miners, sodium fluoride has been considered as a possible agent in osteoporosis. Fluoride is known to substitute for hydroxyl radicals in hydroxyapatite, creating a harder compound, fluorapatite. It also stimulates osteoblast proliferation and stimulation of mesenchymal cells into osteoblasts. Great interest in fluoride's therapeutic use was stimulated in 1982 by the Mayo Clinic study,[45] which showed dramatic decreases in the incidence of vertebral crush fractures.

Sodium fluoride has significant toxicity, most commonly gastrointestinal (GI) (nausea, pain, and rarely bleeding) and musculoskeletal. The latter are due to stress fractures[46] seen early in therapy, before the newly developed osteoid has a chance to mineralize. It is for this reason that calcium must be given to all patients on fluoride to minimize the risk of osteomalacia.

Most studies looking at fluoride have shown an increase in vertebral bone density without an increase in total body calcium. This led to the assumption that perhaps calcium was being redistributed from predominantly cortical to trabecular areas of the body, and some data from current studies[47] indicate a decrease in femoral neck density. There was also concern that although fluorapatite increases compressive strength in vertebrae, it may decrease tensile and torsional strength in bones such as the hip. Small studies indicated that there may be an increased incidence of hip fractures up to 10 times that of normal in patients treated with fluoride.[48,49]

A recent 4-year prospective trial of sodium fluoride versus placebo in postmenopausal women with osteoporosis[50] demonstrated increases in vertebral and femoral bone densities but no decrease in the number of new vertebral fractures. The radial shaft bone density decreased, however, and the number of nonvertebral fractures was higher in the fluoride treatment group. The conclusion of this study was that fluoride therapy increased cancellous but decreased cortical bone mineral density leading to increased skeletal fragility.

Thus, sodium fluoride must still be considered an experimental therapy and used only with caution.

PROGESTINS

Progesterone receptors have been found on bone cells[51] and low progesterone levels have been found in rapid bone losers.[52] Both 19-nortestosterone derivatives and medroxyprogesterone acetate, a 17-acetyl derivative, have been shown to decrease postmenopausal bone loss. Medroxyprogesterone acetate in a dose of 20 mg/day was recently shown to reduce cortical bone loss but was not as effective as conjugated equine estrogen 0.6 mg/day in reducing trabecular bone loss.[53] In the same study, a low dose combination of medroxyprogesterone acetate 10 mg/day plus conjugated equine estrogen 0.3 mg/day was similar in effect to 0.6 mg/day conjugated equine estrogen alone, suggesting a synergistic effect. An adverse effect on serum lipids was not seen with medroxyprogesterone acetate.

ANDROGENS

Stanozolol has been studied in osteoporosis. However, side effects such as hepatic dysfunction, liver tumors, and lipoprotein abnormalities preclude its use. Nandrolone decanoate in doses of 25 to 50 mg every 3 to 4 weeks has recently been shown to significantly increase total body calcium and forearm bone density in women[54] and may prove to be a useful therapy. Minimal or no androgenic side effects should be seen with such doses.

Testosterone replacement in deficient males may be achieved with testosterone cypionate 200 mg every 3 weeks.

THIAZIDES

Pharmacokinetics

Absorption of the thiazides from the gastrointestinal tract is variable. Following oral administration of hydrochlorothiazide, peak effect of diuresis is seen 3 to 6 h after administration with duration of action being 6 to 12 h. Most thiazides are excreted unchanged in the urine.

Use

Hydrochlorothiazide is a member of the benzothiadiazide class of diuretics. The exact mechanism of the possible protective effects of thiazides on bone loss is not clear. Thiazides cause an immediate and sustained reduction in urinary calcium excretion by increasing calcium reabsorption in the early distal tubule of the kidney.[55] This action has been associated with a positive calcium balance. Recent evidence for a renal calcium leak in postmenopausal women,[56] presumably due to the loss of estrogen effect on tubular reabsorption of calcium, might account for the beneficial action of thiazides by correcting this renal leak. Another potential mechanism for the antiresorptive effect of the thiazides might be through their carbonic anhydrase inhibiting activity.[57] Carbonic anhydrase inhibitors can block bone reabsorption,[58] presumably by interfering with the ability of the osteoclast to generate acid. The relative importance of this latter effect of thiazides is unknown.

Many cross-sectional and retrospective studies have suggested a protective effect of thiazide diuretics on the prevention of both bone loss[59] and hip fractures.[60,61] One prospective study of the relation between the use of thiazide diuretics and the risk of hip fracture revealed a relative risk of hip fracture of 0.63 for users of thiazide diuretics.[62] However, a recent case-control study found that thiazide diuretics did not protect against hip fractures. On the contrary, the adjusted relative risk for hip fracture in current thiazide users was 1.6 (95 percent confidence interval, 1.0 to 2.5).[63]

The current role of the thiazides in the prevention and treatment of osteoporosis is therefore unknown, and thiazides cannot be routinely recommended for the treatment of osteoporosis except in the cases due to idiopathic hypercalciuria.[64]

DISODIUM ETIDRONATE AND COHERENCE THERAPY (ADFR)

Pharmacokinetics

Absorption of oral diphosphonates is dependent on both dose and the presence of food in the GI tract. Only approximately 1 percent of a 5-mg/kg dose of disodium etidronate is absorbed on an empty stomach. Following oral administration of disodium etidronate, 50 percent of the absorbed amount is distributed into the bone. The drug is not metabolized, and after 24 h, approximately 50 to 70 percent of the absorbed dose is excreted in the urine. The half-life in bone may be 3 to 6 months or longer.

Animal data on the distribution of intravenous pamidronate sodium suggest that with a 10-mg/kg dose, approximately 50 percent is distributed in bone after 24 h with 20 percent being excreted unchanged in the urine. The half-life in bone is not known.

Use

The concept of coherence therapy of osteoporosis is based upon the work of Frost,[65] who stated that bone resorption and formation occurs in discrete packets (basic multicellular units) which tend to not be in the same phase at all times. Thus therapeutic agents which affect both resorption and formation are not able to have a maximal effect on increasing bone formation. He and others have attempted to get as many units at a time in phase with each other, utilizing understanding of the cycles of normal cell resorption and formation. The bone cells are *activated* using phosphorus, PTH, or fluoride for approximately 1 week, *depressed* with calcitonin or disodium etidronate for about 1 week, then *freed* for 2 months to allow bone formation. The cycle is then *repeated*.

Disodium etidronate, a first-generation biphosphonate, is thought to suppress osteoclastic bone resorption by chemisorbing onto the calcium-hydroxyapatite bone crystal rendering it resistant to osteoclastic hydrolysis. Early studies have shown significant increases in bone formation of up to 8 percent in 1 year[66] and a significant decrease in the rate of new vertebral fractures after 2[67] and 3 years.[68] Disodium etidronate is given in doses of 400 mg/day for the first 2 weeks of a 12-week cycle. It must be given at least 2 h before and after meals since absorption even on an empty stomach is less than 5 percent. Patients must be instructed not to take this drug continuously since prolonged continuous treatment may cause osteomalacia and spontaneous fractures.[69]

Third-generation biphosphonates such as pamidronate sodium (3-amino-1-hydroxypropylidene-1,1-bisphosphonate), which inhibit osteoclastic bone resorption but not mineralization, may prove to be safer and more effective than disodium etidronate. They appear to inhibit resorption by preventing the transformation of monocytic precursors into mature osteoclasts.[70] They are currently being investigated for the treatment of osteoporosis, hypercalcemia of malignancy, and Paget's disease of bone.

TREATMENT OF CORTICOSTEROID-INDUCED OSTEOPOROSIS

Corticosteroids induce osteoporosis through a variety of mechanisms. They directly inhibit osteoblasts, decrease calcium absorption by the gut and increase calcium excretion by the kidney, leading to a net negative calcium loss and resultant secondary hyperparathyroidism,[71] and also appear to decrease sex steroid hormone production.[72,73] An early study seemed to indicate that vitamin D could reverse these effects;[74] however, the results of that study have never been duplicated. Medroxyprogesterone acetate has been shown to prevent steroid-induced osteopenia and resulted in a 17 percent increase in bone mineral density after 1 year in one study.[75] Calcitonin in doses of up to 100 IU on alternate days has been shown to result in significant increases in bone density over a 1-year period in patients with corticosteroid-induced osteoporosis.[76,77] These were small studies, however, and at present, there is no known effective therapy for corticosteroid-induced osteoporosis. Unfortunately, alternate-day corticosteroid administration does not result in less bone loss.[78] Optimization of calcium intake, regular weight-bearing exercise, and replacement of sex steroid hormone if prematurely diminished are conservative and prudent measures.[79] Deflazacort, an oxazoline analog of prednisone, has been shown to induce less bone loss than other corticosteroids[80] and may be just as effective an anti-inflammatory.[81] Further clinical trials of this compound are necessary.

SUMMARY

In summary (Table 19-2), the first steps in the treatment of established osteoporosis involve correcting changeable risk factors such as excessive alcohol and nicotine consumption, sedentary lifestyle, and calcium deficiency. ERT remains the gold

Table 19-2 Therapy of established osteoporosis

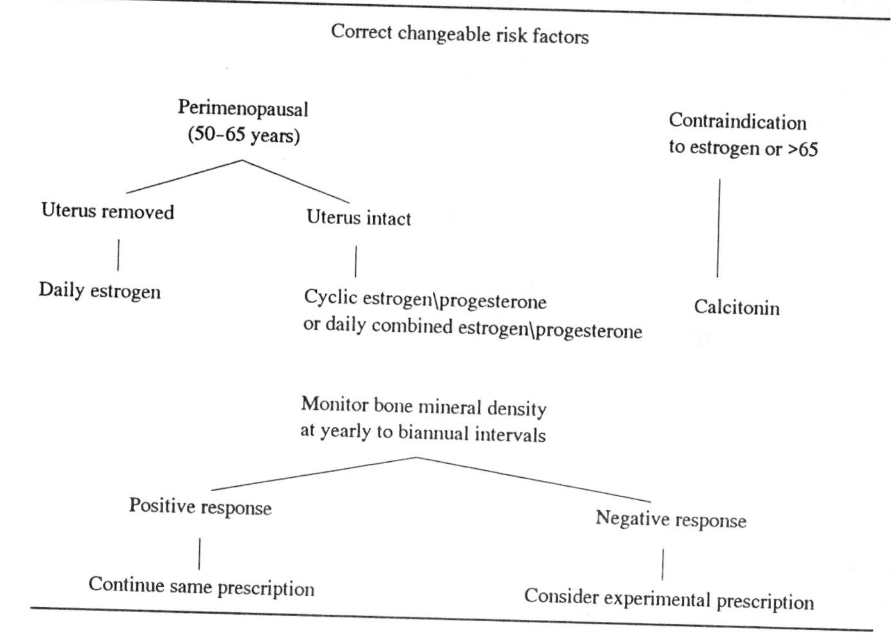

standard for women, at least up to 65 years of age. In older women or women with a contraindication to estrogen, calcitonin is the only other approved drug for osteoporosis. Treatment should be monitored with bone density measurements using DPA or DEXA since not all women will respond to either medication. Cyclical biphosphonate therapy with disodium etidronate may be an alternative but should still be considered experimental. The development of more potent third-generation biphosphonates may prove to be safer and more efficacious. Further clinical trials are necessary to define the exact role of the other medications listed above as well as combination therapy.

REFERENCES

1. NIH Consensus Conference on Osteoporosis. *JAMA* 252(6): 799–802, 1984.
2. Riggs BL, Melton LJ: Involutional osteoporosis. *N Engl J Med* 314: 1676–1684, 1986.
3. Gallagher JC, Melton LJ, Riggs BL, Bergstrath E: Epidemiology of fractures of the proximal femur in Rochester, Minnesota. *Clin Ortho Rel Res* 150: 163–170, 1980.
4. Melton LJ et al: Osteoporosis and the risk of fracture. *Am J Epidemiol* 124: 254–261, 1986.
5. Melton LJ, Riggs BL: Epidemiology of age-related fractures, in Avioli LV (ed): *The Osteoporotic Syndrome*. New York, Grune and Stratton, 1983, pp 45–72.
6. Holbrook TL, Grazier K, Kelsey JL, et al: *The Frequency of Occurrence, Impact and Cost of Selected Musculoskeletal Conditions in the United States*. Chicago, American Academy of Orthopedic Surgeons, 1984.

7. Theigs RD et al: Calcitonin secretion in postmenopausal osteoporosis. *N Engl J Med* 312: 1097–1100, 1985.
8. Marcus R, Madvig P, Young G: Age-related changes in parathyroid hormone and parathyroid action in normal humans. *J Clin Endocrinol Metab* 58: 223–230, 1984.
9. Bullamore JR, Gallagher JC, Wilkinson R, et al: Effect of age on calcium absorption. *Lancet* 2: 535–537, 1970.
10. Tsai K-S, Heath H, Kumar R, Riggs BL: Impaired vitamin D metabolism with aging in women: possible role in the pathogenesis of senile osteoporosis. *J Clin Invest* 73: 1668–1672, 1984.
11. Raisz LG: Local and systemic factors in the pathogenesis of osteoporosis. *N Engl J Med* 318: 818–828, 1988.
12. Nilas L, Christiansen C, Christiansen J: Regulation of vitamin D and calcium metabolism after gastrectomy. *Gut* 26: 252–257, 1985.
13. Compston JE et al: Osteomalacia after small-intestinal resection. *Lancet* 1: 9–13, 1978.
14. Frame B, Parfitt AM: Osteomalacia: Current concepts. *Ann Intern Med* 89: 966–982, 1978.
15. Hahn TJ, Halstead LR: Anticonvulsant drug-induced osteomalacia: Alterations in mineral metabolism and response to vitamin D_3 administration. *Calcif Tissue Int* 27: 13–18, 1979.
16. Jenkins DHR, Roberts JG, Webster D, Williams ED: Osteomalacia in elderly patients with fracture of femoral neck. *J Bone Joint Surg* 55B: 575–580, 1973.
17. Wahner HW, Dunn WL, Riggs BL: Noninvasive bone mineral measurements. *Semin Nucl Med* 13: 282–289, 1983.
18. Mazess RB, Barden H, Ettinger M, Schultz E: Bone density of the radius, spine and proximal femur in osteoporosis. *J Bone Min Res* 3: 13–18, 1988.
19. Richardson ML, Genant HK, Cann CE, et al: Assessment of metabolic bone diseases by quantitative computed tomography. *Clin Orthop* 195: 224–238, 1985.
20. Sartoris DJ, Resnick D: Osteoporosis: update on densitometric techniques. *J Musculoskel Med* 6: 108–123, 1989.
21. Heany RP, Recker RR, Saville PD: Menopausal changes in calcium balance performance. *J Lab Clin Med* 92: 953–963, 1978.
22. Matkovic V, Kostal K, Simunovic I, et al: Bone status and fracture rates in two regions of Yugoslavia. *Am J Clin Nutr* 36: 540–549, 1979.
23. Dawson-Hughes BD, Dallal GE, Krall EA, et al: A controlled trial of the effect of calcium supplementation on bone density in postmenopausal women. *N Engl J Med* 323: 878–883, 1990.
24. Recker RR: Calcium absorption and aclorhydria. *N Engl J Med* 313: 70–74, 1985.
25. Ringe JD: The risk of nephrolithiasis with oral calcium supplementation. *Calcif Tissue Int* 48: 69–73, 1991.
26. Lindsay R, Hart DM, Forrest C, Baird C: Prevention of spinal osteoporosis in oophorectomized women. *Lancet* 1: 1151–1153, 1980.
27. Ettinger B, Genant HK, Cann CE: Long-term replacement therapy prevents bone loss and fractures. *Ann Intern Med* 102: 319–324, 1985.
28. Lindsay R, Tohme JF: Estrogen treatment of patients with established postmenopausal osteoporosis. *Obstet Gynecol* 76: 291–295, 1990.
29. Paganinni-Hill A, Ross RK, Gerkins VR, et al: Menopausal estrogen therapy and hip fractures. *Ann Intern Med* 95: 28–31, 1981.
30. Lindsay R et al: Bone response to termination of oestrogen treatment. *Lancet i*: 1325–1327, 1978.
31. Lufkin EG et al: Estrogen replacement therapy: Current recommendations. *Mayo Clin Proc* 63: 453–460, 1988.
32. Ettinger B, Genant HK, Cann CE: Postmenopausal bone loss is prevented by treatment with low-dosage estrogen and calcium. *Ann Intern Med* 106: 40–45, 1987.
33. Magos AL et al: Amenorrhea and endometrial atrophy with continuous oral estrogen and progestogen therapy in postmenopausal women. *Obstet Gynecol* 65: 496–498, 1985.
34. Weinstein L: Efficacy of a continuous estrogen-progestin regimen in the menopausal patient. *Obstet Gynecol* 69: 929–932, 1987.

35. Civitelli R et al: Bone turnover in postmenopausal osteoporosis: effect of calcitonin therapy. *J Clin Invest* 82: 1268–1274, 1988.
36. DeLignieres B et al: Biological effects of estradiol-17 *B* in postmenopausal women: oral *versus* percutaneous administration. *J Clin Endocrinol Metab* 62: 536–541, 1985.
37. Riis BJ et al: The effect of percutaneous estradiol and natural progesterone on postmenopausal bone loss. Am J *Obstet Gynecol* 156: 61–65, 1986.
38. Ribot C, Tremollieres F, Pouilles JM, et al: Preventive effects of transdermal administration of 17 *B*-estradiol on postmenopausal bone loss: A 2-year prospective study. *Obstet Gynecol* 75: 42–46S, 1990.
39. McDermott MT, Kidd GS: The role of calcitonin in the development and treatment of osteoporosis. *Endo Rev* 8: 377–390, 1987.
40. Gruber HE et al: Long term calcitonin therapy in postmenopausal osteoporosis. *Metabolism* 33: 295–303, 1984.
41. Mazzuoli GF et al: Effects of salmon calcitonin in postmenopausal osteoporosis: A controlled double-blind clinical study. *Calcif Tiss Int* 38: 3–8, 1986.
42. Schwartzman MS, Franck WA: Vitamin D toxicity complicating the treatment of senile, postmenopausal, and glucocorticoid-induced osteoporosis. Four case reports and a critical commentary on the use of vitamin D in these disorders. *Am J Med* 82: 224–230, 1987.
43. Gallagher JC, Goldgar D: Treatment of postmenopausal osteoporosis with high doses of synthetic calcitriol: A randomized controlled study. *Ann Intern Med* 113: 649–655, 1990.
44. Ott SM, Chesnut CH: Calcitriol treatment is not effective in postmenopausal osteoporosis. *Ann Intern Med* 110: 267–274, 1989.
45. Riggs BL et al: Effect of the fluoride/calcium regimen on vertebral fracture occurrence in postmenopausal osteoporosis. *N Engl J Med* 306: 446–450, 1982.
46. O'Duffy DJ et al: Mechanism of acute lower extremity pain syndrome in fluoride treated osteoporotic patients. *Am J Med* 80: 561–566, 1986.
47. Riggs BL: Treatment of osteoporosis with sodium fluoride: An appraisal, in Peck WA (ed): *Bone and Mineral Research, Annual* 2. New York, Elsevier, 1984, pp 366–393.
48. Gutteridge DH et al: Fluoride in osteoporosis: vertebral but not femoral fracture protection. *Calcif Tissue Int* 36: 481, 1984.
49. Hedlund TL, Gallagher JC: Increased incidence of hip fracture in osteoporotic women treated with sodium fluoride. *J Bone Min Res* 4: 223–225, 1989.
50. Riggs BL et al: Effect of fluoride treatment on the fracture rate in postmenopausal women with osteoporosis. *N Engl J Med* 322: 802–809, 1990.
51. Manologas SC, Anderson DC: Detection of high affinity glucocorticoid binding in rat bone. *J Endocrinol* 76: 379–380, 1978.
52. Johnston CC Jr, Norton JA Jr, Khairi RA, Longcope C: Age-related bone loss, in Barzel US (ed): *Osteoporosis II*. New York, Grune & Stratton, 1979, pp 91–100.
53. Gallagher JC, Kable WT, Goldgar D: Effect of progestin therapy on cortical and trabecular bone: Comparison with estrogen. *Am J Med* 90: 171–178, 1991.
54. Need AG, et al: Effects of nandrolone decanoate and antiresorptive therapy on vertebral density in osteoporotic postmenopausal women. *Arch Intern Med* 149: 57–59, 1989.
55. Stier CT, Itskovitz HD: Renal calcium metabolism. *Ann Rev Pharmacol Toxicol* 26: 101–116, 1986.
56. Nordin BEC, Need AG, Morris HA, et al: Evidence for a renal calcium leak in postmenopausal women. *J Clin Endocrinol Metab* 72: 401–407, 1991.
57. Boer AH, Koomans HA, Mees EJ: Acute effects of thiazides with and without carbonic anhydrase inhibiting activity on lithium and free water clearance in man. *Clin Sci* 76: 539–545, 1989.
58. Hall GE, Kenney AS: Effect of acetazolamide on basal and parathyroid hormone-induced bone metabolism. *Calcif Tissue Int* 40: 212–218, 1987.
59. Wasnich R, Davis J, Ross P, Vogel J: Effect of thiazide on rates of bone mineral loss: A longitudinal study. *BMJ* 301: 1303–1305, 1990.
60. Ray WA et al: Long-term use of thiazide diuretics and risk of hip fracture. *Lancet*, April 1, 1989, pp 687–689.

61. Rashiq S, Logan RF: Role of drugs in fractures of the femoral neck. *BMJ* 292: 861–863, 1986.
62. LaCroix AZ et al: Thiazide diuretic agents and the incidence of hip fracture. *N Engl J Med* 322: 286–290, 1990.
63. Heidrich FE, Stergachis A, Gross KM: Diuretic drug use and the risk for hip fracture. *Ann Intern Med* 115: 1–6, 1991.
64. Insagna KL, Broadus AE: Hypercalciuria as a metabolic disease. *Sem Urol* 2: 20–33, 1984.
65. Frost HM: Coherence treatment of osteoporosis. *Orthop Clin North Am* 12: 649–669, 1981.
66. Mallette LE et al: Cyclic therapy of osteoporosis with neutral phosphate and brief, high-dose pulses of etidronate. *J Bone Min Res* 4: 143–148, 1989.
67. Watts NB et al: Intermittent cyclical etidronate treatment of postmenopausal osteoporosis. *N Engl J Med* 323: 73–80, 1990.
68. Storm T, Thamsborg G, Steiniche T, et al: Effect of intermittent cyclical etidronate therapy on bone fracture rate in women with postmenopausal osteoporosis. *N Engl J Med* 322: 1265–1271, 1990.
69. Mautalen C, Gonzalez D, Blumenfeld EL, et al: Spontaneous fractures of uninvolved bones in patients with Paget's Disease during unduly prolonged treatment with disodium etidronate (EHDP). *Clin Orthop Rel Res* 207: 150–155, 1986.
70. Boonekamp PN, v d Wee-Pals LJA, v Wijk-v Lennep MML, et al: Two modes of action of bisphosphonates on osteoclastic resorption of mineralized matrix. *Bone Min* 1: 27–39, 1986.
71. Suzuki Y, Ichikawa Y, Saito E, Homma M: Importance of increased urinary calcium excretion in the development of secondary hyperthyroidism of patients under glucocorticoid therapy. *Metabolism* 32: 151–163, 1983.
72. Crilly RG, Horsman A, Marshall DH, Nordin BEC: Postmenopausal and corticosteroid-induced osteoporosis. *Fron Hormon Res* 5: 53–75, 1978.
73. MacAdams MR, White RH, Chipps BE: Reduction of serum testosterone levels during chronic glucocorticoid therapy. *Ann Intern Med* 104: 648–651, 1986.
74. Hahn TJ, Halstead LR, Teitlbaum SL, Hahn BH: Altered mineral metabolism in glucocorticoid-induced osteopenia: effect of 25-hydroxyvitamin D administration. *J Clin Metab* 64: 655–665, 1979.
75. Grecu EO, Weinshelbaum A, Simmons R: Effective therapy of glucocorticoid-induced osteoporosis with medroxyprogesterone acetate. *Calcif Tissue Int* 46: 294–299, 1990.
76. Ringe JD, Wezel D: Salmon calcitonin in the therapy of corticoid-induced osteoporosis. *Eur J Pharmacol* 33: 35–39, 1987.
77. Luengo M, Picado C, Del Rio L, et al: Treatment of steroid-induced osteoporosis with calcitonin in corticosteroid-dependent asthma: A one-year follow-up study. *Am Rev Resp Dis* 142: 104–107, 1990.
78. Gluck OS, Murphy WA, Hahn TJ, Hahn BH: Bone loss in adults receiving alternate day glucocorticoid therapy. *Arth Rheum* 24: 892–897, 1981.
79. Lukert BP, Raisz LG: Glucocorticoid-induced osteoporosis: pathogenesis and management. *Ann Intern Med* 112: 352–364, 1990.
80. Gennari C, Imbimbo B: Effects of prednisone and deflazacort on vertebral bone mass. *Calcif Tissue Int* 37: 592–593, 1985.
81. Gray RE, Doherty SM, Galloway J, et al: A double-blind study of deflazacort and prednisone in patients with chronic inflammatory disorders. *Arthr Rheum* 34: 287–295, 1991.

CHAPTER

20

PHARMACOLOGIC THERAPY OF RHEUMATIC DISEASES

Eric P. Gall
Martin Higbee

Rheumatologic disease afflicts over 37 million individuals in the United States.[1] There are over one hundred different afflictions which are part of this general classification, including arthritis, related musculoskeletal disorders, and a wide variety of immunologic and vascular abnormalities. Many of these diseases have a predilection for the elderly, and many of them are treated with similar agents. We have chosen to limit our discussions to the most common classes of rheumatic disease afflicting the elderly. These include rheumatoid arthritis (RA), osteoarthritis (degenerative joint disease), the crystalline arthropathies (gout and calcium pyrophosphate dihydrate deposition disease, hydroxyapatite deposition disease), polymyalgia rheumatica, and associated giant cell arteritis. Osteoporosis and Paget's disease are covered in Chap. 19. While many of these diseases can afflict younger individuals as well, they are particularly common in the geriatric population, and the drugs used to treat most of them are applicable to other rheumatic illnesses.

This chapter is divided into two parts. The first discusses the individual diseases, their pathophysiology and the effects of aging, and the rational approach to drug therapy. The second part discusses the clinical pharmacology of the individual drugs used to treat these disorders, with a special emphasis on the effect of aging on the pharmacology, dosing, and toxicity of these drugs.

Arthritis, which stems from the Greek *arthron* (joint) and the suffix "itis" (inflammation), is really classified into two categories. *Noninflammatory arthritis* is best represented by the disease, osteoarthritis. On the other hand, recently there has been some attention paid to aspects of the disease causing some of the classic signs and symptoms of inflammation. *Inflammatory arthritis* is represented in this chapter by the diseases rheumatoid arthritis and the crystalline arthropathies. Polymyalgia rheumatica and giant cell arteritis are examples of primary muscle disorders and inflammatory vessel disease (vasculitis). The primary goal in drug treatment of bone and joint disorders in the elderly is to maintain functional status and independency. Inasmuch as pain and stiffness from such disorders as RA and degenerative joint disease (DJD) are major causes of immobilization, it is imperative that proper diagnosis and drug treatment be initiated. The drug therapy selected must be based upon appropriateness for the diagnosis with due consideration for cost, side effect profile, and compatibility with concomitant diseases and their treatment. Thus, the general goals always stated for these disorders, to "decrease pain and inflammation, preserve joint function, and prevent deformity," have significant impact on maintaining functional status of the elderly patient, and therefore, effecting their level of independence.

RHEUMATOID ARTHRITIS

Rheumatoid arthritis (RA) is a relatively new inflammatory disorder mediated by immune mechanisms. The disease was first described in detail in the early nineteenth century and probably did not occur before the industrial revolution, from the best evidence in skeletal remains. It occurs in a 3 : 1 female-to-male ratio and is most common in the age group between 20 and 40. However, it does have other peaks of incidence which include juvenile and the elderly, often occurring after the age of 60. There is thought to be some correlation between the aging process and an abnormal immune response. There is a high frequency of onset of RA in women 50 to 55 years of age. It is known that the incidence of autoantibodies increases in older patients, presumably due to the decreased functioning of T-suppressor cells.[2] Certainly the incidence of rheumatoid factor, which is an anti-immunoglobulin, occurs with increasing frequency in the elderly whether or not they have arthritis. Rheumatoid factor is seen not only in RA but a variety of chronic inflammatory or postfibrotic diseases, including pulmonary fibrosis, cirrhosis, and tuberculosis.

The criteria for diagnosing RA emanate from a committee of the American College of Rheumatology and were revised in 1987 (Table 20-1).[3] These criteria were designed for epidemiologic purposes and are not absolute. The disease is a systemic chronic inflammatory disease which affects synovial joints and has variable expression. It has a prevalence of about 2 to 3 percent of the population in the United States.[4] The disorder has a wide variety of systemic manifestations including eye disease, pericarditis, pleuritis, rheumatoid nodules, leg ulcerations, Sjögren's syndrome, pulmonary fibrosis, and vasculitis. The disease is often progressive with superimposed exacerbations and partial remissions.

The treatment of RA is related to an understanding of its pathogenesis. There are two major classes of drugs. The first are *nonsteroidal anti-inflammatory drugs*

Table 20-1 American College of Rheumatology criteria for diagnosis of rheumatoid arthritis

1. Morning stiffness for at least 1 hour present for at least 6 weeks
2. Swelling of three or more joints for at least 6 weeks
3. Swelling of wrist, metacarpal phalangeal, or proximal interphalangeal joints for at least 6 weeks
4. Symmetric joint swelling
5. Hand roentgenogram changes typical of RA that must include erosion or unequivocal bony decalcification
6. Rheumatoid nodules
7. Serum rheumatoid factor by a method positive in less than 5 percent of normal individuals

Note: Four or more criteria must be present to diagnose RA.
Source: Modified from Ref. 3.

(NSAIDs), which are used in most arthritic disorders. The second group works by inhibiting the basic immunopathogenic mechanisms of the disease. This group of drugs is called the *disease-modifying antirheumatic drugs* (DMARDs), *second-line agents*, or *remittive agents*. Their anti-inflammatory activity is strictly secondary to their action on the immunologic abnormalities causing the disease and does not occur immediately upon beginning drug therapy. Thus, they have a slow onset of action, often taking weeks or months.

The pathogenesis of RA is complex; it includes many variable mechanisms which intertwine one with another.[5] Many cells are involved: neutrophils, lymphocytes (both T and B cells), macrophages, synovial lining cells, other synovial cells (the dendritic cell), fibroblasts, and the chondrocytes. In addition, a wide variety of inflammatory mediators are involved, including circulating complement and a whole host of cytokines. Synovial fluid is filled with a number of different cells and mediators and is often referred to as *synovial soup.* It is important to note that not all patients have the same pathogenetic mechanisms working at all times. Individual cellular abnormalities and the presence of specific cytokines may lead to a difference in the patient's response to therapy.

While the patient comes to the treating physician for relief of pain, the physician must be more global in his or her approach and attempt to stratify the long-term goals of patient management to include the following:

Inhibition and progression of disease
Relief of inflammation
Maintenance of function
Relief of pain
Improvement of extraarticular problems
Patient education

Older patients are unable to metabolize drugs as well as younger individuals. They are often on multiple drugs for other conditions that might change the pharmacokinetics of the antirheumatic agents and lead to complications. Rheumatoid arthritis is a potentially fatal disease and many causes of fatality may be related to drug therapy. NSAIDs have had an increasing prevalence of gastropathy with increasing prescriptions. Corticosteroids are plagued with many adverse effects and render the patients more susceptible to infection.

The major actions of the two classes of drugs in rheumatoid arthritis are depicted in Table 20-2. The pyramid has depicted the traditional concept for treating rheumatoid arthritis (Fig. 20-1). The base of the pyramid includes diagnosis, rehabilitation, psychosocial planning, and a means of measuring the response to therapy. It includes the NSAIDs. Obviously, the base of the pyramid needs to be maintained as the structure is built above it. The idea of the pyramid is then to add other agents in logical order as the primary agents fail. One uses the least complex, costly, and toxic drugs first and then adds others as primary agents fail. The NSAIDs need to be maintained during the addition of DMARDs.

Recently, the concept of the pyramid approach to treatment of RA has been challenged. Some have suggested the use of an inverted pyramid (Fig. 20-2).[6] The idea led to the concept that more aggressive treatments should be used by clinicians earlier in the disease process. Many patients fail initial therapy and when DMARDs are begun, they often are found to be less than ideally responsive to them. The disease progresses, albeit more slowly, despite the use of these potent agents. There have been some data suggesting that there may be an immunologic trigger which renders the disease irreversible.[7] This idea suggests the abnormal cells, after a period of time, can no longer be suppressed and the disease will be progressive despite the addition of potent agents. It has been thought by some investigators that the point at which erosions are first seen on radiographs may indicate irreversibility and that many patients should be on the remittive agents almost at the onset of disease.[6] In addition, the proponents of this approach suggest that DMARDs are less toxic and NSAIDs probably more toxic than once thought. The latter is because

Table 20-2 Major actions of two classes of drugs to treat rheumatoid arthritis

NSAIDs	DMARDs
Immediate onset of action	Slow onset of action
Dose-related anti-inflammatory activity (reduces swelling)	Anti-inflammatory effects delayed and secondary to immunoregulation
Analgesic	No primary analgesia
Antipyretic	No antipyretic effect
Limited effect on immune system	Immunomodulatory or immunosuppressive
Questionable effect on long-term anatomic and functional outcome of disease	Decrease radiographic erosions, joint destruction, and improve functional outcome
Improve systemic symptoms	Improve systemic symptoms

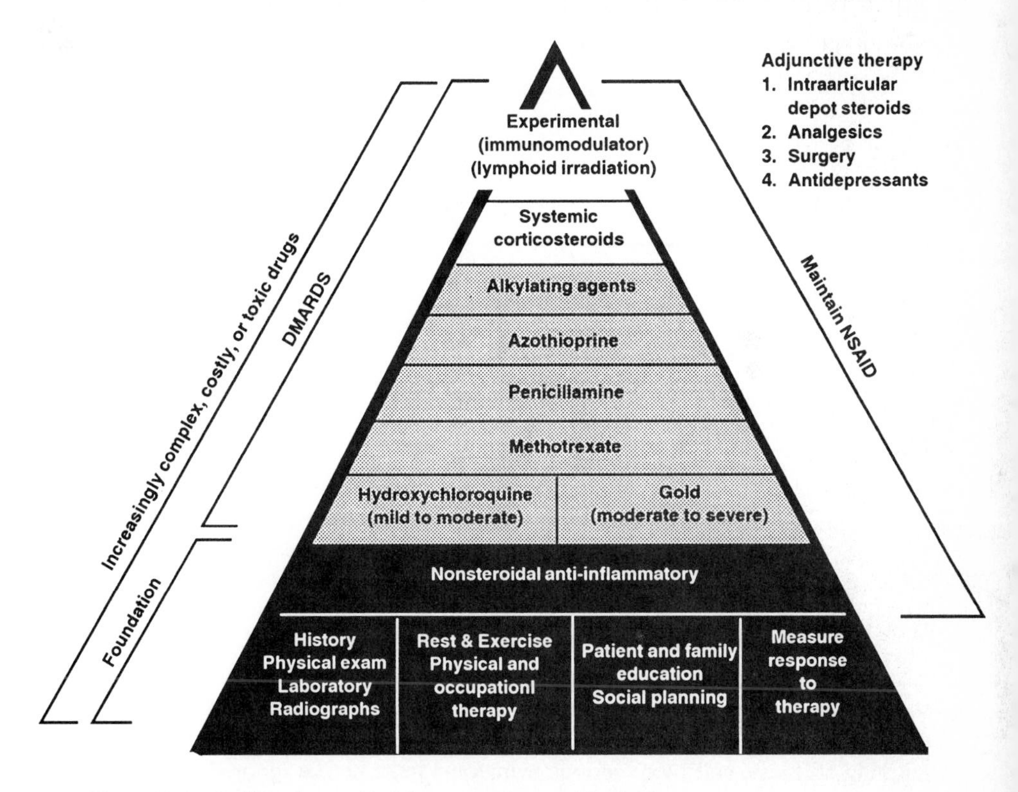

Figure 20-1 Traditional pyramid of therapy for rheumatoid arthritis.

of the gastrointestinal problems as well as renal and other toxicities. Indeed, according to these investigators, there is similar overall toxicity between the group of NSAIDs drugs and the DMARDs. They also argue that the pyramid approach has not improved the outcome of disease, although there has been no direct comparison.

There are arguments, on the other hand, against the use of the inverted pyramid in all patients.[8] We really do not understand what the risk/benefit ratio of early aggressive intervention is. Indeed we are unable to predict which patients will have mild disease not progressing to destructive arthritis. The cost of aggressive treatment in all patients, not only of drugs but of monitoring and toxicity, may be extensive. We also do not know what the long-term toxicity of some of the DMARDs would be in patients whose disease lasts many years. One also worries about the use of a very aggressive program in an elderly individual with many other health problems.

Table 20-3 lists some major errors in the treatment of rheumatoid arthritis. Patients are often put on corticosteroids at the beginning of their disease to attempt to better diagnose this disease and to improve symptoms. It is our opinion that

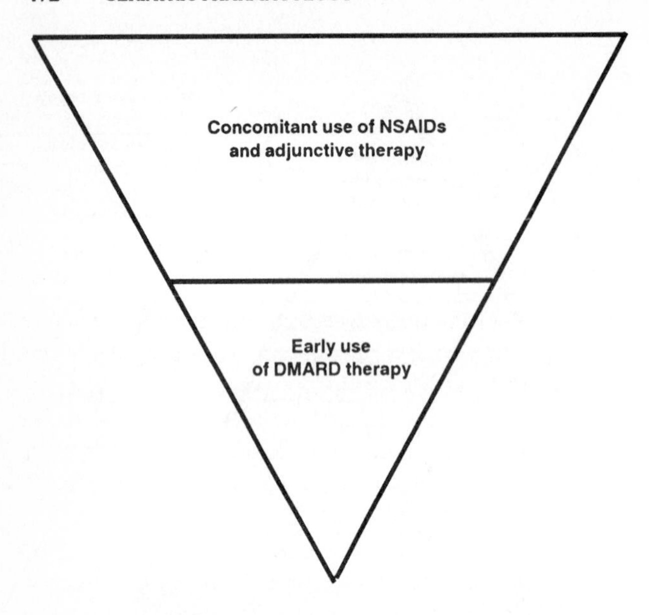

Figure 20-2 Inverted pyramid in treatment of rheumatoid arthritis.

steroids should be used later on in the course of the disease as outlined in the subsequent section. The patient's systemic symptoms, including fatigue, malaise, morning stiffness, and more serious symptoms must not be ignored and are as important as joint symptoms to treat.

All drugs that are used in the treatment of RA, particularly in the elderly, require regular monitoring. Functional problems need to be addressed by other members of the health team. The psychosocial issues may interfere with drug therapy, and the patients require careful education about drugs and the disease. The rheumatologist or other specialists are often able to guide the primary care physician in the appropriate use of drugs, and the pharmacist may also aid the physician

Table 20-3 Major errors in the treatment of rheumatoid arthritis

1. Unnecessary use of steroids
2. Inadequate dose or trial of NSAIDs
3. Failure to treat systemic symptoms
4. Failure to monitor for toxicity
5. Delay use of remittive therapy
6. Failure to address functional joint problems
7. Failure to use physical and occupational therapy and other health professionals
8. Lack of attention to psychosocial issues
9. Failure to educate patient
10. Failure to obtain specialty consultation

in monitoring for toxicity and recognizing potential drug interactions or abnormal drug metabolism.

Nonsteroidal Anti-inflammatory Drugs

The NSAIDs form the basis of anti-inflammatory therapy for rheumatoid arthritis. Aspirin, of course, is the prototype drug and has been in use for the treatment of rheumatoid arthritis since the late-nineteenth century. Unfortunately, no double-blind, placebo-controlled studies have been done to prove efficacy of these agents in altering the course of the disease. It makes ultimate sense, however, that if one suppresses the inflammatory response significantly, one would decrease the rapidity of bone and cartilage destruction. On the other hand, it is known that these drugs may have some adverse effect on cartilage and cartilage metabolism. Thus, in addition to their benefit, in some individuals they may have a detrimental effect.

Most physicians use the newer NSAIDs or enteric-coated aspirin as the agents of choice. In general, higher doses of this class of drugs must be used to treat inflammatory arthritis. These drugs have analgesic effects in low doses but anti-inflammatory levels in high doses. On the other hand, the higher doses may not be well tolerated in elderly individuals who have limited ability to metabolize the drugs because of a decrease in hepatic mass, renal blood flow, and serum albumin. Thus, a careful decision must be made as to a middle ground, and dosage adjustments must be made carefully. Sometimes the drugs must be pushed to the maximum tolerated dose recommended by the package insert in order to achieve an adequate anti-inflammatory response. It usually takes 2 to 3 weeks on an agent at a sufficient dose to ascertain whether or not it is efficacious in controlling RA before switching to another drug.

In trying to choose which agent a physician will use, there are several things that must be taken into consideration. The drugs can be categorized as short- and long-half-life agents (Table 20-4). Short-half-life drugs have the advantage of being more rapidly cleared if there is toxicity. Their disadvantage is that more doses must be taken more frequently and this may lead to a decrease in compliance. Longer

Table 20-4 Long- and short-half-life NSAIDs

Long-half-life	Short-half-life
Aspirin (high dose)	Aspirin (low dose)
Indomethacin SR	Fenoprofen
Naproxen	Flurbiprofen
Phenylbutazone	Ibuprofen
Piroxicam	Indomethacin
Salsalate	Meclofenamate
Sulindac	Tolmetin

half-life drugs may need to be taken less frequently and thus patient compliance is often better. On the other hand, these drugs may have a higher level of toxicity due to cumulative effects, particularly in the elderly individual.

Another area of judgment in choosing NSAIDs is in comparing the toxicity of different agents. For instance, the nonacetylated salicylates have the advantage of not inhibiting platelet function, not inducing exudations in aspirin-sensitive asthmatics, and being less likely to have gastrointestinal and renal toxicity. The nonacetylated salicylates do not inhibit prostaglandin synthesis and thus exert their pharmacologic activity through other means (such as inhibition of neutrophil activation). Other types of individual drug toxicities are outlined in Table 20-5.

Aspirin previously was used as the drug of first choice because of several reasons. It is less expensive, one can measure serum levels, it has excellent efficacy and reasonable safety, and there is extensive experience with this agent. On the other hand, the newer NSAIDs have less gastrointestinal side effects and offer greater patient acceptance. It is clear that every nonsteroidal has anti-inflammatory activity and none are less or more efficacious in patients overall. Thus, choice depends on toxicity, cost, and other issues. Guidelines for choosing these agents are listed in Table 20-6.

It is our opinion that all patients on NSAIDs should be monitored regularly for toxicity. Because of the potential for silent gastrointestinal, renal, and other toxicity, we recommend placing the fact that a patient is taking chronic NSAID therapy on the patient's problem list. In addition, the patient should be evaluated 2 to 4 weeks after starting on a new NSAID. The patient should be questioned about toxic side effects and screened with a urinalysis, blood count, and renal function test. With the increasing reports of hepatotoxicity, screening for liver function abnormalities should be done as well. It is recommended that all patients be monitored every 6 to

Table 20-5 Drug toxicity specific to certain agents

Side effect	Less frequent or severe	More frequent or severe
Aplastic anemia	Other agents	Phenylbutazone
Asthma	Nonacetylated salicylates	ASA, other NSAIDs
CNS toxicity	Low-dose ASA, other NSAIDs	Indomethacin, phenylbutazone, high-dose ASA
Diarrhea	Other NSAIDs	Meclofenamate with or without sulindac
Peptic ulcer disease	Enteric-coated ASA, new NSAIDs	Phenylbutazone, indomethacin, uncoated aspirin
Platelet dysfunction	Nonacetylated salicylate short-acting NSAIDs	Aspirin (Permanent for life of platelet)
Renal toxicity	Nonacetylated salicylates, sulindac (?)	Long-acting NSAIDs, all NSAIDs
Salt retention and congestive heart failure	Aspirin, other NSAIDs	Indomethacin, phenylbutazone

Table 20-6 Guidelines for choosing NSAIDs

Clinical setting, problem	Preferred NSAID (approach)
Efficacy versus toxicity	Newer NSAIDs
Poor compliance	Aspirin (measure serum levels), long-acting NSAIDs (fewer doses less often)
Age	Consider individual drug metabolism
Cardiovascular disease (congestive failure)	NSAID with low sodium retention (not indomethacin or phenylbutazone)
Peptic disease	Salsalate, enteric-coated preparations, newer NSAIDs, concomitant H_2 blockers, misoprostal
Diarrhea	Avoid meclofenamate, sulindac
Renal disease	Nonacetylated salicylate, sulindac, drugs metabolized by liver if in renal failure
Bleeding (hemophilia)	Nonacetylated salicylate
Surgery (elective)	Short-half-life (stop three half-lives before surgery), nonacetylated salicylate
Adult-onset asthma (aspirin sensitive)	Nonacetylated salicylate; avoid all other NSAIDs

12 months. Should they have underlying organ pathology which renders them more susceptible to side effects, testing should be done more frequently.

In general, NSAIDs should be administered with meals. Some of the gastric toxicity is due to direct contact of the drug with the gastric mucosa, and drug absorption is not altered when taken with food. No nonsteroidal drug is safe with active ulcer disease. In the sensitive patient all nonsteroidals cause asthma with the exception of nonacetylated salicylates; in this patient other nonsteroidals, with the above exception, should not be used. The efficacy of NSAIDs is equal but toxicity and individual patient preference are variable and individual in nature.

The usual reasons for NSAID failure include inadequate dosage to achieve anti-inflammatory effect drug interaction, insufficient time for judging efficacy, noncompliance, or actual inefficacy of the drug. Multiple nonsteroidals taken concomitantly will usually lower serum levels by competitive inhibition and by displacing each other from albumin binding sites.[9] Other problems include toxicity and a reverse placebo effect (the doctor downplaying the potential efficacy of the drug to the patient).

Usually, patients are begun on NSAID therapy at the time of first diagnosis, and if the drugs are not completely effective somewhere between 3 and 6 months after the onset of adequate anti-inflammatory therapy, a decision is made regarding starting the patient on DMARDs. At any time during the course of therapy adjunctive treatment may be used. Adjunctive treatment can include the use of interarticular steroids, soft-tissue injections, additional analgesic therapy, surgery, and antidepressant drugs.

DISEASE-MODIFYING ANTIRHEUMATIC DRUGS (REMITTIVE AGENTS)

Disease-modifying antirheumatic drugs (DMARDs) are currently used much earlier in rheumatoid arthritis than in the past. The major factor influencing the decision to use DMARDs includes the presence of persistent active disease. One must ask whether the disease is susceptible to drug intervention. In other words, if the disease is inactive with only the pain and deformity being present, it is unlikely that DMARDs will be effective. The patient must be informed as to the reason for utilizing the drugs and the need to monitor toxicity and maintain drug dosage. One must assess the patient for any contraindications to the use of the drug, either due to other pharmacotherapy or concomitant disease. There is no specific contraindication of age to the use of these drugs.

The remittive agents have nonspecific anti-inflammatory effect, and they are all characterized by a delayed onset of action. While NSAIDs have an immediate effect as soon as therapeutic blood levels are reached, the DMARDs may not show any results for 6 weeks to 6 months. All of these drugs treat the underlying disease by their effect on various cellular and humoral immune mechanisms. They modify the disease from the clinical, serologic, and radiologic standpoint if they are maximally effective. They are tissue protective and are all either immunosuppressive or immunomodulatory.

The DMARDs approved by the Federal Drug Administration (FDA) include hydroxychloroquine and oral and intramuscular gold, penicillamine, methotrexate, and azathioprine. Other disease-modifying agents which are used but are not FDA approved include cyclophosphamide and chloroquine. Since corticosteroids are not DMARDs, they are discussed separately.

Hydroxychloroquine

Hydroxychloroquine is best used in relatively early mild-to-moderate disease. It is useful in active RA not responsive to adequate doses of NSAIDs alone and is almost always used concomitantly with them in rheumatoid disease. It has also been used successfully in combination with gold, methotrexate, and other DMARDs and may have additive activity when used in combination.

The mechanism of action of hydroxychloroquine is not well understood. The toxicity of the drug is minimized by limiting the dose to a maximum of 400 mg/day and by careful follow-up including ophthalmologic examination every 6 months with Red Amsler Grid testing (central visual fields with a colored object). The drug should not be used as a sole DMARD in severe aggressive active RA because of inadequate potency. The initial dose is 200 mg twice daily for 8 to 12 weeks. If this dose is ineffective, the drug should be discontinued, since it is unlikely to be effective. If effective, the dose is maintained between 200 and 400 mg/day (maintain the minimum effective dose). Doses higher than 400 mg/day increase ocular toxicity and should not be used. Ocular toxicity is cumulative and the patient should report visual symptoms.

Gold

Parenteral gold has been the standard against which other remittive agents are compared in the treatment of RA. Gold is available for oral use and intramuscular injection. The IM preparation has been shown to prevent radiographic progression of erosions over a 2-year period.[10] Recent controversies over its true remittive efficacy are centered around uncontrolled epidemiologic surveys, not controlled trials.[11] Most rheumatologists consider gold thiomalate and gold thioglucose to be potent remittive agents. The problems of administration, particularly in the elderly patient, include the inconvenience of a weekly injection in a physician's office and the cost of the drug, laboratory monitoring, and physician visits. Many rheumatologists now utilize methotrexate before parenteral gold in the pyramid of therapy for these reasons.

Auranofin is the oral form of gold, and while effective, it lacks the potency of the parenteral preparations. It has less toxicity, but loose stools and diarrhea are a problem in up to 40 percent of patients and can be particularly annoying in the older individual. This may be lessened with concomitant use of psyllium. The potency of oral gold is similar to hydroxychloroquine, and it should not be used in aggressive disease.

Administration Injectable gold is administered first in a test dose of 10 mg (deep IM in the buttock). If tolerated, 25 mg is given the following week and then 50 mg every week until 1 g total dose is reached, toxicity occurs, or therapeutic efficacy is reached. If 1 g total dose is reached without amelioration of symptoms, one can try higher doses or continue on 50 mg/week for a few more months before abandoning the drug as inefficacious. If toxicity occurs, the clinician must determine whether it is drug related and how serious it is. Mild reactions (slight skin rash, mild proteinuria) may be managed with temporary cessation or reduction of drug dose and/or frequency. Serious toxicity (thrombocytopenia, aplastic anemia, severe desquamative dermatitis, nephrotic syndrome) require permanent cessation of drug and often symptomatic therapy. If the drug is effective without toxicity, gradual reduction of frequency of dose should be attempted. Too often the clinician precipitously decreases the frequency from weekly to monthly with a resulting relapse in disease and perceived drug failure. The injections should be gradually decreased from weekly, biweekly, every 3 weeks, and monthly with several months between each dose reduction. Tapering the dosage, for instance, to every 2 weeks should be carried out for 8 to 12 doses without a flare before proceeding to 3-week intervals. Many patients, however, will require long-lasting weekly or biweekly therapy.

Monitoring requires a clinician to query patients with every dose about toxicity. We recommend a urine *dipstick* every visit for protein and hemoglobin with a full urinalysis being done every fourth injection. Complete blood counts (CBCs) and platelet counts should be done every second to fourth injection. Periodic renal function tests are recommended every 6 months. Oral gold, when it is used, is given as 3 mg two to three times a day. Monitoring is required monthly and should include blood counts and urinalysis.

Penicillamine

The use of penicillamine for RA has decreased markedly since the advent of newer remittive agents. It was first used because of its beneficial effect in decreasing rheumatoid factor in seropositive patients and because of its ameliorative effects on vasculitis. Penicillamine was shown to be equal in efficacy to gold.[12] Long-term usage by rheumatologists, however, has been disappointing due to a perceived less-than-optimal effect and because of some of the more common serious side effects. These include nephrotic syndrome, hematologic toxicity, autoimmune disease, frequent nausea, and dysgeusia. Because of poor absorption, it is taken on an empty stomach. However, penicillamine appears to be particularly effective in reducing rheumatoid nodules, which may worsen on some patients on methotrexate. It continues to be useful in patients with vasculitis.

The administration of penicillamine can be best described as "go low, go slow." The initial dose is 125 or 250 mg once a day on an empty stomach. After 12 to 16 weeks the dose can be titrated upward by 125 to 250 mg at a time. Doses up to 500 mg/day can be taken as a single dose; doses above that are split. The maximum dose is 1000 mg/day. Monitoring includes monthly complete stool count, platelet counts, and full urinalysis as well as periodic physician follow-up visits and renal function tests.

Immunosuppressive (Cytotoxic) Agents

Cytotoxic agents, particularly methotrexate, are now used earlier in the course of RA than in the past. Azathioprine and methotrexate are FDA approved for use, while cyclophosphamide and chlorambucil are not FDA approved but are used on occasion if other drugs fail or for serious systemic disease.

Toxicity of all these agents is increased in the elderly. These drugs should be used only in active disease. The patient should not be able to conceive children and should not have active infection, and both the physician and patient must be knowledgeable both about expectations and toxicity.

Toxicity may be common to all cytotoxic agents or may be unique (Table 20-7). Recommended doses should be reduced when initiating therapy in the elderly

Table 20-7 Toxicity immunosuppressive agents (0–4 +)

	Azathioprine	Methotrexate	Cyclophosphamide	Chlorambucil
		Common to all agents		
Dose-related marrow toxicity	++	+	++	++
Susceptibility to infection	+	+	++	++
Gastrointestinal intolerance	++	+	++	++
Rash	+	+	+	+
Pulmonary fibrosis	+/–	+/–	+/–	+/–
		Toxicity not shared by all drugs		
Hepatic				
Abnormal LFT	+	++	–	–
Cirrhosis, fibrosis	+	+	–	–
Stomatitis	+	+	–	–
Hair loss	–	+	+	+
Amenorrhea/azoospermia	–	+		+
Cystitis (fibrosis)	–	–	+++	+
Teratogenesis	?	+++	?	?
Allergic pneumonitis	–	++	–	–
Neoplasia	+/–	–	+	+/–

because of altered kinetics, other concomitant diseases and organ involvement, and the presence of other drugs.

Methotrexate (Rheumatrex) Methotrexate, an anticancer agent, has been proven to be effective in RA.[13] Its relatively rapid effect, good efficacy, and ease of administration as well as its tolerable toxicity profile have led to its common use in treating this disease. This drug is administered in low-dose *pulse* therapy and is usually given by mouth once a week. In patients with poor compliance or who experience severe nausea, the drug may be given parenterally.

The indications for methotrexate are active rheumatoid arthritis not satisfactorily responsive to NSAIDs alone and/or not responsive to other agents preferred by the clinician. The dose is usually begun at 7.5 mg (three 2.5-mg tablets) once a week. In the elderly or debilitated patient one may begin a reduced dose of 5 mg/week; this is prescribed on a specific day for clarity (i.e., 3 tablets on Monday morning). Usually at the onset of therapy only enough drug is given until the patient returns for a follow-up visit to check on compliance. We do not recommend a liver biopsy before therapy or during therapy unless the patient is at high risk for hepatotoxicity. Abstinence from alcohol is recommended. If nausea occurs, the dose may be split into three equal doses given every 12 h over a 24-h period.

Toxicity is monitored by monthly CBC, platelet count, and liver and renal function tests. Periodic urinalysis should be done and the patient should be seen every 2 to 3 months. Doses may be titrated as high as 15 or even 20 mg weekly. Higher doses are associated with increased toxicity. The average patient takes approximately 10 mg/week. The response is seen in 8 to 10 weeks and dose changes upward are made every 3 to 4 months. While arthritis is relieved in 60 to 80 percent of patients, rheumatoid nodules are usually not improved or may worsen. The response to methotrexate seems to be sustained over a long period of time,[13] and discontinuation is often associated with a disease flare. Pulmonary toxicity is seen in 3 to 5 percent of patients; this toxicity presents as a dry cough and shortness of breath. Hepatic cirrhosis is, on the other hand, exceedingly rare (<0.1 percent).[14] It should not be used in patients with chronic liver disease and should be used with caution in patients with renal failure or pulmonary fibrosis.

Azathioprine This purine antagonist is an effective agent in treating rheumatoid arthritis. It is usually used in patients who have failed two or three other remittive agents and is preferred in older patients because of the remote possibility of causing a neoplasm. Bone marrow suppression, including leukopenia and thrombocytopenia is usually the limiting toxicity. Azathioprine is begun in a dose of 1 mg/kg (50 to 100 mg) orally per day. The dose is gradually titrated upward by 25-mg increments until a response occurs or toxicity ensues. An early sign of toxicity is often a WBC dropping below 3000 to 4000/mm^3. Monitoring includes monthly CBC and platelet counts as well as periodic function tests. Concomitant allopurinol requires a two-thirds reduction in azathioprine.

Cyclophosphamide and chlorambucil Cyclophosphamide and chlorambucil are rarely used in rheumatoid arthritis and require the same monitoring as in other diseases. They are used in daily oral doses (Cytoxan 1 to 2 mg/kg/day; chlorambucil 2 to 4 mg/day). This drug is sometimes used in high-dose intravenous bolus (750 mg/m^2 body surface area) in necrotizing vasculitis.

Corticosteroids

These drugs are often misused in RA because of the dramatic symptomatic relief they offer. Their toxicity, however, particularly in the elderly (osteoporosis, glucose intolerance, salt retention, skin fragility, susceptibility to infection, avascular osteonecrosis) makes their use of concern. In addition, these drugs have been shown to be anti-inflammatory but have no remittive properties.[15] Joint destruction continues irrespective of treatment, while functional capacity may improve in the short term. Some have recommended the use of low-dose oral prednisone (5 to 10 mg/day) in elderly patients as a safe alternative to DMARDs or as a bridge therapy between drugs[16]; it is our opinion that such use has some danger.

The indications for use of oral corticosteroids in RA are as follows:

1. When a fast-acting anti-inflammatory drug is needed and NSAIDs are contraindicated (i.e., bleeding peptic ulcer) and analgesics alone are ineffective
2. When serious systemic disease occurs (vasculitis, pericarditis, etc.)
3. After all other means are exhausted and the disease is still active
4. For short periods of time for humane reasons (e.g., important trip)

The use of high doses, or "dose packs," to "cool down disease" is to be decried because this leads to steroid dependency and denotes a failure in first-line therapies. Likewise, there is no rationale for the use of adrenocorticotropic hormone (ACTH), which also inhibits the pituitary-adrenal axis.

Steroids should be started, when used for arthritis, at a low dose (2 to 5 mg prednisone in a single dose/day). Every other day therapy may be tried but usually is less effective. A maximum dose of 10 mg daily is used for arthritis, while higher doses may be needed for systemic problems. One should constantly try to maximize alternative treatments and attempt to slowly withdraw prednisone by decreasing the dose 1 mg at a time every few weeks. Females should be on estrogen replacement if not contraindicated as well as calcium supplements to lessen osteopenia. Careful monitoring of steroid therapy is needed.

Other Therapy

Specific immunomodulator therapy holds great promise for the future. Currently studied experimental therapies include apheresis, pulse high-dose steroids, combination therapy, cyclosporine a, sulfasalazine, interferon, dapsone, retinoids, Omega-3 fatty acids, humanized monoclonal antibodies, tilomisole, therafectin, new immunosuppressive drugs, new NSAIDs, and bisphosphonates.

OSTEOARTHRITIS (DEGENERATIVE JOINT DISEASE)

Osteoarthritis is a disorder which is generally considered to be noninflammatory in nature and to be associated with wear and tear of the joints and with aging. The British refer to this disease as *osteoarthrosis* to connote its noninflammatory nature. The common name used in this country is *degenerative joint disease* (DJD).

Osteoarthritis has been identified in prehistoric remains and is ancient, even occurring in subprimate animals. It is the most common rheumatic disease in prevalence, afflicting over 40 million Americans alone. While thought to be caused by overuse of the joint, recent work has suggested that genetic and metabolic abnormalities may predispose some patients to this disorder.[17] The joint pathology demonstrates loss of cartilage matrix and abortive attempts of chondrocytes to proliferate and repair damage to the cartilage. Eventually, cartilage fissuring and loss occurs with underlying reactive new bone and osteophyte formation. In some patients inflammatory changes are seen in addition to the degenerative abnormalities. The latter are felt to be due to crystal deposition (calcium hydroxyapatite and pyrophosphate).

NSAIDs are the mainstay of therapy for this disorder. Since they have no effect on progression of the disease and since analgesia is the desired result, lower doses of NSAIDs are usually used initially in DJD. The dose is increased if there are inflammatory signs or if low doses are ineffective. There is no clear indication that one nonsteroidal or class of nonsteroidals is more effective than any other in the treatment of DJD.

Obviously, most patients with DJD are older, and thus increased medication toxicity is expected. This is particularly true in those NSAIDs with a long half-life. Another peculiar but rare side effect of these agents seen in patients with osteoarthritis is the sudden massive loss of cartilage (cartilage melt) in an arthritic joint. The cause of this phenomenon is unknown, and if it occurs, the offending NSAID should be discontinued.

Other therapy for DJD includes occasional intraarticular depot steroid injections (no more than one or two times per year in an individual joint), physical therapy, and surgery. Systemic corticosteroids and remittive agents have no place in the treatment of this disease. Pure analgesics such as acetaminophen may substitute for NSAIDs.

CRYSTAL ARTHROPATHY

There are three basic types of crystal arthritis commonly seen in elderly patients: gout, calcium pyrophosphate deposition disease (CPPD), and hydroxyapatite deposition disease (apatite arthropathy). Deposition of the particular crystal occurs within the joint, and the resultant inflammatory arthritis may lead to joint destruction.

Gout Gout is caused by sodium urate crystals. Uric acid levels are elevated in the serum due to either increased production or decreased excretion by the kidney. The crystals then deposit into tissues (synovium and cartilage) causing both acute attacks and chronic destructive arthritis. In synovial tissue the crystal is sodium urate because of the approximate pH of 7.4; in urine it is uric acid because of the low pH. Crystals may deposit in other tissues of the body, particularly the kidney, and lead to systemic disease such as urinary calculi and interstitial nephritis. Table 20-8 depicts some more common causes for hyperuricemia and Table 20-9 shows drug effects on serum uric acid levels. The diagnosis of gout is made by aspirating joint fluid and identifying sodium urate crystals under polarized light microscopy. These crystals are bright, needle-shaped, negatively birefringent material.

The treatment of gout requires that, if present, the acute attack be completely treated first. The treatment of choice, if possible, is the use of NSAIDs. Aspirin is not recommended because of its effects on serum uric acid levels. Unless peptic ulcer disease or other contraindications are present, high doses of NSAIDs are used.

Table 20-8 Causes of abnormalities in uric acid metabolism

Overproduction of uric acid	Underexcretion of uric acid
Congenital (enzyme defect)	Intrinsic renal disease
Hemolytic disorders	Lead poisoning
Myeloproliferative disease	Competition for renal uric acid secretion
	Drugs
	Acidosis (lactic, ketotic)
Psoriasis	Idiopathic
Cytotoxic drugs	

Phenylbutazone and indomethacin, although potent and effective, are not recommended in elderly patients, particularly if cardiac or renal disease is present. High doses of other NSAIDs (i.e., 3200 to 3600 mg ibuprofen/day in divided doses with meals) are used for the first day or two followed by moderate to high doses until the acute attack has resolved.

Oral colchicine may be used at a dose of 1 tablet (0.5 or 0.65 mg) every hour until efficacy or toxicity is reached or until 10 tablets have been consumed. While colchicine has some diagnostic specificity, it may be effective in other disorders such as pseudogout. In general, the gastrointestinal toxicity is so common because of colchicine's narrow therapeutic window, it has largely been abandoned in favor of newer NSAIDs. IV colchicine may be used when oral drugs cannot be taken. Two milligrams is infused IV in saline or dextrose over 30 min with care not to extravasate. Doses of 1 mg may be repeated every 6 h until a total dose of 4 mg has been reached in 24 h, if necessary. Patients do not suffer gastrointestinal side effects and marrow toxicity may occur without warning if the recommended dose is exceeded.

When these agents are contraindicated, corticosteroids in doses equivalent to 60 to 100 mg of prednisone per day will also ameliorate the acute attack. Likewise, ACTH 40 IU parenterally twice a day may be used.

Table 20-9 Drug effects on uric acid excretion by kidney

Increased excretion (lower serum level)	Decreased excretion (higher serum level)
Aspirin, high dose	Aspirin, low dose
Clofibrate	Alcohol
Phenylbutazone	Diuretics
Radiologic contrast agents	Ethambutol
Sulfinpyrazone	Levodopa
Warfarin	Phenytoin
Probenecid	

Drugs to treat the acute attack should be utilized until it is completely resolved. Uric-acid-lowering drugs should not be administered until the acute attack is resolved because they will exacerbate or prolong the acute attack. Once the painful inflammation ceases, the patient is given 0.5 mg of colchicine two or three times a day to reduce the incidence of recurrence while the serum uric acid is being lowered. Colchicine is continued for 6 weeks after the appropriate serum uric acid level has been attained (≤6 mg/dL).

The drug of choice for hyperuricemia depends on whether overproduction or underexcretion of uric acid occurs. Overproducers (greater than 800 mg urine uric acid/day) should be treated with allopurinol in a dose high enough to lower the serum uric acid below the pK (6.0 mg/100 mL). This usually requires 100 to 300 mg allopurinol once a day. The need for higher doses may suggest noncompliance or an enzyme disorder. Allopurinol is also preferentially used with tophaceous gout, renal calculi, and renal failure. Lower doses are usually the rule in the elderly. Underexcretors (<600 mg urine uric acid/day) without the above complications may be treated with probenecid 500 mg twice daily. In either case, doses are titrated upward until a serum uric acid <6 mg/dL is reached. Adequate hydration is requisite with uricosuric agents, and alkalinization of the urine may be needed to prevent renal calculi. The patient is monitored periodically to assure normal uric acid levels and recurrent attacks are treated with NSAIDs. The patient must realize that this treatment is a lifelong commitment, even when asymptomatic. Allopurinol toxicity (vasculitis, rash, hepatitis, etc.) precludes its use in everyone, and thus, uricosurics are recommended when possible. Dietary restrictions are unnecessary due to the potency of the uric-acid-lowering agents.

Finally, the area of treatment of asymptomatic hyperuricemia is controversial. We recommend treating this in patients who have had urinary calculi or who have increased production of uric acid (> 1000 mg/day urinary excretion) or in patients who have a single kidney.

Calcium pyrophosphate deposition disease(CPPD) CPPD was described by McCarty in 1962.[18] The deposition of crystals in the joint is frequently visible on the radiograph (knee, wrist, pelvis, hip most commonly) and is called chondrocalcinosis. The acute attack of arthritis caused by these crystals is called pseudogout. A chronic destructive arthropathy may ensue which may resemble RA or DJD. The diagnosis is made by radiography (chondrocalcinosis) and fluid aspiration identifying the crystal with polarized light microscopy (pseudogout).

CPPD is associated with a variety of underlying disorders, including hyperparathyroidism, hemochromatosis, acromegaly, neuropathic arthropathy, gout, diabetes mellitus, ochronosis, Wilson's disease, and hypophosphatasia.

The long-term treatment is centered around identifying and treating, when possible, the underlying disorder. There is no specific prophylactic or curative therapy otherwise. For acute therapy one uses high doses of NSAID therapy similar to that described with gout. Fluid aspiration and injection with depot corticosteroids will also help.

Hydroxyapatite arthropathy Acute inflammatory arthritis, periarthritis, calcific tendonitis, and bursitis have all been attributed to the calcium hydroxyapatite crystal, which is the same material present in normal bone. The reason that this crystal deposits in nonosseous areas, where it excites anti-inflammatory response, is not known. Indeed, often such depositions are not symptomatic. While this disorder is seen frequently, it is particularly common in patients with chronic renal failure and in patients incapacitated with neurologic problems.

In addition to the syndrome described above, some patients with osteoarthritis have moderate to severe inflammation in the proximal and distal interphalangeal joints of their hands, a condition called erosive osteoarthritis. Finally, some elderly women have a severe resorptive arthritis of the shoulder, the so-called Milwaukee shoulder.[19] Both of these clinical entities are caused by hydroxyapatite deposition.

Treatment of this class of crystal arthropathy is with NSAIDs used as needed to relieve symptoms. There is no prophylactic therapy other than surgically removing the crystalline material when necessary. This is done occasionally in recurrent severe calcific tendonitis of the shoulder.

POLYMYALGIA RHEUMATICA AND GIANT CELL ARTERITIS (TEMPORAL ARTERITIS)

Polymyalgia rheumatica (PMR) is a syndrome characterized by proximal myalgias of the shoulder and hip girdle regions without true inflammatory muscle disease, atrophy, or weakness. It is almost exclusively a disease of patients older than 55 years and is associated with a markedly increased sedimentation rate (the Westergren, frequently over 100 mm/h). Serum levels, muscle enzymes, electromyograms, and muscle biopsies are normal.

PMR is frequently associated with a more serious disorder, temporal arteritis. This disease is a giant-cell granulomatous arteritis usually of extracranial vessels, particularly the temporal artery, but also involving branches of the aorta and the ciliary artery of the eye.

These patients may have unilateral headaches, transient diplopia, or visual loss as well as jaw claudication and other neurologic symptoms. The most serious sequela of the disease is permanent blindness, resulting from retinal artery occlusion and stroke.

The etiology of these diseases is unknown. The diagnosis of PMR is a clinical one. The diagnosis of temporal arteritis is made by biopsy of one or both temporal arteries. Occasionally a clinical diagnosis alone may be the deciding factor in treatment.

Treatment of PMR requires low-dose corticosteroids in the range of 5 to 10 mg prednisone daily. Temporal arteritis, however, is a medical emergency and requires immediate treatment with approximately 60 mg/day of prednisone as soon as the disorder is suspected. Failure to institute therapy promptly can result in permanent blindness. The biopsy of the temporal artery is then performed within

24 to 48 h to verify diagnosis. Maintenance therapy for both diseases is the lowest daily dose of steroid needed to control both symptoms and the sedimentation rate (if it can be established that the elevation is due to the disease). Alternate-day steroids should not be used. Attention should be given to osteoporosis aggravated by steroids as well as other side effects in these individuals. If the patient is maintained on long-term corticosteroids, supplementation with calcium, estrogens, and possibly vitamin D may prevent long-term difficulties with osteoporosis. PMR has been treated with nonsteroidal anti-inflammatory drugs alone, but this therapy has not been as effective as low-dose steroid therapy.

Both diseases have an average span of 3 years duration, but some patients will have a much shorter period of time and some patients will go on for many years. The only way to determine whether the disease will exacerbate is by gradually reducing the steroids every 3 to 6 months by 1-mg/day increments to determine whether the sedimentation rate begins to climb or the symptoms return.

Salicylates

Salicylates have been used since the late 1800s after Felix Hoffman, a German chemist, used salicylates to treat his father's arthritis. Salicylates are the least expensive, most widely used, and best studied of all the analgesic, antipyretic, and anti-inflammatory agents.[20,21]

Pharmacologic actions Salicylates exert analgesic, antipyretic, and anti-inflammatory actions. Analgesia is produced primarily through inhibition of prostaglandin synthesis, with the recognition that prostaglandins have the ability to sensitize pain receptors. Aspirin and other nonacetylated salicylates are considered mild analgesics. However, the type of pain must be considered since location and type of pain is important to efficacy. In postoperative pain, salicylates can be superior to opioid analgesics, while "hollow-organ" (visceral) pain is poorly treated with salicylates. Antipyretic action is the result of both hypothalamic suppression of pyrogen-stimulated prostaglandin synthesis and peripheral vasodilation. Anti-inflammatory action is also thought to be secondary to prostaglandin synthesis inhibition. However, inflammation is a complex phenomena involving a number of enzyme systems and mediators. The exact role of salicylates in ameliorating inflammation is not well defined, especially in regard to the nonacetylated salicylates which exert minimal prostaglandin synthesis inhibition. Other mechanisms of action may explain salicylate effects such as lysosomal stabilization, kinin and leukotriene production, alteration of chemotactic factors, and most importantly, inhibition of neutrophil activation, which appears to play a major role in anti-inflammatory action.[21,22]

Pharmacokinetics Salicylates are rapidly and completely absorbed after oral administration, with the majority of absorption occurring in the upper small intestine and minimal absorption through the gastric mucosa. Measurable serum levels of drug are found within 30 min after ingestion, and in most preparations, maximum serum concentrations are achieved in 2 h.[21] Bioavailability and rate of absorption depend upon dosage form, presence of food, gastric emptying time, presence of antacids, gastric pH, and ionization of the salicylate molecule. Enteric-coated salicylates in the past had erratic absorption, but newer agents are much more reliable. Aspirin suppositories have erratic and incomplete absorption due to aspirin's low pK_a and the neutral pH of the lower bowel resulting in a large proportion of ionized, nonabsorbable aspirin. Food slows the absorption of salicylate, but with chronic, continual dosing, the rate of absorption of any drug is unimportant clinically. Complete absorption eventually occurs in the presence of food. Antacids increase the ionization but also increase solubility and, therefore, have little appreciable effect on absorption. Salicylates are readily and rapidly distributed through all body tissues with the highest concentrations found in plasma, liver, heart, lungs, and renal cortex. Aspirin is rapidly hydrolyzed by mucosal and hepatic esterases and is transformed to salicylic acid. Hydrolyzed salicylate is 90 percent bound to plasma albumin.[21] In hypoalbuminemic states such as rheumatoid arthritis or in elderly patients with malnutrition or other disease states affecting albumin concentrations, higher free salicylate serum concentrations occur. Indeed, there is a known age-related decline in serum albumin concentrations, which may explain increased dose-related toxicity in this population.[23]

Salicylate biotransformation occurs in many tissues but is primarily metabolized in hepatic tissue with subsequent urine elimination of metabolites. Both linear (first-order) and nonlinear (zero-order) metabolism occurs, which greatly influences the pharmacokinetics of salicylates. Linear metabolism produces gentisic acid (<1 percent), salicylic acid (10 percent), and salicyl acyl glucuronide (5 percent). Nonlinear metabolism encountered in the production of salicyluric acid (75 percent) and salicyl phenolic glucuronide (10 percent) can become saturated and, therefore, cause dramatic changes in serum/tissue concentrations and half-life of salicylate. The plasma half-life for aspirin is approximately 15 to 20 min. However, salicylate half-lives, as a result of the two nonlinear elimination pathways, are dose dependent. With low doses, metabolism is linear and salicylate half-life is 2 to 4 h, whereas with high doses, the nonlinear pathways are saturated and half-lives of 15 to 30 h can be encountered.[21] In therapeutic anti-inflammatory doses, half-lives generally range from 6 to 12 h. With renal impairment, the dose-response curve becomes markedly changed and is a factor to consider when administering salicylates to elderly patients.[21,24] In general, given the variable pharmacokinetics encountered from individual to individual, one must monitor closely the efficacy and side-effect potential. In many cases, serum concentration determinations will be helpful to maximize the use of salicylates and avoid toxicity.

Administration Doses of salicylate used will, of course, depend upon therapeutic effect desired (see individual diseases above). For analgesia and antipyresis, doses of aspirin required are low (650 mg, which may be given three to four times daily). However, to achieve anti-inflammatory effects, daily doses of 3.2 g (10 tablets) to 3.9 g (12 tablets) need to be initiated with increases of not more than 325 mg to 650 mg (1 to 2 tablets) every 5 to 7 days to achieve therapeutic serum concentrations between 15 and 30 mg/dL. Serum concentrations should not be obtained for at least 5 days after initiation of salicylate therapy or after a dose increase since steady state is not reached until after five half-lives have past. Additionally, collecting blood for serum concentration determinations should be obtained at the end of a dosing interval, just prior to the next dose or 4 h postdose to allow for adequate distribution to occur.

A wide variety of dosage formulations are available: plain tablets, enteric-coated tablets, suppositories, gums, and buffered (antacid combination), timed-release, controlled-release, and effervescent tablets. Cost, ease of administration, and acute gastrointestinal irritation must be considered when selecting a preparation. Plain tablets offer low cost. Enteric-coated and timed-release preparations offer decreased acute, direct gastric irritation but increased cost. Timed-release formulations may also increase compliance due to fewer administrations per day. Suppositories can cause rectal irritation and should be avoided as an alternative route of administration. Buffered tablets do not contain enough antacid to provide gastric protection but do increase their dissolution. Likewise, effervescent tablets offer the advantage of drug already in solution and, therefore, are less likely to cause acute, direct gastric irritation. However, the increased potential problems with sodium and alkali ingestion (sodium bicarbonate) make these preparations undesirable, especially in the elderly. In general, it is best to advise patients or their caregivers to administer salicylates, especially aspirin, with meals and a snack at bedtime. Another consideration to decrease direct gastric irritation would be the use of a nonacetylated salicylate. These agents have been reported to have decreased gastric irritation as compared with aspirin. Magnesium salicylate should be used with caution since many elderly have reduced renal function which may lead to magnesium toxicity.

Adverse drug reactions Salicylates are capable of causing a large variety of side effects affecting many organ systems. These side effects are well known but need special consideration in elderly patients due to the increased morbidity and mortality associated with drugs and disease in the elderly.

Gastrointestinal side effects include gastritis, peptic ulceration, and bleeding with resultant iron deficiency. Gastrointestinal side effects are the result of either direct or systemic (indirect) effects. Gastritis is due to direct irritant action of the salicylates upon the gastric mucosa. The administration of concomitant H_2 blocker or sucralfate will not affect this process and increases cost of therapy. Additionally, there is no evidence to suggest that superficial damage (gastritis) correlates with more serious complications such as peptic ulceration and hemorrhage nor is it a precursor to such side effects.[25]

Peptic ulceration and hemorrhage is due to systemic effects of salicylates and other NSAIDs through prostaglandin synthesis inhibition. Prostaglandins are responsible for maintaining the integrity of the gastric mucosal protective barrier through prostaglandin-stimulated production of mucus, bicarbonate, and phospholipid layers as well as maintaining the *tight junction* of epithelial cells and mucosal blood flow. Given this mechanism for development of these potentially serious side effects, it is understandable why the use of H_2 blockers and sucralfate is not effective in preventing these side effects.[25,26] The use of misoprostol [synthetic prostaglandin E (PGE) analog] is effective in preventing such complications.[26,27]

In the elderly, peptic ulceration and hemorrhage represent a more serious and subtle problem. The elderly are a high-risk population for these side effects and they frequently, up to 60 percent, develop these problems asymptomatically.[26,28,29] The analgesia produced by salicylates and other NSAIDs is suspected to play a role in diminishing symptoms. Also, the elderly often have other risk factors for ulceration and hemorrhage such as concomitant ulcerogenic drug use (corticosteroids) and smoking.

Hepatic injury has been reported with aspirin and other salicylates, especially in patients with salicylate serum concentrations above 25 mg/dL, lupus, or Still's disease. Salicylate is a direct hepatotoxin resulting in asymptomatic transaminase elevations. In most cases, a dose reduction results in normalization of transaminases, and discontinuation of therapy is seldom necessary.[30] Monitoring serum salicylate concentrations is recommended with discontinuation of salicylate therapy should transaminases continue to rise or the patient develop anorexia, nausea, or jaundice.

Renal toxicity attributed to salicylates is related to situations in which renal blood flow (RBF) and, therefore, glomerular filtration rate (GFR) diminish as a result of decreased PGE_2 and prostacyclin synthesis. These two prostaglandins are responsible for maintaining RBF and GFR in patients who have reduced renal function as a result of elevated angiotensin II and catecholamines found in such conditions as congestive heart failure, nephrotic syndrome, liver cirrhosis with ascites, hypovolemia, and persons over 60 years old.[30] Clinicians should monitor patients at risk for salicylate-induced renal toxicity for increases in edema, weight, blood urea nitrogen (BUN), serum creatinine, and potassium.[30]

The most common central nervous system (CNS) side effect to salicylates is tinnitus, which occurs when serum concentrations approach 30 mg/dL. However, this sign of toxicity may be an unreliable indicator of toxicity in elderly due to age-related hearing loss, and accelerated levels should be monitored.[30] Salicylate serum concentrations exceeding 30 mg/dL can be associated with other CNS side effects such as confusion, agitation, slurred speech, hallucinations, and even seizures and coma.[21,30] Clinicians should not allow aging bias in dementia or institutionalized individuals to cause them to dismiss these symptoms.

Allergy to aspirin is seen in some adults, particularly if they exhibit the classic triad: nasal polyposis, steroid-dependent asthma, and vasomotor rhinitis. It is postulated that aspirin and other NSAIDs inhibit cyclooxygenase, therefore decreasing synthesis of bronchodilating prostaglandins precipitating bronchospasm. Patients exhibiting this syndrome should not take aspirin and other NSAIDs.

Nonacetylated salicylates which have no effects on prostaglandins may be given safely to those patients. Aspirin also causes, in some, urticaria and angioedema, which is not a result of prostaglandin blockade but is true allergy.[21,30]

Hematologic adverse effects to acetylated salicylates are due to irreversible inhibition of platelet function through acetylation of cyclooxygenase, thereby blocking production of thromboxane A_2 necessary for platelet activation and aggregation.[21,30] Since platelets lack mitochondria, they do not have the ability to synthesize new cyclooxygenase and are, therefore, inactivated for the life of the platelet.[30] This reaction does not occur with nonacetylated salicylates, which therefore may be the drugs of choice in patients with coagulopathies or who need surgery. Aspirin should be discontinued at least 1 week prior to surgery.[30] Caution should also be exercised with elderly receiving anticoagulants, as platelet dysfunction may predispose to bleeding and easy bruising, commonly encountered normally in aged skin. Patients with chronic salicylism may exhibit neurologic dysfunction and appear demented. In severe salicylate intoxication, pulmonary edema and renal failure may occur.

Drug interactions Salicylates have potentially serious drug-drug interactions with several drugs frequently used in the geriatric population.[31]

Oral anticoagulants and heparin. Therapeutic doses of salicylates reduce plasma prothrombin concentrations, displace coumarin from protein binding sites, and impair platelet aggregation.

Corticosteroids. These drugs decrease serum salicylate concentrations. The mechanism for this action is not well understood. However, the decrease in salicylates may be due to increased GFR on hepatic metabolism induced by corticosteroids. Difficulty may arise when steroids are tapered and discontinued and salicylates doses become elevated. Also, the risk of gastrointestinal ulceration is increased if corticosteroids and aspirin are used concomitantly. The use of corticosteroids alone has not been proven to cause gastrointestinal ulceration.[32]

Methotrexate. Salicylates block the renal tubular secretion of methotrexate and may also displace this drug from protein binding sites, thus resulting in increased free drug.

Other NSAIDs. Salicylates, through plasma protein binding competition, may result in increased renal clearance of these agents due to increased free drug available for excretion. A single aspirin per day may however be taken with NSAIDs for therapeutic antiplatelet effects.

Angiotensin converting enzyme inhibitors. The antihypertensive effect of these agents may be decreased, possibly secondary to prostaglandin inhibition.

H_2 blockers. Increases in salicylate serum concentrations have been reported when used concomitantly.

Uricosurics (probenecid and sulfinpyrazone). Salicylates in low doses, less than 2 g/day, inhibit the uricosuric action of these drugs.

Sulfonylureas and exogenous insulin. Salicylates in doses greater than

2 g/day exhibit a hypoglycemic effect. Also, competition for plasma protein binding may enhance oral hypoglycemic action through displacement.

Nonsteroidal Anti-inflammatory Agents

A large number of nonsalicylate NSAID drugs are now available. These agents include the propionic acid derivatives (fenoprofen, flurbiprofen, ibuprofen, ketoprofen, and naproxen), indole derivatives (indomethacin, sulindac, and tolmetin), pyrazolone derivatives (phenylbutazone and oxyphenbutazone), fenamates (meclofenamate and mefenamic acid), oxicams (piroxicam), and phenylacetic acids (diclofenac). The newer NSAIDs have been developed to decrease the toxicity, particularly gastrointestinal toxicity, associated with older agents (indomethacin and pyrazolone derivatives).

Pharmacologic action The nonsalicylate NSAIDs exhibit pharmacologic action similar to the salicylate. Drug trials have not shown one agent superior to another in treatment of arthritis, and a significant intersubject variability exists in regard to response to these agents. For this reason, when an agent has been selected for a proper indication, is given a sufficient trial (2 to 3 weeks) at a proper dose, and fails to result in resolution, another NSAID should be selected. There exists no indicators for clinicians to use in predicting who will respond to which agent.[33] Some clinicians prefer to switch agents by initiating new therapy with an agent from another chemical class, e.g., change from a propionic acid to an oxicam. There are no scientific data to support this idea. However, it is an acceptable method of selection. Like salicylate, these agents are analgesic in low doses and are anti-inflammatory with higher doses (see Table 20-10).

The mechanism of action of NSAIDs is the same as that of salicylates. Mechanisms other than cyclooxygenase inhibition are suggested by some incongruities observed with other drugs. For example, other prostaglandin synthesis inhibitors (such as tricyclic antidepressants or α-tocopherol) fail to ameliorate inflammation, nonacetylated salicylates exhibit minimal prostaglandin inhibition, and gold increases prostaglandin E and F production yet decreases inflammation. Actions of NSAIDs include inhibition of neutrophil activation, superoxide free radicals, lipoxygenase and leukotrienes, phosphodiesterase, cell-mediated immunity, and histamine.[21,22,30]

Pharmacokinetics All NSAIDs are rapidly and extensively absorbed. In general, food delays absorption but does not affect the extent of absorption. Administering with food is often recommended to decrease or minimize direct gastric irritation. Protein (albumin) binding is greater than 90 percent for all NSAIDs, and their elimination is primarily through hepatic biotransformation with metabolites excreted in the urine. The plasma half-lives range from 2 to 86 h (see Table 20-10). Those agents with long half-lives offer the advantage of once or twice daily dosing, thereby affording better compliance, more convenience, and less nursing time in

Table 20-10 Comparison of anti-inflammatory agents

	Aspirin	Fenoprofen	Ibuprofen	Indomethacin	Meclofenamate	Naproxen	Phenylbutazone
Strength	Many	300-mg tablets	300-,400-, 600-,800-mg tablets	25-, 50-mg capsules 75 mg sustained release	50-100-mg capsules	250-, 375-, 500-mg tablets	100-mg tablets
Anti-inflammatory dose range (day)	3-6 g	2400-3200 mg	1600-3200 mg	75-150 mg	200-400 mg	500-1000 mg	300-800 mg
Plasma half-life (dosage)	2 h or dose	3 h (qid related) (qid or more)	1.8-2 h	4.5 h (tid, qid)	2-3 h	13 h (bid)	72 h (tid)
Analgesic effect	+	+	+	+	+	+	+
Antipyretic effect	+	+	+	+	+	+	+
Platelet inhibition	++	+	+	+	+	+	+
Asthma (aspirin sensitive)	+	+	+	+	?	+	?
Safe for active ulcer	No	No	No	No	No	No	No
Gastrointestinal effects	++	+	+	+++	++	+	+++
Rash	+	+	+	+	+	+	+
CNS effects	+ (dose related)	+	+	++	+	+	++
Ocular effects	-	-	+	+	+/-	-	+
Na^+ retention	-	+	+	+	+	+	++
Marrow suppression	-	+/-	+/-	+	-	+	+++
Hepatic dysfunction	+	?	-	+	+	-	+

administering. Due to altered results of drugs in the elderly, caution is advised (see salicylates).

Administration When selecting a NSAID for use in an elderly patient, four considerations need attention. First, a clear indication should exist, since the elderly have a high incidence of asymptomatic gastrointestinal ulceration and hemorrhage.[28,29] The second consideration must be expected therapeutic outcome. If analgesia is the therapeutic goal, then one needs to consider if a NSAID is indicated. If desired, then low analgesic doses should be selected. If anti-inflammatory action is desired, then one must assure appropriate doses are administered (see Table 20-10). Dose adjustments based on renal function must be considered in the elderly. Naproxen and ketoprofen require administering 25 percent reduction of the recommended dose in elderly and 50 percent reduction in renal disease. Tolmetin and piroxicam have recommendations for dose reduction when creatinine clearance is

Sulindac	Tolmetin	Flurbiprofen	Ketoprofen	Piroxicam	Diclofenac
150-, 200-mg tablets	200, 400 mg	50-, 100-mg tablets	25-, 50-, 75- mg tablets	10, 20 mg	25-, 50-, 75-mg tablets
300–400 mg	600–2000 mg	100–300 mg	150–300 mg	10–20 mg	100–200 mg
16.8 h (bid)	1 h (qid)	5.7 h	2–4 h	30–86 h	2 h
+	+	+	+	+	+
+	+	+	+	+	+
+	+	+	+	+	+
?	+	+	+	+	+
No	No	No	No	No	No
+	+	+	++	+	+
+	+	+	+	+	+
+	+	+	+	+	+
+	–	+	+	?	?
+/–	+/–	+	+	+	+
–	–	+/–	+/–	+/–	+/–
+	–	–	+	?	?

less than 50 mL/min. Indomethacin and sulindac require dose reduction when creatinine clearance is less than 10 mL/min. The third consideration is proper monitoring for adverse effects (see RA). Also, one needs to consider significant drug-drug interactions and monitor for changes in disease control for those drugs. The fourth and last consideration is the end point of therapy.

Adverse drug reactions The side effects of NSAIDs may be classified as those that are extensions of their pharmacologic action (gastrointestinal ulceration, sodium retention), those that are dose related (CNS effects), and those that are allergic in nature. Some adverse reactions are, of course, similar to those encountered with salicylates and only differ quantitatively where others are unique to this group of drugs or individual agent.

Gastrointestinal side effects are the most common side effects reported for the nonsalicylate NSAIDs. These side effects range from dyspepsia, nausea, and vomiting to frank hemorrhage, ulceration, and perforation. These adverse effects are the result of either direct irritation (dyspepsia, nausea) or systemic action (ulceration, hemorrhage). The propionic acid derivatives and sulindac have comparatively fewer gastrointestinal side effects than aspirin, whereas the pyrazolone derivatives and indomethacin have more. As mentioned above, the elderly are at higher risk for NSAID-induced gastrointestinal side effects which are frequently asymptomatic.[26,28,29] Direct irritation may be minimized by administering with food or antacids. For those at high risk for ulceration, hemorrhage, and perforation, the concomitant use of misoprostol will prevent such complications. The use of H_2 blockers or sucralfate may provide ineffective prophylaxis and should be used with caution in order to avoid a false sense of security. Meclofenamate results in as much as one-third of patients developing diarrhea.

Hepatic enzyme elevations have been noted in some patients. Toxic hepatitis has been reported, and deaths have occurred due to cumulative toxicity in long-half-life drugs and combined renal and liver failure.

Renal adverse effects are primarily due to the renal prostaglandin synthesis inhibition, resulting in diminished RBF and subsequent decreased GFR. Additionally, fluid and sodium retention are extensions of NSAID pharmacologic action.

CNS adverse effects are frequently encountered in the elderly who receive NSAIDs. Somnolence, dizziness, tinnitus, tremor, confusion, and other CNS symptoms are usually mild but may require discontinuation of drug or changing to another NSAID. These reactions, particularly confusion, are more common with indomethacin and the pyrazolone derivatives. Skin rashes and pruritus may be seen with these agents. Patients who exhibit allergic reactions to aspirin will cross-react with these agents as well.

Hematologic side effects are similar to those encountered with aspirin. However, with the nonaspirin NSAIDs, platelet inhibition is reversible once the agent is discontinued as compared to the irreversible reaction aspirin induces. Bone marrow suppression (aplasia, thrombocytopenia, and agranulocytosis) is an idiosyncratic reaction that could occur with any NSAID but is particularly feared with phenylbutazone. For this reason, pyrazolone derivatives are seldom used today and are recommended for short courses of anti-inflammatory therapy (7 days). The elderly are reported to be at higher risk.

Drug interactions Drug interactions stated above for salicylates are found also with the nonsalicylate NSAIDs. A few differences exist[31]:

Antihypertensives. Antihypertensive effects may diminish, particularly with indomethacin. The mechanism is not clearly understood, but it is suggested that prostaglandins and related compounds may be involved in beta-adrenergic blocker antihypertensive action.

Diuretics. Natriuretic and antihypertensive effects may be reduced. Also, potassium, especially with potassium-sparing diuretics, may become elevated.

Phenytoin. Displacement from albumin is possible, resulting in enhanced pharmacologic effects.

Corticosteroids

The use of corticosteroids is particularly discouraged for elderly patients with arthritis. When one is considering the benefits and risks of these agents, the serious side effects tend to make one lean toward omitting these agents, using them for short courses of therapy, or administering them locally. These agents are ineffective in the treatment of osteoarthritis.

Pharmacologic action Corticosteroids exhibit a variety of actions which help control inflammation. Steroid action is mediated through a specific cell surface receptor site. It is transported as a steroid-receptor complex to the nucleus, where a reaction with nuclear chromatin takes place. Messenger RNA causes formation of specific cytoplasmic proteins, which then mediate the biologic effects caused by the corticosteroids. Corticosteroids inhibit leukocyte migration to the inflammatory site. Also, they are potent inhibitors of prostaglandins by a mechanism different than NSAIDs. Capillary permeability is reduced. These drugs also cause lymphopenia, probably through redistribution of cells. All lymphocytes are depressed, but T cells are more affected than B cells. Specific antibody response is decreased, however. Suppression of cell-mediated immunity is probably also mediated indirectly by inhibition of the access of macrophages and monocytes to site of inflammation.

These effects are beneficial to patients with immune disorders (e.g., rheumatoid arthritis), but they also inhibit normal immune response. The magnitude of these pharmacologic actions is dependent on dose, duration of action, and interval between doses.[21,34]

Short-acting drugs include cortisone, prednisone, prednisolone, methylprednisolone; intermediate-acting drugs include triamcinolone; and long-acting drugs include dexamethasone. The longer the action, the more likely adrenal suppression will occur. For this reason, prednisone and prednisolone are more frequently used. Also, administering steroids daily in the morning minimizes adrenal suppression since this more closely simulates the normal diurnal cortisol cycle.

Pharmacokinetics Corticosteroids are well absorbed in the upper jejunum with peak plasma concentrations obtained in 1 to 2 hours. Corticosteroids are 80 percent bound to transcortin-corticosteroid binding globulin and the remainder to corticosteroid binding albumin. The albumin-bound corticosteroids dissociate more readily and diffuse into extravascular fluids. Metabolism to inactive compounds occurs in the liver with the intermediates undergoing conjugation to glucuronic acid or sulfate. These products are then excreted (99 percent metabolized) by the kidney. Also, one should clearly recognize that biologic action does not correlate well with and greatly exceeds plasma half-lives.

Administration See specific diseases.

Adverse drug reactions Corticosteroids affect fluid and electrolyte balance, cardiovascular and muscle function, the nervous system, lymphoid tissue, and

Table 20-11 Steroid adverse reactions

Accelerated atherogenesis	Hypertension
Acne	Infection
Allergic reaction	Menstrual disorder
Avascular necrosis	Myocardial infarction
Cataract	Myopathy
Congestion failure	Osteoporosis
Depression	Pancreatitis
Early death	Peptic ulcer
Ecchymosis	Perspiration
Edema	Psychosis
Electrolyte disorder (NA ↑, K↓)	Pulmonary embolus
Glaucoma	Skin fragility
Hirsutism	Striae
Hot flashes	Thrombosis
Hyperlipidemia	Vasculitis

carbohydrate, fat, and protein metabolism as well the lenses in eyes, intraocular pressure, and bone and skin changes (Table 20-11). The use of corticosteroids needs to be approached cautiously in the elderly, where these side effects are more serious.

Drug interactions *Hypoglycemics* cause increases in blood glucose, thus countering their effects.

NSAIDs may enhance ulcerogenic potential or other ulcerogenic drugs.

Digitalis may cause hypokalemia, thus increasing toxicity to digitalis drugs.

Diuretics: When corticosteroids are used with diuretics, severe hypokalemia may occur.

Gold

Gold is available in parenteral and oral preparations. Gold sodium thiomalate, aurothioglucose, and the oral auranofin are slow acting anti-inflammatory compounds constituting one of the classes of drugs that have been shown to inhibit radiographic erosions in rheumatoid arthritis.[29] These agents can suppress or prevent arthritis but do not cure rheumatoid arthritis.

Pharmacologic action The exact mechanism of action of gold is not known. Gold is taken up by macrophages, which results in inhibition of phagocytosis and lysosomal membrane stabilization. This action, therefore, suppresses immune responsiveness. Also, decreased serum concentrations of rheumatoid factor and immunoglobulins have been observed. Other mechanisms of action have been proposed but are not well documented or accepted: interference with complement activation, prostaglandin synthesis inhibition, and interference with lysosomal enzyme activity.[21]

Pharmacokinetics Parenteral gold preparations deliver 50% gold content and result in peak serum concentrations in 2 to 6 h. Serum protein (albumin) binding is 95 to 99 percent with these preparations; excretion is 70 percent in urine and 30 percent in feces. Oral gold delivers 29% gold content and is only 25 percent absorbed. Oral gold reaches peak concentration in serum between 1 and 2 h and is 60 percent bound to albumin. Oral gold is excreted via urine and feces as well. Due to low bioavailability, fecal excretion of oral gold is 85 to 95 percent where that which is absorbed (15 percent) is 60 percent excreted in urine.[21]

Gold distributes widely in body tissues, but the highest concentrations are found in the reticuloendothelial system and both adrenal and renal cortices. Arthritic joints have more gold accumulation than normal joints. Although oral gold results in similar serum concentrations to parenteral, the accumulation of gold over a 6-month period of treatment is only 20 percent of that seen parenterally.[21] There is no correlation to response or toxicity with serum concentrations. The excretion of gold is augmented by dimercaprol and penicillamine, which may be used to speed removal if toxicity is encountered.

Adverse drug reactions About 35 percent of patients receiving gold therapy experience toxicity. A majority of toxic effects are minor, such as skin rash, mouth ulceration, and abnormal urinalysis. These adverse reactions may not require discontinuation of gold therapy.

Skin rashes include maculopapular, petechial, exfoliative, lichen planus, and pityriasis rosealike rashes. Most are pruritic. Some patients experience a metallic taste. For some patients, gold therapy can be reinstituted in low doses without recurrence of rashes.

Since gold causes bone marrow suppression, immune thrombocytopenia, agranulocytosis, anemia, and aplastic anemia are possible as well as potentially fatal. Fortunately, thrombocytopenia occurs in only 1 to 3 percent of patients, and other bone marrow effects are less common.

Proteinuria is common and is usually mild. Nephrotic syndrome and glomerulitis with proteinuria and hematuria may develop. Mild problems respond to readjustments in dose, whereas more severe reactions require discontinuation of the drug.

Rare side effects in the form of interstitial pneumonitis and fibrosis can occur. Patients who develop fever, cough, shortness of breath, rash, and mouth ulcers may have widespread interstitial infiltrates. Pulmonary symptoms may not resolve with drug discontinuation. Other reported toxicity includes deposition of gold in eyes and skin (chrysiasis), hepatitis, and peripheral neuropathy. Nitroid reactions resemble anaphylactoid effects with flushing, dizziness, sweating, and occasionally syncope. Rarely, true anaphylaxis occurs. Studies have shown that patients given aqueous solutions of gold have more common nitroid reactions, skin eruptions, and albuminuria. Use of the oil suspension of aurothioglucose may decrease these reactions.

Drug interactions The use of gold with immunosuppressants, phenylbutazone, oxyphenbutazone, and antimalarials is discouraged since the agents all may cause bone marrow suppression. Gold is chelated by penicillamine and, therefore, not given concomitantly in treatment.

Penicillamine

Penicillamine is an agent which has been used to chelate copper in Wilson's disease but has been proven effective in rheumatoid arthritis. This agent is used as a second-line drug in the therapy of rheumatoid arthritis. However, it is commonly considered after a course of gold therapy has been intolerable or has failed.[35]

Pharmacologic action The mechanism of action of penicillamine is poorly understood. This agent affects the immune system by decreasing IgM rheumatoid factor. Other serum immunoglobulins are unaffected. Also, penicillamine selectively inhibits T-lymphocyte function, thereby decreasing cell-mediated immune response. Response may take 2 to 3 months.

Pharmacokinetics Penicillamine is well absorbed from the gastrointestinal tract, with peak serum concentrations reached within 2 to 3 hours. Penicillamine is 80 percent bound to albumin. Steady-state serum concentrations rise slowly with prolonged therapy as well as decline slowly after discontinuation of penicillamine therapy, suggesting extensive tissue distribution.[35]

Penicillamine is extensively metabolized with little unchanged drug excreted in the urine. A biphasic elimination exists with a rapid elimination half-life of 1 to 5 h and a slow elimination phase with a half-life of 4 to 8 days.[35] This helps explain the reason one observes a slow rise in steady-state serum concentrations over prolonged therapy.

Adverse drug reactions Mild renal toxicity occurs in 10 to 30 percent of patients. Proteinuria may be mild and self-limited but should necessitate discontinuation of the drug if it is greater than 2 g/24 Bu. Hematuria may also occur. Proteinuria may be prolonged after discontinuation of the drug. Nephrotic syndrome has been relatively common. Renal toxicity is caused by an immune complex glomerulonephritis. Leukopenia (2 percent), thrombocytopenia (4 percent), and aplastic anemias (<0.1 percent) are potential serious side effects. A white blood cell (WBC) count of less than 3500/mm^3 or an absolute neutrophil count below 2000/mm^3 requires permanent withdrawal of the drug.

Mild skin rashes have frequently been reported with penicillamine. Should these reactions become persistent or serious, the drug should be discontinued. Hypogeusia, a decrease in taste perception, usually occurs during the first 6 weeks of therapy. Rashes and taste abnormalities occur more frequently in elderly than in younger adults, whereas leukopenia, thrombocytopenia, and proteinuria appear equally in young and old adults.[36] Since toxicity appears dose related, it is recommended not to exceed a dose of 750 mg/day in the elderly.

Other autoimmune adverse effects have been reported, including Goodpasture's syndrome, thyroiditis, pemphigus, systemic lupus erythematosus, myasthenia gravis, and obliterative bronchiolitis. Approximately 10 percent of patients with hypersensitivity to penicillin will have a cross-reaction with penicillamine. However, a history of penicillin allergy is not a contraindication to penicillamine use.

Drug interactions Penicillamine chelates heavy metals. Food may inhibit its absorption due to this action. Also, iron deficiency anemia may be precipitated. This drug should be used cautiously with other bone marrow suppressants. Due to the drug's interaction with pyridoxine (vitamin B_6), isoniazid peripheral neuritis is more frequent since both drugs react with the vitamin.

Immunosuppressives

A brief summary of pharmacologic actions, pharmacokinetics, and adverse effects of immunosuppressive drugs is presented here in that their use in the elderly is essentially no different than in younger adults.

Pharmacologic action The mechanisms of action of these agents remains unknown in regard to their pharmacologic action in rheumatoid arthritis. Azathioprine, which is metabolized to 6-mercaptopurine, inhibits purine synthesis and inhibits nucleotide interconversion in nucleic acid synthesis. Cyclophosphamide and chlorambucil bind to cellular macromolecules and cross-link DNA strands, thereby impairing DNA replication. Methotrexate, a folic acid antagonist, binds to folate reductase, which inhibits DNA synthesis. Obviously, tissues most susceptible to the cytotoxic effects of these agents are those undergoing rapid cellular turnover: Bone marrow, hair, bladder, and intestinal and buccal mucosal cells.

Pharmacokinetics Azathioprine is well absorbed with peak serum concentrations occurring within 2 h. It is 30 percent bound to plasma proteins and has a half-life of 1 to 1½ h. The drug is hepatically metabolized by xanthine oxidase, and its metabolites are excreted in the urine. Patients receiving allopurinol should have their azathioprine dose reduced by two-thirds to avoid serious toxicity due to inhibition of xanthine oxidase by allopurinol.[36]

Methotrexate absorption after oral administration appears to be dose dependent, indicating a saturable absorption mechanism. Doses at or below 30 mg/m^2 are well absorbed with an approximate bioavailability of 60 percent. Up to 35 percent of methotrexate administered orally may be degraded in the gastrointestinal tract. Peak methotrexate serum concentrations are reached 1 to 2 h following oral or IM administration. Methotrexate undergoes hepatic and intracellular biotransformation to polyglutamated forms which can be converted back to methotrexate by hydrolysis. Elimination is primarily renal (80 to 90 percent of administered dose) in unchanged form, but biliary (approximately 10 percent) and fecal eliminations contribute to excretion. Plasma half-life is dose dependent. With doses less than 30 mg/m^2, the half-life range is 3 to 10 h.[21,35,37]

Adverse drug reactions (Table 20-7) Bone marrow suppression is a common toxicity with all cytotoxic drugs. Leukopenia and thrombocytopenia are the most common expressions of toxicity and often occur together.[37] Susceptibility to infection is increased with cytotoxic agents, which is attributable to their impact in the immune system: Alterations in both humoral and cell-mediated immunity as well as suppression of granulocytes and inflammatory response.[37] Infection rates increase for both normal and unusual bacterial infections. There is a significant increase in the incidence of herpes zoster infections with these agents. Given the decline in cell-mediated immunity with age, one should be cautious when initiating cytotoxic therapy in the elderly.

Rashes may occur with cytotoxic agents. These are usually mild and generally do not require discontinuation of therapy.

Gastrointestinal side effects are common. The most frequent and common symptoms are nausea, vomiting, and diarrhea. Pancreatitis has been reported with azathioprine.[37]

Chronic pulmonary fibrosis is an insidious but rare adverse effect which may occur with cytotoxic agents. Patients will present with a dry cough, dyspnea, fever, and malaise.[35,37]

Hepatic damage is most commonly encountered with the use of azathioprine and methotrexate. Azathioprine causes a hypersensitivity hepatitis manifested by cholestasis and jaundice. Methotrexate causes a hepatic fibrosis or cirrhosis. Abnormal, transient elevations of liver function tests occur with methotrexate in patients with or without fibrosis or cirrhosis. Unfortunately, the fibrosis or cirrhosis occurs without clinical or laboratory signs of the disease. This had led some clinicians to suggest liver biopsy when cumulative methotrexate doses reach 1.0 to 1.5 g, although we do not follow this procedure except in high-risk patients.[37] Oral ulceration and stomatitis occur most frequently with methotrexate and will generally resolve with dose reduction or discontinuation of the agent. Azathioprine has also been shown to produce oral side effects but at a rate of 5 percent or less.[37]

Alopecia most commonly occurs with cyclophosphamide followed by chlorambucil and methotrexate in this order. Hair loss may be complete or incomplete, and hair growth will return after discontinuation of the agent. Cystitis is a common adverse effect to cyclophosphamide and appears primarily limited to this cytotoxic agent. As many as one-third of patients receiving cyclophosphamide orally on a daily basis develop hemorrhagic cystitis. This complication is thought to be due to the metabolite acrolein rather than the parent drug itself. Also, bladder fibrosis and carcinoma have been associated with this agent but at a lower incidence. These adverse effects could be reduced by administering the dose in the morning and having the patient drink large amounts of fluids (10 to 12 glasses) daily. This will not only dilute the offending metabolite but cause frequent voiding, thereby decreasing bladder exposure.[37] Mesna has also been used concomitantly to decrease the toxicity.

An acute pneumonitis which begins abruptly and without warning occurs early with methotrexate therapy. This is not a dose-related disease. Histologically, infiltrates of mononuclear cells in association with eosinophils and plasmacytes are found in interstitial spaces and in alveolar spaces. Usually prompt recovery occurs with methotrexate discontinuation. However, up to 10 percent with or without corticosteroid treatment die as a result of this complication. Less than 10 percent will develop the reaction again upon rechallenge.[37]

Azoospermia is observed with chlorambucil and cyclophosphamide. This could be a concern for a few older males with young, childbearing-age, female partners. Neoplasia is a potential and major concern with the use of cytotoxic agents. Methotrexate appears to lack evidence for carcinogenesis, whereas the others have documented neoplastic adverse effects, primarily in the hematopoietic and lymphatic systems. There exists a controversy since some studies indicate an increased risk for Hodgkin's and non-Hodgkin's lymphoma, multiple myeloma, and leukemia in rheumatoid arthritis patients untreated with cytotoxic agents. Azathioprine and cyclophosphamide appear to have the highest risk for the development of non-Hodgkin's lymphoproliferative disorders, with a relative risk of 13.5 for azathioprine and 13.0 for cyclophosphamide.[37]

Drug interactions These agents should not be administered with other bone-marrow-suppressing agents or immunosuppressants. Azathioprine should have its dose reduced one-half to two-thirds its usual dose when administered with allopurinol due to the latter's inhibition of xanthine oxidase. Also, allopurinol may be associated with increased frequency of bone marrow suppression due to cyclophosphamide when given concomitantly with this cytotoxic. The mechanism for this enhancement is not understood.[31] Methotrexate renal tubular secretion may be blocked by salicylates. This reaction may also occur with diuretics.[31]

Antimalarials

Chloroquine phosphate and hydroxychloroquine sulfate are useful treatments of RA as well as joint and skin manifestations of systemic lupus erythematosus.

Pharmacologic action The mechanism of action of these agents is not fully understood. Proposed mechanisms of action are inhibition of nucleic acid and protein synthesis, prostaglandin inhibition, stabilization of lysosomal membranes, inhibition of phagocytosis and chemotaxis, alterations in antibody production, and depression of lymphocyte and monocyte function.

Pharmacokinetics These agents are readily absorbed from the gastrointestinal tract and are about 55 percent bound to plasma protein. Considerable tissue deposition occurs in the retina, liver, spleen, kidneys, lungs, and leukocytes. Lesser amounts are concentrated in the CNS. Degradation to carboxyl acid derivatives and other metabolic products occurs, but 70 percent of the drug is excreted unchanged in the urine. With single doses, the half-life approaches 3 days, but with daily doses, the half-life increases to 6 to 7 days or longer. Small amounts are present in the urine for years after long-term treatment.

Adverse drug reactions The most feared side effect is ocular damage. This includes ciliary dysfunction (with blurred vision caused by accommodation defects), corneal edema, punctate opacities (deposition of drug), macular edema and pigmentation, increased recovery time to bright-light exposure, increased threshold to red light in the macula, optic disc pallor, retinal deposits, and visual field defects. The symptoms include blurred vision, reading difficulties, scotomas, and blindness. For these reasons, baseline and periodic eye examination should be done, especially since elderly have significant eye changes which occur with aging. One would not want to discount an adverse effect to aging changes.

Skin rash and bleaching of the hair are common. Aplasia of the bone marrow or single-element cellular suppression occurs rarely. Patients with glucose-6-phosphate dehydrogenase deficiency react to these drugs with hemolytic anemia. Gastrointestinal side effects of anorexia, nausea, vomiting, diarrhea, and abdominal cramps are not uncommon. Because antimalarials may flare the skin disease itself, they should usually not be used in the treatment of psoriatic arthritis.

Drug interactions Antimalarial diseases may potentiate marrow suppressants and folic acid antagonists. Cimetidine may reduce the clearance and metabolism of chloroquine. Kaolin and magnesium trisilicate may decrease the absorption of these agents.

Colchicine

Colchicine has been used to treat gout since 1763.

Pharmacologic action The exact mechanism of action for its use in gout is unknown. Proposed mechanisms of action include inhibition in leukocyte migration, disappearance of microtubules resulting in decreased lactate production therapy decreasing uric acid crystal deposition, interference with kinin production, and reduction of phagocytosis.

Pharmacokinetics Colchicine is rapidly absorbed after oral administration. Metabolism by deacetylation occurs in the liver, and the metabolites are excreted in the bile and undergo enterohepatic cycling. IV colchicine leaves the blood within minutes and is widely distributed within a 30-min period. Serum concentrations of single doses decrease after 60 min and then increase due to reabsorption from enterohepatic circulation. Excretion in urine is variable, and most of the drug is excreted in the stool.

Adverse drug reactions Colchicine appears to be more toxic in aged or debilitated patients, particularly those with renal, gastrointestinal, or cardiac disease. The most predictable and common side effects of the oral drug are gastrointestinal: vomiting, abdominal pain, and nausea, especially at maximum doses. This provides the clinician with a margin of safety since gastrointestinal toxicity usually denotes therapeutic concentrations of the drug and occurs before more serious side effects appear. Thus, if one discontinues colchicine at this point, bone marrow suppression will be avoided. The onset of toxicity after IV colchicine may be delayed. Again, gastrointestinal difficulties may be apparent and may be followed by vascular damage, shock, and occasionally death. Bone marrow suppression is manifested by agranulocytosis, thrombocytopenia, and aplastic anemia. Other reported side effects are peripheral neuritis, purpura, myopathy, hair loss, dermatoses, and rarely hypersensitivity.

Drug interactions Colchicine induces a reversible malabsorption of pyridoxine (vitamin B_6) by altering the function of the ileal mucosa. Also, in general, colchicine may enhance the sensitivity to CNS depressants. Additionally, colchicine may elevate alkaline phosphatase and serum aminotransferases.

Uricosurics

The idea to use agents to increase uric acid secretion began in 1877, when it was noted that high doses of aspirin enhanced loss of uric acid into the urine. Many agents are uricosuric in action, but the most commonly used is probenecid.

Pharmacologic action Both probenecid and sulfinpyrazone block postsecretory reabsorption of uric acid by the renal tubule, thereby increasing the excretion of secreted urate. Probenecid also inhibits tubular secretion of most penicillins and cephalosporins, resulting in a twofold increase in serum antibiotic concentrations.

Pharmacokinetics Probenecid is well absorbed from the gastrointestinal tract and produces peak serum concentrations in 2 to 4 hours. Uricosuric action begins as early as 40 min after a single oral dose. At therapeutic levels, the drug is approximately bound 90 percent to albumin. Serum half-life is 4 to 12 h, which is dose dependent, since doses over 2 g exhibit half-lives over 8 h, in contrast with lower doses having a half-life of approximately 4 to 5 h. This indicates a saturable metabolic pathway. Probenecid is metabolized by hydroxylation to active metabolites which are excreted in the urine.

Adverse drug reactions Probenecid is well tolerated and free of serious side effects. The most common complaints are gastrointestinal disturbances, anorexia, nausea, and vomiting. These occur in approximately 5 percent of patients taking probenecid and 10 to 15 percent of those receiving sulfinpyrazone. Many of these side effects may be lessened if taken with food or antacids. Other, less frequent side effects are rash, fever, anemia, leukopenia, agranulocytosis, thrombocytopenia, and renal failure.

Urate nephrolithiasis can occur with the use of uricosurics. In order to minimize this problem, patients who are hyperuricemic secondary to excessive uric acid production should be identified. As described in gout, all patients utilizing these drugs should be well hydrated.

Drug interactions In general, any drug which is secreted into renal tubules could interact with these agents. Probenecid is known to interfere with tubular excretion of salicylates, pyrazinamide, methotrexate, penicillins, cephalosporins, sulfonylureas, naproxen, indomethacin, rifampin, para-aminosalicylic acid (PAS), dyphylline, dapsone, and clofibrate. Therefore, to minimize potential toxicities of these drugs due to increased serum concentrations, close monitoring and dose reduction may be necessary.

Allopurinol

For patients who produce excess uric acid from purine metabolism, allopurinol and its active metabolite, oxypurinol, are indicated to prevent gout and calcium oxalate calculi. Also, the drug is used to prevent acute rises in uric acid in the treatment of malignancies.

Pharmacologic action Allopurinol and its metabolite, oxypurinol, competitively inhibit xanthine oxidase. Allopurinol is 5 to 10 times as potent as oxypurinol. However, xanthine oxidase metabolizes allopurinol to oxypurinol. Allopurinol is bound to xanthine oxidase more avidly (15 times) than is xanthine. Administration of allopurinol results in a significant reduction in both serum and urinary uric acid concentrations within 2 to 3 days. The magnitude of decline is dose dependent, and a week or more may be required before full therapeutic effect is noted.[21]

Pharmacokinetics Allopurinol is well absorbed from the gastrointestinal tract with a 90 percent bioavailability. Peak serum concentrations are achieved in 2 to 3 h for allopurinol and 4.5 h for oxypurinol. Allopurinol has a half-life of 1 to 2 h, but its active metabolite, oxypurinol, has a half-life of approximately 15 to 30 h. Allopurinol is excreted primarily by renal filtration. However, oxypurinol is filtered and subsequently reabsorbed in the renal tubule. Interestingly, uricosurics enhance the clearance rate of oxypurinol.

Since this drug and its active metabolite are renally cleared, it is imperative to adjust the dose based upon creatinine clearance. This is particularly important in the elderly, who frequently have age-related decline in creatinine clearance (Cl_{cr}).[38] In general, most elderly will only require 100 to 150 mg daily. Should one fail to take into account creatinine clearance, toxicity may result from accumulation. A severe life-threatening toxicity syndrome has been reported consisting of an erythematous desquamative skin rash, fever, hepatitis, eosinophilia, and worsening renal function.[38]

Adverse drug reactions Allopurinol is generally well tolerated with the most common problem being precipitation of acute gouty attacks. This initial effect may be minimized by treating with reduced doses and using prophylactic colchicine. Maculopapular, pruritic rashes occur in 5 to 10 percent of patients taking allopurinol. Gastrointestinal symptoms occur at the same rate and generally include nausea, diarrhea, gastritis, dyspepsia, and abdominal pain. Other side effects occur but are uncommon or rare.

Drug interactions *Thiazide diuretics*: The mechanism is unclear, but these diuretics may enhance allopurinol toxicity.[31]

6-MP or azathioprine: Xanthine oxidase inhibition results in decreased clearance of the cytotoxic agents. Dose of cytotoxic agent should be reduced one-fourth to one-third usual dose.

Ampicillin/Amoxicillin: Concomitant administration with allopurinol results in increased skin rash incidence.

REFERENCES

1. Gall EP: Introduction and classification of rheumatic diseases, in Gall EP (ed): *Symposium on Rheumatic Diseases—Primary Care*, Vol 11. Philadelphia, Saunders, 1984, pp 201-209.
2. Ruffatti A, Rossi L, Calligaro A, et al: Autoantibodies of systemic rheumatic diseases in the healthy elderly. *Gerontology* 36:104-111, 1990.
3. Arnett FC, Edworthy SM, Bloch DA: The 1987 Revised American Rheumatism Association Criteria for the Classification of Rheumatoid Arthritis. *Arthritis Rheum* 31: 315-324, 1988.
4. Wolfe AM: The epidemiology of rheumatoid arthritis: A review. *Bull Rheum Dis* 19: 518-521, 1968.
5. Yocum DE: Pathogenesis in rheumatoid arthritis, in Schumacher HR, Gall EP (eds): *Rheumatoid Arthritis, An Illustrated Guide To Pathology, Diagnosis and Management*. Philadelphia, Lippincott, 1988, chap 5, pp 5.1-5.20.
6. Wilski KR, Healy LA: Remodeling the pyramid—a concept whose time has come. *J Rheumatol* 16: 565-567, 1989.
7. Wilder RL, Case JP, Croford LJ, et al: Endothelial cells and the pathogenesis of rheumatoid arthritis in humans and streptococcal cell wall arthritis in Lewis rats. *J Cell Biochem* 45: 162-166, 1991.
8. Hess EV, Luggen ME: Remodeling the pyramid—a concept whose time has not yet come. *J Rheumatol* 16: 1175-1176, 1989.
9. Schlegel SI: General characteristics of nonsteroidal antiinflammatory drugs, in Paulus HE, First DE, Dromgoole SH (eds): *Drugs for Rheumatic Disease*. New York, Churchill, Livingstone, 1987, pp 203-226.
10. Sigler JW, Bluhm GB, Duncan H: Gold salts in the treatment of rheumatoid arthritis, a double blind study. *Ann Int Med* 80: 21-26, 1974.
11. Epstein W, Hewke CJ, Yelin EH, Katz PP: Effect of parenterally administered gold therapy on the course of adult rheumatoid arthritis. *Ann Intern Med* 114: 437-444, 1991.
12. Huskisson EC, Gibson TJ, Balme HW, et al: Penicillamine and gold in rheumatoid arthritis. *Ann Rheum Dis* 33: 532-535, 1974.
13. Kremer JM, Lee JK: A long term prospective study of the use of methotrexate in rheumatoid arthritis: update after a mean of 53 months. *Arthritis Rheum* 31: 577-584, 1988.
14. Aponte J, Petrelli M: Histopathologic findings in the liver of rheumatoid arthritis patients treated with long term bolus methotrexate. *Arthritis Rheum* 31: 1457-1464, 1988.

15. Bersten CA, Freyberg RH: Rheumatoid patients after 5 or more years of corticosteroid treatment: A comparative analysis of 183 cases. *Ann Intern Med* 54: 938–953, 1961.
16. Harris ED: Management of rheumatoid arthritis, in Kelley WM, Harris ED, Ruddy S, Sledge CB (eds): *Textbook of Rheumatology*, 3d ed. Philadelphia, W.B. Saunders, 1989, pp 982–992.
17. Knowlton RG, Katzenstein PL, Moskowitz RW, et al: Genetic linkage of a polymorphism in the type II procollagen gene to primary osteoarthritis associated with mild chondroplasia. *N Engl J Med* 322: 526–530, 1990.
18. McCarty DJ, Kohn NN, Faires JS: The significance of calcium phosphate crystals in synovial fluid of arthritis patients: "The pseudogout syndrome" I: Clinical aspects. *Ann Intern Med* 56: 711–737, 1962.
19. McCarty DJ et al: Milwaukee shoulder: Associating of mirrospheroids containing hydroxyapatite crystals, active collagenase and neutral protease with rotator cuff defects. *Arthritis Rheum* 24: 464–473, 1981.
20. Stankebaum GA, Wilkens RF: Treatment of arthritis in the elderly, in Vestal RE (ed): *Drug Treatment in the Elderly*. Sidney, Australia, ADIS Health Science, 1984, pp 175–186.
21. Flower RJ, Moncada S, Vane JR: Analgesic-antipyretics and anti-inflammatory agents: drugs employed in the treatment of gout, in Gilman AG, Goodman LS, Wall TW, Murad F (eds): *The Pharmacologic Basis of Therapeutics*, 7th ed. New York, McMillan, 1985, pp 674–715.
22. Weismann G. Aspirin. *Sci Am* 264: 84–90, 1991.
23. Wallace S, Whiting B, Runcie J: Factors affecting drug binding in plasma of elderly patients. *Br J Clin Pharmacol* 3: 327–330, 1976.
24. Davies DF, Shock NW: Age changes in glomerular filtration rate, effective renal plasma level and tubular excretory capacity in adult males. *Clin Invest* 29: 496–501, 1950.
25. Graham DY: Prevention of gastroduodenal injury induced by chronic nonsteroidal anti-inflammatory drug therapy. *Gastroenterology* 96: 675–681, 1989.
26. Knodel LC: Preventing NSAID-induced ulcers: the role of misoprostol. *Consult Pharm* 4: 37–41, 1989.
27. Silverstein FE, Kimmey MB, Saunders DR, et al: Gastric protection by misoprostol against 1399 mg of aspirin: An endoscopic study. *Drug Dis Sci* 31(2 suppl): 137S–141S, 1989.
28. Clinch D, Banerjee AK, Ostick G: Absence of abdominal pain in elderly patients with peptic ulcer. *Age Aging* 13: 120–123, 1984.
29. Pounder R: Silent peptic ulceration: deadly silence or golden silence? *Gastroenterology* 96: 626–631, 1989.
30. Schlegel SI: General characteristics of nonsteroidal anti-inflammatory drugs, in Paulus HE, Furst DE, Dromgoole SH (eds): *Drugs for Rheumatic Disease*. New York, Churchill Livingstone, 1987, pp 203–226.
31. Hansten PD, Horn JR: *Drug Interactions*, looseleaf edition. Philadelphia, Lea & Febiger, 1990, pp 519–595.
32. Conn HO, Blitzer BL: Nonassociation of adrenocorticosteroid therapy and peptic ulcer. *N Engl J Med* 294: 473–478, 1976.
33. Hurt DF, Huskisson EC: Nonsteroidal anti-inflammatory drugs: Current status and rational therapeutic use. *Drugs* 27: 232–255, 1984.
34. Farici AS, Dole DC, Balow JE: Glucocorticosteroid therapy: mechanisms of action and clinical considerations. *Ann Intern Med* 84: 304–314, 1976.
35. Schuna AA, Vejraska BD: Rheumatoid arthritis and the seronegative spondyloarthropathies, in Dipiro JT, Talbert RL, Hayes PE, et al (eds): *Pharmacotherapy: A Pathophysiologic Approach*. New York, Elsevier Science, 1989, pp 881–898.
36. Stein HB, Patterson AC, Offer RC, et al: Adverse effects of D-penicillamine in rheumatoid arthritis. *Ann Intern Med* 92: 24–29, 1980.
37. Clements PJ: Cytotoxic immunosuppressive drugs, in Paulus HE, Furst DE, Dromgoole SH, (eds): *Drugs for Rheumatic Disease*. New York, Churchill Livingstone, 1987, pp 135–155.
38. Hande KR, Noone RM, Stone WJ: Severe allopurinol toxicity: description and guidelines for prevention in patients with renal insufficiency. *Am J Med* 76: 47–56, 1984.

CHAPTER

21

DRUG THERAPY OF AIRWAYS OBSTRUCTIVE DISEASES

John W. Bloom
Alan D. Barreuther

As one grows older, a relatively subtle decline in lung function occurs as part of the normal aging process. The effects of aging on the respiratory system in the adult result in a loss of elastic recoil of the lung, changes in the subdivisions of lung volume [decrease in the forced expiratory volume in 1 s (FEV_1) and vital capacity], a decrease in the maximum expiratory flow, and a decrease in the arterial P_{O_2}.[1] The decrease in the vital capacity with aging was first described in 1846 by John Hutchison. From cross-sectional and longitudinal studies of lung function, a picture of the growth and decline in lung function with age is apparent.[1] As shown in Fig. 21-1, the vital capacity increases in early life, reaching a peak at about age 20. For the next two decades, there is a plateau in the vital capacity followed by a decline that is apparent at about 40 years of age. After this point, vital capacity continues to decline at a rate that increases as one ages. The decline in the FEV_1 over time follows a similar pattern as the vital capacity. The changes that occur as a result of aging are similar to the changes that occur with disease. Nevertheless, the changes that occur with aging alone do not produce respiratory symptoms unless there are disease-associated decreases in lung function. However, in the elderly the lung function changes associated with respiratory disease have a greater impact when superimposed on the normal decline associated with aging.

Airways obstruction is the most common chronic respiratory problem in the elderly. Airways obstructive diseases have been divided into broad categories based primarily on the degree of reversibility. Reversible disorders are generally classified as asthma, and those that are more persistent or progressive, primarily chronic

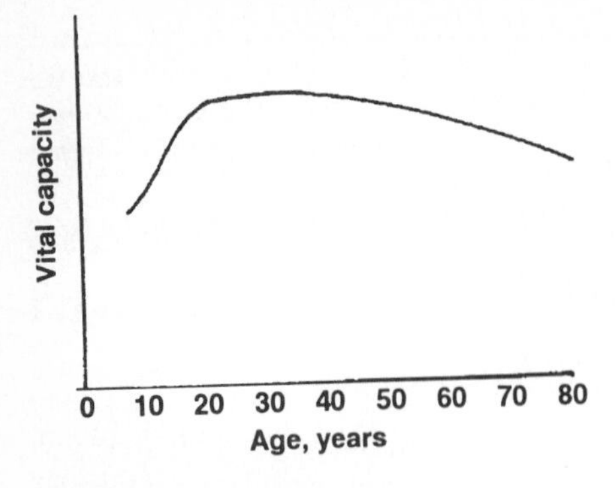

Figure 21-1 Change in vital capacity with age. (From Knudson RJ: Physiology of the aging lung, in Crystal RG, West JB, et al (eds): *The Lung: Scientific Foundations*. New York, Raven, 1991, pp 1749–1759. Used with permission.)

obstructive bronchitis and emphysema, are termed chronic obstructive pulmonary disease (COPD). The hallmark of asthma is bronchial hyperresponsiveness to various nonspecific stimuli. There is a relationship between the degree of bronchial hyperresponsiveness and the severity of asthma. It has recently been recognized that chronic asthma involves a characteristic inflammatory response in the airways.[2,3] The current belief is that bronchial hyperresponsiveness is a consequence of this inflammatory response in the airways which may be the result of allergic mechanisms. A major risk factor for asthma is the serum immunoglobulin E (IgE) level.[4] The overall prevalence of asthma is related closely to the serum IgE level, even in individuals with negative skin tests for common aeroallergens. In contrast, COPD results from irritant-induced irreversible damage. Destruction of lung parenchyma leading to loss of lung recoil and secondary persistent airflow limitation is diagnosed as emphysema. Chronic obstructive bronchitis is often used to describe persistent airflow limitation resulting from extensive inflammatory and obliterative changes in the small airways. Because emphysema and chronic obstructive bronchitis usually coexist in an individual patient, the term COPD is commonly used. The major risk factor for COPD is cigarette smoking. Smoking causes an acceleration in the usual rate of decline in the FEV_1 associated with aging. There is a close relationship between the degree of decrease in FEV_1 and the pack-years of smoking.[5]

It is often difficult to determine whether the practitioner is dealing with a persistent form of asthma or with a partially reversible form of COPD. This is an especially important problem in the elderly. Chronic asthma can progress to irreversible airway obstruction even in nonsmokers.[6] This irreversible obstruction is possibly the result of long-standing inflammation associated with asthma that leads to subepithelial fibrosis in the airways.[7] The degree of airway obstruction in asthmatic patients is related to the severity and duration of asthma. Indeed, elderly asthmatics have been shown to have severe disease with more marked ventilatory impairment than younger asthmatics.[8] Furthermore, in the elderly asthmatic patient, the degree of impairment is related to the duration of disease. Thus, long-standing asthma in the elderly patient commonly results in persistent airway obstruction that mimics COPD.[9] Therapeutically, the distinction between asthma and COPD may be important because of the current emphasis on anti-inflammatory treatment of asthma.[10] It has been suggested that the regular use of anti-inflammatory agents in asthma may lead to a reduction in the morbidity associated with this disease.[11] In addition, it is clear that the rate of progression and mortality are much less in patients with typical asthma compared to those with COPD associated with cigarette smoking.[12]

A large proportion of patients with airways obstructive diseases are elderly. The diagnosis of COPD is usually not made until the sixth or seventh decade, unless there is some underlying host risk factor such as $alpha_1$-antitrypsin deficiency. The mean age of individuals with chronic airway obstruction in a large study of a general population was over 65 years.[13] Although the onset of asthma often occurs in childhood or early adult life, asthma is not uncommon in the geriatric population. In a longitudinal study of a general population sample in Tucson, Arizona, asthma was present in 3.8 percent of men and 7.1 percent of women over age 65.[8] An additional 4.1 percent of men in this age group reported having asthma, but they had smoked heavily and were diagnosed as having emphysema also. The age of onset of asthma was over 40 years in 52 percent of the cases. Although the study in Tucson may overestimate the prevalence of asthma because of in-migration of individuals with respiratory disease, it does demonstrate that the prevalence of asthma in the adult population is constant and does not decline in the elderly. In another population survey in Wales,[13] 2.9 percent of individuals over age 70 had current symptomatic asthma and an additional 3.6 percent had mild asthma or a history of asthma. Recent data from the Tucson study show that it is not uncommon for the diagnosis of asthma to be made in the elderly.[14] Of 1185 subjects who denied ever having asthma on enrollment, 40 (3.4 percent) reported a new diagnosis of asthma after age 60 (average age 71 years).

This chapter focuses on pharmacologic therapy of airways obstructive diseases in the elderly. Obviously, an accurate diagnosis is necessary, and evaluation should include a chest radiograph and pulmonary function testing. In the elderly patient with new onset of wheezing or dyspnea, causes other than asthma (e.g., congestive heart failure, pulmonary embolism, or mechanical obstruction of the airways) or COPD should also be considered. In addition to drug therapy, treatment should be comprehensive and should include exercise and rehabilitation, smoking cessation, weight control, and education for adjustment to limitations.

BRONCHODILATORS

Drugs for airways obstructive diseases can be divided into broad categories of bronchodilators and anti-inflammatory agents. Bronchodilators, which include β-adrenergic agonists, theophylline, and anticholinergic agents, act primarily to relax airway smooth muscle, although theophylline may have minor anti-inflammatory effects in the airways and β-adrenergic agonists stabilize mast cells.

β-Adrenergic Agonists

β-Adrenergic agonists are effective bronchodilators and are the cornerstone of therapy in asthmatic patients. These agents act by stimulating β_2-adrenergic receptors in airway smooth muscle.[15] This stimulation activates adenyl cyclase, which results in an increase in cyclic adenosine monophosphate (AMP), activation of protein kinase A, and relaxation of airway smooth muscle. In addition, β-adrenergic agonists may inhibit release of mediators from mast cells in the airways by activating β_2 receptors on these cells and increasing mucociliary clearance in the airways. Their activity is facilitated by corticosteroids possibly by up-regulation of β_2 receptors. Because the therapeutic effects of these agents are mediated entirely through β_2-adrenergic receptors, there is no indication for the use of the nonselective β-adrenergic agonists, such as isoproterenol, which are associated with cardiovascular side effects due to stimulation of β_1-adrenergic receptors in the heart. The β_2-adrenergic receptor agonists are only relatively selective; at larger doses, β_1 receptors are also activated. Selective β_2-adrenergic agonists (see Table 21-1) have an onset of action within minutes when given by inhalation and are effective for 3 to 6 h. The rapid onset of action with these agents makes them the choice for therapy of acute episodes of wheezing and dyspnea. β-Adrenergic agonists are also useful in prevention of bronchoconstriction resulting from exercise and other stimuli.

The mode of administration of β-adrenergic agents is extremely important. The inhaled route is preferable to oral administration. When the oral route of administration was compared to inhaled using a metered-dose inhaler (MDI), the inhaled route produced more rapid and more effective bronchodilation with fewer

Table 21-1 β_2-Adrenergic bronchodilators available in United States

Drug	Dosage form	Strengths
Metaproterenol (Alupent)	Tablets	10 mg and 20 mg
	Oral solution	10 mg/5 mL
	MDI	650 μg/spray
	Nebulizer solution	5%
Terbutaline (Bricanyl, Brethaire)	Tablets	2.5 mg and 5 mg
	MDI	200 μg/spray
	Injection	1 mg/mL
Albuterol (Proventil, Ventolin)	Tablets	2 mg and 4 mg
		4-mg extended release
	Oral solution	2 mg/5 mL
	MDI	90 μg/spray
	Dry Powder Rotohaler	200 μg/capsule
	Nebulizer solution	0.5% (5 mg/mL)
Bitolterol (Tornolate)	MDI	370 μg/spray
Pirbuterol (Maxair)	MDI	200 μg/spray

systemic side effects such as tremor, nervousness, and palpitations.[16] A theoretical problem with the inhaled route of administration is that the bronchodilating agent may not reach the peripheral airways, especially if acute bronchospasm is present. However, even in acute asthma, there is no difference in the effectiveness between inhaled and intravenous terbutaline.[17]

A major problem with the use of MDIs is improper inhalation technique. This is a particularly important problem in the elderly. Allen and Prior[18] studied the use of MDIs in 30 elderly patients and found that only 60 percent used appropriate technique and only 10 percent ideal technique. The most frequent errors noted were failure to breath-hold after inhalation, not continuing to inhale after actuation of the canister, lack of any coordination whatsoever between inhalation and actuation, and inhalation through the nose. In a study of inhaler technique in 595 patients who attended a chest clinic, the elderly were less likely to use correct technique and more likely to be responsive to teaching. In a test of the ability of elderly patients to trigger MDIs, over one-third were unable to generate sufficient force to trigger any of the inhalers tested and less than a one-third could trigger all of the inhalers.[19]

Spacer devices such as a reservoir bag (InspirEase) or tube space (Aerochamber) are helpful for elderly patients who have difficulty coordinating the inhalation/activation step with MDIs (see Table 21-2). In a study of elderly patients with airways obstruction, the use of a spacer when inhaling β-adrenergic agonist from an MDI produced a greater bronchodilating effect.[20] For patients who are unable to generate sufficient force to activate the MDI, a simple plastic adaptor (Ventease) makes activation possible by a simple hand grip motion.

Patients must be instructed carefully in the use of the MDI. Observation of MDI technique is essential to ensure correct procedure.[21] The MDI should be shaken prior to each activation. Patients should breathe out slowly to a volume just below their normal resting volume; they should not exhale forcibly. The mouthpiece should be placed in the mouth with the opening between the teeth and directed over the tongue. The head should be tilted back slightly. Patients should begin to inhale slowly through the mouth and then activate the inhaler. Inhalation should continue to total lung capacity and breath should be held for at least 10 s. Ongoing

Table 21-2 Aerosol delivery devices and ancillary aids

Device	Type
Aerochamber	Tube spacer with universal fit with audible inhalation flow warning
InhalAid	Portable reservoir delivery device with audible inhalation flow warning
InspirEase	Compact, portable reservoir delivery device with audible inhalation flow warning
Vent-ease	Squeeze grip activator adapter for certain MDIs; allows "squeezing" motion rather than "push" motion to activate MDI

education in the proper MDI technique is necessary. Improper MDI technique is a major reason for the failure of therapy in patients with airways obstruction.[21]

Dry-powder inhalers may be easier to use for patients who have difficulty synchronizing activation and inhalation. Medication delivery with dry-powder inhalers is activated by patient inhalation, and synchronization of activation and inhalation is unnecessary. β-Adrenergic agonists may also be inhaled using a small-volume nebulizer in patients who are unable to successfully use MDIs or dry-powder inhalers.

Tremor and palpitations are the most common side effects of β-adrenergic agonists.[15] Tremor results from stimulation of β_2-adrenergic receptors in skeletal muscle and palpitations from stimulation of β_2-adrenergic receptors in the peripheral vasculature resulting in vasodilatation with reflex increase in the force and rate of cardiac contraction. Tolerance to these side effects usually develops quickly with regular use, but they may be a particular problem in the elderly. Tremor and palpitations are more common for any degree of bronchodilatation when the drug is given orally or by injection than when inhaled.[22] This is the result of the far greater plasma concentrations of drug when given by the oral or parenteral route. When a β-agonist is inhaled from an MDI using proper technique, no significant plasma concentration is achieved.[23] Therefore, side effects such as tremor after inhalation using an MDI may indicate poor technique, leading to larger deposition in the mouth and oropharynx with subsequent gut absorption producing higher plasma concentrations. Use of a spacer or reservoir device may resolve these side effects. When β-agonists are administered by aerosol using a small-volume nebulizer, side effects can be reduced by using a smaller dose. At higher doses, β-adrenergic agonists can produce hypokalemia.[24,25] This effect could be especially severe if superimposed on preexisting hypokalemia secondary to diuretic or corticosteroid therapy or associated with hypoxemia during an acute exacerbation of airways obstruction. Cardiac arrhythmias secondary to β-adrenergic agonist therapy are thought to be rare, especially when the drug is given by the inhaled route, but this question has not been extensively studied in the elderly. There are isolated reports of arrhythmias in elderly patients with COPD following inhaled β-agonist administered in large doses using a small-volume nebulizer.[26] In addition, an increased incidence of arrhythmias has been reported in patients who were treated with a combination of theophylline and β-agonists.[27]

Theophylline

Although theophylline is a relatively ineffective bronchodilator and is associated with a high incidence of unwanted effects, it has been considered by many physicians in the United States as first-line therapy for patients with asthma or COPD. At present, there is much controversy regarding the role of theophylline, and there appears to be a trend toward using theophylline as a second- or third-line choice for therapy. Part of the popularity of theophylline has undoubtedly resulted from the relatively long duration of action of the oral sustained-release preparations along with aggressive marketing of a plethora of preparations. This was particularly true several years ago when the U.S.-marketed β-adrenergic agonist aerosols were nonselective and comparatively short acting.

Although theophylline has been in use for over 50 years, the mechanism of its action remains unclear.[28] The classical teaching has been that theophylline produces bronchodilatation by inhibiting phosphodiesterase, thereby increasing cyclic AMP levels in airway smooth muscle cells. This has been discarded as a possible mechanism because the theophylline levels necessary to inhibit phosphodiesterase greatly exceed the generally accepted therapeutic range of 10 to 20 μg/mL in humans. It has also been proposed that the action of theophylline is the result of antagonism of adenosine receptors. Although antagonism of adenosine receptors occurs at theophylline levels in the therapeutic range, a related drug that is a potent bronchodilator, enprofylline, is not an adenosine receptor antagonist.[29] Other possible mechanisms are alteration of cellular calcium metabolism and epinephrine release. Even though theophylline is a relatively weak bronchodilator, there are patients with both asthma and COPD that appear to benefit from it. Possible beneficial effects other than bronchodilation that could explain this clinical finding are an increase in mucociliary clearance, heightened respiratory drive, improvement in cardiovascular function, increase in diaphragmatic contractility, decrease in dyspnea, and improvement in exercise capacity.[29]

Theophylline is well absorbed from the gastrointestinal tract, and bioavailability is not affected by increasing age.[30] Dozens of oral theophylline preparations are available in the United States. For acute therapy, aminophylline (the ethylenediamine salt of theophylline) or theophylline itself may be given intravenously. The volume of distribution for theophylline is relatively constant between individuals at 0.5 L/kg, so that 1 mg/kg theophylline will raise the serum level 2 μg/mL.[31] Thus, 5 mg/kg of theophylline (or 6 mg/kg aminophylline, 1 mg aminophylline = 0.80 mg theophylline) will result in a serum concentration of approximately 10 μg/mL. Although the volume of distribution is relatively constant among individuals, resulting in a standardized loading dose, the clearance ($t_{1/2}$) of theophylline not only varies markedly between individuals but also may vary in the same individual over time.[29] Only about 10 percent of theophylline is excreted unchanged through the kidneys. The major route of clearance is metabolism by the cytochrome microsomal enzyme system in the liver. Thus, any of several drugs or related conditions that affect hepatic metabolism may alter theophylline clearance (Table 21-3). Factors that decrease theophylline clearance are especially important because they may result in toxic serum concentrations. The physician must be particularly careful not to give an antibiotic during an exacerbation of symptoms that reduces theophylline clearance (e.g., erythromycin or ciprofloxacin) without checking serum theophylline levels and adjusting the dose appropriately.

Whether theophylline clearance is reduced in the elderly is unclear, with equal numbers of studies demonstrating either decreased clearance in the elderly or no effect with age.[31-38] Interpretation of these studies is difficult because of confounding factors such as associated illnesses, cigarette smoking, and the presence of other

Table 21-3 Factors reported to decrease theophylline clearance (increase $t_{1/2}$)

Liver disease
Cor pulmonale
Congestive heart failure
Fever, viral illness, flu shots
Erythromycin, cimetidine, ciprofloxacin
Low-protein / high-CHO diet

medications. Certainly, associated illnesses and medication interactions may explain the widespread clinical impression that theophylline clearance is decreased by approximately one-third in the elderly population. Although obesity does not affect theophylline metabolism directly, it must be taken into account when maintenance dose calculations are made. Dose calculations should be made on the basis of ideal body weight because of limited distribution of theophylline to fat.

The major drawback to theophylline therapy is the high incidence of toxic effects, and risk of toxicity is thought to be increased in the elderly. Common side effects are nausea, tremor, headache, agitation, and insomnia. These side effects are especially common when therapy is begun and may be reduced by gradually increasing the dose when initiating therapy. Recent studies have demonstrated that asthmatic children treated with theophylline may have learning and behavior problems and perform poorly on psychologic testing.[39,40] These studies raise the possibility that theophylline may have similar adverse effects in the elderly, especially those who are neurologically compromised.[41]

Of particular concern are severe toxic effects including seizures and cardiac arrhythmias that may be life threatening.[42] Although seizures are usually associated with high serum concentrations, theophylline-associated arrhythmias may occur at therapeutic serum concentrations.[43] In 15 patients with COPD (mean age 66 years), oral theophylline administration was associated with a significant increase in ventricular ectopic beats from 43 to 72 per hour.[44] In 16 elderly patients, multifocal atrial tachycardia (MAT) was found to be a toxic effect of theophylline.[45] The theophylline levels in 25 percent of these patients were in the therapeutic range. When theophylline was discontinued, the atrial rate decreased and MAT resolved. In 5 patients who were rechallenged with intravenous aminophylline, MAT recurred at serum levels between 16 and 25 μg/mL; in 3 patients MAT recurred at levels in the therapeutic range. Similarly, in a recent study of 100 hospitalized patients with airways obstruction, the authors concluded that theophylline causes tachycardia and serious arrhythmias even at serum theophylline concentrations considered to be therapeutic.[46] In addition, elderly patients in this study were more likely to develop theophylline-associated arrhythmias.

Because theophylline toxicity in the elderly may be associated with serum theophylline concentrations in the accepted therapeutic range of 10 to 20 μg/mL, it may be reasonable to keep the serum concentration closer to 10 μg/mL in the elderly patient. The rationale for the accepted therapeutic range of 10 to 20 μg/mL has been challenged by Rogers and coworkers.[47] The accepted approach is based on the belief that the dose-response curve for theophylline is linear over the range of serum concentrations from 5 to 20 μg/mL. This belief is derived from data obtained from a study of six young asthmatics.[48] In this study, the data from the six asthmatic patients were plotted on a log scale. If these data are plotted on a linear scale as shown in Fig. 21-2, it is clear that the improvement in FEV_1 reaches a plateau in the range of 10 μg/mL with relatively little improvement between 10 and 20 μg/mL. This finding was confirmed by Klein and coworkers[49] in a study of nine stable adult asthmatic patients. In these patients, the FEV_1 increased significantly as the mean theophylline level increased from 6.4 to 12.8 μg/mL but there was no further significant improvement at a mean value of 19.2 μg/mL.

Theophylline, usually in an oral sustained-release preparation, is used by many physicians in the United States as first-line therapy for chronic asthma. Relative to the inhaled β-adrenergic agonists, theophylline is a weak bronchodilator. When optimal doses of inhaled β-adrenergic agonists are used, there is little or no additional benefit adding theophylline to the regimen.[50,51] Furthermore, in the elderly theophylline may be a less effective bronchodilator than in younger asthmatics.[52] The bronchodilator effect of increasing serum theophylline concentrations was studied in 10 young (mean age 26 years) and 10 elderly (mean age 68 years) asthmatics. The elderly individuals demonstrated a lower bronchodilator response to theophylline than the younger patients. Although this result may be the consequence of more severe airways obstruction in the older patients, it demonstrates that theophylline may be less effective in the more severely impaired elderly patient.

For acute exacerbations of asthma, intravenous aminophylline or theophylline is commonly given. Siegel and coworkers[53] evaluated the efficacy of intravenous aminophylline in patients seen in the emergency department with acute asthma. All patients were treated with the β-adrenergic agonist metaproterenol by inhalation from a small-volume nebulizer (15 mg hourly for 3 h) and were randomly assigned to receive intravenous aminophylline or placebo. Pulmonary function improved to

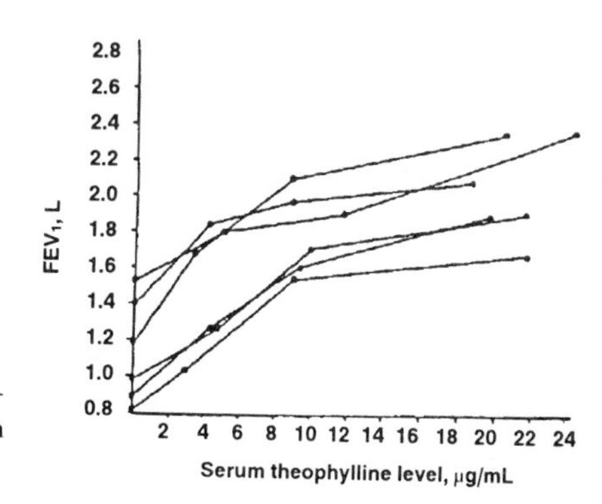

Figure 21-2 Improvement in FEV_1 with increasing theophylline level. (From Ref. 47, with permission.)

a similar degree in the placebo and aminophylline groups. There was no additional benefit of aminophylline, even in asthmatics with more severe obstruction. Furthermore, there were significantly more side effects in the aminophylline-treated patients than those receiving only β-adrenergic agonists. A recent meta-analysis evaluated the efficacy of intravenous aminophylline therapy for acute exacerbations of asthma.[54] Analysis of 13 clinical trials judged to be of acceptable design demonstrated no benefit of adding aminophylline to sympathomimetic bronchodilators. Again, toxic effects were more common in aminophylline-treated patients.

Oral theophylline is widely used as maintenance therapy for patients with COPD, especially in combination with inhaled β-adrenergic agents. Use of theophylline in patients with COPD is controversial, and the available clinical trials do not demonstrate a clear benefit of adding theophylline.[50,51] A recent randomized, controlled trial of theophylline in patients with severe COPD demonstrated that theophylline reduced the sensation of dyspnea and improved gas exchange and pulmonary function.[55] Although this study showed a definite effect of theophylline, the comparison group was treated with placebo only. In other studies demonstrating a beneficial effect of theophylline when added to inhaled β-adrenergic agonists or anticholinergic agents in patients with COPD, the major deficiency has been that the dose of the inhaled bronchodilator was not optimal.[56] Nevertheless, some studies do demonstrate a small additional benefit of theophylline, which may be important in the severely obstructed patient. Because of the poor risk/benefit ratio of theophylline, especially in the elderly patient, the advantage of adding theophylline should be demonstrated objectively (e.g., significant improvement in pulmonary function or a decrease in the amount or frequency of medication use). Guyatt and colleagues[57] have suggested using an "N-of-1" trial in the individual patient to determine optimal therapy.

Rice and coworkers[58] have recently addressed the question of whether theophylline was beneficial in acute exacerbations of COPD. Patients with severe COPD were studied during hospitalization for acute exacerbation. In addition to inhaled metaproterenol, intravenous methylprednisolone, and antibiotics, patients received either intravenous aminophylline in a dose adjusted to achieve a therapeutic level or placebo. After 72 h of treatment, there was no difference in subjective or objective improvement between the aminophylline and placebo groups. Importantly, almost 50 percent of the aminophylline group experienced side effects associated with theophylline therapy, even though drug levels were within the therapeutic range.

Anticholinergics

Anticholinergics have been used to treat respiratory disorders for centuries.[59] They were derived from the *Atropa belladonna* and *Datura stramonium* plants and consisted primarily of the alkaloid atropine. The therapeutic usefulness of atropine was limited by side effects. Because it was well absorbed, even when administered by inhalation, atropine caused systemic effects such as tachycardia, blurred vision, dry mouth, and urinary retention. Over the past two decades, quaternary ammonium analogs of atropine, such as ipratropium bromide, have been developed.[60] Because of the quaternary ammonium group, ipratropium carries a charge and is poorly absorbed across membranes. Therefore, when inhaled into the lung, ipratropium is not absorbed into the systemic circulation and has no side effects in other organs.

Cholinergic control of airway smooth muscle tone is mediated by nerves that travel in the vagus.[60] Cholinergic nerves release acetylcholine, which acts on muscarinic receptors in airway smooth muscle, causing contraction. This pathway can be activated through reflex mechanisms by stimulation of irritant receptors in the airway lumen. Anticholinergic drugs block muscarinic receptors in airway smooth muscle, inhibit vagally mediated cholinergic tone, and cause bronchodilation. Because anticholinergics block only bronchoconstriction mediated through cholinergic nerves, they are not extremely protective against some bronchoconstrictor stimuli.[61] They provide only partial protection against allergen challenge, do not block mediator release from mast cells, and are not useful in preventing exercise-induced bronchoconstriction. Anticholinergics do not block the direct effects of various allergic mediators, such as histamine, on airway smooth muscle. They block only the effect mediated by acetylcholine released from cholinergic nerves. In contrast, β-adrenergic agonists directly stimulate β_2-adrenergic receptors in airway smooth muscle to relax airway smooth muscle and produce bronchodilatation regardless of the bronchospastic stimulus. Because of this, β-adrenergic agonists are more effective in patients with asthma than are anticholinergic agents. The onset of bronchodilation with anticholinergics is relatively slow (requiring 15 to 30 min with peak effect at 1 to 2 h) but long lasting (6 to 8 h). For this reason, β-adrenergic drugs are more effective than anticholinergic drugs for reversing acute attacks of bronchospasm. Anticholinergic agents are second-line bronchodilators in asthmatic patients and should be used in combination with a β-adrenergic agent. Anticholinergics may be especially useful in the older asthmatic or those with primarily bronchitic symptoms,[62] but they have not been evaluated specifically in elderly patients. These agents have also been shown to be useful in asthmatics with nocturnal symptoms.

Although anticholinergics are less effective bronchodilators than β-adrenergic agonists in patients with asthma, they have been shown to be as effective or more effective than β-adrenergic agonists in patients with COPD.[60] They appear to be particularly effective in those patients with the most severely compromised pulmonary function.[63] Thus, in contrast to patients with asthma, the only reversible component in patients with COPD appears to be vagal tone.

The available anticholinergic agents are listed in Table 21-4. Atropine is unsuitable because of side effects, as noted above. The quaternary analogue ipratropium bromide is available in MDI formulation. Because the drug is poorly absorbed from the airways, the side effects common with atropine (tachycardia, dry mouth, blurred vision, and urinary retention) do not occur. The only important side effect appears to be cough in a small percentage of patients.[62] The recom-

Table 21-4 Anticholinergic agents

Preparation	Chemical type	Available in United States	FDA approved as bronchodilator	Optimal dosage
Atropine sulfate	Tertiary	Yes	No	NA
Glycopyrrolate (Robinul)	Quaternary	Yes	No	NA
Ipratropium bromide (Atrovent)	Quaternary	Yes	Yes	3–4 times/day

mended dose, 2 puffs (36 μg) three to four times daily is probably too small to produce optimal effect in many patients with severe obstruction. Many patients appear to respond only if given 4 to 8 puffs at each administration. These higher doses have been shown to be much more effective in blocking nocturnal symptoms in asthmatics.[64] Because ipratropium is so well tolerated, there is no reason to avoid administering larger doses. At the present time, the only quaternary agent available in the United States capable of administration as a solution for nebulization, but not approved for use by the Federal Drug Administration (FDA), is glycopyrrolate injection. Glycopyrrolate has been shown to be effective,[65] but the dose required for nebulization of this injectable drug is prohibitively expensive.

Because of its relative lack of side effects, inhaled ipratropium is a good choice as a bronchodilator in elderly patients with airways obstruction. In addition, no drug interactions have been reported with inhaled ipratropium.

ANTI-INFLAMMATORY AGENTS

Anti-inflammatory drugs, such as corticosteroids and cromolyn sodium, do not have an immediate bronchodilator effect and are not useful for rapid relief of symptoms. Anti-inflammatory agents must be given on a long-term basis as prophylactic therapy, with the goal of suppressing the chronic inflammation thought to be involved in the pathogenesis of asthma.

Corticosteroids

Corticosteroids have had a primary role in the treatment of asthma for the past 40 years. They are extremely effective for suppressing the inflammation that appears to play a key role in producing the bronchial hyperresponsiveness of asthma. The introduction of inhaled corticosteroids over the past decade is an important advance in asthma therapy.[66-68] The role of corticosteroid therapy in COPD is less clear, as discussed below.

Although corticosteroids decrease the inflammatory response in asthma, the exact mechanism of action is unknown. Corticosteroids reduce sputum and blood eosinophilia and block the release of mediators from eosinophils and macrophages but not from mast cells.[69] Corticosteroids may have a direct effect on vascular endothelial cells to reduce the effects of inflammatory mediators, producing microvascular leakage in the airways. They do not block the immediate response to allergen challenge but inhibit the influx of inflammatory cells into the lung after exposure to allergen and prevent the development of bronchial hyperresponsiveness. At the molecular level, corticosteroids induce the synthesis of lipocortin, which prevents phospholipase-A_2 production and the release of arachidonic acid from cell membranes, thus decreasing the synthesis of leukotrienes, prostaglandins, and platelet activating factor.[70] Corticosteroids appear to reverse the desensitization of β-adrenergic receptors in airway smooth muscle and may prevent the development of tachyphylaxis to β-adrenergic agents.[71]

Several corticosteroid preparations with different properties are available for systemic administration (Table 21-5). The most commonly used preparation in the United States is prednisone. Prednisone must be activated by conversion to prednisolone in the liver. Theoretically, in patients with severe liver impairment, prednisone may be less effective than the other agents listed which do not require liver activation. Otherwise, prednisone and prednisolone are equivalent agents. Methylprednisolone has slightly less mineralocorticoid effect than prednisone, and methylprednisolone is considered by some to be more effective in the treatment of asthma because it is better secreted into alveoli. Prednisone, prednisolone, and methylprednisolone are relatively short acting and suppress plasma adrenocorticotropic hormone (ACTH) activity for only 24 to 36 h compared to the longer acting preparations triamcinolone and dexamethasone. These shorter acting oral agents are usually given as a single dose early in the morning. This once daily regimen appears to reduce the likelihood and severity of suppression of the hypothalamic pituitary axis (HPA).[72] A single morning dose is as effective as divided doses for

Table 21-5 Corticosteroid preparations for systemic administration

Drug	Equivalent pharmacologic dose, mg	Mineralocorticoid activity	Plasma half-life, h	Duration of HPA suppression, days
Hydrocortisone	20	2+	1.5	1.25–1.5
Prednisone	5	1+	2.7	1.25–1.5
Prednisolone	5	1+	2.75	1.25–1.5
Methylprednisolone	5	0	3.0	1.25–1.5
Triamcinolone	4	0	4.2	2.25
Dexamethasone	0.75	0	5.0	2.75
Betamethasone	0.6	0	5.0	3.25

treatment of most patients with airways obstructive diseases. Hydrocortisone and methylprednisolone can be given intravenously in acute situations.

For patients who require prolonged oral corticosteroid therapy, alternate-day therapy may be as effective as daily therapy. Alternate-day therapy is associated with a decrease in HPA suppression and corticosteroid-associated side effects.[73] Obviously, one of the shorter acting agents, such as prednisone, must be used to achieve the benefits of alternate-day therapy. In patients who have been treated with long-term corticosteroid therapy, HPA suppression is likely. These patients can develop adrenal insufficiency on the off day of alternate therapy. Therefore, the switch to alternate-day therapy should be gradual. Many clinicians double the dose on the "on day" of alternate-day therapy and gradually taper the "off day." When the patient is stable on alternate-day therapy, the dose can be slowly tapered to the lowest alternate-day dose tolerated.

Corticosteroids given by inhalation have proven to be effective in the management of asthma.[67] The inhaled corticosteroids available in the United States are shown in Table 21-6. There appears to be little difference between these inhaled preparations except that inhaled dexamethasone may be associated with greater systemic toxicity. A newer agent, budesonide, has the highest topical activity but is not available in the United States at present. Beclomethasone dipropionate has been the most extensively studied.[74] After inhalation, beclomethasone is not inactivated in the lung but is absorbed from the airways into the systemic circulation and can have systemic effects if given in high doses. Only about 15 percent of the inhaled dose reaches the airways. The amount that is deposited in the mouth can be reduced by use of a spacer or reservoir. The portion of the dose that is swallowed is metabolized in the first pass through the liver and has negligible systemic effects.[74] Initially, the recommendation was to give inhaled corticosteroid four times a day, but recent studies show no significant differences in respiratory symptoms or pulmonary function between twice daily and four times daily dosing regimens.[66,75] Because patient compliance is better on the twice daily schedule, this regimen is recommended for most patients.[75]

The efficacy of corticosteroids in acute attacks of asthma is well documented. Exacerbations resolve more rapidly with corticosteroid therapy than with bronchodilator therapy alone, but there are no exact guidelines for the dose and route of administration. In one study of hospitalized asthmatic patients with

Table 21-6 Inhaled corticosteroid preparations

Drug	Dosage form
Beclomethasone diproprionate (Vanceril, Beclovent)	50 μg/spray
Triamcinolone acetonide (Azmacort)	100 μg/spray
Flunisolide (AeroBid)	250 μg/spray
Dexamethasone (Decadron)	100 μg/spray

severe bronchospasm, methylprednisolone 125 mg every 6 h was more effective than 40 mg every 6 h during the first 48 h of hospitalization.[76] But the data from other studies suggest that doses higher than the equivalent of 100 mg of prednisone daily have little if any additional effect on the rate of improvement.[77] Nevertheless, for severe acute obstruction requiring hospitalization, most physicians give larger doses by the intravenous route initially with the goal of achieving high concentrations in the lung. For acute exacerbations managed on an outpatient basis, high-dose oral corticosteroids (equivalent to prednisone 30 to 60 mg daily) are effective.[61] The initial dose should be continued until improvement occurs followed by a tapering regimen. The initial dose and duration depend on the severity of the obstruction, but usually improvement occurs in 1 to 2 weeks, and most patients can be tapered rapidly when function has returned to baseline. When the dose has been tapered to the range of 15 to 20 mg of prednisone daily, inhaled corticosteroids should be started and the oral corticosteroid tapered completely. Inhaled corticosteroids can be discontinued temporarily during acute attacks if they aggravate acute bronchospasm. In addition, the effectiveness of inhaled corticosteroids in acute asthma has not been documented.

Inhaled corticosteroids have been shown to be very effective in reducing the bronchial hyperresponsiveness of asthma without the side effects associated with oral corticosteroid therapy. An attempt should be made to switch all patients requiring oral corticosteroids to inhaled corticosteroid therapy.[61,66] For patients who require oral corticosteroids for management of asthma, the addition of inhaled corticosteroid allows oral therapy to be withdrawn or reduced in dose while symptoms are controlled and lung function is maintained. Some patients with severe oral-corticosteroid-dependent asthma require inhaled daily doses in the range of 2000 μg daily of beclomethasone dipropionate to allow a reduction in the oral corticosteroid dose while maintaining control of asthma. In some patients, a linear relationship between inhaled corticosteroid dose and improvement in lung function has been demonstrated. The beclomethasone dipropionate inhalers available in the United States (Table 21-6) deliver only 50 μg/puff. In Europe, *high-dose* inhalers (BecloForte) are available which deliver 250 μg/puff, which allows a high dose to be given much more easily, since fewer inhaler puffs are necessary.

The efficacy of corticosteroids in patients with COPD is unclear. There is no consensus in the literature in regard to this question. For patients with acute exacerbations of COPD, the usual practice is to treat with corticosteroids. This practice is supported by a controlled trial in patients that required hospitalization for an acute exacerbation of COPD.[78] These patients were randomized to receive either methylprednisolone (0.5 mg/kg every 6 h for 3 days) or placebo in addition to usual treatment with bronchodilators and antibiotics. The methylprednisolone group showed a greater improvement in pulmonary function at 12 h and throughout the 3 days of therapy. The statistical analysis of this study has been criticized,[79] but 55 percent of the patients in the methylprednisolone treatment group had a 40 percent or greater improvement in pulmonary function compared to 14 percent in the placebo group. Another study of the efficacy of corticosteroids during acute COPD exacerbations compared improvement in patients during the first 5 h in the emergency department treated with methylprednisolone or placebo in addition to standard bronchodilator therapy.[80] No effect of treatment on pulmonary function was seen in the first 5 h. Thus, the effect of corticosteroids in acute exacerbations is delayed for up to 12 h.

A more controversial issue is whether clinically stable patients with COPD benefit from oral corticosteroid therapy. At least 33 clinical studies have attempted to answer this question with varying conclusions. It appears that for the majority of patients with clinically stable COPD, oral corticosteroid therapy is not effective in improving pulmonary function or exercise tolerance. But a minority of patients do have a favorable response that can be documented objectively. In one study 6 of 46 patients had greater than 50 percent improvement in FEV_1.[81] The data from the available studies have been evaluated recently in a meta-analysis.[82] For this analysis, a favorable response to therapy was defined as 20 percent or greater improvement in FEV_1. All study treatments were similar, usually the equivalent of 40 mg of prednisone daily for 2 weeks. The conclusion drawn from this analysis was that patients with stable COPD receiving oral corticosteroid therapy have an improvement in FEV_1 approximately 10 percent more often than COPD patients receiving placebo. Several of these studies attempted to determine the patient characteristics associated with a response to corticosteroids. Some have demonstrated that corticosteroid responders also respond to β-adrenergic agonist bronchodilators, but some patients respond to corticosteroids in the absence of a β-adrenergic response. Sputum or peripheral blood eosinophilia have also been associated with a favorable response to corticosteroids, but this has not been confirmed by others.[83,84] Thus, it appears that if COPD patients show a marked response to β-adrenergic bronchodilator or eosinophilia, they may be more likely to have a favorable response to corticosteroids. However, a lack of bronchodilator response or eosinophilia does not preclude a response to corticosteroids.

Although inhaled corticosteroids are extremely effective in asthma, the effectiveness of inhaled corticosteroids in COPD patients is unclear. Several studies have evaluated the response to inhaled beclomethasone compared to oral prednisone or prednisolone.[85-87] Generally, the inhaled route was less effective than the oral but the oral doses were probably equivalently larger (30 to 40 mg of prednisone compared to 400 to 1500 μg of beclomethasone). In one study,[86] inhaled corticosteroid was as effective as oral drug in inpatients but less effective in outpatients, suggesting that close supervision and technique are important. In a study of 12 COPD patients that had a response to oral prednisone, 5 of the 12 had a response to 400 μg of inhaled beclomethasone, which was at least 50 percent of that achieved by prednisone.[85] These results suggest that in COPD patients who respond to oral corticosteroids, inhaled corticosteroids may allow the oral dose to be discontinued or tapered.

Chronic oral corticosteroid therapy is associated with adrenal insufficiency following withdrawal of therapy and multiple other serious side effects, some of which are listed in Table 21-7. These side effects of corticosteroid therapy

Table 21-7 Adverse effects of chronic (oral) systemic glucocorticoid administration

Hypothalamic-pituitary-adrenal suppression	Inhibition of leukocyte and monocyte function
Myopathy	Osteoporosis/compression fractures
Weight gain	Pancreatitis
Hyperglycemia	Psychiatric disturbances
Sodium retention	Hypokalemia alkalosis
Hypertension	Skin fragility
Impaired wound healing	Glaucoma
Subcutaneous tissue atrophy	Cushingoid appearance
Hypokalemia	Hyperlipidemia
Posterior subcapsular cataract	

appear to be more common and more serious in the elderly. Corticosteroid-related osteoporosis, vertebral compression fractures, cataracts, glaucoma, hyperglycemia, and hypertension are especially common in the elderly. In a study of elderly patients (mean age 77 years) with COPD receiving oral corticosteroid therapy (prednisolone 2.5 to 12.5 mg/day), the incidence of serious side effects was increased 40 percent over those in a matched control group and appeared to be dose related.[88] Because of the high incidence of corticosteroid-induced osteoporosis in the elderly, physical activity to stimulate bone formation and calcium supplementation are recommended. Serious infectious complications have also been reported in elderly patients treated with oral corticosteroid therapy for COPD.[89] These included invasive pulmonary aspergillosis, septicemia, cryptococcal meningitis, and cytomegalovirus pneumonia. Although reactivation of tuberculosis associated with corticosteroid therapy has not been documented in the elderly population, the current practice is isoniazid prophylaxis in patients with a positive tuberculin skin receiving chronic systemic corticosteroid therapy.

In contrast to orally administered corticosteroids, inhaled corticosteroids are associated with few side effects.[66,68] The major side effects are oropharyngeal candidiasis and dysphonia. These side effects are uncommon at relatively low doses (400 μg or less of beclomethasone daily), but the incidence is dose related at higher doses. The incidence of these effects can be reduced by using a spacer or reservoir device, as shown in Fig. 21-3. In addition, patients are instructed to rinse their mouth with water following inhaled corticosteroid administration. Although adrenal suppression may be an important side effect of low doses of inhaled corticosteroid in children, a very high dose (1500 μg of inhaled beclomethasone) causes little or no adrenal suppression in adults.[66]

Because of the marked absence of serious side effects with inhaled compared to oral corticosteroid therapy, every effort should be made to substitute inhaled corticosteroid for oral therapy. When oral corticosteroids are necessary, the risk of

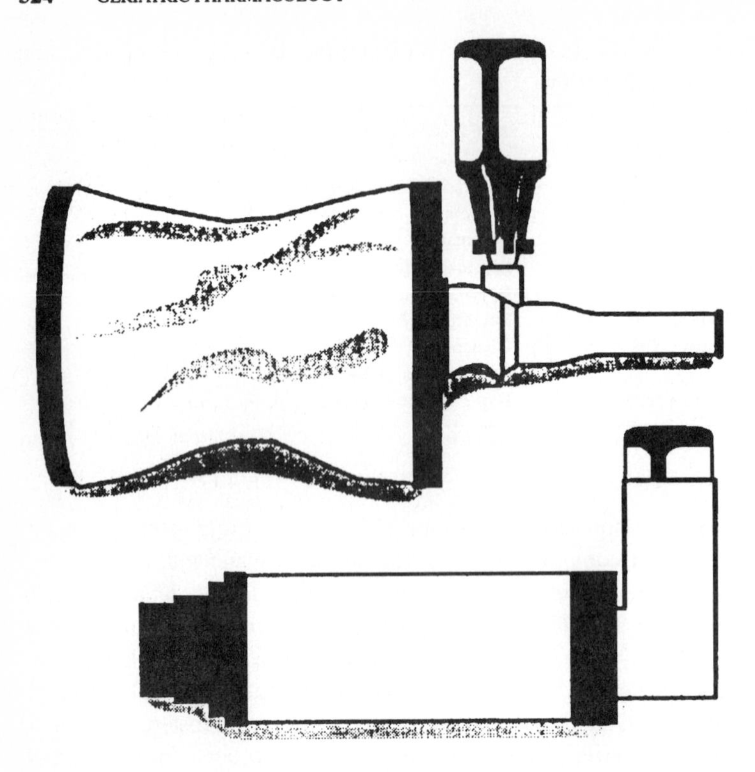

Figure 21-3 Spacer and reservoir devices for use with metered dose inhalers. (Adapted from Ref. 21.)

side effects, especially adrenal suppression, may be reduced by administering the total dose once a day in the morning and by switching to alternate-day therapy, if possible.

Cromolyn Sodium

Inhaled cromolyn sodium [disodium cromoglycate (DSCG)] is less effective than inhaled corticosteroid for asthma but is the first-line anti-inflammatory agent used in children because it has virtually no major side effects. Cromolyn inhibits both the early and late bronchoconstrictor response to allergen challenge and the subsequent increase in bronchial hyperresponsiveness.[90] Cromolyn also is effective in preventing exercise-induced asthma. Long-term treatment with cromolyn in asthma produces a decrease in bronchial hyperresponsiveness. The mechanism of action of cromolyn is unknown, but because of its ability to block the early response to antigen, cromolyn was initially thought to inhibit release of mediators from mast cells by stabilizing cells. Because cromolyn also inhibited the late response to antigen, it was thought that it might also stabilize inflammatory cells involved in the late response, possibly eosinophils and macrophages. Also, cromolyn may have an effect on the C-fiber afferent sensory nerves in the airways and may prevent irritant-induced bronchoconstriction.

Children with allergic asthma are thought to have a better response to cromolyn than adult asthmatics. Although cromolyn has been used predominantly to treat asthma in children, cromolyn may be effective in adult asthmatics.[91] In a study of adults with chronic asthma, 18 to 76 years of age, cromolyn improved symptoms, reduced the use of other medications, and improved pulmonary function compared to placebo in a 4-month trial. Also, bronchial hyperresponsiveness was decreased in the cromolyn group. Thus, cromolyn can be effective in adult asthmatics who are usually not regarded as candidates for cromolyn therapy. Although the anti-inflammatory drug of choice in the adult asthmatic is inhaled corticosteroid, cromolyn might be a useful adjunct in the adult patient who does not have satisfactory control of symptoms with inhaled corticosteroid. Also, cromolyn could be used before an anticipated allergen exposure, such as exposure to a dog or cat. If effective in the elderly asthmatic patient, cromolyn would be a very useful agent because the only side effects are cough or throat irritation associated with administration. Cromolyn is available for inhalation from a metered-dose inhaler, as solution for nebulization, and as a powder for administration from a dry-powder inhaler (Spinhaler). Cromolyn is given four times a day or prior to allergen exposure.

Other Anti-inflammatory Agents

Methotrexate and gold salts, both used in the management of chronic rheumatoid arthritis, have been advocated as steroid-sparing agents to reduce the dose of oral corticosteroid in patients with severe asthma. The use of methotrexate has been in vogue since Mullarkey and coworkers[92] showed that a low dose (15 mg per week) allowed a reduction in the dose of oral corticosteroids in patients with severe asthma without deterioration in pulmonary function. A subsequent report of a double-blind, placebo-controlled study has not confirmed this finding.[93] This discordance suggests that the steroid-sparing effect of methotrexate is, at best, small. Because of the risk of serious toxicity with methotrexate, it should be used with caution only in severe asthmatics requiring high-dose oral corticosteroids on a chronic basis.

APPROACH TO THERAPY

The patient should be educated concerning the nature of the disease and the goals of therapy. Education should include an awareness of the warning signs of an exacerbation of disease such as appearance of nocturnal symptoms and increased bronchodilator requirements. For patients with asthma, avoidance of allergens and bronchospastic triggers is important. Pneumococcal vaccine should be given on one occasion and influenza vaccine given on a yearly basis. Medications that aggravate bronchospasm should be avoided, especially β-adrenergic blocking

Table 21-8 β-Adrenergic blocker eye drops

Drug	Trade name	Blocking activity
Betaxolol	Betoptic	β_1
Levobunolol	Betagan	β_1 and β_2
Metipranol	OptiPranolol	β_1 and β_2
Timolol	Timoptic	β_1 and β_2

agents. Oral beta blockers, regardless of their selectivity, should not be used for treatment of hypertension or angina in patients with airways obstruction. Many elderly patients are treated with β-adrenergic blocker eye drops for glaucoma, and these may cause severe bronchospasm in sensitive patients. The β-adrenergic blocker eye drop preparations used in the United States are listed in Table 21-8. The cardioselective beta blocker, betaxolol, may be tolerated by asthmatics who require a beta-blocker eye drop for treatment of glaucoma.[94] Some patients with asthma are sensitive to aspirin and nonsteroidal anti-inflammatory drugs (NSAIDs). These agents may cause life-threatening bronchospasm in these patients. Due to the increased frequency of arthritis in the elderly, the physician must be alert to the possibility of worsening of airways obstruction due to aspirin or NSAIDs.

Therapy of Asthma

The most effective bronchodilators in asthmatic patients are β-adrenergic agonists given by the inhaled route. All asthmatic patients should use a β-adrenergic agonist such as albuterol from a metered-dose inhaler for episodes of bronchospasm or for prevention of symptoms such as exercise-induced asthma. Although patients have been instructed in the past to use β-adrenergic agonist inhalers on a regular basis, many asthmatics have used them only *as needed.* Use only when needed may be preferable. This approach allows early detection of worsening asthma by an increase in inhaler use. In addition, there is some evidence that administration of β-adrenergic agonists on a scheduled rather than prn basis may result in worsening of asthma.[95] For patients with mild asthma who have infrequent symptoms or only exercise-induced asthma, therapy in addition to prn inhaled β-adrenergic agonist is probably unnecessary. As discussed above, the use of a spacer or reservoir device for the elderly patient improves the effectiveness of beta agonists administered by an MDI.

If it is necessary for the patient to use the β-agonist inhaler on a daily basis because of symptoms, additional therapy is necessary. In the elderly asthmatic, inhaled corticosteroid would be the next step. A relatively low dose of beclomethasone, 400 μg daily, causes no systemic corticosteroid effects. The only side effects are oral candidiasis and hoarseness, and these can be minimized or eliminated by use of a spacer and rinsing the mouth after inhalation. Inhaled corticosteroid must be given on a regular basis and a twice daily regimen (beclomethasone 50 μg/puff as 4 puffs twice daily) is adequate for most patients. In addition, administration twice daily improves compliance. For patients who are not controlled on inhaled corticosteroids, as indicated by the continued frequent use of many inhalations from a β-agonist inhaler, a larger dose of inhaled corticosteroid should be given. Doses of up to 2 mg (2000 μg) of beclomethasone a day are associated with little or no adrenal suppression in the adult. The major difficulty with this therapy is the number of puffs required because the *high-dose* inhalers available in Europe are not yet available in the United States. Therapy with a combination of inhaled beta agonist and inhaled corticosteroid will control symptoms in most asthmatics. The low dose of inhaled beclomethasone (400 μg/day, 8 puffs) is as effective as 7.5 to 10 mg of prednisone daily for most patients, while higher doses may be equivalent to therapy with 20 mg or more of prednisone daily. Patient education is essential and is an ongoing process. Patients must be educated to realize that the inhaled corticosteroids are preventative therapy and must be used on a regular basis. If symptoms are optimally controlled on inhaled corticosteroids, the dose can be tapered very slowly (2 puffs every 7 to 10 days) to determine the minimal dose necessary for control of symptoms.

If symptoms are not controlled on a combination of inhaled beta agonist and inhaled corticosteroids, additional therapy is necessary. Another anti-inflammatory agent such as inhaled cromolyn could be added, but it would probably be of little benefit in the elderly patient. Cromolyn is not as effective as inhaled corticosteroids but is relatively more effective in children or the younger atopic asthmatic. In the asthmatic child, many physicians would add cromolyn before inhaled steroids or certainly before high-dose inhaled steroids. A reasonable approach at this point would be additional bronchodilator therapy. In the younger patient, many physicians would add theophylline to the regimen. Because of the narrow therapeutic window and the increased risk of serious toxicity with theophylline in the elderly (arrhythmias, seizures, and death), a more reasonable approach would be a trial of anticholinergic therapy with inhaled ipratropium bromide. In contrast to oral theophylline, inhaled ipratropium has essentially no important side effects. Because of the relatively slow onset of bronchodilatation with anticholinergic agents, they should be used on a regular basis "like a pill" (2 to 4 puffs qid). The patient should continue to use the more rapid acting inhaled β-agonist prn for acute episodes of bronchospasm. Obviously, the patient must have a clear understanding of how these inhaled medications differ and how they should be used. Patient education is essential and must be repeated on several occasions.

For patients who continue to have symptoms on the regimen outlined above, oral corticosteroids are necessary. Oral corticosteroids are recommended last because of the serious side effects associated with long-term administration. As outlined above, the elderly are especially susceptible to the adverse effects of chronic oral corticosteroid therapy. Therapy should be begun with prednisone in a dose of approximately 40 mg daily until symptoms are controlled. When control has been achieved, the dose should be tapered rapidly to 15 to 20 mg daily and then more slowly (2.5 to 5 mg every week) to determine the minimum amount of corticosteroid necessary. When stable, a switch to alternate-day therapy should be attempted by giving double the minimum dose every other day. If the patient does well, attempts should be made on an intermittent basis to eliminate the oral corticosteroid from the regimen.

Although chronic administration of oral corticosteroids should be avoided if possible, a short course of oral corticosteroid therapy is recommended for an acute exacerbation of asthma and should not be delayed. This is especially important in the elderly population who are at a greater risk of death from asthma than the younger adult population. The adverse effects of a short course of oral prednisone are less dangerous than the frequent use of β-adrenergic agonist inhalers in the elderly patient who may be hypoxemic in the setting of severe bronchospasm and may have underlying ischemic heart disease. Prednisone should be started in a dose of 30 to 60 mg daily. Many physicians "hold" inhaled corticosteroids during acute exacerbations because they aggravate bronchospasm in some patients and may be associated with a higher incidence of oral candidiasis in the patient receiving a high dose of oral corticosteroid. When symptoms stabilize (usually in 7 to 10 days), prednisone can be tapered rapidly. The inhaled corticosteroid is restarted when the oral dose has been tapered to 15 to 20 mg daily.

Therapy of Chronic Obstructive Pulmonary Disease

For the symptomatic patient with COPD, first-line therapy is a bronchodilator. Whether the bronchodilator should be inhaled anticholinergic or inhaled β-adrenergic agonist is controversial. In studies of patients with COPD, anticholinergic agents are either as effective or more effective bronchodilators than β-adrenergic agonists. Ipratropium bromide, the only anticholinergic agent available by MDI in the United States, is poorly absorbed and virtually free of any side effects. Ipratropium does not cause tremor or cardiovascular effects, side effects that are especially important in the elderly. The duration of bronchodilatation is longer with ipratropium than the available beta agonists. Tachyphylaxis does not occur with continued anticholinergic use. A drawback to the use of ipratropium is the relatively slow onset of action compared to beta agonists. Because of the slow onset of action, ipratropium should be administered on a regular basis, 2 to 4 puffs three or four times a day. For patients who have attacks of bronchospasm, inhaled β agonists provide more rapid relief. Our approach in the elderly COPD patient is to begin therapy with ipratropium administered on a regular basis and to increase the dose if necessary. An increase in dose is not associated with side effects. If patients have attacks of shortness of breath and wheezing, an inhaled β-adrenergic agonist should be added to the regimen for use on a prn basis because of its rapid onset of action. Although theophylline is widely used as bronchodilator therapy in the COPD patient, it is a less effective bronchodilator than the anticholinergics and β-adrenergic agonists in COPD patients, and its use in the elderly is associated with an increased risk of serious toxicity.

The risk of toxicity may be especially great in patients with severe COPD and associated cor pulmonale or congestive heart failure. In these patients, theophylline levels are likely to increase during an exacerbation of disease due to decreased hepatic clearance. Because of the poor risk/benefit ratio of theophylline, we feel that the use of theophylline in the elderly COPD patient is rarely indicated. If theophylline is used in these patients, the dose should be adjusted to maintain the serum theophylline level in the range of 8 to 12 μg/mL rather than the usually accepted therapeutic range of 10 to 20 μg/mL. In addition, the benefit of adding theophylline to the regimen should be demonstrated objectively.

For patients with severe disease who continue to be severely disabled despite the therapeutic regimen described above, a trial of corticosteroids may be warranted. Only 10 to 15 percent of patients will benefit from corticosteroid therapy, and the side effects of chronic therapy may be devastating in the elderly patient. Therefore, the effectiveness should be documented objectively as a significant increase in the FEV_1, in the range of at least 20 percent. A trial of 40 mg of prednisone daily for 2 weeks should be sufficient. If improvement occurs, the dose should be tapered and attempt made to substitute inhaled corticosteroids for oral therapy. If inhaled corticosteroids are ineffective in maintaining the improvement, a switch to alternate-day therapy should be attempted.

For acute exacerbations of COPD, a short course of oral corticosteroid therapy may speed improvement in pulmonary function and resolution of symptoms. Systemic corticosteroid therapy has been demonstrated to benefit some patients with COPD with severe acute exacerbations requiring hospitalization. For outpatient management of exacerbations, prednisone in a dose of 40 to 60 mg daily is usually given until improvement occurs and then tapered as rapidly as tolerated. Most physicians would also treat with a 10 to 14-day course of antibiotic therapy, such as amoxicillin or trimethoprim-sulfamethoxazole, if the patient complains of increased amounts of purulent sputum in addition to dyspnea.[96]

Long-term oxygen therapy will benefit hypoxemic patients with COPD by decreasing pulmonary hypertension and erythrocytosis and improving exercise tolerance and neuropsychologic function. For patients with a P_{O_2} of 55 torr or less on room air or P_{O_2} of 59 or less with evidence of cor pulmonale or erythrocytosis, mortality is significantly decreased with continuous oxygen therapy.[97]

REFERENCES

1. Knudson RJ: Physiology of the aging lung, in Crystal RG, West JB et al (eds): *The Lung: Scientific Foundations.* New York, Raven, 1991, pp 1749–1759.
2. Beasley R, Roche WR, Roberts JA, et al: Cellular events in the bronchi in mild asthma and after bronchial provocation. *Am Rev Respir Dis* 139: 806–817, 1989.
3. Kirby JC, Hargreave FE, Gleich GJ, O'Byrne PM: Bronchoalveolar cell profiles of asthmatic an nonasthmatic subjects. *Am Rev Respir Dis* 127: 413–416, 1983.
4. Burrows B, Martinez FD, Halonen M, et al: Association of asthma with serum IgE levels skin-test reactivity to allergens. *N Engl J Med* 320: 271–277, 1989.

5. Burrows B, Knudson RJ, Cline MG, et al: Quantitative relationships between cigarette smoking and ventilatory function. *Am Rev Respir Dis* 115: 195-205, 1977.
6. Brown PJ, Greville HW, Finucane KE: Asthma and irreversible airflow obstruction. *Thorax* 39: 131-136, 1984.
7. Roche WR, Beasley R, Williams JH, Holgate ST: Subepithelial fibrosis in the bronchi of asthmatics. *Lancet* 1: 520-524, 1989.
8. Burrows B, Barbee RA, Cline MG, et al: Characteristics of asthma among elderly adults in a sample of the general population. *Chest* 100: 935-942, 1991.
9. Lee HY, Stratton TB: Asthma in the elderly. *Br MJ* 4: 93-95, 1972.
10. Barnes PJ: New concepts in the pathogenesis of bronchial hyperresponsiveness and asthma. *J Allergy Clin Immunol* 83: 1013-1026, 1989.
11. Sears MR: Increasing asthma mortality—fact or artifact? *J Allergy Clin Immunol* 82: 957-960, 1988.
12. Burrows B, Bloom JW, Traver GA, et al: The course and prognosis of different forms of chronic airways obstruction in a sample from the general population. *N Engl J Med* 317: 1309-1314, 1987.
13. Burr ML, Charles TJ, Roy K, Seaton A: Asthma in the elderly: An epidemiological survey. *Br MJ* 1: 1041-1049, 1979.
14. Burrows B, Lebowitz MD, Barbee RA, Cline MG: Findings prior to diagnoses of asthma among the elderly in a longitudinal study of a general population sample. *J Allergy Clin Immunol* 88: 870-877, 1991.
15. Nelson HS: Adrenergic therapy of bronchial asthma. *J Allergy Clin Immunol* 77: 771-785, 1986.
16. Shim C, Williams MH Jr: Bronchial response to oral versus aerosol metaproterenol in asthma. *Ann Intern Med* 93: 428-431, 1980.
17. Williams SJ, Winner SJ, Clark TJ: Comparison of inhaled and intravenous terbutaline in acute severe asthma. *Thorax* 36: 629-632, 1981.
18. Allen SC, Prior A: What determines whether an elderly patient can use a metered dose inhaler correctly? *Br J Dis Chest* 80: 45-49, 1986.
19. Armitage JM, Williams SJ: Inhaler technique in the elderly. *Age Ageing* 17: 275-278, 1988.
20. Thompson A, Traver GA: Comparison of three methods of administering a self-propelled bronchodilator. *Am Rev Resp Dis* 125: 140, 1982.
21. Traver GA, Tremper-Mitchell J, Flodquist-Priestley G: *Respiratory Care—A Clinical Approach.* Gaitherburg, Aspen, 1991, pp 87-93.
22. Newhouse MT, Dolovich MB: Control of asthma by aerosols. *N Engl J Med* 315: 870-874, 1986.
23. Popa VT: Clinical pharmacology of adrenergic drugs. *J Asthma* 21: 183-207, 1984.
24. Gelmont DM, Balmes JR, Yee A: Hypokalemia induced by inhaled bronchodilators. *Chest* 94: 763-766, 1988.
25. Martelli A, Otero C, Gil B, Gonzalez S: Fenoterol and serum potassium. *Lancet* 1: 1197, 1989.
26. Higgins RM, Cookson WOCM, Lane DJ, et al: Cardiac arrhythmias caused by nebulized beta-agonist therapy. *Lancet* 2: 863-864, 1987.
27. Stibolt TB, Youtsey DJ, Buist AS: Cardiac toxicity of theophylline, albuterol and the combination in severe COPD. *Am Rev Respir Dis* 139(4, part 2): A14, 1989.
28. Bukowskyj M, Nakatsu K, Munt PW: Theophylline reassessed. *Ann Intern Med* 101: 63-73, 1984.
29. Persson CG: Overview of effects of theophylline. *J Allergy Clin Immunol* 78: 780-787, 1986.
30. Vestal RE, Cusack BJ, Mercer GD, et al: Aging and drug interactions—effect of cimetidine and smoking on the oxidation of theophylline and cortisol in healthy men. *J Pharmacol Exp Ther* 241: 488-500, 1987.
31. Jusko WJ, Koup JR, Vance JW, et al: Intravenous theophylline therapy: nomogram guidelines. *Ann Intern Med* 86: 400-404, 1977.
32. Powell JR, Vozeh S, Hopewell P, et al: Theophylline disposition in acutely ill hospitalized patients. The effect of smoking, heart failure, severe airway obstruction, and pneumonia. *Am Rev Respir Dis* 118: 229-238, 1978.

33. Cusack B, Kelly JG, Lavan J, Noel J, O'Malley: Theophylline kinetics in relation to age: the importance of smoking. *Br J Clin Pharmacol* 10: 109-114, 1980.
34. Bauer LA, Blouin RA: Influence of age on theophylline clearance in patients with chronic obstructive pulmonary disease. *Clin Pharmacokinet* 6: 469-477, 1981.
35. Au WYW, Dutt AK, DeSoyza N: Theophylline kinetics in chronic obstructive airway disease in the elderly. *Clin Pharmacol Ther* 37: 472-478, 1985.
36. Talseth T, Kornstad S, Boye NP, Bredesen JE: Individualization of oral theophylline dosage in elderly patients. *Acta Med Scand* 210: 489-492, 1981.
37. Ramsay LE, MacKay A, Eppel ML, Oliver JS: Oral sustained-release aminophylline in medical inpatients: factors related to toxicity and plasma theophylline concentrations. *Br J Clin Pharmacol* 10: 101-107, 1980.
38. Antal EJ, Kramer PA, Mercik SA, et al: Theophylline pharmacokinetics in advanced age. *Br J Clin Pharmacol* 12: 637-645, 1981.
39. Rachelefsky GS, Wo J, Adelson J, et al: Behaviour abnormalities and poor school performance due to oral theophylline use. *Pediatrics* 78: 1133-1138, 1986.
40. Furukawa CT, Shapiro GG, Duhamel T: Learning and behavior problems associated with theophylline therapy. *Lancet* 1: 621, 1984.
41. Fanta CH: Asthma in the elderly. *J Asthma* 26: 87-97, 1989.
42. Sessler CN: Theophylline toxicity: Clinical features of 116 consecutive cases. *Am J Med* 88: 567-576, 1990.
43. Zwillich CW, Sutton FD, Neff TA, et al: Theophylline-induced seizures in adults. *Ann Intern Med* 82: 784-787, 1975.
44. Patel AK, Skatrud JB, Thomsen JH: Cardiac arrhythmias due to oral aminophylline in patients with chronic obstructive pulmonary disease. *Chest* 80: 661-665, 1981.
45. Levine JH, Michael JR, Guarnieri T: Multifocal tachycardia: A toxic effect of theophylline. *Lancet* 1: 12-14, 1985.
46. Bittar G, Friedman HS: The arrhythmogenicity of theophylline. *Chest* 99: 1415-1420, 1991.
47. Rogers RM, Owens GR, Pennock BE: The pendulum swings again—toward a rational use of theophylline. *Chest* 87: 280-282, 1985.
48. Mitenko PA, Ogilvie TI: Rational intravenous doses of theophylline. *N Engl J Med* 289: 600-603, 1973.
49. Klein J, Lefkovitz M, Spector S, Cherniak R: Relationship between serum theophylline levels and pulmonary function before and after inhaled beta-agonist in "stable" asthmatics. *Am Rev Respir Dis* 127: 413-416, 1983.
50. Lam A, Newhouse MT: Management of asthma and chronic airflow limitation. Are methylxanthines obsolete? *Chest* 98: 44-52, 1990.
51. Hill NS: The use of theophylline in "irreversible" chronic obstructive pulmonary disease. *Arch Intern Med* 148: 2579-2584, 1988.
52. Chandler MHH, Clifton GD, Burki NK, et al: Pulmonary function in the elderly: response to theophylline bronchodilation. *J Clin Pharmacol* 30: 330-335, 1990.
53. Siegel D, Sheppard D, Gelb A, Weinberg PF: Aminophylline increases the toxicity but not the efficacy of an inhaled beta-adrenergic agonist in the treatment of acute exacerbations of asthma. *Am Rev Respir Dis* 132: 283-286, 1985.
54. Littenberg B: Aminophylline treatment in severe asthma. A meta-analysis. *JAMA* 259: 1678-1684, 1988.
55. Murciano D, Auclair M-H, Pariente R, Aubier M: A randomized, controlled trial of theophylline in patients with severe chronic obstructive pulmonary disease. *N Engl J Med* 320: 1521-1525, 1989.
56. Newhouse MT: Is theophylline obsolete? *Chest* 98: 1-3, 1990.
57. Guyatt GH, Townsend M, Nogradi S, et al: Acute response to bronchodilator. An imperfect guide for bronchodilator therapy in chronic airflow limitation. *Arch Intern Med* 148: 1949-1952, 1988.
58. Rice KL, Leatherman JW, Duane PG, et al: Aminophylline for acute exacerbations of chronic obstructive pulmonary disease—a controlled trial. *Ann Intern Med* 107: 305-309, 1987.

59. Gandevia B: Historical review of the use of parasympatholytic agents in the treatment of respiratory disorders. *Postgrad Med J* 51(suppl 7): 13-20, 1975.
60. Gross NJ, Skorodin MS: Anticholinergic, antimuscarinic bronchodilators. *Am Rev Respir Dis* 129: 856-870, 1984.
61. Barnes PJ: A new approach to the treatment of asthma. *N Engl J Med* 321(22): 1517-1527, 1989.
62. Gross NJ: Ipratropium bromide. *N Engl J Med* 319: 486-494, 1988.
63. Braun SR, McKenzie WN, Copeland C, et al: A comparison of the effect of ipratropium and albuterol in the treatment of chronic obstructive airway disease. *Arch Intern Med* 149: 544-547, 1989.
64. Hughes DTD: The use of anticholinergic drugs in nocturnal asthma. *Postgrad Med J* 63(suppl): 47-51, 1987.
65. Johnson BE, Suratt PM, Gal TJ, Wilhoit SC: Effect of inhaled glycopyrrolate and atropine in asthma. *Chest* 85: 325-328, 1984.
66. Toogood JH, Jennings B, Baskerville JC: Aerosol corticosteroids, in Weiss EB, Segal MS, Stein M (eds): *Bronchial Asthma: Mechanisms and Therapeutics,* 2d ed. Boston, Little, Brown 1985, pp 698-713.
67. Cockcroft DW, Hargreave FE: Outpatient management of bronchial asthma. *Med Clin North Am* 74(3): 797-809, 1990.
68. Konig P: Inhaled corticosteroids—their present and future role in the management of asthma. *J Allergy Clin Immunol* 82: 297-306, 1988.
69. Morris HG: Mechanisms of action and therapeutic role of corticosteroids in asthma. *J Allergy Clin Immunol* 75: 1-13, 1985.
70. Flower RJ: Lipocortin and the mechanism of action of the glucocorticoids. *Br J Pharmacol* 94: 987-1015, 1988.
71. Stiles GL, Caron MG, Lefkowitz RJ: B-adrenergic receptors: Biochemical mechanisms of physiological regulation. *Physiol Rev* 64: 661-743, 1984.
72. Spector SL: The use of corticosteroids in the treatment of asthma. *Chest* 87(suppl): 73S-79S, 1985.
73. Ackerman GL, Nolan CM: Adrenocorticortical responsiveness after alternate day corticosteroid therapy. *N Engl J Med* 278: 405-409, 1968.
74. Williams MH: Beclomethasone dipropionate. *Ann Intern Med* 95: 464-467, 1981.
75. Meltzer EO, Kemp JP, Welch MJ, Orgel HA: Effect of dosing schedule on efficacy of beclomethasone dipropionate aerosol in chronic asthma. *Am Rev Respir Dis* 131: 732-736, 1985.
76. Haskell RJ, Wong BM, Hansen JE: A double-blind, randomized clinical trial of methylprednisolone in status asthmaticus. *Arch Intern Med* 143: 1324-1327, 1983.
77. Woolcock AJ, Jenkins CR: Clinical responses to corticosteroids, in Kaliner MA, Barnes PJ, Persson CGA (eds): *Asthma—Its Pathology and Treatment.* New York, Dekker, 1991, chap 23, pp 633-665.
78. Albert RK, Martin TR, Lewis SW: Controlled clinical trial of rmethylprednisolone in patients with chronic bronchitis and acute respiratory insufficiency. *Ann Intern Med* 92: 753-758, 1980.
79. Glenny RW: Steroids in COPD. The scripture according to Albert. *Chest* 91: 289-290, 1987.
80. Emerman CL, Connors AF, Lukens TW, et al: A randomized controlled trial of methylprednisolone in the emergency treatment of acute exacerbations of COPD. *Chest* 95: 563-567, 1989.
81. Mendella LA, Manfreda J, Warren CPW, Anthonisen NR: Steroid response in stable chronic obstructive pulmonary disease. *Ann Intern Med* 96: 17-21, 1982.
82. Callahan CM, Dittus RS, Katz BP: Oral corticosteroid therapy for patients with stable chronic obstructive pulmonary disease—a meta-analysis. *Ann Intern Med* 114: 216-223, 1991.
83. Blair GP, Light RW: Treatment of chronic obstructive pulmonary disease with corticosteroids. *Chest* 86: 524-528, 1984.
84. Shim C, Stover DE, Williams MH: Response to corticosteroids in chronic bronchitis. *J Allergy Clin Immunol* 62: 363-367, 1978.
85. Shim CS, Williams MH Jr: Aerosol beclomethasone in patients with steroid-responsive chronic obstructive pulmonary disease. *Am J Med* 78: 655-658, 1985.

86. Harding SM, Freedman S: A comparison of oral and inhaled steroids in patients with chronic airways obstruction—features determining response. *Thorax* 33: 214-218, 1978.
87. Robertson AS, Gove RI, Wieland GA, Sherwood Burge P: A double blind comparison of oral prednisone 40 mg/day with inhaled beclomethasone dipropionate 1500 μg/day in patients with adult onset chronic obstructive airways disease. *Eur J Resp Dis* 69(suppl 146): 565-569, 1986.
88. Thomas TPL: The complications of systemic corticosteroid therapy in the elderly. *Gerontology* 30: 60-65, 1984.
89. Wiest PM, Flanigan T, Salata RA, et al: Serious infectious complications of corticosteroid therapy in COPD. *Chest* 95: 1180-1184, 1989.
90. Bernstein IL: Cromolyn sodium in the treatment of asthma: Coming of age in the United States. *J Allergy Clin Immunol* 76: 381-388, 1985.
91. Petty TL, Rollins DR, Christopher K, et al: Cromolyn sodium is effective in adult chronic asthma. *Am Rev Respir Dis* 139: 694-701, 1989.
92. Mullarkey MF, Blumenstein BA, Andrade WP, et al: Methotrexate in the treatment of corticosteroid-dependent asthma: A double-blind crossover study. *N Engl J Med* 318: 603-607, 1988.
93. Erzurum SC, Leff JA, Evans Cochran J, et al: Lack of benefit of methotrexate in severe, steroid-dependent asthma. *Ann Intern Med* 114: 351-360, 1991.
94. Dunn TL, Gerber MJ, Shen AS, et al: The effect of topical ophthalmic instillation of timolol and betaxolol on lung function in asthmatic subjects. *Am Rev Respir Dis* 133: 264-268, 1986.
95. Sears MR, Taylor DR, Print CG, et al: Regular inhaled beta-agonist treatment in bronchial asthma. *Lancet* 336: 1391-1396, 1990.
96. Anthonisen NR, Manfreda J, Warren CPW: Antibiotic therapy in exacerbations of chronic obstructive pulmonary disease. *Ann Intern Med* 106: 196-204, 1987.
97. Nocturnal Oxygen Therapy Trial Group: Continuous or nocturnal oxygen therapy in hypoxemic chronic obstructive lung disease. *Ann Intern Med* 93: 391-398, 1980.

CHAPTER

22

CANCER CHEMOTHERAPY

Robert T. Dorr
William S. Dalton

The association between aging and the development of cancer is inextricable. In patients 65 years of age and older, cancer is the second leading cause of death, with heart disease being first. The overall incidence in mortality due to cancer increases progressively with increased age with no obvious plateau (Fig 22-1). Over 50 percent of all cancers occur in 11 percent of the population, which consists of individuals older than 65.[1] At age 25 the probability of developing cancer is 1 in 700, versus 1 in 14 at age 65. In men, cancer incidence is four times greater in patients older than 65 compared to that of the 45-to-64-year-old age group. The incidence of prostate cancer increases tenfold in patients older than 65, compared to those 45 to 64 years of age. Patients 65 years and older have a threefold greater incidence of lung cancer, kidney cancer, and non-Hodgkin's lymphoma compared to patients aged 45 to 64. Seventy percent of breast cancers are diagnosed in woman aged 50 and older.

Because cancer risk is associated with increasing age, the overall incidence of cancer will likely increase as the population ages. The absolute number of elderly patients will double in the next few decades.[2] In 1990, 31 million U.S. citizens were 65 years of age or older, and this number will increase to approximately 65 million by the year 2030. In 1965, one out of every nine Americans was 65 years of age or older. By 2030, one in five people will be considered elderly.[3] Obviously, medical professionals in all specialties will be dealing with more and more elderly patients

Supported in part by Grants 17094 and 31078 from the Department of Health and Human Services, National Institutes of Health, Bethesda, Maryland.

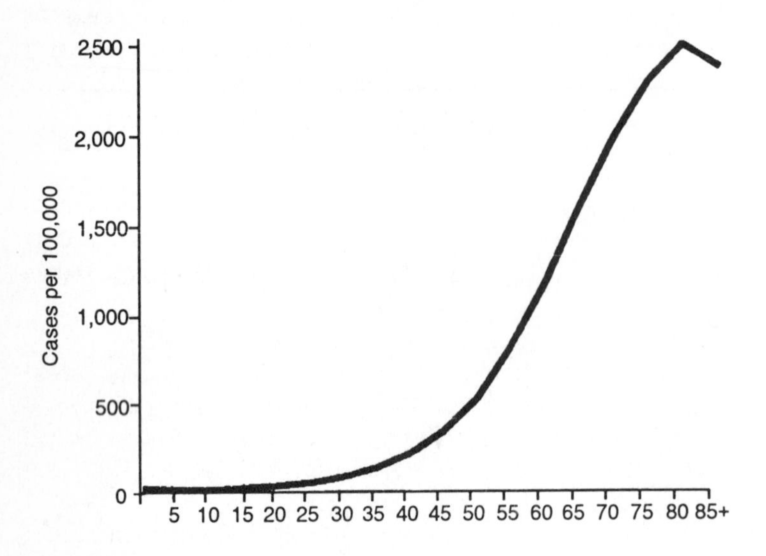

Figure 22-1 United States cancer incidence rates by 5-year age groups including all groups, races, and sexes. From the NCI SEER Program, 1983–1987, as described in Yancik and Ries.[1]

with cancer. Management of elderly patients is challenging due to problems of comorbid diseases and possible decline of organ function due directly to age.

Choices of therapy also vary with the age of the patient.[4] A study of over 20,000 cases by this group examined the relationship between age and the use of potentially curative therapy for specific cancers. For cancers of most sites, either local or regional stage, the proportion of cases receiving potentially curative therapy declined with age. Overall mortality rates during the first year after diagnosis were much higher for local stage cases without treatment than for those who received treatment. These data demonstrated that cancer therapy varies with age and suggest that decision making regarding therapy is influenced by the presence of other diseases. Physicians and patients alike are less willing to take risks in the treatment of elderly patients who have comorbid diseases.

Cancer chemotherapy has had a significant impact on both survival and quality of life for many patients with various cancers. These advances have occurred primarily in patients with hematologic diseases such as leukemias and malignant lymphomas, but advances have also been made in the treatment of certain solid tumors such as ovarian cancer, small cell lung cancer, and early breast cancer.[5] Unfortunately, the more common tumors such as nonsmall cell lung cancer, colon cancer, pancreatic cancer, and prostate cancer remain relatively resistant to chemotherapy, and the main modality of therapy for these diseases is surgery or hormone therapy.

Drugs used in the treatment of cancer are generally the most toxic used in medicine. The therapeutic index for most chemotherapeutic drugs is very narrow, and life-threatening toxicity may occur with only slight modifications in dose or drug handling. A thorough understanding of clinical pharmacology is imperative when administering chemotherapy and several steps must be considered:

1. Choice of appropriate dose and route of administration
2. Awareness of any organ of dysfunction which may alter the physiologic disposition of drugs or enhance organ toxicity
3. Knowledge of potential drug interactions which may alter drug effectiveness or toxicity

Each elderly patient brings unique disease-related or preexsisting medical conditions which may influence choice of drugs and dosages. Every effort should be made to use the best drug(s) at the maximum dose in order to achieve the best response, but adjustments may be necessary depending on the clinical circumstance.

The treating physician must also have a clear therapeutic goal when treating the cancer patient. If the disease treated has a significant chance of cure, then the risk-benefit ratio may favor an aggressive, albeit more toxic, approach; on the other hand, if the disease is regarded as incurable and the goal of therapy is palliation, then the patient should not be exposed to treatment which will impair quality of life and may even shorten survival. Quality-adjusted survival analysis is now recommended for studies involving toxic anticancer drug regimens in an elderly population.[6]

A number of malignancies, including high-grade lymphomas, breast cancer, and small cell lung cancer, when treated with adequate doses of chemotherapy, are responsive and in certain cases even cured. In a study conducted by the Southwest Oncology Group, patients age 65 or older appeared to have a worse prognosis for advanced malignant lymphoma than did younger patients; however, treatment guidelines included an initial automatic dose reduction of 50 percent for patients 65 or older.[7] Thus, dose reductions for these patients may have been the prime factor in their inferior outcome. It obviously would be advantageous to identify beforehand which elderly patients would tolerate standard doses of chemotherapy or how doses should be modified for optimal management of elderly cancer patients.

Intuitively, decreased tolerance to cancer chemotherapy might be expected in the elderly patient. Renal and pulmonary function both decrease with age, bone marrow cellularity decreases, and pharmacokinetics of some drugs may be altered.[8] However, in a retrospective study completed by Begg et al.,[9] elderly patients treated for lung, breast, and colorectal carcinoma fared no worse with regard to chemotherapeutic toxicity. A number of problems exist with this study which makes extrapolation to the entire elderly population difficult. The investigators admit a selection bias stating "some selectivity of elderly cases for these studies (may exist), since the prevalence of elderly patients in oncology clinics is higher than the prevalence of elderly patients enrolled in studies." It is clear from these clinical trials that more attention is needed on the treatment of older patients with cancer.

The purpose of this chapter is to review the commonly used chemotherapeutic drugs in elderly cancer patients considering (1) drug absorption, distribution, metabolism, and excretion in an elderly population with diminished capacity for drug clearance and (2) limited capacity for compensatory responses to drug excesses. When sufficient data are available, specific recommendations for individual drugs are made.

CHEMOTHERAPY DRUG MONOGRAPHS

Bleomycin Sulfate

Bleomycin sulfate is a complex antibiotic product produced from *Streptomyces verticillius*. There are 13 different glycopeptide fractions which make up the commercial drug.[10] The main component of bleomycin ($\geq$ 50% content) is the A2 fragment with a molecular weight of approximately 1400. Bleomycin has demonstrated significant antitumor activity in a number of malignancies including squamous cell carcinoma of the head and neck, cervix, vulva, vaginal area, skin, penis, and rectum.[11] The drug is also active in both Hodgkin's and non-Hodgkin's lymphomas including the T-cell cutaneous disease mycosis fungoides.[11] As part of combination regimens, bleomycin is also active in the treatment of advanced testicular cancer and lung cancer.

Mechanism of action Bleomycin has a unique mechanism among the anticancer drugs. The drug binds to iron using six structural nitrogens to form a bleomycin-iron complex. This complex is capable of ferric oxidase activity which ultimately produces deoxyribonucleic acid (DNA) strand breaks.[12] The DNA strand breaks actually result from oxygen-free radicals which are generated in a stepwise process from the bleomycin-iron-oxygen complex. Thus, the cytotoxicity from bleomycin is dependent on the availability of both iron and oxygen. There may also be some intercalation of the bithiazole rings of bleomycin between guanine-cytosine-based pairs in DNA.[13] The overall cytotoxic activity is cell cycle phase specific with predominant effects expressed in late G_2 and early M phases.

Toxicity Bleomycin can cause immediate life-threatening anaphylactic-type reactions. This has a high incidence in patients with lymphoma, although a more common presentation is a fever with or without chills which can occur with each dose of the drug. The fever may involve excessive sweating and dehydration especially in patients with lymphoma and can result in hypotension leading to renal failure and/or death. Bleomycin is unusual in that it is primarily nonmyelosuppressive. Bleomycin can produce dose-limiting skin toxicity which involves a severe erythema, thickening, and hyperpigmentation. Mild stomatitis may also occur following bleomycin therapy.

Late effects of the drug are more serious and involve a cumulative dose-related pulmonary toxicity. This toxicity typically presents as pneumonitis with a dry cough, dyspnea, and diffuse infiltrates in the pulmonary fields. It can progress steadily over weeks and in many cases is fatal. Histologically there is a shift of the type I to type II pneumonocytes in the lung. There appear to be two forms of this disease: An acute pulmonary toxicity which is responsive to glucocorticosteroids and drug discontinuation and a cumulative pulmonary toxicity which results in diffuse fibrosis which does not respond to medical therapy. Of particular importance, this pulmonary toxicity is much more common in patients over 70 years of age and those who have received prior pulmonary radiation.[14] It is also much more common when total cumulative lifetime doses exceeding 400 units have been given.

Pharamacokinetics Bleomycin has a short terminal half-life between 2 and 4 h.[15,16] Although there is significant metabolism of the drug, approximately half of the dose can be recovered in the urine at 24 h. Approximately 20 to 40 percent of this urinary drug is the unmetabolized parent compound. Enzymatic inactivation of the drug appears to be avid in the liver, kidney, and bone marrow.[17] Such enzymatic inactivation is significantly absent in the skin and lung.[18] In patients with renal dysfunction, bleomycin pharmacokinetics may be altered when the estimated serum creatinine is above 35 mL/min.[19] Furthermore, the prior use of nephrotoxic drugs such as cisplatin can similarly reduce bleomycin clearance with an increase in the clinical toxicity of the drug.[20] The drug appears to be well absorbed following IM or SC injection, and it is known in some cases to localize in a number of tumor sites. When given by intracavitary administration, approximately half the dose of bleomycin may be systemically available.[21] Nonetheless, bleomycin is highly useful for the control of both intraperitoneal and intrapleural metastases.

Dosing Typical doses for bleomycin as a single agent range from 10 to 20 units/m^2 given one or two times per week. In combination with other agents, a lower dose is typically used. For continuous-infusion therapy doses of 30 units/day for 4 or 5 days have been used without undue toxicity. Except for the dose adjustments for renal failure and for cumulative dosing (<400 units) there are no dose adjustments recommended based on age.

Bleomycin has also been administered by a number of intracavitary routes of relevance to an elderly patient population. For superficial bladder tumors, doses of 30 to 120 units have been administered in 30 to 60 mL of water and retained for 2 h.[22] For the control of malignant infusions intracavitary doses of about 15 to 240 units total dose are used. For pleural effusions the drug is typically diluted in 100 mL of saline and is instilled into the pleural cavity via thoracotomy tube which is clamped for 24 h. Doses exceeding 100 units appear to be required for adequate therapy in these settings. Intraperitoneal metastases have been treated with doses of 60 to 150 mg and appear to produce a response rate of approximately 47 percent.[23]

Carmustine (BCNU)

Carmustine is a nitrosourea-based antitumor agent which is chemically characterized by high lipid solubility and a low molecular weight. The drug is active in primary brain cancer and in other tumors metastatic to the central nervous system. It also has activity in multiple myeloma in second-line drug combinations as well as in regimens for refractory Hodgkin's and non-Hodgkin's lymphomas. High-dose carmustine has also been a mainstay in autologous bone marrow transplantation preparatory regimens.

Mechanism of action Carmustine acts primarily as a DNA alkylating agent via a variety of microsomal metabolites.[24] In addition, the drug is known to block a number of enzymatic reactions which result in prolonged inhibition of DNA synthesis. Carmustine shares some cross resistance to classical alkylating agents. Resistance is partially mediated by an enzyme known as O^6-alkyltransferase (the MER^+ phenotype).[25] Other cytotoxic mechanisms for BCNU include inhibition of DNA repair possibly by carbamoylation of cellular proteins.[26] Cytotoxic effects of carmustine are cell-cycle phase-nonspecific, although a preferential arrest in G_2 phase has been noted.[27]

Toxicity The primary dose-limiting toxicity of BCNU is delayed and includes panmyelosuppression.[28] Leucopenia and sometimes severe thrombocytopenia peak with an uncharacteristically delayed nadir of 3 to 5 weeks after administration. Myelotoxicity can also persist for longer periods.[29] Thus, carmustine has a much longer and more severe myelotoxicity than other agents. This is believed to be due to cellular damage directed at the pluripotential stem cell level in the bone marrow.

Carmustine can also cause some immediate reactions on administration characterized by a burning sensation in the vein or extremity used for infusion. Thrombophlebitis and extravasation necrosis are quite rare with this drug. Significant dilution of the drug is recommended if administered through peripheral veins. Carmustine causes a moderate to high degree of nausea and vomiting, and prophylactic antiemetics are highly recommended with the drug. Rare toxicities with BCNU include liver and renal dysfunction, although these are uncommon at lower doses and tend not to be cumulative. Liver damage is noted by elevation of serum aspartate aminotransferase (SGOT), alkaline phosphatase, and serum bilirubin and this may have a delayed onset.[30] Renal toxicity tends to be cumulative with all of the nitrosoureas including carmustine. Another long-term chronic toxicity of the drug is pulmonary fibrosis.[31] This is associated with a very high mortality rate and does not appear to be dose related. However, the more common pulmonary toxicity with carmustine is an acute pulmonary reaction which is highly responsive to corticosteroids and drug discontinuation.

Pharmacokinetics Carmustine has a very short half-life of about 11 to 16 min in vivo.[32] The drug is highly metabolized principally in the liver via the microsomal enzyme system. This metabolism appears to be necessary for both the elimination of the drug and for the formation of active (alkylating) metabolites. A relatively small amount of carmustine is excreted in the urine, typically 30 percent or less as intact drug or metabolites. Up to 60 to 70 percent of a radiolabeled drug dose can be recovered in the urine as metabolites within 96 h. An uncommon characteristic of carmustine is the ability to achieve high drug levels in the central nervous system (CNS). CNS levels of carmustine tend to be approximately 50 to 60 percent of those simultaneously measured in the plasma.[33]

Dosing For standard (non-ABMT) dosing regimens carmustine is usually given every 6 to 8 weeks to compensate for the greater degree of myelotoxicity. Typical doses call for 75 to 100 mg/m^2 IV daily for two consecutive days or up to 200 mg/m^2 as a single injection. In high-dose autologous bone marrow transplantation programs carmustine doses range from 450 to 600 mg/m^2.[34] This dose would be fatal without the subsequent administration of normal bone marrow to the patient.

There are relatively few studies which suggest that age per se is a factor in the dosing of carmustine. However, because of the greater degree of myelotoxicity directed at the stem cell population, some dose de-escalation may be needed in elderly patients either with intrinsic limited bone marrow reserve or who have received extensive prior radiotherapy and/or cytotoxic therapy. Clearly, elderly patients with a poor performance status are poor candidates for high-dose carmustine therapy. Similarly, there do not appear to be any studies relating age as a factor in the pharmacokinetic disposition of the drug. Because of the relatively small fraction excreted in the urine, significant dose adjustments are not needed in the case of renal dysfunction. Similarly there are no nomograms for adjusting doses based on hepatobiliary function. Indeed, the best indicator for drug clearance would be tests of the cytochrome P-450 mixed-function oxidase system which are not currently available.

Drug interactions A number of drugs may interact with carmustine based on competition for hepatic enzymatic pathways. In this regard the H_2 antagonist cimetidine has been shown to potentiate carmustine toxicities in preclinical systems[35] and in cancer patients receiving carmustine and cimetidine simultaneously.[36,37] Conversely, experimental studies have shown that microsomal enzyme inducers such as phenobarbital can block experimental carmustine toxicities in animals. Because of the use of multiple drugs in the elderly population, it may be prudent to temporarily discontinue any other highly metabolized drugs when carmustine is administered to avoid a potentially toxic interaction.

Chlorambucil

Chlorambucil is a nitrogen mustard derivative with an aminophenyl butyric acid side chain. It has anticancer activity in a variety of human malignancies although it is primarily used in the treatment of chronic lymphocytic leukemia (CLL).[38,39] The drug has also been used in a variety of other cancers including Hodgkin's and non-Hodgkin's lymphoma,[40] ovarian carcinoma,[41] and breast carcinoma.[42] In the treatment of CLL chlorambucil is most often used in the long-term maintenance phase of the disease.

Mechanism of action Chlorambucil is a classic alkylating agent which cross-links adjacent DNA strands similarly to the prototype drug nitrogen mustard. This activity is cell cycle non-phase specific. A difference between chlorambucil and nitrogen mustard is the relatively slow rate of activation of the bischloroethylamine side chains on chlorambucil. This facilitates oral administration of the drug, which is then slowly activated chemically (nonenzymatically) to the alkylating moieties.

Toxicity Chlorambucil is one of the better tolerated oral alkylating agents, especially in an elderly population. Bone marrow depression, principally neutropenia, is the primary dose-limiting effect. Rarely, irreversible bone marrow damage is reported, and in very high doses (>144 mg/m^2) seizures and coma have been described. Oddly, the CNS effects may be less common in elderly patients and have typically been seen only in children.[43]

Chlorambucil occasionally causes gastrointestinal nausea and vomiting and this is typically well managed by antiemetics such as metoclopramide.[44] Liver and renal toxicity is very rarely reported with this drug. Another rare toxicity with chlorambucil is pulmonary fibrosis, which typically follows long-term use.[45] This is noted by alveolar dysplasia and evidence of diffuse pulmonary fibrosis on chest radiographs. Prolonged continuous dosing with chlorambucil is not recommended due to the well-known propensity to cause chromosomal damage and with a tenet increased risk of secondary acute leukemia.[46] This has typically been noted in breast cancer patients receiving continuous chlorambucil for over 4 years.[46]

Pharmacokinetics Chlorambucil appears to have good oral bioavailability of approximately 76 percent even if taken with food. However, the bioavailability can range from 56 to 105 percent.[47] The half-life of the parent molecule chlorambucil in humans is approximately 109 min, and about half of the dose is excreted in the urine. The primary metabolite is phenylacetic acid mustard, which has a half-life of 145 min and urinary fraction excretion of approximately 25 percent.[48] This high degree of urinary excretion would suggest that dose alterations be considered for patients with severely compromised renal function (see Table 22-1).

Dosing The usual oral dose of chlorambucil in CLL is 0.1 to 0.2 mg/kg daily for 3 to 6 weeks. The drug can also be administered on an intermittent basis at a dose of 0.4 mg/kg every 4 weeks.[49] This usually results in a total dose of 6 to 12 mg for remission induction therapy. Maintenance therapy in CLL is usually given in doses of 2 to 6 mg daily. Prolonged continuous daily dosing of solid tumors such as breast cancer is not recommended due to the markedly enhanced risk of developing secondary acute leukemia.

Chlorambucil is a relatively easy compound to use in the elderly population since it is well tolerated orally and generally produces consistent bone marrow suppressive effects.

Cisplatin

Cisplatin is a planar inorganic platinum coordination compound chemically known as *cis*-diamminedichloroplatinum (CDDP) (II). Cisplatin is known to have a wide spectrum of antitumor activity.[50] This includes activity in potentially curative testicular cancer regimens combined with etoposide or vinblastine and bleomycin.[51] The drug is also active in patients with advanced non-Hodgkin's lymphoma[52] and ovarian carcinoma.[53] A variety of other solid tumors may also respond including squamous carcinoma of the head and neck,[54] nonsmall cell lung cancer,[55] bladder cancer,[56] and to some degree advanced breast cancer.[57] In head and neck cancer cisplatin is typically combined with infusion 5-fluorouracil, although there is some question whether this combination is superior to cisplatin alone.[58] The activity in ovarian cancer is high as a single agent, but, again, cisplatin is typically used in combinations to overcome resistance to single agents.

Mechanism of action Cisplatin interacts with DNA in a fashion unique from that of the classic alkylating agents. Thus, while cisplatin does form some interstrand DNA-DNA crosslinks,[59] there is also intrastrand crosslinking which may comprise the primary cytotoxic lesion.[60] This activity is cell cycle phase nonspecific.

Toxicity Cisplatin can be difficult to use in elderly patients who may have preexisting renal dysfunction or hearing impairment.

The primary dose-related toxicity of cisplatin is damage to the renal tubules manifested by an elevation in the blood urea nitrogen (BUN) or serum creatinine.[61] The peak effect is usually noted between the tenth and twentieth days after treatment, and fortunately this damage is typically reversible. Patients receiving other concomitant nephrotoxic drugs such as gentamicin and possibly cephalosporins may be at greater risk for developing acute renal failure following cisplatin.[62] Strategies to avoid a significant renal tubular damage include administration of the drug as a dilute solution as part of a total hydration program and the concomitant administration of diuretics, including the osmotic diuretic mannitol and/or a loop diuretic such as furosemide.

Ototoxicity is another toxic effect of cisplatin and is noted by a high-frequency hearing loss usually above the frequency of normal speech. It can be seen in up to 30 percent of patients treated.[63] Occasional tinnitus without vestibular dysfunction has also been observed. Both ototoxicity and nephrotoxicity can be prevented or completely ameliorated by adequate hydration. Of note, older patients and especially those who have lower than average hearing threshold prior to chemotherapy with cisplatin are more likely to experience a greater hearing threshold shift following administration of the drug. Thus, elderly patients with hearing impairment who require cisplatin therapy should be forewarned of this potential decrease in hearing.

Severe emesis is a typical effect of cisplatin therapy.[64] With any cisplatin regimen, extensive antiemetic premedication is required. This can involve either combinations of dexamethasone, metoclopramide, lorazepam, and prochlorperazine[65] or the use of the newer serotonin type 3 receptor antagonist ondansetron or granisetron.[66] Another feature of cisplatin-induced emesis is a prolonged duration of nausea and anorexia following therapy. Thus, while symptoms are usually most severe in the immediate administration time period, it is not uncommon for nausea and anorexia to persist for several days following administration of the drug. Repeat doses of antiemetics may be important for such susceptible patients. Finally, there are a variety of other less common reactions with cisplatin. These include anaphylactic hypersensitivity reactions seen in over 5 percent of patients and a cumulative dose-limiting peripheral neuropathy.[67] This is noted by a stocking glove type of neuropathy with numbness, tingling, and sensory loss found distally in the arms and legs. This toxicity tends to be cumulative with cisplatin but is not noted with the related platinum-containing agent carboplatin. Cisplatin may also induce a symptomatic hypomagnesemia, which can be reduced but not prevented with prophylactic magnesium supplementation.[68] This is due to a renal loss of magnesium reabsorption capacity and can become cumulatively more severe with prolonged regimens.

Myelosuppression is fortunately not a principal dose-limiting effect of the drug and is typically only seen with very high dose therapy (>200 mg/m^2).[69] It can, however, be more severe in an elderly population with limited bone marrow reserve. Anemia due to renal dysfunction is also seen with cisplatin. Fortunately, cisplatin-induced anemia has been shown to respond to recombinant erythropoietin.[70]

Pharmacokinetics Cisplatin is a highly bound agent and very little free drug (<5 percent) is ever present in the plasma. Thus, the overall half-life of platinum can be artificially prolonged due to a slow release of free drug from the deep-tissue compartment. It has been reported that cisplatin has a triphasic disappearance curve with half-lives of 20 min, 48 to 70 min, and 24 h for the alpha, beta, and gamma half-lives, respectively.[71] The first two phases of elimination probably represent clearance of unbound free drug while the third phase represents the slow release of drug from tissue and plasma protein-binding sites. About 90 percent of the drug is removed by renal processes including both glomerular filtration and tubular secretion. Less than 10 percent of the drug is removed by biliary secretion.[72,73] The drug does appear to distribute reasonably well into the CNS wherein plasma and intracerebral tumor platinum concentrations may be comparable.[74]

Dosing Typical cisplatin dosing regimens include 20 mg/m^2 daily for 5 days repeated every 3 weeks in testicular cancer[51], and for solid tumors, 100 to 120 mg/m^2 IV every 3 to 4 weeks.[75] Alternatively, a dose of 100 mg/m^2 can be repeated on days 1 and 8 of a 20-day treatment cycle.[76] Overall, there is a controversy over whether cisplatin is truly a dose-intensive compound.[77]

Cisplatin dose adjustments specifically for the elderly population are not recommended. However, dosing considerations should include renal function and the presence of preexisting severe myelosuppression.

Cyclophosphamide

Cyclophosphamide is an oxazaphosphorine type of alkylating agent. It has a wide spectrum of clinical use with activity as part of combination regimens for induction therapy of non-Hodgkin's lymphoma,[78] adult leukemia,[79] and occasionally as a replacement for mechlorethamine in the MOPP regimen for Hodgkin's disease.[80] As a single agent it is potentially curative in Burkitt's lymphoma[81] and is frequently used in conjunction with doxorubicin in the management of advanced breast cancer[82] or endometrial carcinoma.[83]

Mechanism of action Cyclophosphamide is unique among the alkylating agents in that it requires activation by hepatic microsomal enzymes before cytotoxic activity is produced. Ultimately, two active metabolites are produced, acrolein and phosphoramide mustard.[84] Acrolein does not have antitumor cytotoxic activity but is associated with specific binding and damage to the urinary bladder. Conversely, phosphoramide mustard appears to comprise the active alkylating moiety from the drug and is relatively unstable once formed. The activity of cyclophosphamide is primarily to crosslink adjacent DNA strands to block the synthesis of macromolecules including DNA and RNA. This activity is cell cycle phase nonspecific.

Toxicity The primary dose-limiting toxicity of cyclophosphamide is leukopenia with a nadir of approximately 8 to 14 days and recovery by 18 to 25 days. There is less thrombocytopenia with cyclophosphamide than with other alkylating agents and the compound has been called "platelet sparing." This may be of benefit in elderly patients with consistently low platelet counts. One manifestation of high-dose cyclophosphamide therapy is acute sterile hemorrhagic cystitis. Rarely is this toxicity dose limiting, and it is usually preventable by adequate hydration prior to therapy. Alternatively, the thiol agent, mesna, can be administered concurrently with cyclophosphamide. The sulfhydryl group in mesna acts to bind acrolein in the urinary bladder before toxicity is produced. Other toxicities which are common with cyclophosphamide include alopecia and a moderate degree of nausea, vomiting, and anorexia. Rare toxicities include a pneumonitis, which may be fatal, and the syndrome of inappropriate antidiuretic hormone release (SIADH).[85]

Pharmacokinetics Studies using radiolabeled cyclophosphamide have shown that oral bioavailability ranges from 31 to 66 percent of a dose.[86] Others have reported an oral bioavailability of 90 percent for unmetabolized cyclophosphamide with a first-pass (hepatic extraction) effect of only 8 percent. A latter study by

Struck et al.[87] showed that levels of alkylating metabolites following IV administration are slightly higher but roughly comparable to those following oral administration of the drug. Approximately 15 percent of the dose is excreted unchanged in the urine, and the remainder is excreted in the urine as metabolites.[88] Thus, dose adjustments for renal dysfunction are unnecessary.[89] The plasma half-life of intact cyclophosphamide ranges from 4-7 h.[86,89] The mean renal clearance of intact drug is approximately 11 mL/min or 15 percent of creatinine clearance. Of interest, body weight may affect the elimination of the compound.[90] In high-body-weight (obese) women, cyclophosphamide clearance was low, about 20 mL/min/m^2 and the plasma half-life was correspondingly long (>8 h). Conversely, lower body weight women had cyclophosphamide clearance values of 40 to 100 mL/min with plasma half-lives of over 8 h. Neither group showed changes in the volume of distribution, which averaged approximately 36 L (range from 19 to 62 L).[90]

There are no studies which suggest that cyclophosphamide elimination or pharmacokinetics differ in the elderly. However, because of the use of multiple drugs in this population, several drug interactions should be kept in mind when dosing cyclophosphamide in an elderly population. The agent allopurinol has been reported to prolong the half-life of cyclophosphamide, although this could not be demonstrated in a follow-up trial in 143 patients with lymphoma.[91] One interaction of potential clinical significance is the combination of the H_2 antagonist cimetidine with cyclophosphamide. This interacton has been shown to increase the alkylating metabolites and toxicity in an animal model.[92] Of interest, the related H_2 antagonist ranitidine does not alter cyclophosphamide activity in mice[93] or in human cancer patients.[94] A similar mechanism of hepatic enzyme down regulation may occur when alpha-interferon is combined with cyclophosphamide. In a preclinical system, interferon combined with cyclophosphamide has shown positive antitumor results. However, in myeloma patients relatively low alpha-interferon doses of 3×10^6 units significantly increased the myelosuppressive effects of cyclophosphamide.[95] Thus, patients receiving alpha-interferon with cyclophosphamide should have close monitoring for potential increased myelotoxicity.

Dosing Two general schedules of cyclophosphamide dosing are used: A single dose given every 3 to 4 weeks or several divided doses over a period of 2 to 4 days repeated at 3-to-4-week intervals. The maximal dose of cyclophosphamide given as a single injection is 500 to 1500 mg/m^2 of body surface area or 30 to 40 mg/kg/treatment course. These courses are repeated at 3-to-4-week intervals. With the four times daily or five times daily schedule, doses of 60 to 120 mg/m^2 of body surface area (1 to 2.5 mg/kg/day) are used. All doses require careful assessment of myelosuppression, and there is one study to suggest that dosing should be altered in the elderly (>65 years old) based on renal function.[96] In this trial, elderly patients with breast cancer received standard doses of the combination "CMF" unless their creatinine clearance was less than 70 mL/min. In patients with reduced renal function, the oral cyclophosphamide doses given on days 1 to 14 were adjusted according to the following formula:

$$\text{Cyclophosphamide dose} = 100\ \text{mg/m}^2 \times \frac{\text{pretreatment creatinine clearance}}{70}$$

The use of this adjusted dose schema for cyclophosphamide and methotrexate resulted in no significant differences in the toxicities of the CMF regimen in the elderly population compared to the younger patient population.[96] Response and survival were similarly unaffected by the renal-based dose modification. Of interest, this method resulted in higher drug doses in 24 percent of the elderly population over 60 years who would have otherwise received an arbitrary one-third dose reduction.[96]

Cytarabine (ARA-C)

Cytarabine is a nucleoside analog of deoxycytidine which differs by the substitution of arabinose for deoxyribose. It is most useful clinically in hematologic malignancies usually in combination with other cytotoxic agents. The principal use of the drug is in the induction and maintenance therapy for acute myeloid leukemia (AML).[97] Recent clinical advances in the use of cytarabine include high-dose chemotherapy for patients with refractory AML.[98] It has also shown some activity as a differentiating agent in some myelodysplastic syndromes.

Mechanism Cytarabine requires metabolism to its ultimate active form, the triphosphorylated nucleotide ARA-C-CTP.[99] This metabolite acts as a competitive inhibitor of DNA polymerase, and after incorporation onto the growing DNA chain, further DNA synthesis is halted. Cytarabine is highly cell cycle phase specific for S-phase and is relatively inactive in nonproliferating cells.[100]

Toxicity The primary toxicity of cytarabine is hematopoietic depression, although high cumulative doses can also lead to permanent CNS damage. Bone marrow damage following cytarabine typically involves leukopenia and thrombocytopenia although anemia may rarely occur. Gastrointestinal toxicity is usually not dose limiting and can include stomatitis, anorexia, and rarely, gastrointestinal hemorrhage. A flulike syndrome has also been reported to follow cytarabine and is noted by fevers, arthralgias, and sometimes a rash on the palms, soles, neck, and chest. Hepatic and renal toxicities are generally not severe with this agent, although liver enzymes may be transiently elevated in approximately one-third of patients given standard or high-dose therapy.

With high-dose therapy (>200 mg/m^2) cerebellar dysfunction can be seen with an onset of approximately 6 to 8 days. There is some suggestion that this is related to cumulative doses of the drug with toxicity relatively rare at total doses <30 g/m^2.[101] Another retrospective analysis also suggested that age exceeding 50 years was a risk factor for CNS toxicity from cytarabine.[102] Finally, renal insufficiency has also been correlated to high-dose cytarabine neurotoxicity.[103] In this trial, 76 percent of patients with a creatinine clearance less than 60 mL/min developed neurotoxicity. In contrast, only 8 percent of patients with good renal function as estimated by creatinine clearance above 60 mL/min developed CNS toxicities. Therefore, dose reductions were recommended in this trial for any patient receiving high-dose cytarabine if renal insufficiency was present.[103] The use of infusion periods longer than 3 h may also reduce cytarabine CNS toxicity.[104]

One explanation for the correlation between renal function and neurotoxicity is the potential accumulation of the deaminated metabolite uracil arabinoside which has been found to be a direct neurotoxin when administered into the cerebral spinal fluid of primates.[105] Other rare toxicities of high-dose therapy include noncardiogenic pulmonary edema which can occasionally be fatal. Finally, ocular toxicity from high-dose cytarabine is noted in most patients and may be ameliorated by prophylactic glucocorticosteroid eye drops. Signs and symptoms include excessive tearing, photophobia, pain, and blurred vision.[106] This toxicity may directly relate to the secretion of relatively high concentrations of cytarabine-activated metabolites into the tear fluid following high-dose chemotherapy.

Pharmacokinetics Cytarabine is primarily metabolized to the inactive agent uracil arabinoside. This metabolite is extensively excreted into the urine, and at 24 h 90 percent of the dose can be recovered in the urine. A small percentage of drug is excreted in the bile. The levels of drug in the CNS are approximately 40 to 50 percent of simultaneous plasma levels. These high levels presumably result from the lack of the inactivating enzyme cytidine deaminase in the CNS. The half-life of the parent compound is extremely short at approximately 15 min, and this is due to extensive deamination to uracil arabinoside.[107]

Dose The standard dose of cytarabine for remission induction therapy in the treatment of acute nonlymphocytic leukemia ranges from 100 to 150 mg/m^2/day for 5 to 10 days given either as a continuous 24-h infusion or in divided doses every 6 to 12 h.[97] The high-dose regimen of cytarabine calls for 2 to 3 g/m^2 given as a 1-to-2-h infusion every 12 h for 8 to 12 doses.[98] Both the low- and high-dose cytarabine regimens can be combined with DNA intercalators such as doxorubicin.

Dosing modifications are recommended for patients receiving high-dose cytarabine with renal dysfunction (creatinine clearance <60 mL/min). In addition, patients with severe hepatic dysfunction may require lower doses, although specific nomograms for either setting are not well described. There is no current dose adjustment recommended based on age.

Daunorubicin HCl

Daunorubicin is an anthracycline analog of doxorubicin which has a hydroxyl group at the 9 position on the a ring of the aglycone (daunomycinone). The amino sugar daunosamine is glycosidically lined at the number 7 carbon and is identical to doxorubicin.[108] Daunorubicin has antitumor activity primarily in acute nonlymphocytic leukemia (ANLL).[109] It is typically combined with other cytotoxic agents such as cytarabine, prednisone, and a thiopurine such as 6-mercaptopurine or 6-thioguanine.[110]

Mechanism of action Daunorubicin produces a number of biochemical effects which contribute to the antitumor activity of the compound. As with doxorubicin, daunomycin generates oxygen-free radicals due to a redox cycling of the quinone moiety. This activity is dependent upon molecular oxygen, a reducing equivalent or enzyme such as cytochrome P-450 reductase, and the availability of divalent metals, especially iron. The iron-daunomycin complex can form superoxide species which degrade into highly reactive hydroxyl radicals and act to peroxidize membrane lipids in many cells, including the heart. The iron-chelating agent ICRF-187 (cardioxane) has been shown to block the production of heart toxicity from daunomycin without altering the antitumor activity. Other free radical scavengers and antioxidants such as vitamin E and glutathione have been effective in a variety of experimental systems but have not shown conclusive activity in preclinical animal models nor in clinical studies.

Toxicity Myelosuppression is the major toxicity of daunorubicin, with leukocyte, and platelet nadirs generally occur 10 to 14 days following drug administration.[111] Bone marrow recovery is usually evident in the peripheral blood within 3 weeks after administration. A second toxicity which is occassionally dose limiting is severe stomatitis and/or mucositis which may affect the entire gastrointestinal tract. This can result in severe gastrointestinal toxicity occasionally leading to gastrointestinal perforations and death especially with repeated dosing or dose-intensive daunorubicin therapy. Of note, this toxicity may be more severe in an elderly patient population. As with the other cytotoxic agents, alopecia may be produced and the compound is a severe vesicant if inadvertently extravasated. Transient elevations in serum bilirubin or other liver enzymes may occasionally be noted, but this is rarely associated with dose-limiting toxicity. However, as with doxorubicin, impairment of hepatobiliary function as noted by elevated serum bilirubin does require significant dose reduction. Daunorubicin also colors the urine red due to excretion of up to 15 percent of a dose in the urine. This does not represent toxicity. Finally, cardiotoxicity is a significant risk with cumulative doses of daunorubicin above 500 mg/m^2. Of interest, in the initial clinical survey of daunorubicin cardiotoxicity, the cumulative dose associated with a 5 percent incidence of cardiotoxicity was much higher than the official 500 mg/m^2 dose limit. It may be close to 650 mg/m^2.[112] There is also some evidence from this trial that children and infants were more susceptible to daunorubicin-induced congestive heart failure (CHF). Several predisposing factors may increase the likelihood or the severity of daunorubicin-induced cardiomyopathy. These include preexisting arrhythmias, longstanding hypertension or preexisting CHF, and finally, prior use of radiotherapy involving the chest.

Because of decreased cardiac reserve, age probably lowers the cumulative dose but not the individual dose in an antileukemic regimen.

Pharmacokinetics Daunorubicin primarily undergoes hepatobiliary secretion in the feces as the predominant route of elimination as with doxorubicin. Both parent drug and a large number of hydroxylated metabolites and conjugates to glucuronide or sulfate have been noted in the bile and feces. However, a larger fraction of a daunorubicin dose is excreted in the urine. This approaches 15 percent of a daunorubicin dose in contrast to the more than 5 percent for doxorubicin. The major metabolite of daunorubicin is the alcohol doxorubicinol, which has greater polarity but much less antitumor efficacy compared to the parent molecule.[113] Of the urinary fraction, only about 3 percent of the dose is excreted as doxorubicinol, and other daunorubicin metabolites are recovered in small amounts in the urine including 7-deoxydaunorubicin and daunorubicinol aglycones.

Dose Typical doses for ANLL remission induction therapy are 45 mg/m^2/day for three consecutive days when used in combination with other agents. Dose reductions are required for patients with elevated serum bilirubin and/or reduced renal function (see Table 22-2, following the drug monographs). Of interest, however, these dose reductions have not been prospectively evaluated and should be used as a general guide to therapy. High-dose therapy with daunorubicin is complicated by the onset of severe gastrointestinal toxicity which limits the amount of drug that can be safely administered as a large single dose. Furthermore, the gastrointestinal toxicities of daunorubicin may be worsened with more frequent administration. Thus, dose intensification with daunorubicin in any age population is difficult. The effect of age on tolerance to daunorubicin has been evaluated in several leukemia trials, and at present there is no convincing evidence that dose reductions are required in patients over 60 years of age. Indeed, response rates are consistently lower in studies in which arbitrary dose reductions were allowed for older patients who otherwise had normal hepatobiliary and renal function.

Doxorubicin

Doxorubicin is an anthracycline antibiotic obtained from *Streptomyces* microorganisms. The four-membered anthracycline ring of doxorubicin is believed to intercalate between base pairs of DNA, particularly in guanine-cytosine-rich areas. This intercalation blocks both ribonucleic acid (RNA) and especially DNA synthesis. In addition, doxorubicin blocks the activity of topoisomerase II enzymes leading to protein-linked double-strand breaks in DNA.[114]

Doxorubicin has been shown to form oxygen free radicals in the presence of a reducing milieu such as with a cytochrome P-450 reductase and NADPH.[115] This process appears to be enhanced in the presence of oxygen and is catalyzed by divalent metals such as Fe(II). This forms the basis of the intriguing interaction between doxorubicin and ICRF-187 (cardioxane) as an inhibitor of doxorubicin-induced cardiotoxicity. By chelating divalent iron, cardioxane is believed to block doxorubicin-induced oxygen free-radical formation in the heart. This prevents peroxidation of membrane lipids in the myocyte and has reduced cardiac toxicity in vitro.[116] A clinical trial has shown significant enhancement of dose intensity for doxorubicin combined with cardioxane.[117]

Toxicity The primary dose-limiting toxicity of doxorubicin is myelosuppression, principally leukopenia with a nadir of 10 to 14 days after administration of the drug. Other hematologic toxicities such as anemia and thrombocytopenia are less common. The recovery from myelosuppression is usually prompt with resolution approximately 3 weeks following administration of the drug. Doxorubicin can also produce severe local tissue damage if extravasated. These ulcers may result in up to one-third of extravasations and the lesions undergo a slow, indolent expansion which may ultimately involve deep-seated structures such as tendons and nerves. Numerous pharmacologic antidotes have been evaluated but few have demonstrated unequivocal efficacy.[118] However, the topical administration of 99 percent (v/v) dimethylsulfoxide (DMSO) has been shown to have good clinical efficacy in a nonrandomized trial.[119] The specific regimen involved the application of 1.5 mL of DMSO every 6 h for 14 days. In addition, several experimental studies have shown efficacy for the topical administration of cold packs.[120,121] Nonetheless, prevention of extravasation reactions by the use of central venous catheters or very scrupulous intravenous technique is highly recommended. This may be especially important in older patients with more fragile peripheral veins.

A less common intravenous reaction involves the so-called venous flare resulting from the local release of histamine from the vein.[122] This is noted by an erythematous streak up the vein usually associated with delayed pruritis but not with loss of vein patency. Prophylactic antihistamines and glucocorticosteroids may be helpful, although the interaction is variable among different patient populations.

The major chronic dose-limiting toxicity of doxorubicin is cardiomyopathy, which is particularly noted at cumulative doses above 550 mg/m^2.[123] This total lifetime dose limit is reduced in patients who have received prior mediastinal irradiation exceeding 2000 rads or those patients over 70 years of age and/or who have preexisting cardiovascular diseases such as a history of myocardial infarction or long-standing hypertension.[124] Rarely, anthracycline-induced cardiac toxicity has been noted after only the first or second dose of the drug.[125] Overall, though, the best predictor for heart failure is the cumulative dose of the drug. Evaluation of cardiac function by nuclear scanning (MUGA scan) or two-dimensional echocardiography is recommended in elderly patients prior to beginning doxorubicin treatment.

Pharmacokinetics Intravenously administered doxorubicin is rapidly distributed in body tissues with about 75 percent of the drug bound to plasma proteins, primarily albumin.[126] In blood the free fraction is also dependent upon the hematocrit.[127] Patients with anemia may need to be transfused prior to administering doxorubicin to prevent enhanced toxicity. The elimination of doxorubicin occurs primarily in the liver, and a number of metabolites have been identified. Overall, most of the drug is eliminated in the bile, which accounts for about 40 percent of the administered dose.[128] Slightly less than half of the total biliary drug is doxorubicin and about a quarter is doxorubicinol.[128] Very little drug, only 5 to 10, is excreted in the urine, and the majority of this is as doxorubicin.

Alterations in doxorubicin pharmacokinetics Patients with cholestasis will have delayed doxorubicin clearance and can experience increased toxicity from standard doses.[129] This has mandated the reduction in dosing based on serum bilirubin levels. In contrast, Chan et al,[130] could find no significant alterations in the pharmacokinetics of the drug given to patients with either cirrhosis or simple hepatocellular enzyme elevations. As an index of plasma clearance, indocyanine green may be administered, and this has been shown to correlate to both hepatobiliary function and doxorubicin clearance.[131] Thus, delayed clearance of an indocyanine green dose from the plasma is associated with higher bilirubin levels and reduced doxorubicin clearance. This test could be useful in older patients in whom hepatobiliary function may be compromised.

Obesity may also reduce the clearance of doxorubicin in cancer patients.[132] Mildly obese patients (115 to 130 percent of ideal body weight) and obese patients with greater than 130 percent body weight experience significantly delayed clearance of doxorubicin. This can lead to increased systemic exposure and a prolonged elimination half-life.[132] The half-life of doxorubicin in nonobese patients in this study was 13 h, 15 h in the mildly obese, and 20 h in the obese patients . The area under the plasma concentration curve (AUC) also increased proportionally in the three groups. There were no changes in the volume of distribution of doxorubicin nor in the disposition of doxorubicinol in the obese population in this study.

Age may be another significant factor for altered clearance of doxorubicin. One trial has shown that the highest clearances of doxorubicin may be observed in younger patient populations.[133] In this trial the early phase clearance of the drug was altered in the population above 50 years of age. The early phase clearances in the older population were all below 50 $L/h/m^2$. This compares to early phase drug clearances in the younger population, which ranged from 35 to 200 $L/h/m^2$. The best correlations between age and doxorubicin clearance were found in breast cancer and lymphoma patients.

These observations suggested that higher peak doxorubicin levels were achieved in the population older than 50. This finding is also compatible with those of Piazza et al.[127]

Dose adjustments are recommended for patients with elevated serum bilirubin and/or evidence of reduced indocyanine green clearance. However, dose adjustments are not firmly indicated in elderly patients without some predisposing factor such as elevated bilirubin or preexisting heart disease or prior radiotherapy involving the chest cardiac silhouette. Of interest, there are no studies that suggest that mild impairments of bone marrow function necessitate dose reduction with doxorubicin. The most conclusive dosing information involves the cumulative nature of the cardiac damage which requires a maximum lifetime cumulative dose of 500 mg/m^2. Age does appear to be a factor which lowers this dose limit.[123] Conversely, the administration of doxorubicin by continuous infusion appears to increase this maximum lifetime dose limit and is useful in older populations if central venous access can be assured. Although firm endpoints are not available, doxorubicin doses up to 750 mg/m^2 have been safely administered as a 4-day continuous infusion. These doses appear to be equieffective to bolus administration and do not lead to greater myelosuppression, although mucositis may be enhanced.[134]

Etoposide (VP-16)

Etoposide is a semisynthetic epipodophyllotoxin derived from *Podophyllum peltatum* or the mayapple herb. The principal antitumor activity of etoposide is in small cell lung cancer, in certain non-Hodgkin's lymphomas, in testicular cancer, and in ANLL. The mechanism of action of etoposide is unique and differs from that of the parent molecule podophyllotoxin.

Mechanism of action Unlike the anthracycline and anthracene type of agents, etoposide does not intercalate to DNA and indeed does not bind to DNA at all. Etoposide inhibits DNA topoisomerase II (TOPO-II) enzymes which produces protein-linked DNA strand breaks in cells. This process involves stabilizing the otherwise "cleavable complex" between a TOPO-II homodimer protein and double-stranded DNA.[135] The inhibitory activity is maximal in the G_2 phase due to the high expression of TOPO-II during this premitotic phase of division.

Toxicity The dose-limiting toxicity of etoposide is leukopenia, although thrombocytopenia may also occur. The nadir for leucocyte suppression is about 16 days, and generally recovery is complete after 20 to 22 days. Gastrointestinal toxicity is also described but usually involves only mild to moderate nausea, vomiting,and anorexia.[50] The drug also can induce alopecia in up to 90 percent of patients, but it is less severe than the anthracenes or anthracyclines. Stomatitis is occasionally reported, and there is a relatively high incidence of allergic reactions to the drug when given IV.[136] These are felt to be due to the lipophilic solvent system, and this may explain some of the phlebitis associated with the drug. Bronchospasm with wheezing has also been rarely observed and is usually responsive to antihistamines and glucocorticosteroids. Rare neurotoxicity is described with etoposide. This is primarily a CNS depression characterized by somnolence and fatigue. Peripheral neuropathy has been reported in less than 1 per cent of patients. In this latter regard, age appears to be a predisposing factor along with both impaired nutritional status and prior therapy with other neurotoxic drugs such as vincristine.[137]

Etoposide is relatively rapidly cleared from the plasma with an elimination half-life on the order of 7 h.[138] This half-life does not appear to be dependent upon the dose, route, or method of administration. About one-third of the drug is eliminated renally of which about two-thirds is parent etoposide.[139] Very little drug is detectable after standard doses in the cerebral spinal fluid, and even with doses of 400 to 800 mg/m^2 cerebrospinal fluid (CSF) levels are below 2 percent of concurrent plasma levels.[140] Biliary secretion of the parent drug accounts for less than 2 percent of the dose, although fecal recovery of drug and metabolites may account for up to 16 percent of drug elimination.[139] The major metabolites of etoposide are the cis trans, and picro-hydroxy acids and the cis (picro) lactone.[141, 138] The major urinary metabolite is 4′-dimethylepipodophilic acid-O-(4,6-ethylidene-β-deglucopyranoside).[142] All of these metabolites have much less activity, and most of the metabolites have much less activity or are inactive compared to the parent molecule. A large fraction of etoposide is bound to plasma proteins. This may approach 95 percent in patients with normal hepatic function.[143] The unbound fraction of the drug may comprise only less than 5 percent of the total plasma concentration. Patients with increased bilirubin and/or decreased albumin may have an increase in this free fraction even though drug clearance is unaltered.[143] Age has not been reported to affect etoposide clearance. However, a number of other conditions may lower the clearance of the drug including prior or concurrent cisplatin therapy,[144] obesity, and elevated alkaline phosphatase levels.[145] The concomitant use of other nephrotoxic drugs such as ifosfamide and cisplatin have consistently been associated with reduced etoposide clearance by up to 27 percent. This may reduce etoposide clearance from a normal value of 26 $mL/min/m^2$ to 19 $mL/min/m^2$ as noted after three ifosfamide/VP-16 courses.[146] Similarly, cyclosporin A infusions of 18 mg/kg/day have also been shown to decrease etoposide clearance.[147]

Etoposide is also given by the oral route in a gelatin capsule form. The absolute oral bioavailability of this preparation ranges from 25 to 74 percent with a mean oral bioavailability of 48 percent.[148] There is a controversy over whether the daily oral dose should be divided, with some reports describing better bioavailability for split daily doses.[149] Other groups have not reported a consistent enhancement in bioavailability with split dosing. However, there may be a nonlinear increase in the AUC with single oral doses exceeding 200 mg. Of note, oral etoposide bioavailability and general pharmacokinetics appear to be highly variable showing both intra- and interpatient variations. Furthermore, neither the coingestion of food nor the administration of other chemotherapy agents appears to consistently alter etoposide absorption.[150] Thus, the drug may demonstrate altered disposition both within a given patient and independent of the route of administration or other known pharmacokinetic features.

Dosing A general principle for dosing etoposide calls for frequent drug administration schedules to take advantage of cell cycle-dependent cytotoxicity. In addition, a rough doubling of the oral dose over that given intravenously is recommended to account for the 50 percent bioavailability. Finally, significant etoposide dose reductions may be required if other myelosuppressive drugs are used or if a patient has had significant prior myelotoxic therapy and has poor bone marrow reserve and/or poor performance status. Age does not appear to be a variable for dosing etoposide. In general, etoposide doses can be repeated every 3 to 4 weeks depending upon the leucocyte count. Continuous oral daily regimens have recently been explored involving 21 days on and 21 days off.[151] For short IV infusions, single doses of 200 to 250 mg/m^2 have been administered in lung cancer. For testicular cancer a dose of 50 to 100 mg/m^2/day for 5 days has been utilized. These latter doses were repeated at 3-to-4 week intervals. Finally, continuous IV administration of etoposide has been explored using doses of 80 to 125 mg/m^2/day for 5 days repeated at 4 weeks. Continuous oral etoposide has been administered in small cell lung cancer at doses ranging from 160 mg/m^2 for 5 days to 50 mg/m^2 /day for up to 21 days. In each instance the dosing interval is repeated at 4 weeks.[152,153] The theoretic advantage of the continuous oral therapy is that it allows for prolonged outpatient administration of the cell cycle specific agent. This may have significant other advantages in elderly patients since multiple injections are avoided and the daily oral dose can be individualized to each patient's bone marrow reserve and overall performance status.

5-Fluorouracil (5-FU)

5-Fluorouracil is a modified pyrimidine which differs from the normal base uracil by the presence of a fluorine in the number 5 position. Fluorouracil has antitumor activity in the elderly in a variety of solid tumors, principally those involving various adenocarcinomas of the gastrointestinal tract. The drug is also active in head and neck cancer, renal cell carcinoma, and squamous cell carcinoma of the esophagus. In colorectal cancer 5-fluorouracil is typically given as an extended infusion to capitalize on the DNA-specific (S-phase-specific) activity of the compound.[154] Newer uses of 5-fluorouracil in colorectal cancer include combinations with levamisole[155] or leucovorin[156] in order to enhance the antitumor activity.

Mechanism of action Leucovorin appears to modulate 5-fluorouracil activity by enhancing the binding of the molecule with the enzyme thymidylate synthetase. This complex is known to involve a ternary structure involving reduced folates, 5-fluorouracil nucleotide, and a sulfhydryl residue on thymidylate synthetase. Another potential mechanism of 5-FU which may be important for gastrointestinal toxicity involves the conversion of 5-fluorouracil to the triphosphate for nucleotide which is incorporated into RNA and DNA. However, the main cytotoxic activity of 5-FU appears to be mediated by its active metabolite, 5-fluorodeoxyuridylate monophosphate (FdUMP). This is the moiety which binds to thymidylate synthetase to halt DNA synthesis in the S phase.

Toxicity The primary dose-limiting effect of 5-fluorouracil is myelosuppression, principally granulocytopenia and thrombocytopenia with a nadir of 9 to 14 days for the granulocytes and 7 to 14 days for the platelets. Fluorouracil-induced myelosuppression is dramatically lessened with continuous infusion therapy (e.g., over 5 days). Another toxicity which is occasionally dose limiting involves the gastrointestinal tract. While nausea and vomiting may occur, it is usually of low intensity. However, diarrhea can be dose limiting, particularly with the combinations of 5-FU with leucovorin.[157] Stomatitis may also be more severe with the prolonged infusions of 5-FU. With these infusions another unusual toxicity is palmar-plantar erythrodysethesias. This has been noted following long-term infusions of 5-FU and is progressive, necessitating therapy discontinuation. Treatment with 50 to 100 mg of pyridoxine per day may help alleviate the syndrome.[158]

Pharmacokinetics 5-Fluorouracil has a relatively short half-life due to extensive hepatic and nonhepatic conversion to both active and inactive metabolites. Age does not appear to be a factor in the clearance of this drug. However, the elimination of 5-FU may occur in a nonlinear fashion whereby a doubling of the dose may be accompanied by a decrease in the nonrenal clearance of the drug and an elevation in steady-state drug levels. In other words, the drug half-life may be twice as long at high doses as with low doses.[159] Up to 80 percent of 5-FU is metabolized in the liver, although there is no evidence that patients with an impaired liver function require dose reductions.[160] About 15 percent of a dose may be found intact in the urine 6 h after administration, and 90 percent of this is excreted in the first hour. Nonetheless, renal dysfunction does not generally require dose adjustment. The primary metabolite eliminated in the urine is alpha-fluoro-beta-alanine, which accounts for about 60 to 90 percent of an administered dose. Biliary excretion only amounts to 2 to 3 percent of 5-FU clearance. The terminal half-life of 5-FU following a standard dose of 500 mg/m2 given as an IV bolus is approximately 13 min.[161]

Dosing There are a large number of reported regimens for 5-fluorouracil dosing. These include the use of a loading dose, weekly IV bolus, or continuous infusion over 4 to 5 days. With the loading dose scheme, an initial dose of 12 mg/kg (maximum 800 mg) is given daily for 4 days either as a single daily bolus injection or as a 4-day infusion. However, the loading dose regimen has been associated with significant morbidity, and therefore alternate schemas are currently favored. One of the most common is to administer 370 mg/m^2/day of 5-FU as an IV bolus for 5 days with oral leucovorin. Alternatively, a 5-day continuous infusion can be used at a dose of 500 mg/m^2 beginning 24 h before 5-FU and continuing for 12 h afterward.[162] With prolonged infusions, doses of 1 g to 2 g of 5-FU per day may be administered for up to 5 days with 4-week intervals between repeat doses. There does not appear to be strong rationale for dose modification based either on altered hepatic or renal function, or on age per se as a dose-modifying factor.

Topical 5-FU cream (Efudex) is used frequently in elderly patients for the treatment of various neoplastic keratoses.[163] The drug appears to only achieve penetration into damaged skin areas with an onset of action in the range of 2 to 3 days. The use of an occlusive dressing can accelerate the desired inflammatory reaction.

Ifosfamide

Ifosfamide is a close chemical congener of the DNA-alkylating agent cyclophosphamide. It is most useful in treating refractory testicular carcinoma and for soft tissue sarcomas.

Mechanism of action Ifosfamide is metabolized by cytochrome P-450 enzymes to the cytotoxic moiety ifosforamide mustard and the urinary bladder toxin, acrolein. Crosslinking of DNA by ifosforamide mustard leads to cell death whereas acrolein lacks antitumor activity.

Pharmacokinetics Contrary to early reports, ifosfamide does not exhibit dose-dependent elimination.[164] However, the clearance of the drug does appear to increase with five daily infusions of 1.5g/m^2/day from about 65 mL/min on day 1 to 115 mL/min on day 5.[164] This effect was not seen with continuous 24-h infusions of a 5-g/m^2 dose.

Age has also been reported to alter ifosfamide pharmacokinetics by increasing the drug's half-life.[165] The normal half-life for the parent compound of 5 to 6 h was slightly but significantly longer in the aged population whereas clearance remained unchanged. This appeared to be due to a larger volume of distribution associated with an increase in the ratio of body fat to lean weight (i.e., obesity) in the elderly population.

Toxicity The primary dose-limiting toxicity of ifosfamide is neutropenia and urinary tract irritation. The sulfhydryl compound mesna can prevent and alleviate the hemorrhagic cystitis and does not alter the hematologic toxicity or the antitumor efficacy. Ifosfamide also produces CNS toxicities characterized mainly as depression, somnolence, and rarely, coma. These effects may be mediated by the minor chloroacetaldehyde metabolite which can accumulate to toxic levels in the presence of significant renal dysfunction.

Dosage The usual dose of ifosfamide is 1.5 to 2.0 g/m^2/day for five consecutive days. Continuous infusion doses average 5 g/m^2/24 h × 1 day but may be associated with greater renal toxicity. All ifosfamide regimens include the simultaneous use of mesna given in three divided doses each at 20 per cent of the ifosfamide dose: 15 min before ifosfamide and again at 4 and 8 h after ifosfamide. Specific dose adjustments for reduced renal function and/or age have not been reported.

Interferon Alpha

Alpha-interferons comprise a group of up to 17 chemically related proteins.[166] The recombinant molecules are produced in *Escherichia coli* and have a molecular weight of approximately 19,000 (about 165 amino acids). Commercial formulations of alpha-interferon include Intron A (alpha-interferon 2b, Schering Corporation) and Roferon-A (alpha-interferon 2a, Roche Laboratories). A recent multispecies natural human leucocyte interferon has also recently become available under the generic name alpha N3 interferon (Alferon, Purdue Frederick).

Activity The alpha-interferons have a broad spectrum of antitumor activity. However, their official FDA approval is limited to the treatment of hairy cell leukemia,[167] AIDS-associated Kaposi's sarcoma, venereal warts (Condylomata acuminata), and certain forms of chronic viral hepatitis. Responses in hairy cell leukemia are characterized by prolonged normalization of bone marrow function with dramatic restoration of normal red blood counts, white blood counts, and platelet counts. This peaks 3 to 4 months after the initiation of therapy. Alpha-interferon therapy is not curative in hairy cell leukemia, and a certain number of patients may relapse on the drug. In some cases it is associated with the development of a neutralizing serum antibody. Nonetheless, over 80 per cent of responding patients typically remain in prolonged, continuous remissions of their disease for years. This has had a major impact on life prolongation in this disease. Other hematologic malignancies which are common in the elderly and are responsive to alpha-interferon include chronic myelogenous leukemia,[168] non-Hodgkin's lymphomas, and multiple myeloma wherein the drug is used to maintain remissions induced by cytotoxic drug combinations. Certain solid tumors are also sensitive to the drug. These include AIDS-related Kaposi's sarcoma,[169] malignant melanoma,[170] and renal cell carcinoma.[171] Some other cancers are also responsive to local applications of the drug including ovarian carcinoma treated with high-dose IP therapy[172] and malignant melanoma.[173]

Mechanism of action Aplha-interferon is taken up into cells by high-affinity cell surface receptors (about 100 to 10,000 per cell[174]). Following binding, the protein-receptor complex is internalized and may be partially processed before interacting with specific sites in the nucleus. A large number of genes are known to be activated by alpha-interferon. These result in the enhanced expression of certain antiviral enzymes, including 2′, 5′-oligoadenylate synthetase (2′, 5′-A), an enzyme which forms long strands of polyadenylylated nucleotide and is associated with response to the drug in patients with chronic myelogenous leukemia and certain viral diseases. Alpha-interferon also induces a specific protein kinase which blocks elongation/intitiation factor eIF-2. This leads to a blockade in the delivery of RNA to the ribosome, thereby markedly reducing protein synthesis.[175]

The overall inhibition of protein synthesis may indeed explain many of the antitumor effects and some of the drug interactions with alpha-interferon. Cellular division is slowed through all phases of the cell cycle, and in some cases such as multiple-myeloma, tumor cells are believed to accumulate in the G_0 (resting phase) of growth. Other indirect mechanisms of alpha-interferon action involve stimulation of host immunologic responses to tumor cells by enhancement of natural killer (NK) cell activity and release of other cytokines from macrophages such as interleukin 2 (IL-2) and tumor necrosis factor (TNF). In addition, there is enhanced antigen expression in some tumor cells, causing an increase in the major histocompatibility proteins to be expressed on the surface and thereby rendering the cells more susceptible to immunologic attack.

Toxicity The primary dose-limiting toxicity of alpha-interferon is a flulike syndrome comprising fever, chills, malaise, myalgia, and headache.[176] Chills usually precede the fever in up to 40 percent of the patients and the febrile reaction may peak about 4 to 6 h after dosing. For severe flulike symptoms indomethacin may be useful,[177] although acetaminophen is most commonly used to reduce these toxicities. Fortunately, the incidence and severity of the flulike syndrome decreases as the drug is continually administered (tachyphylaxis). In older patients, fatigue may be the most common dose-limiting toxicity of the drug. In this population some tolerance may be achieved with late night administration of doses and with intermittent (nonconsecutive daily) dosing schedules.[176]

Other toxicities of alpha-interferon are usually not dose-limiting and are only severe when high-dose therapy is administered. These include gastrointestinal toxicity and rare hepatic or renal toxicities. About one-third of patients may have a slight and temporary elevation in liver transaminase levels. A smaller percentage of patients may experience proteinuria following administration of the drug, but frank renal toxicity is rare with interferon. Fortunately, the alpha-interferons do not produce significant myelosuppression at standard doses. A very mild and transient leucopenia may be noted in approximately 50 percent of patients. Fortunately the granulocyte levels recover briskly within days after drug discontinuation. Both central and peripheral nervous system toxicities have been described with alpha-interferon but are only significant at doses above 15 to 20 $\times 10^6$ IU/day.

Pharmacokinetics Alpha-interferons are rapidly eliminated from the plasma following parenteral administration.[178] The drug is well absorbed from either subcutaneous or intramuscular sites, although peak levels are delayed by approximately 4 and 7 h after the IM and subcutaneous routes, respectively.[178] The terminal elimination half-life of the drug varies between 3 and 6 h with a clearance value of greater than that for creatinine (approximately 2.8mL/min/kg[178]).

Alpha-interferon does not distribute into the CNS to any appreciable amount unless extremely high doses of the drug are administered. The major route of clearance for alpha-interferon involves renal catabolism to inactive peptide fragments which are excreted into the urine.[179] This process does not appear to involve glomerular function per se, and patients with chronic renal failure have similar alpha-interferon pharmacokinetics to those with normal renal function.[180] Hemodialysis also does not effect alpha-interferon pharmacokinetics.

Dosing The approved dose levels for hairy cell leukemia range from 2 to 3 $\times 10^6$ IU/m^2/day given subcutaneously or intramuscularly from 3 to 7 times per week. Higher doses have been explored in solid tumor therapy. However, there is not a clear dose-response relationship for doses exceeding 5×10^6 IU/m^2 in most human cancers.[181] The single indication for high-dose alpha-interferon therapy is AIDS-related Kaposi's sarcoma and possibly lymphoma. In Kaposi's sarcoma clinical response rates are maximal after doses of 10 to 20×10^6 IU/m^2 are administered. This high dose level requires gradual escalation from a starting dose of 3×10^6 IU/m^2/day. Doses are then increased over several weeks with immediate dose reduction by 50 per cent when serious toxicities are encountered. Fixed doses of 3×10^6 IU/m^2 three times weekly have been found to be effective in the treatment of non-A non-B hepatitis (hepatitis C).[182]

Pharmacodynamic studies suggest that a single therapeutic dose of alpha-interferon provides for 2 to 3 days of antiviral activity in normal volunteers.[183] There are no known dose adjustments based on age. However, it should be kept in mind that fatigue may be a typical dose-limiting toxicity of the drug in any population. Thus, patients with a poor performance status and/or fatigue from other causes prior to therapy may tolerate much lower doses of this agent. In the elderly population no specific dose adjustments need to be made for reduced hepatic or renal function.

Drug interactions Because of the potential for polypharmacy in the elderly population, there are few drug interactions which may require dose adjustments in patients receiving alpha-interferon. Indeed, alpha-interferon has been shown to reduce the quantity of hepatic microsomal enzymes.[184] Highly metabolized compounds which may require dose reductions in patients receiving alpha-interferon include cyclophosphamide, theophylline, warfarin, and barbiturate-type sedative/hypnotic agents. While these reactions have not yet been confirmed in humans, the animal data are persuasive that patients receiving alpha-interferon should be carefully titrated while receiving other highly metabolized compounds. Indeed, interferon is experimentally synergistic with cyclophosphamide and doxorubicin,[185] and in humans increased anticancer drug toxicities are noted. There is also a suggestion that alpha-interferon may modulate either the toxicity and/or the pharmacokinetics of the fluoropyrimidine antimetabolite 5-fluorouracil. The combination of 5-fluorouracil and alpha-interferon has been found to be active in pilot clinical trails in colorectal cancer, but a significant increase in 5-FU toxicities may result. It has also been difficult to duplicate the initial positive results in this trial[186] However, toxic synergy can clearly be obtained with significant enhancement in 5-FU myelotoxicity and gastrointestinal toxicity when alpha-interferon is administered. Some studies have also shown a reduction in the clearance of 5-fluorouracil with alpha-interferon therapy, although this requires further confirmation.

Melphalan

Melphalan is a DNA-alkylating agent which combines the amino acid L-phenylalanine with a nitrogen mustard type of alkylating group. It has thus been typically labeled L-PAM (L-phenylalanine mustard). Melphalan has significant antitumor activity in multiple myeloma[187] usually in combination with prednisone.[188] In addition, it has been used extensively in the adjuvant therapy of breast cancer.[189] Other solid tumors which are sensitive to melphalan include malignant melanoma, rhabdomyosarcoma and other sarcomas, and ovarian cancer.

Mechanism of action Melphalan is a DNA-alkylating agent which slowly activates via the loss of chloride ions. This ultimately results in bifunctional alkylation of DNA with crosslinking of the two complimentary DNA strands. The rate of crosslink formation is slower with melphalan than with nitrogen mustard, and removal of melphalan crosslinks is also slower. An unusual component of melphalan's activity is that cellular uptake is mediated via the specific amino acid receptor for L-phenylalanine.

Toxicity Myelosuppression is the primary dose-limiting toxicity of melphalan. It is characterized by leucopenia and thrombocytopenia with a nadir of approximately 14 and 21 days following dosing, respectively. Thus, the hematologic toxicity of melphalan has a more delayed onset than with most other alkylating agents. This may often produce an apparent cumulative myelosuppression which in some older patients may cause the leucopenic nadir to be extended to 5 to 6 weeks. Importantly, melphalan has a high leukemogenic activity which is typically noted following long-term therapy. It is heralded by a preleukemic pancytopenia. Other occasional toxicities include alopecia, dermatitis, and rarely, pulmonary fibrosis.

Pharmacokinetics Oral melphalan tablets are very poorly and erratically absorbed. The peak plasma level is achieved within 2 h of ingestion. Absolute bioavailability in one trial ranged from 25 to 89 percent with a mean of 56 percent. Importantly, when melphalan is taken with food, absorption is dramatically lessened due to drug degradation in the small bowel prior to absorption.[190] The drug is eliminated primarily by nonenzymatic hydrolysis to mono- and dihydroxy (inactive) derivatives.[191] There may also be some conjugation to glutathione via glutathione transferase enzymes. The pharmacokinetic elimination of the drug is biphasic with half-lives of 6 to 8 min for the alpha phase and about 1 h for the terminal beta phase.[192] Although the majority of the drug is cleared nonrenally, about 21 to 34 percent of drug may be excreted in the urine.[193] Thus, myelosuppression is greatly enhanced in patients with renal dysfunction.[194] Therefore, dose adjustments are probably required in patients with renal dysfunction (see Table 22-1).

Dosing In multiple myeloma melphalan is given intermittently for 4 to 7 days at single doses up to 10 mg/m^2. These doses are usually repeated at 4-to-6-week intervals depending on the resolution of bone marrow toxicity. In breast cancer, a dose of 0.15 mg/kg/day for 5 days is repeated at 5-to-6-week intervals.[189] See Table 22-1 for suggested dose reduction considerations in elderly patients with renal dysfunction.

Methotrexate

Methotrexate is an analog of folic acid which is active in a variety of malignant and nonmalignant diseases characterized by hyperplastic cell growth. It is a commonly used agent in elderly populations due to its oral activity and low toxicity. As an antitumor agent it is commonly included in regimens for the treatment of acute lymphoblastic and myeloblastic leukemia and also for trophoblastic cancer.[195] Methotrexate is also active in high doses in several solid tumors, especially osteogenic sarcoma,[196] head and neck cancer, lung cancer, breast cancer and ovarian cancer. In nonmalignant diseases, methotrexate is typically used for refractory psoriasis and rheumatoid arthritis.[197]

Mechanism of action Methotrexate binds tightly to the enzyme dihydrofolate reductase, thereby blocking the conversion of dihydrofolic to tetrahydrofolic acid.[198] Reduced cellular folates are thereby depleted, ultimately blocking a number of biochemical processes requiring one-carbon transfer reactions. Thus, methotrexate inhibits DNA, RNA, and protein synthesis, although the most sensitive enzyme blockade appears to be thymidylate synthetase. This inhibitory activity is cell cycle specific for S phase, although the drug is active in most other phases of division as well.

Pharmacokinetics Orally administered methotrexate is incompletely absorbed with a bioavailability of approximately 33 percent.[199] About 50 percent of the drug is bound to plasma proteins, and otherwise, methotrexate is widely distributed throughout the total body water. In conventional doses, methotrexate is primarily excreted unchanged in the urine, and only a small amount of a partially active 7-hydroxy methotrexate metabolite is noted following high-dose therapy.

The half-lives of methotrexate are about 20 min for an alpha phase and between 3 and 4 h for the terminal beta phase elimination of the drug. An unusual characteristic of methotrexate is its propensity to accumulate in third-space body fluids such as the effusions in the peritoneal and especially pleural cavity.[200] In these situations, methotrexate can accumulate and slowly leach back into the systemic circulation long after the drug would otherwise be eliminated from the plasma. This has been associated with excess toxicity. Management of this syndrome requires removal of such third-space fluids prior to dosing.

Toxicity The dose-limiting toxicity of methotrexate is leucopenia and thrombocytopenia. Anemia can rarely occur. The nadir for leucocyte suppression varies between 4 and 7 days with recovery usually complete by 21 days. A similar platelet nadir is recorded. Methotrexate causes relatively little nausea and vomiting, although it does produce a higher incidence of stomatitis than some other agents. With long-term dosing, hepatotoxicity has been reported and may be noted by a rise in SGOT levels. In addition there may be a synergistic hepatic toxicity with chronic long-term use and the ingestion of ethanol. Rare toxicities include rashes, pruritus or urticaria, and pneumonitis, which may respond to corticosteroids. With high-dose therapy renal failure has been reported to occur, especially if the urine is at an acid pH. This favors precipitation of methotrexate crystals in the renal tubules. This can be prevented by prophylactic alkalinization of the urine and the use of copious hydration during high-dose methotrexate therapy.

Dosing There are a large number of dosing regimens for methotrexate as an antitumor agent. Conventional doses typically involve 30 to 50 mg/m^2 given orally or intravenously each week. Higher doses of 0.5 to 1 g/m^2 have been given as an infusion over 36 to 48 h. These higher doses require leucovorin rescue to prevent potentially fatal myelosuppression.

Dose adjustments are required with methotrexate in the presence of renal dysfunction (Table 22-1). There may also be adjustments required in any patient over the age of 65 who is receiving therapy for breast cancer with a methotrexate-containing regimen. Based on a Eastern Cooperative Oncology Group Study, the methotrexate dose in milligrams in patients older than 65 may be adjusted according to the following formula:

$$\text{Methotrexate dose in milligrams} = 40\ \text{mg/m}^2 \times \frac{\text{creatinine clearance}}{70}$$

This equation assumes an "ideal" pretreatment creatinine clearance of 70 mL/min. Typically this dose is given on days 1 and 8 of the "CMF" (cyclophosphamide, methotrexate, and fluorouracil) regimen.[96] Alternatively, the Anderson formula may be used to adjust methotrexate doses in renal dysfunction as suggested in Table 22-1.

Mitomycin C

Mitomycin is an antibiotic streptomyces-derived antibiotic which has activity in a variety of adenocarcinomas of gastrointestinal origin.[201] It is also useful in breast cancer typically as part of a salvage regimen. Other solid tumors which are responsive to mitomycin C include nonsmall cell lung cancer and transitional cell carcinoma of the urinary bladder.[202]

Mechanism of action Mitomycin C is a bioreductive alkylating agent which crosslinks DNA strands to halt cell division.[203] In addition to alkylation of DNA, mitomycin C may also produce DNA strand breaks mediated by oxygen free radicals. These effects appear to involve the cyclic reduction of the quinone portion of the drug to yield hydrogen peroxide.[204] The cytotoxic action of mitomycin C is not cell cycle phase specific.

Toxity The principal dose-limiting toxicity of mitomycin C is myelosuppression principally reflected as reduced leucocytes and platelets. A usual characteristic is occasional delayed and possibly cumulative myelosuppression. In some cases the nadir following mitomycin C may occur at 2 to 3 weeks and approximately 6 to 8 weeks may be needed between repeat doses. Anemia can also occur with mitomycin C, and this may be related to high cumulative doses of at least 50 to 60 mg/m^2. The potent nature of mitomycin-induced bone marrow toxicity can make this agent difficult to use at full doses in an elderly population.

Other acute effects of mitomycin C include mild to moderate nausea and vomiting and stomatitis which is typically not severe. Rarely, renal toxicity may occur,[205] and high cumulative doses can produce a microangiopathic hemolytic anemia syndrome.[206] With high-dose therapy veno-occlusive disease of the liver has also been reported.[207]

Other rare effects include alopecia and soft tissue necrosis if the drug extravasates.[208] Interstitial pneumonia has also been reported.[209]

Pharmacokinetics Mitomycin C is eliminated primarily by nonrenal metabolism. The half-lives following an IV bolus injection have mean values of about 8 min for the alpha phase and 52 min for the beta (terminal) phase of elimination.[210] Less than 10 percent of a mitomycin dose is excreted into the urine, and this is generally maximal within a few hours of drug administration. Relatively small amounts of the drug have been recovered in bile and feces. There do not appear to be significant changes in mitomycin C pharmacokinetics in patients with altered hepatic function.[210] The drug appears to exhibit linear pharmacokinetics with no evidence of accumulation following higher dose therapy. Unfortunately the hepatic extraction rate of mitomycin C is 23 percent, which is too low to use arterial administration as a viable treatment option.[211]

Dosing The recommended dose of mitomycin C when used as a single agent is 20 mg/m^2 given intravenously every 6 to 8 weeks. When combined with other myelosuppressive drugs a maximal dose of 10 mg/m^2 is administered every 6 to 8 weeks. Again, no dose reductions are recommended for patients with altered renal or hepatic function.

Mitoxantrone HCl

Mitoxantrone is an anthracenedione-based agent which has aminoethylamino side chains that are believed to facilitate binding interactions with DNA. The drug is principally used for remission induction therapy in acute nonlymphocytic leukemia, but it also has significant activity in advanced breast cancer and malignant lymphona.[212]

Mechanism of action Mitoxantrone has several potential mechanisms of action which may explain the antitumor activity. First, it is known to intercalate into DNA in a process similar to that of anthracyclines such as doxorubicin.[213] In addition, mitoxantrone inhibits the activity of DNA topoisomerase II (TOPO-II) enzymes.

This results in the formation of a cleavable complex between the enzyme and DNA leading to protein-linked DNA double-strand breaks.[214] Topoisomerase activity is maximal in the G_2 phase in which mitoxantrone's activity is also maximal. Overall, though, mitoxantrone is a cell cycle nonspecific agent with the majority of activity in the late S phase and early G_2 phase.

In contrast to anthracyclines like doxorubicin, mitoxantrone does not appear to undergo the cyclic oxidation reduction (redox) reactions. Mitoxantrone is very difficult to reduce, and as such it has not been shown to produce oxygen free radicals which are believed to be responsible for cardiotoxicity. Nonetheless, the chelating agent ICRF-187 has been shown to partially ameliorate mitoxantrone heart toxicity by a mechanism which probably involves iron metal chelation.

Toxicity The major dose-limiting toxicity of mitoxantrone is myelosuppression denoted primarily as leucopenia.[212] The drug rarely produces pancytopenia, and leucocyte suppression with a nadir between 10 and 14 days is more common. As with other DNA intercalating agents, bone marrow recovery is generally complete by day 21. Other toxicities are both less frequent and less severe with mitoxantrone compared to the anthracyclines. This includes mild nausea and vomiting in less than one-half of treated patients. Mucositis also tends to be mild to moderate even with the every-3-week dosing schedule seen in breast cancer patients. However, mucositis from mitoxantrone may be more prominent with a three consecutive daily dose schedule as used in ANLL therapy. Nonetheless, less than 10 percent of patients on these courses will develop serious mucositis. Similarly, alopecia is very limited and mitoxantrone does not appear to be a consistent vesicant if inadvertently extravasated.[118]

The major cumulative effect of the drug is cardiac damage, which is manifest by severe CHF. The pattern is typical to that of anthracycline agents, and the cumulative dose limit for mitoxantrone used as a single agent is reported to be 160 mg/m^2.[212] Patients who have received prior anthracycline therapy should not receive cumulative mitoxantrone doses above 120 mg/m^2. The diagnostic indications for halting mitoxantrone therapy include either endomyocardial biopsies with evidence of characteristic histopathologic changes or a significant drop in the ejection fraction.[215]

Dosing For acute nonlymphocytic leukemia the recommended mitoxantrone dose is 12 mg/m^2 daily for three consecutive days (total dose 36 mg/m^2). These doses can be combined with cytarabine (ARA-C) in either a high-dose (2 to 3 g/m^2) or a standard-dose (300 mg/m^2) regimen. For solid tumors a dose of 12 to 14 mg/m^2/week every 3 weeks has been recommended.[212]

Pharmacokinetics Mitoxantrone is highly bound to plasma proteins (78 percent), and this binding is not affected by the presence of other highly bound drugs such as doxorubicin, phenytoin, or aspirin. The drug appears to undergo at least three phases of elimination with an alpha half-life of 2.4 to 15 min, a beta half life of 17 min to 3 h, and a terminal gamma half-life of 2.9 to 298 hours with a median value reported to be in the range of 12 days.[216] The major route of elimination of mitoxantrone is hepatobiliary secretion and very little drug is excreted in the urine. Nonetheless, the small fraction (<10 percent) that is excreted in the urine may be sufficient to color the urine green since the drug is bright blue. The bone marrow is known to be a major site of distribution of the drug,[217] and large amounts of the drug may be retained in the bone marrow and other organs for prolonged periods. This may account for up to 15 percent of an administered dose. Other tissues with high drug concentrations include the liver, pancreas, thyroid, spleen, and interestingly, the heart. There are at least two minor metabolites for mitoxantrone which have been described. These are the mono- and dicarboxylic acids.

Patients with reduced hepatobiliary function may require decreased doses of the drug (see Table 22-2).[218] Again as with doxorubicin, mitoxantrone dose adjustments do not need to be made for patients with elevated liver function tests without elevation of serum bilirubin.[219] Indeed, Chlebowski et al.[219] have suggested that full-dose therapy (14 mg/m^2) can be given to patients with moderate bilirubinemia (1.3 and 3.5 mg/dL), and a dose of 8 mg/m^2 can be safely given to patients with severe hyperbilirubinemia (>3.5 mg/dL). Dose adjustments based on age alone are not recommended for mitoxantrone.

Tamoxifen

Tamoxifen (Nolvadex) is a nonsteroidal antiestrogenic analog of clomiphene. The primary indication for tamoxifen is in the treatment of estrogen receptor-positive breast cancer. Advanced breast cancer in postmenopausal women is the most common clinical indication; however, it is also effective as adjuvant treatment of primary breast cancer.[220] The most common dose schedule calls for 10 mg orally twice a day on a continuous basis. There is no evidence that higher doses are more effective. The majority of tamoxifen and metabolites are excreted in the feces at a slow rate. Dosage adjustments for impaired hepatic function do not appear to be necessary.

Toxicity A thorough evaluation of side effects associated with tamoxifen treatment in postmenopausal women has been reported by Love et al.[221] Tamoxifen treatment most frequently caused vasomotor symptoms (hot flashes) and gynecologic complaints. A quality-of-life assessment showed virtually no difference between tamoxifen recipients and placebo recipients in general quality-of-life scores. Importantly, antiestrogen therapy with tamoxifen for 2 years did not lessen bone mineral density.

Clinical trials A study reported in 1985 by Allan et al.[222] evaluated tamoxifen as primary treatment of breast cancer in elderly or frail patients. These investigators found that 68 percent of patients had a reduction in their tumor when treated with tamoxifen alone. The actuarial survival at 5 years was 52 percent. The investigators felt that tamoxifen was effective therapy in elderly patients with primary breast cancer. Presumably, elderly patients who are considered too frail for surgery or primary radiotherapy may benefit from the use of tamoxifen as primary treatment of breast cancer.

Results of a study by Taylor et al.[223] comparing tamoxifen to chemotherapy (cyclophosphamide, methotrexate, fluorouracil) as initial therapy for metastatic breast cancer in elderly women found that survival rates tended to favor the use of tamoxifen. The investigators concluded that initiation of hormone therapy rather than chemotherapy was justified for elderly patients with metastatic breast cancer but that chemotherapy was useful in patients who did not have hormone-responsive disease.

Pharmacokinetics Tamoxifen is highly metabolized to active antiestrogenic compounds with long plasma half-lives. The primary *N*-desmethyl metabolite has a terminal elimination half-life of 10 to 14 days compared to 7 days for the parent compound.[224] Up to 75 per cent of a radiolabeled drug dose is recovered in the feces as glucuronide and/or sulfate conjugates.[225] There is no drug accumulation in patients with renal dysfunction.[226] However, patients with liver obstruction may experience elevated exposure to tamoxifen and its related metabolites.[227] Toxicity was not increased in this case, and at present no specific dose adjustments are recommended in the presence of hepatobiliary dysfunction.

Vinblastine

Vinblastine is an alkaloid isolated from the periwinkle plant (*Vinca rosea*). It is active in a variety of solid tumors including testicular carcinoma, Kaposi's sarcoma, and breast cancer.[51,228] Vinblastine also has activity in Hodgkin's and non-Hodgkin's lymphomas.[229]

Mechanism of action Vinblastine binds to the protein tubulin, which forms microtubular assemblies within cells.[230] The cytotoxic mechanism is believed to involve blocked polymerization of tubulin causing cell cycle arrest in the metaphase portion of mitosis.[231] Vinblastine is thus a cell cycle–specific agent.

Pharmacokinetics Vinblastine has a large apparent volume of distribution consistent with a high degree of protein and tissue binding. There are three elimination phases with half-lives of 25 min, 53 min, and 19 to 25 h, respectively.[232] The drug does not pass effectively into the blood-brain barrier but is partially metabolized in the liver and largely excreted as both intact drug and metabolites into the bile.

Toxicity The major dose-limiting effect of vinblastine is bone marrow suppression reflected primarily as leukopenia. The nadir for leukopenia is approximately 4 to 10 days with recovery occurring after another 2 weeks. Vinblastine also produces thrombocytopenia, although it is generally much less serious than leukopenia. Erythrocytes are typically only slightly depressed.

Vinblastine also causes nausea and vomiting in a small percentage of patients. This is usually well handled by antiemetics. With extremely high dose therapy vinblastine can produce peripheral neurotoxicity characterized by constipation, adynamic ileus, and abdominal pain.

Other side effects of vinblastine include a reversible mild alopecia, rashes, and stomatitis. Rarely the drug has caused jaw pain and an unusual complaint of pain overlying a solid tumor mass. Raynaud's phenomenon has also been reported when vinblastine is combined with bleomycin in testicular cancer.

Dosing Vinblastine can be given by a variety of dosing schemes, and the dose is dependent on the bone marrow reserve of the patient, the performance status, and to some degree, liver function. Typically, doses are not given more frequently than once weekly, and the dose range is 4 to 20 mg/m^2 repeated at 3-week intervals. Patients are usually started at a lower dose, which is increased at 0.05-mg/kg increments depending on the degree of leukopenia. For continuous infusions a dose of 1.5 to 1.7 mg/m^2/day for 5 days produced mild to moderate myelosuppression, whereas a 2-mg/m^2/day dose produced severe life-threatening myelosuppression.[228]

Because of the high degree of biliary secretion of this compound, dose reductions are recommended for patients with hepatic dysfunction as reflected by elevated serum bilirubin and/or elevated alkaline phosphatase levels (see Table 22-2). There are no reported effects of age on the pharmacokinetics or toxicity of vinblastine. However, because of the high degree of specific myelotoxicity with this drug, doses in an elderly population with poor bone marrow reserve and/or poor performance status should be lower.

Vincristine Sulfate (Oncovin)

Vincristine is an alkaloid obtained from the periwinkle plant. It is structurally similar to vinblastine. Vincristine has a broad spectrum of antitumor activity in human cancers.[233] Significant antitumor effects have been noted in breast carcinoma, sarcomas, and Hodgkin's and non-Hodgkin's lymphomas.

Mechanism of action Vincristine acts similarly to vinblastine in causing mitotic inhibition and an arrest of cell division in metaphase. This occurs due to binding of the drug to tubulin, which constitutes the major structural protein of the microtubules. Because microtubules make up the mitotic spindle structure, cell division is halted following exposure to vincristine. Thus, this agent is considered cell cycle–specific for mitosis.

Pharmacokinetics The pharmacokinetics of vincristine are similar to vinblastine, although a larger percentage of a dose may be excreted by the hepatobiliary tract. Vincristine also has a triphasic elimination with a very long terminal half-life of up to 25 h. Approximately two-thirds of a dose can be recovered from the feces within 72 h, and a much smaller component (5 to 10 percent) from the urine in 72 h. Approximately half of the eliminated drug can be recovered as the intact compound.

Toxicity The major dose-limiting toxicity with vincristine is peripheral neuropathy which can be reflected as jaw pain or more commonly as tingling paresthesias in the extremities, particularly in the feet. Other manifestations of the peripheral neuropathy include constipation due to a paralytic or adynamic ileus. This can be managed with laxatives, enemas, and metoclopramide. Fortunately, vincristine has much less myelotoxicity than most other agents and can be typically employed at full doses with other myelosuppressive drugs. This drug is a known vesicant which must be carefully administered to avoid severe extravasation necrosis. Inadvertent extravasations of the drug can be managed by hyaluronidase, and for prolonged vincristine infusions, peripheral veins must not be used.

Dosing The typical dose in adults is 1.4 mg/m^2, and generally doses above 2.5 to 3 mg are not administered at a single time. For IV infusions a tolerable dose was found to be 0.5 $mg/m^2/day$ for 5 days or 0.25 $mg/m^2/day$ for patients with poor performance status or preexisting neurologic complications.[234]

There are no specific dose reductions indicated in the elderly population. However, patients with moderate hepatobiliary dysfunction manifested by elevated serum bilirubin and/or elevated serum alkaline phosphatase levels should receive reduced doses of the drug. In addition, patients with preexisting peripheral nerve damage whether from prior vinca alkaloids or from other causes should also have reduced doses considered (see Table 22-2).

CANCER DRUG DOSE ADJUSTMENTS BASED ON ALTERED RENAL AND HEPATIC FUNCTION

Compromises in renal and hepatic function may be much more common in an elderly cancer population due to other preexisting diseases or intercurrent illnesses. For most chemotherapy agents, dosing will be unaffected by such factors. However, some agents have predominant elimination by renal or hepatic routes, and their effects may be significantly enhanced in patients with altered organ function. For these few agents, dose modification should be considered with the understanding that prospective studies validating specific dosing schemes are generally unavailable.

For renally eliminated drugs the important considerations are (1) the fraction of a dose excreted renally as active drug or active metabolite(s) and (2) the degree of renal impairment in the individual patient. These terms can be combined to yield

Table 22-1 Suggested dosing guidelines for anticancer agents excreted renally

		Percentage of normal dose based on patient's creatinine clearance[a]		
Agent	Fraction of dose excreted in urine	65 mL/min	35 mL/min	15 mL/min
Bleomycin	0.62	70	50	NR
Carmustine	0.43	80	70[b]	NR
Cisplatin	0.8	75	50[b]	NR
Cytarabine (high-dose only)	0.8	60	NR	NR
Etoposide	0.3	85	75	70
Melphalan (IV)	0.34	85	75	70[b]
Methotrexate	0.77	70	45	NR

[a]NR, dosing is not recommended.
[b]Less nephrotoxic agent should be used if possible.

an equation which is used to estimate the fraction F of a normal dose to administer to a patient with reduced renal function[235]:

$$F = \text{ND} \times f(k - 1) + 1$$

where ND is the normal dose, f the fraction of the drug dose excreted renally as the parent compound and as any active metabolites, and k the patient's creatinine clearance divided by a "normal" creatinine clearance of 120 mL/min. Alternatively, the factor k can be represented by a normal serum creatinine of 1 to 1.2 divided by the patient's serum creatinine. Thus, for a drug such as methotrexate, for which 77 percent of a dose is eliminated renally in a patient with a creatinine clearance of 40 mL/min, the calculation becomes

$$\begin{aligned} F &= \text{ND} \times (0.77(40/120 - 1) + 1) \\ F &= \text{ND} \times (0.77(-0.33) + 1) \\ F &= \text{ND} \times (-0.26 + 1) \\ F &= 0.74\ \text{ND} \end{aligned}$$

or 74 percent normal dose

Table 22-1 summarizes the results of this estimation technique for the renally excreted anticancer agents reviewed earlier. Again, the recommendations in Table 22-1 have not been prospectively evaluated and should be used only as a general guide to dosing a patient with renal dysfunction. Also, the guidelines in Table 22-1 do not take into account the effects of other relevant clinical factors such as hepatic function, performance status, and preexisting myelotoxicity. The suggested doses in Table 22-1 show that unless at least 30 percent of a drug dose is excreted renally, the dose adjustment suggested by the formula is trivial.

Cyclophosphamide does not require dose adjustments in the presence of renal failure despite its known genitourinary toxicity. This may be due to the 24-h urinary excretion of only 10 percent of a dose as parent compound and only about 7 to 17 percent of a dose as active alkylating metabolites.[86,236] Indeed, there is only one report of severe cyclophosphamide hematologic toxicity in a single patient with moderate renal impairment.[86] However, the markedly elevated peak level of active metabolites in this patient suggests that hepatic drug metabolism may have been significantly enhanced.

Melphalan has also had severe myelotoxicity described in nephrectomized dogs even though a relatively low drug fraction (0.34) is excreted renally.[48] Similar effects have been observed with IV melphalan in elderly cancer patients with impaired renal function.[48,237] Dosage adjustment of orally administered melphalan should be considered, keeping in mind the low relative bioavailability of melphalan tablets (see melphalan monograph).

Several of the drugs in Table 21-1 produce nephrotoxic metabolites which can acutely damage the kidneys and ultimately impair renal function. Cisplatin is known to bind to the renal tubular epithelium leading to a loss of concentrating ability and commensurate elevation of BUN and serum creatinine. This requires aggressive prophylactic hydration, the use of diuretics, and possible dose reduction for preexisting renal impairment.

With nitrosoureas such as carmustine, lomustine (CCNU), or methyl CCNU, a cumulative nephropathy develops after doses of 1200 to 1500 mg/m^2 are administered. Of note, these nephrotoxic effects appear to be enhanced with age. Therefore, total dose limits should be considered for nitrosoureas when used in an elderly population. Similarly, dose adjustments for cytarabine are only recommended for high-dose antileukemic therapy wherein impaired renal function may predispose patients to irreversible cerebellar toxicity. Importantly, the toxic effect may be similarly enhanced in patients greater than 60 years of age although definitive prospective studies are not available.

Dose adjustments for some antitumor agents should be based on hepatic function, specifically hepatobiliary function. For these agents, minimal amounts are excreted renally and the predominant means of clearance is hepatic. This may involve hepatic metabolism and conjugation to glucuronide and/or sulfate for ultimate biliary secretion into the bile. Table 22-2 lists the antitumor agents which are principally eliminated by hepatic clearance. As with dose adjustments for renal dysfunction, there are no prospective trials to validate the suggested dose modifications in patients with altered hepatobiliary function. Furthermore, for the hepatically excreted drugs, few diagnostic tests are available to quantitatively estimate hepatic function in an elderly patient population. For doxorubicin, mild to moderate hepatic enzyme and serum bilirubin elevation does not appear to alter drug elimination.[130] Similarly Gisselbrecht et al.[239] reported that alkaline phosphatase elevation and prolonged BSP retention did not produce altered doxorubicin elimination. Indeed, Bern et al.[240] suggested that the doxorubicin guidelines in Table 22-2 may overestimate dose reductions necessary to prevent severe toxicity. One

Table 22-2 Antitumor agents with altered pharmacokinetics in patients with hepatobiliary dysfunction

Agent	Fraction of a dose cleared hepatically	Pharmacokinetic effects on hepatic dysfunction[a]			Fraction of normal dose to administer for different serum bilirubin levels, mg/dL		
		$t_{1/2}$	Cl	V_d	<1.2	1.2–3.0	>3.0
Daunorubicin	0.85	↑	↓	NC	1.0	.75	0.5[b]
Doxorubicin	0.95	↑	↓	NC[c]	1.0	.75	0.5
Etoposide	0.70	↑	↓	Unknown	None currently recommended		
Mitoxantrone	0.8	↑	↓	↓	1.0	1.0	0.5–0.75[b]
Tamoxifen	0.75	↑	↓	Unknown	None currently recommended		
Vinblastine	0.8	↑	↓	NC	1.0	1.0	0.6[b]
Vincristine	0.75	↑	↓	NC	1.0	1.0	0.6[b]

[a] $t_{1/2}$ = plasma half life; Cl = total body clearance; V_d = volume of distribution; NC = no change.
[b] Official package insert recommendation.
[c] Based on pharmacokinetic studies; effects on clinical antitumor activity and toxicity unknown.
Source: Adapted from Ref. 238.

trial has suggested that doxorubicin clearance correlates with indocyanine green clearance (ICG) but not with increased serum bilirubin or elevated hepatic enzyme levels in the serum.[131]

For mitoxantrone, several groups have recommended reduced doses in patients with hepatic dysfunction. In one trial two patients with hepatic dysfunction had a prolonged half-life of 69 h compared to 37 h in normals.[218] Total body clearance was reduced from 239 mL/kg/h in patients with normal hepatic function compared to 160 mL/kg/h in the two patients with hepatic dysfunction. Urinary excretion of mitoxantrone was also reduced from 6.8 percent of a dose to 3.6 percent of a dose over 24 h in one trial[218] and from 13 percent to 4 percent over 5 days in another study.[241]

As Table 22-2 indicates, the vinca alkaloids are also eliminated principally by nonrenal mechanisms. Up to 72 percent of a radiolabeled vincristine dose is recovered in the feces 72 h after IV administration. Half of this amount is recovered as metabolites.[242] Another study reported that 50 percent of a dose is recovered in the bile over the same time period.[243] Substantially less vinblastine (10 to 30 percent of a dose) is recovered in the feces 42 h after administration.[231,232]

Based on this high degree of hepatobiliary elimination, several groups have reported increased vinca toxicities in patients with hepatic dysfunction noted by elevated serum enzyme levels. In one trial patients with elevated alkaline phosphatase levels experienced a threefold increase in the AUC for vincristine with a plasma elimination half-life extended from a normal 5.1 h to 13 h.[244] Furthermore, Mueller and Flaherty[245] described increased vincristine neurotoxicity in patients with hepatic dysfunction. Ratain et al[246] have also reported that albumin levels may correlate with nonlinear vinblastine clearance (lower clearance with low albumin) and that overall clearance decreases with repeated dosing. This trend for lower clearance was also associated with rising serum bilirubin, alkaline phosphatase, and SGOT, although the statistical correlation was not significant. The same clinical trend has also been observed with vinblastine[247] and the related compound vindesine.[248] Thus, hepatic dysfunction probably requires dose reductions for vinca alkaloids. The tentative guidelines presented in Table 22-2 may be used as a rough dosing approximation until more definitive studies are available.

REFERENCES

1. Yancik R, Ries LG: Cancer in the aged. *Cancer* 68: 2502–2510, 1991.
2. Holmes R, Hearne E: Cancer stage-to-age relationship: implications for cancer screening in the elderly. *J Am Geriat Soc* 29: 1009–1014, 1981.
3. Spencer G: Projections of the population of the United States by age, sex and race, U.S. Bureau of the Census, Current Population Reports, Series P-25, No. 1018. Washington, D.C., U.S. Government Printing Office, 1989,pp. 1988–2080.
4. Samet J, Hunt WC, Key C, et al: Choice of cancer therapy varies with age of patient. *Jama*255: 3385–3390, 1986.
5. Bonadonna G: Does chemotherapy fulfill its expectations in cancer treatment. *Ann Oncol* 1: 11–21, 1990.
6. Goldhirsch A, Gelber RD, Simes RJ, et al: Costs and benefits of adjuvant therapy in breast cancer: A quality-adjusted survival analysis. J Clin Oncol 7: 36–44, 1989.
7. Coltman CA, Dahlberg S, Jones SE, et al: CHOP is curative in thirty percent of patients with large cell lymphoma. A twelve-year Southwest Oncology Group followup. *Advances in Chemotherapy: Update on Treatment for Diffuse Large Cell Lymphoma.* New York, Wiley, 1986, pp. 71–77.
8. Phister JE, Jue SG, Cusack BJ: Problems in the use of anticancer drugs in the elderly. *Drugs* 37: 551–565, 1989.
9. Begg CB, Cohen JL, Ellerton J: Are the elderly predisposed to toxicity from cancer chemotherapy. *Cancer Clin Trials* 3: 369–376, 1980.
10. Umezawa H: Chemistry and mechanism of action of bleomycin. *Fed Proc* 33: 2296–2302, 1974.
11. Blum RH, Carter SK, Agre K: A clinical review of bleomycin—a new, antineoplastic agent. *Cancer* 31: 903–914, 1973.
12. Crooke ST, Bradner WT: Bleomycin: A review. *J Med* 7: 333–428, 1976.
13. Kasai H, Naganawa H, Takita T, et al: Chemistry of bleomycin. XXII. Interaction of bleomycin with nucleic acids, preferential binding to guanine base and electrostatic effect of the terminal amine. *J Antibiot (Tokyo)* 31: 1316, 1978.
14. Samuels ML, Johnson DE, Holoye PY, et al: Large-dose bleomycin therapy and pulmonary toxicity. A possible role of prior radiotherapy. *JAMA* 35: 1117–1120, 1976.
15. Hall SW, Broughton A, Strong JE, Benjamin RS: Clinical pharmacology of bleomycin by radioimmunoassay. *Clin Res* 25: 407A, 1977.
16. Alberts DS, Chen HSG, Liv R, et al: Bleomycin pharmacokinetics in man. *Cancer Chemother Pharmacol* 1: 1–5, 1978.
17. Ohnuma T, Holand JF, Masuda H, et al: Microbiological assay of bleomycin: inactivation, tissue distribution and clearance. *Cancer* 33: 1230–1238, 1974.

18. Chabner BA, Myers CE, Oliverio VT: Clinical pharmacology of anticancer drugs. *Semin Oncol* 4: 165–191.
19. Crooke ST, Friedrich L, Broughton A, et al: Bleomycin serum pharmacokinetics as determined by a radio-immunoassay and a microbiologic assay in a patient with compromised renal function. *Cancer* 399: 1430–1434, 1977.
20. Yee GC, Crom WR, Champion JE, et al: Cisplatin-induced changes in bleomycin elimination. *Cancer Treat Rep* 67: 587–589, 1983.
21. Alberts DS, Chen HSG, Mayersohn M, et al: Bleomycin pharmacokinetics in man. II. Intracavitary administration. *Cancer Chemother Pharmacol* 2: 127–132, 1979.
22. Bracken RB, Johnson DE, Rodriquez L, et al: Treatment of multiple superficial tumors of the bladder with intravesical bleomycin. *Urology* 9 (2): 161–163, 1977.
23. Ostrowski MJ, Halsall GM: Intracavitary bleomycin in the management of malignant effusions: multicenter study. *Cancer Treat Rep* 66: 1903–1907, 1982.
24. Wheeler GP, Chumley S: Alkylating activity of 1,3-bis(2-chloroethyl)-1-nitrosourea and selected compounds. *J Med Chem* 10: 259–265, 1980.
25. Erickson LC, Laurent G, Sharkey N, et al: DNA crosslinking and monoadduct repair in nitrosourea-treated human tumour cells. *Nature* 288: 727–729, 1980.
26. Kann HE Jr, Kohn KW, Lyles TM: Inhibition of DNA repair by the 1,3-bis (2-chloroethyl)-1-nitrosoureas breakdown product, 2-chloroethyl isocyanate. *Cancer Res* 34: 398–402, 1974.
27. Tobey RA, Crissman HA: Comparative effects of three nitrosourea derivatives on mammalian cell cycle progression. *Cancer Res* 25: 460–470, 1975.
28. DeVita VT, Carbone PP, Owens AB, et al: Clinical trials with 1,3-bis(2-chloroethyl)-1-nitrosourea, NSC-409962. *Cancer Res* 25: 1876–1881, 1965.
29. Oliverio VT: Toxicology and pharmacology of the nitrosoureas. *Cancer Chemother Rep* (part 3) 4: 13–20, 1973.
30. Lokich JJ, Drum DW, Kaplan W: Hepatic toxicity of nitrosourea analogues. *Clin Pharmacol Ther* 16: 363–367, 1874.
31. Holoye PY, Jenkins DE, Greenberg SD: Pulmonary toxicity in long-term administration of BCNU. *Cancer Treat Rep* 60: 1691–1693, 1976.
32. Levin VA, Hoffman W, Weinkam RJ: Pharmacokinetics of BCNU in man: preliminary study of 20 patients. *Cancer Treat Rep* 62: 1305–1312, 1978.
33. DeVita VT, Denham C, Davidson J, et al: The physiological disposition of carcinostatic 1,3-bis (2-chloroethyl)-1-nitrosourea (BCNU) in man and animals. *Clin Pharmacol Ther* 8: 566–577, 1967.
34. Peters WP, Eder JP, Henner WD, et al: High-dose combination alkylating agents with autologous bone marrow support: phase I trial. *J Clin Oncol* 115: 41–46, 1989.
35. Dorr RT, Soble MJ: H2-antagonists and carmustine. *J Cancer Res Clin Oncol* 115: 41–46, 1989.
36. Volkin RL, Shadduck RK, Winklstein A, et al: Potentiation of carmustine-cranial irradiation-induced myelosuppression by cimetidine. *Arch Intern Med* 142: 243–245, 1982.
37. Selker RG, Moore P, LeDolce D: Bone-marrow depression with cimetidine plus carmustine. *N Engl J Med* 299 (15): 834, 1978.
38. Han T, Ezdinli EZ, Shimaoka K, Desai DV: Chlorambucil vs. combined chlorambucil-coricosteroid therapy in chronic lymphocytic leukemia. *Cancer* 31: 502–512, 1973.
39. Knospe WH, Loeb V Jr, Huguley CM Jr: Bi-weekly chlorambucil treatment of chronic lymphocytic leukemia. *Cancer* 33: 555–561, 1974.
40. Ezdinli EZ, Stutzman L: Chlorambucil therapy for lymphomas and chronic lymphocytic leukemia. *JAMA* 189: 23–26, 1965.
41. Williams CJ, Mead GM, Macbeth FR, et al: Cisplatin combination chemotherapy versus chlorambucil in advanced ovarian carcinoma: mature results of a randomized trial. *J Clin Oncol* 3: 1455–1462, 1985.
42. Freckman HA, Fry HL, Mendez FL, et al: Chlorambucil-prednisone therapy for disseminated breast carcinoma. *JAMA* 189: 23–26, 1964.

43. Williams SA, Makker SP, Grupe WE: Seizures—a significant side effect of chlorambucil therapy in children. *J Pediatr* 93: 516–518, 1978.
44. Blumenreich MS, Woodcock TM, Sherrill EJ, et al: A phase I trial of chlorambucil administered in short pulses in patients with advanced malignancies. *Cancer Invest* 6 (4): 371–375, 1988.
45. Cole SR, Myers JJ, Klatsky AU: Pulmonary disease with chlorambucil therapy. *Cancer* 41: 455–459, 1978.
46. Lerner HJ: Acute myelogenous leukemia in students receiving chlorambucil as long-term adjuvant chemotherapy for stage II breast cancer. *Cancer Treat Rep* 62 (8): 1135–1138, 1978.
47. Adair CG, Bridges JM, Desai ZR: Can food affect the bioavailability of chlorambucil in patients with haematological malignancies? *Cancer Chemother Pharmacol* 17: 99–102, 1986.
48. Alberts DS, Chang SY, Chen H-SG, et al: Comparative pharmacokinetics of chlorambucil and melphalan in man. *Rec Results Cancer Res* 74: 124–131, 1980.
49. Sawitsky A, Rai KR, Glidewell O, et al (Cancer and Leukemia Group B): Comparison of daily versus intermittent chlorambucil and prednisone therapy in the treatment of patients with chronic lymphocytic leukemia. *Blood* 50 (6): 1049~-1059, 1977.
50. Rozencweig M, Von Hoff DD, Henney JE, Muggia FM: VM-26 and VP-16-213: A comparative analysis. *Cancer* 40: 334–342, 1977.
51. Einhorn LH, Donahue J: *Cis*-diamminedichloroplatinum, vinblastine and bleomycin combination chemotherapy in disseminated testicular cancer. *Ann Intern Med* 87: 293–298, 1977.
52. Rossoff AH, Slayton RE, Perlia CP: Preliminary clinical experience with *cis*-diamminedichloroplatinum (II) (NSC119875, CACP). *Cancer* 30 (6): 1451–1456, 1972.
53. Wiltshaw E, Kroner T: Phase II study of *cis*-dichlorodiammineplatinum (NSC 119875) in advanced adenocarcinoma of the ovary. *Cancer Treat Rep* 60: 55–60, 1976.
54. Hill JM, Loeb E, MacLellan A, et al: Clinical studies of platinum coordination compounds in the treatment of various malignant diseases. *Cancer Chemother Rep* 59: 647–659, 1975.
55. Ruckdeschel JC, Finkelstein DM, Mason BA, Creech RH: Chemotherapy for metastatic non-small-cell bronchogenic carcinoma: EST 2575, Generation V—a randomized comparison of four cisplatin-containing regimes. *J Clin Oncol* 3 (1): 72–79, 1985.
56. Loehrer PJ, Elson P, Kuebler JP, et al: Advanced bladder cancer: prospective intergroup trial comparing single agent (COOP) versus M—VAC combination therapy (INT 0078). *Proc Am Soc Clin Oncol* 9: 132, 1990.
57. Cox EB, Burton GV, Olsen GA, Vugrin D: Cisplatin and etoposide: An effective treatment for refractory breast carcinoma. *Am J Clin Oncol* 12 (1): 53–56, 1989.
58. Campbell JB, Dorman EB, McCormick M, et al: A randomized phase III trial of cisplatinum, methotrexate, cisplatinum + methotrexate, and cisplatinum + 5-fluorouracil in end-stage head and neck cancer. *Acta Otolaryngol (Stockh)* 103 (5–6): 519–528, 1987.
59. Zwelling LA, Anderson T, Koln KW: DNA-protein and DNA interstrand cross linking by *cis-/* and *trans*-platinum (II) diamminedichloride in L1210 mouse leukemia cells and its relation to cytotoxicity. *Cancer Res* 39: 365–369, 1979.
60. Poirier MC, Lippard SJ, Zwelling LA, et al: Antibodies elicited against *cis* dis-amminedichloroplatinum (II)-DNA adducts formed in vivo and in vitro. *Proc Natl Acad Sci USA* 79: 6443–6447, 1982.
61. Hardaker WT, Stone RA, McCoy R: Platinum nephrotoxicity. *Cancer* 34: 1030–1032, 1974.
62. Gonzalez Vitale JC, Hayes DM, et al: Acute renal failure after *cis*-dichlorodiammineplatinum (II) and gentamicin cephalothin therapies. *Cancer Treat Rep* 62(5): 693–698, 1978.
63. Piehl IJ, Meyer D, Perlia CP, Wolfe VI: Effects of *cis*-diammine dichloroplatinum (NSC-119875) on hearing function in man. *Cancer Chemother Rep* 58: 871–875, 1974.
64. Higby DJ, Wallace HJ, Albert DJ, Holland JF: Diamminedichloroplatinum: phase I study showing responses in testicular and other tumors. *Cancer* 33: 1219–1225. 1974.
65. Carr BI, Doroshow JH, Morgan RJ, et al: Combination antiemetic therapy based on high doses of either prochlorperazine or metoclopramide given complete protection against platinum-induced emesis. *Proc Am Soc Clin Oncol* 8: 325, 1989 (abstract).

66. Hesketh PJ, Murphy WK, Lester EP, et al: GR 38032F (GR-C507/75): A novel compound effective in the prevention of acute cisplatin-induced emesis. *J Clin Oncol* 7 (6): 700–705, 1989.
67. Kedar A, Cohen ME, Freeman AL: Peripheral neuropathy as a complication of *cis*-dichlorodiammineplatinum (II) treatment: A case report. *Cancer Treat Rep* 62(5): 819–821, 1980.
68. Schilsky RL, Anderson T: Hypomagnesemia and renal magnesium wasting in patients receiving cisplatin. *Ann Intern Med* 90: 929–931, 1979.
69. Ozols RF, Corden BJ, Jacob J, et al: High-dose cisplatin in hypertonic saline. *Ann Intern Med* 100: 19–24, 1984.
70. Henry D, Keller A, Kugler J, et al: Treatment of anemia in cancer patients on cisplatin chemotherapy with recombinant human erythropoietin (RHUEPO). *Proc Am Soc Clin Oncol* 9: 182, 1990.
71. Smith PHS, Taylor DM: Distribution and retention of the antitumor agent^{195M} Pt-*cis*-diamminedichloroplatinum (II) in man. *J Nucl Med* 15: 349–351, 1974.
72. Casper ES, Kelsen DP, Alcock NW, Young CW: Platinum concentrations in bile and plasma following rapid and six hour infusions of *cis*-dichlorodiammineplatinum (II). *Cancer Treat Rep* 63: 2023–2025.
73. Jacobs C, Kalman SM, Tretton M, Weiner MW: Renal handling of *cis*-diamminedichloroplatinum (II). *Cancer Treat Rep* 64: 1223–1266, 1980.
74. Stewart DJ, Molepo M, Hungerholtz H, et al: Concentrations of platinum in intracerebral vs extracerebral human tumors following intravenous cisplatin. *J Neurooncol* 71: 527, 1989.
75. Bonomi P, Blessing JA, Stehman FB, et al: Randomized trial of three cisplatin dose schedules in squamous-cell carcinoma of the cervix: A Gynecologic Oncology Group study. *J Clin Oncol* 3(8): 1079–1085, 1985.
76. Gandara DR, Wold H, Perez EA, et al: Cisplatin dose intensity in non-small cell lung cancer: phase II results of a day 1 and day 8 high-dose regimen. *J Natl Cancer Inst* 81: 790–794, 1984.
77. Livingston RB: Cisplatin in the treatment of solid tumors: effect of dose and schedule. *J Natl Cancer Inst* 81: 724–725, 1989 (editorial).
78. Skarin AT, Rosenthal DS, Moloney WC, Frei E, III: Combination chemotherapy of advanced non-Hodgkin's lymphoma with bleomycin, adriamycin, lyclophosphamide, vincristine, and prednisone (BACOP). *Blood* 49(5): 759–770, 1977.
79. Whitecar JP, Bodey GP, Freireich EJ, et al: Cyclophosphamide, vincristine, cytosine arabinoside and prednisone (COAP) combination chemotherapy for acute leukemia in adults. *Cancer Chemother Rep* 56:453–550, 1972.
80. DeVita VT, Serpick AA, Carbone PP: Combination chemotherapy in the treatment of advanced Hodgkin's disease. *Ann Intern Med* 73 (6): 881–895, 1970.
81. Ziegler JL, Morrow RH, Fass L, et al: Treatment of Burkitt's tumor with cyclophosphamide. *Cancer* 26: 474–484, 1970.
82. Jones SE, Durie BGM, Salmon SE: Combination chemotherapy with adriamycin and cyclophosphamide for advanced breast carcinoma. *Cancer* 36: 90–97, 1975.
83. Muggia FM, Chia G, Reed LJ, Romney SL: Doxorubicin-cyclophosphamide. Effective chemotherapy for advanced endometrial adenocarcinoma. *J Obstet Gynecol* 128: 314–319, 1977.
84. Colvin M, Padgett CA, Fenselau C: A biologically active metabolite of cyclophosphamide. *Cancer Res* 33: 915–918, 1973.
85. Steele TH, Serpick AA, Block JB: Antidiuretic response to cyclophosphamide in man. *J Pharmacol Exp Ther* 185: 245–253, 1973.
86. Bagley CM, Bosllick FW, DeVita VT: Clinical pharmacology of cyclophosphamide. *Cancer Res* 33: 226–233, 1973.
87. Struck RF, Horne K, Phillips JG, et al: Plasma levels and AUC data for the antitumor-active metabolites of cyclophosphamide (CPA) in cancer patients treated intravenously (i.v.) or orally (p.o.) with cyclophosphamide. *Proc Am Assoc Cancer Res* 27: 167, 1986 (Abstr 663).
88. Jardine I, Brundett R, Colvin M, et al: Approaches to the pharmacokinetics of cyclophosphamide (NSC-26271): quantitation of metabolites. *Cancer Treat Rep* 60: 403–408, 1976.

89. Juma FD, Rogers HJ, Trounce JR: Effect of renal insufficiency on the pharmacokinetics of cyclophosphamide and some of its metabolites. *Eur J Clin Pharmacol* 19: 443-451, 1981.
90. Powis G, Reece P, Ahmann DL, Ingle JN: Effect of body weight on the pharmacokinetics of cyclophosphamide in breast cancer patients. *Cancer Chemother Pharmacol* 20: 219-222.
91. Stolbach L, Begg C, Bennett JM, et al: Evaluation of bone marrow toxic reaction in patients treated with allopurinol. *JAMA* 247: 334-336, 1982.
92. Dorr RT, Alberts DS: Cimetidine enhancement of cyclophosphamide antitumor activity. *Br J Cancer* 45: 35-43, 1982.
93. Dorr RT, Soble MJ, Alberts DS: Interaction of cimetidine but not ranitidine with cyclophosphamide in mice. *Cancer Res* 46: 1795-1799, 1986.
94. Alberts DS, Mason-Liddil NM, Plezia P: Lack of ranitidine effects on cyclophosphamide bone marrow toxicity or metabolism: A placebo controlled clinical trial. *J Natl Cancer Inst* 83: 1739-1743, 1991.
95. Durie BGM, Clouse L, Braich T, et al: (1986) Interferon alfa-2b-cyclophosphamide combination studies: in vitro and phase I-II clinical results. *Sem Onc*-XIII (3 Suppl 2): 84-88, 1986.
96. Gelman RS, Taylor SG, IV: Cyclophosphamide, methotrexate, and 5-fluorouracil chemotherapy in women more than 65 years old with advanced breast cancer: the elimination of age trends in toxicity by using doses based on creatinine clearance. *J Clin Oncol* 2: 1404-1413, 1984.
97. Bodey GP, Coltman CA, Hewlett JS, Freireich EJ: Progress in the treatment of adults with acute leukemia. *Arch Intern Med* 136: 1383-1388, 1976.
98. Rudnick SA, Cadman EC, Capizzi RL, et al: High dose cytosine arabinoside (HDARAC) in refractory acute leukemia. *Cancer* 44: 1189-1193, 1979.
99. Momparler RL: Kinetic and template studies with 1-β-D-arabinofuranosylcytosine-5′-triphosphatase and mammalian deoxyribonucleic acid polymerase. *Mol Pharmacol* 8: 362-370, 1972.
100. Skipper HE, Schabel FM, Wilcox WS: Experimental evaluation of potential anticancer agents. XXI. Scheduling of arabinosyl cytosine to take advantage of its S-phase specificity against leukemic cells. *Cancer Chemother Rep* 51: 125-141, 1967.
101. Herzig RH, Hines JD, Herzig GP, et al: Cerebellar toxicity with high-dose cytosine arabinoside. *J Clin Onc* 5(6): 927-932, 1987.
102. Graves T, Hooks MA: Drug-induced toxicities associated with high-dose cytosine arabinoside infusions. *Pharmacotherapy* 9(1): 23-28, 1989.
103. Damon LE, Mass R, Linker CA: The association between high-dose cytarabine neurotoxicity and renal insufficiency. *J Clin Onc* 7(10): 1563-1568, 1989.
104. Capizzi RL, Poole M, Cooper MR, et al: Treatment of poor risk acute leukemia with sequential high-dose ARA-C and asparaginase. *Blood* 63: 694-700, 1984.
105. Lopez JA, Agarwal RP: Acute cerebellar toxicity after high-dose cytarabine associated with CNS accumulation of its etabolite, uracil arabinoside. *Cancer Treat Rep* 68 (10): 1309-10, 1984.
106. Ritch PS, Hansen RM, Heuer DK: Ocular toxicity from high-dose cytosine arabinoside. *Cancer* 51: 430-432, 1983.
107. Van Prooijen R, Kleijn E, Haanen C: Pharmacokinetics of cytosine arabinoside in acute myeloid leukemia. *Clin Pharmacol Ther* 21(6): 774-750, 1977.
108. Grein A, Spalla C, DiMarco A: Decrizione e classificazione di un attinomycete *(Streptomyces peucetius* sp. Nova) Produttore di una sostavia and affivita antitumorale: la dawnomicina. *G Microbiol* 11: 19-115, 1963.
109. Greene W, Huffman D, Wiernik PH, et al: High-dose daunorubicin therapy for acute nonlymphocytic leukemia. *Cancer* 30: 1419-1427.
110. Gale RP: Advances in the treatment of acute myelogenous leukemia. *N Engl J Med* 300: 1189-1199, 1979.
111. Jones B, Holland JF, Morrison AR, et al: Daunorubicin (NSC-82151) in the treatment of advanced childhood lymphoblastic leukemia. *Cancer Res* 31: 84-90, 1971.
112. Von Hoff DD, Rozencweig M, Layard M, et al: Daunomycin-induced cardiotoxicity in children and adults. *Am J Med* 62: 200-208, 1977.

113. Chauvergne J, Carton M, Berlie J, et al: Essau de chimotherapie anticancereuse par la duborimycine. Analyse de 151 observations. *Bull Cancer* 63: 41-58, 1976.
114. Tewey KM, Chen GL, Nelson EM, et al: Intercalative drugs interfere with the breakage-reunion reaction of mammalian DNA topoisomerase II. *J Biol Chem* 259: 9182-9187, 1984.
115. Handa K, Sato S: Stimulation of microsomal NADPH oxidation by quinone group containing anticancer chemicals. *Gann* 67: 523, 1976.
116. Doroshow JH: Prevention of doxorubicin-induced killing of MCF-7 human breast cancer cells by oxygen radical scavengers and iron chelating agents. *Biochem Biophys Res Commun* 135: 330-335, 1986.
117. Speyer JL, Green MD, Kramer E, et al: Protective effect of the bispiperazinedione ICRF-187 against doxorubicin-induced cardiac toxicity in women with advanced breast cancer. *N Engl J Med* 319: 745-752, 1988.
118. Dorr RT: Antidotes to vesicant chemotherapy extravasations *Blood Rev* 4: 41-60, 1990.
119. Olver IN, Aisner J, Hament A, et al: A prospective study of topical dimethyl sulfoxide for treating anthracycline extravasation. *J Clin Oncol* 6: 1732-1735, 1988.
120. Dorr RT, Alberts DS, Stone A: Cold protection and heat enhancement of doxorubicin skin toxicity in the mouse. *Cancer Treat Rep* 69(4): 431-437, 1985.
121. Harwood KVS, Bachur NR: Evaluation of dimethylsulfoxide and local cooling as antidotes for doxurubicin extravasation in a pig model. *Oncol Nurs Forum* 14: 39-44, 1987.
122. Souhami L, Feld R: Urticaria following intravenous doxorubicin administration. *JAMA,* 240 (15): 1624-1626, 1978.
123. Von Hoff DD, Layard MW, Basa P, et al: Risk factors for doxorubicin-induced congestive heart failure. *Ann Intern Med* 91: 710-717, 1979.
124. Minow RA, Benjamin RS, Gottlieb JA: Adriamycin (NSC-123127) cardiomyopathy—an overview with determination of risk factors. *Cancer Chemother Rep* Part 3 6(2): 195-210, 1975.
125. Bristow MR, Billingham ME, Mason JW, Daniels JR: Clinical spectrum of anthracycline antibiotic cardiotoxicity. *Cancer Treat Rep* 62(6): 873-879, 1978.
126. Eksborg S, Ehrsson H, Ekqvist B: Protein binding of anthraquinone glycosides, with special reference to adriamycin. *Cancer Chemother Pharmacol* 10: 7-10, 1982.
127. Piazza E, Broggini M, Trabattoni A, et al: Adriamycin distribution in plasma and blood cells of cancer patients with altered hematocrit. *Eur J Cancer Clin Oncol* 17: 1089-1096, 1981.
128. Riggs CE Jr, Benjamin RS Serpick AA, et al: Biliary disposition of adriamycin. *Clin Pharmacol Ther* 22: 234-241, 1977.
129. Benjamin RS: A practical approach to adriamycin (NSC-123127) toxicology. *Cancer Chemother Rep* Part 3 6: 191-194, 1975.
130. Chan KK, Chlebowski RT, Tong M, et al: Clinical pharmacokinetics of adriamycin in hepatoma patients with cirrhosis. *Cancer Res* 40: 1263-1268, 1980.
131. Doroshow J, Chan K: Relationship between doxorubicin (D) clearance and indocyanine green dye (ICG) pharmacokinetics (PK) in patients with hepatic dysfunction. *Proc Am Soc Clin Oncol* 1: 11, 1982.
132. Rodvold KA, Rushing DA, Tewksbury DA: Doxorubicin clearance in the obese. *J Clin Oncol* 6: 1321-1327, 1988.
133. Robert J, Hoerni B: Age dependence of the early-phase pharmacokinetics of doxorubicin, *Cancer Res* 43: 4467-4469, 1983.
134. Legha SS, Benjamin RS, Mackay B, et al: Reduction of doxorubicin cardiotoxicity by prolonged continuous intravenous infusion. *Ann Intern Med* 96: 133-139, 1982.
135. Ross W, Towe T, Glisson B, et al: Role of topoisomerase II in mediating epipodophyllotoxin-induced DNA cleavage. *Cancer Res* 44: 5857-5860, 1984.
136. Creaven PJ, Newman SJ, Selawry OS, et al: Phase I clinical trial of weekly administration of 4′-demethylepiposophyllotoxin 9-(4,6-O-ethylidene-β-D-glucopyranoside) (NSC-141540; VP-16-213). *Cancer Chemother* Rep 58: 901-907, 1974.

137. Thant M, Hawley RJ, Smith MT, et al: Possible enhancement of vincristine neuropathy by VP-16. *Cancer* 49: 859–864, 1982.
138. Evans WE, Sinkule JA, Crom WR, et al: Pharmacokinetics of teniposide (VM-26) and etoposide (VP16-213) in children with cancer. *Cancer Chemother Pharmacol* 7: 145–150, 1982.
139. Creaven PJ, Allen LM: EPEG, a new antineo-plastic epipodophyllotoxin. *Clin Pharmacol Ther* 18: 221–226, 1975.
140. Hande KR, Wedlund PJ, Noone RM: Pharmacokinetics of high dose etoposide (VP16-213) administered to cancer patients. *Cancer Res* 44: 379–382, 1984.
141. Creaven PJ: The clinical pharmacology of VM26 and VP16-213: Brief overview. *Cancer Chemother Pharmacol* 7: 133–140, 1982.
142. Allen LM, Marcks C, Creaven PJ: 4′ Demethyl-epipodophyllic acid-9-(4,6-O-ethylidene-β-D-glucopyranoside), the major urinary metabolite of VP-16-213 in man. *Proc Am Assoc Cancer Res* 17: 15, 1976.
143. Stewart CF, Arbuck SG, Fleming RA, Evans WE: Changes in the clearance of total and unbound etoposide in patients with liver dysfunction. *J Clin Oncol* 8: 1874–1879, 1990.
144. Saito H, Brown, NS, Ho DH, et al: Pharmacokinetic study of 72-hour continuous infusion of cisplatin and etoposide in patients with non-small cell lung cancer. *Proc Am Assoc Cancer Res* 32: 173, 1991.
145. Pfluger K-H, Schmidt L, Merkel M, et al: Drug monitoring of etoposide (VP16-213). Correlation of pharmacokinetic parameters to clinical and biochemical data from patients receiving etoposide. *Cancer Chemother Pharmacol* 20: 59–66, 1987.
146. Crom WR, Kearns CM, Meyer WH, Rodman JH: Changes in etoposide pharmacokinetics during combination chemotherapy with ifosfamide in Ewing sarcoma patients. *Proc Am Assoc Cancer Res* 32: 174, 1991.
147. Lum BL, Kaubisch S, Gosland MP, et al: The effect of cyclosporine (CSA) on etoposide (E) pharmacokinetics in a phase I trial of E with CSA as a modulator of multidrug resistance (MDR). *Proc Am Soc Clin Oncol* 10: 102, 1991.
148. Smyth RD, Pfeffer M, Scalzo A, Comis RL: Bioavailability and pharmacokinetics of etoposide (VP-16). *Sem Oncol* XII: 348–51, 1985.
149. Harvey VJ, Slevin ML, Joel SP, et al: The pharmacokinetics of oral etoposide. (VP16-213). *Proc Am Soc Clin Oncol* 3: 24, 1984.
150. Harvey VJ, Slevin ML, Joel SP, et al: The effect of food and concurrent chemotherapy on the bioavailability of oral etoposide. *Br J Cancer* 52: 363–367, 1985.
151. Hainesworth JD, Johnson DH, Frazier SR, Greco FA: Chronic daily administration of oral etoposide—a phase I trial. *J Clin Oncol* 7: 396–401, 1989.
152. Carney DN, Grogan L, Smit EF, et al: Single-agent oral etoposide for elderly small cell lung cancer patients. *Semin Oncol* 17: 49–53, 1990.
153. Greco A, Johnson DH, Hainsworth JD: Chronic daily administration of oral etoposide. *Semin Oncol* 17: 71–74, 1990.
154. Hansen RM, Quebbeman E, Anderson T: 5-Fluorouracil by protracted venous infusion. A review of current progress. *Oncology* 46(4): 245–250, 1989.
155. Moerel CG, Fleming TR, MacDonald JS, et al: Levamisole and fluorouracil for adjutant therapy of resected colon carcinoma. *N Engl J Med* 322(6): 352–358, 1990.
156. Laufman LR, Krzeczowski KA, Roach R, Sesal M: Leucovorin plus 5-fluorouracil: An effective treatment for metastatic colon cancer. *J Clin Oncol* 5(9): 1394–1400, 1987.
157. Grem JL, Hoth DF, Hamilton M, et al: Overview of current status and future directions of clinical trials with 5-fluorouracil in combination with folinic acid. *Cancer Treat Rep* 71: 1249–1264, 1987.
158. Fabian CJ, Molina R, Slavik M, et al: Pyridoxine therapy for palmar-plantar erthrodysesthesia associated with continuous 5-fluorouracil infusion. *Invest New Drugs* 8(1): 57–63, 1990.
159. Schaaf LJ, Dobbs BR, Edwards IR, Perrier DG: Nonlinear pharmacokinetic characteristics of 5-fluorouracil (5-FU) in colorectal cancer patients. *Eur J Clin Pharmacol* 32: 411–418, 1987.
160. Floyd FA, Hornbeck CL, Byfield JE, et al: Clearance of continuously infused 5-fluorouracil in

adults having lung or gastrointestinal carcinoma with or without hepatic metastases. *Drug Intell Clin Pharm* 16: 665–667, 1982.

161. Heggie GD, Sommadossi J, Cross D, et al: Clinical pharmacokinetics of 5-fluorouracil and its metabolites in plasma, urine, and bile. *Cancer Res* 47: 2203–2206, 1987.
162. Doroshow JH, Leong L, Margolin K, et al: Refractory metastatic breast cancer: salvage therapy with fluorouracil and high-dose continuous infusion leucovorin calcium. *J Clin Oncol* 7(4): 439–444, 1989.
163. Klein E, Stoll HL, Miller E, et al: The effects of 5-fluorouracil (5FU) ointment in the treatment of neoplastic dermatoses. *Dermatologica* 140(Suppl I): 21–33, 1970.
164. Lewis LD: Ifosfamide pharmacokinetics. *Invest New Drugs* 9: 305–311, 1991.
165. Lind MJ, Margison JM, Cerny T, et al: Prolongation of ifosfamide elimination half-life in obese patients due to altered drug distribution. *Cancer Chemother Pharmacol* 25: 139–142, 1989.
166. Sehgal PB: The interferon gene. *Biochem Biophys Acta* 695: 17–33, 1982.
167. Quesada JR, Hersh DM, Rueben J, Gutterman JV: α-Interferon for induction of remission of hairy cell leukemia. *N Engl J Med* 310: 15–18, 1984.
168. Talpaz M, McCredie KB, Mavligit GM, Gutterman JU: Leukocyte interferon induced myeloid cytoreduction in chronic myelogenous leukemia. *Blood* 62: 689–692, 1983.
169. Groopman JE, Gottlieb MS, Goodman J, et al: Recombinant alfa-2 interferon therapy for Kaposi's sarcoma associated with acquired immunodeficiency syndrome. *Ann Intern Med* 100: 671–677, 1984.
170. Goldstein D, Laszlo J: Interferon therapy and cancer: from imaginon to interferon. *Cancer Res* 46: 4315–4329, 1986.
171. Quesada JR, Rios A, Swanson D, et al: Antitumor activity of recombinant-derived interferon alpha in metastatic renal cell carcinoma. *J Clin Oncol* 3: 1522–1528, 1985.
172. Berek JS, Hacker NF, Lichtenstein A, et al: Intraperitoneal recombinant α-interferon for "salvage" immunotherapy in Stage III epithelial ovarian cancer: A gynecologic oncology group study. *Cancer Res* 45: 4447–4453, 1985.
173. von Wussow P, Block B, Hartmann F, Deicher H: Intralesional interferon-alpha therapy in advanced malignant melanoma. *Cancer* 61: 1071–1074, 1988.
174. Aguet M, Mogenson KE: Interferon receptors, in Gresser (ed), *Interferon, I.* London, Academic Press, 1983, pp. 1–22.
175. Samuel CE: Mechanisms of interferon action: phosoporylation of protein synthesis initiation factor eIF-2 in interferon-treated cells by a ribosome-associated kinase possessing site specificity similar to hemin-regulated rabbit reticulocyte kinase. *Proc Natl Acad Sci (USA)* 76: 600–607.
176. Quesada JR, Talpaz M, Rios A, et al: Clinical toxicity of interferons in cancer patients: A review. *J Clin Oncol* 4: 234–243, 1986.
177. Miller RL, Steis RG, Clark JW, et al: Randomized trial of recombinant α2b-interferon with or without indomethacin in patients with metastatic malignant melanoma. *Cancer Res* 49: 1871–1876, 1989.
178. Wills RJ, Dennis S, Spiegel HE, et al: Interferon kinetics and adverse reactions after intravenous, intramuscular, and subcutaneous injection. *Clin Pharmacol Ther* 35(5): 722–727, 1984.
179. Bino T, Madar F, Gertler A, Rosenberg H: The kidney is the main site of interferon degradation. *J Interferon Res* 2: 301–308, 1982.
180. Hirsch MS, Tolkoff-Rubin NE, Kelly AP, Rubin RH: Pharmacokinetics of human and recombinant leukocyte interferon in patients with chronic renal failure who are undergoing hemodialysis. *J Infect Dis* 148(2): 335, 1983.
181. Goldstein D, Laszlo J: Interferon therapy in cancer: from imaginon to interferon. *Cancer Res* 46:4315-4329, 1986.
182. Davis GL, Balart LA, Schiff ER, et al: Treatment of chronic hepatitis C with recombinant interferon alfa: A multicenter randomized, controlled trial. *N Engl J Med* 321: 1501–1506, 1989.
183. Barouki FM, Witter FR, Griffin DE, et al: Time course of interferon levels, antiviral stage, 2′,5′-oligoadenylate synthetase and side effects in healthy men. *J Interferon Res* 7: 29–39, 1987.

184. Singh G, Renton KW: Interferon-mediated depression of cytochrome P-450-dependent drug biotransformation. *Molec Pharmacol* 20: 681-684, 1981.
185. Balkwill FR, Moodie EM: Positive interactions between human interferon and cyclophosphamide or adriamycin in a human tumor model system. *Cancer Res* 44: 904-908, 1984.
186. Wadler S, Schwartz EL, Goldman M, et al: Fluorouracil and recombinant alfa-2a-interferon: An active regimen against advanced colorectal carcinoma. *J Clin Oncol* 7(12): 1769-1775, 1989.
187. Alexander R, Bergsagel DE, Migliore PJ, et al: Melphalan therapy for plasma cell myeloma. *Blood* 31: 1, 1968.
188. Costa G, Engle RL Jr, Schilling A, et al: Melphalan and prednisone: An effective combination for the treatment of multiple myeloma. *Am J Med* 54: 589-599, 1973.
189. Fisher B, Carbone P, Economou SG, et al: 1-Phenylalanine mustard (L-PAM) in the management of breast cancer: A report of early findings. *N Engl J Med* 292: 117-122, 1975.
190. Alberts DS, Peng YM, Fisher B: Minimal melphalan (L-PAM) systemic availability (SA): A potential cause for failure of adjuvant breast cancer trials *Proc Am Soc Clin Oncol* 3: 38, 1984. (Abstract C-149).
191. Evans TL, Chang SY, Alberts DS, et al: In vitro degradation of L-phenylalanine mustard (L-PAM). *Cancer Chemother Pharmacol* 8: 175-178, 1982.
192. Alberts DS, Chang SY, Chen H-SG, et al: Kinetics of intravenous melphalan. *Clin Pharmacol Ther* 26(1): 73-80, 1979.
193. Reece PA, Hill HS, Green RM, et al: Renal clearance and protein binding of melphalan in patients with cancer. *Cancer Chemother Pharmacol* 22: 348-352, 1988.
194. Cornwell GG, III, Pajak TF, McIntyre OR, et al: Influence of renal failure on myelosuppressive effects of melphalan: Cancer and Acute Leukemia Group B experience. *Cancer Treat Rep* 66: 475-481, 1982.
195. Smith EB, Weed JC Jr, Tyrey L, Hammond CB: Treatment of nonmetastatic gestational trophoblastic disease: results of methotrexate alone versus methotrexate—folinic acid. *Am J Obstet Gynecol* 144: 88-92, 1982.
196. Frei E, Jaffe N, Tattersal M, et al: New approaches to cancer chemotherapy with methotrexate. *N Engl J Med* 292(16): 846-851, 1975.
197. Weinblatt ME, Coblyn JS, Fox DA, et al: Efficacy of low-dose methotrexate in rheumatoid arthritis. *N Engl J Med* 312: 818-822, 1985.
198. Goldman ID: Analysis of the cytotoxic determinants for methotrexate (NSC-740): role for "free" intracellular drug. *Cancer Chemother Rep* 6: 51-61, 1975.
199. Campbell MA, Perrier DG, Dorr RT, et al: Methotrexate: Bioavailability and pharmacokinetics. *Cancer Treat Rep* 69(7-8): 833-838, 1985.
200. Evan WE, Pratt CB: Effect of pleural effusion on high-dose methotrexate kinetics. *Clin Pharmacol Ther* 24(1): 68-72, 1978.
201. Doll DC, Weiss RB, Issell BF: Mitomycin: ten years after approval for marketing. *J Clin Oncol* 3(2): 276-286, 1985.
202. DeFuria MD, Bracken RB, Johnson DE, et al: Phase I-II study of mitomycin C topical therapy for low-grade, low-stage transitional cell carcinoma of the bladder: An interim report. *Cancer Treat Rep* 64: 225-230, 1980.
203. Iyer V, Szybalski N: Mitomycin and porfiromycin: Chemical mechanism of activation and cross-linking of DNA. *Science (Wash., D.C.)* 145: 55-58, 1964.
204. Tomasz M: $H_2 O_2$ generation during the redox cycle of mitomycin C and DNA-bound mitomycin C. *Chem-Biol Interact* 13: 89-97, 1976.
205. Hanna WT, Krauss S, Regester RF, Murphy WM: Renal disease after mitomycin C therapy. *Cancer* 48: 2583-2588, 1982.
206. Liu K, Mittelman A, Sproul EE, Elias EG: Renal toxicity in man treated with mitomycin C. *Cancer* 28(5): 1314-1320, 1971.
207. Lazarus HM, Gottfried MR, Herzig RH, et al: Veno-occlusive disease of the liver after high-dose mitomycin C therapy and autologous bone marrow transplantation. *Cancer* 49: 1789-1795, 1982.

208. Argenta LC, Manders EK: Mitomycin C extravasation injuries. *Cancer* 51: 1080–1082, 1983.
209. Orwoll ES, Kiessling PJ, Patterson JR: Interstitial pneumonia from mitomycin. *Ann Intern Med* 89: 352–355, 1978.
210. van Hazel GA, Scott M, Rubin J, et al: Pharmacokinetics of mitomycin C in patients receiving the drug alone or in combination. *Cancer Treat Rep* 67(9): 805–810, 1983.
211. Hu E, Howell SB: Pharmacokinetics of intraarterial mitomycin C in humans. *Cancer Res* 43: 4474–4477, 1983.
212. Shenkenberg TD, Von Hoff DD: Mitoxantrone: A new anticancer drug with significant clinical activity. *Ann Intern Med* 105: 67–81, 1986.
213. Durr FE: Biologic and biochemical effects of mitoxantrone. *Semin Oncol* 11(3 Suppl 1): 3–10, 1984.
214. Bowden GT, Roberts R, Alberts DS, et al: Comparative molecular pharmacology in leukemic L1210 cells of the anthracene anticancer drugs mitoxantrone and bisantrene. *Cancer Res* 45: 4915–4920, 1985.
215. Benjamin RS, Chawla SP, Ewer MS, et al: Evaluation of mitoxantrone cardiac toxicity by nucler angiography and endomyocardial biopsy. *Proc Am Soc Clin Oncol* 3: 40, 1984 (abstract).
216. Alberts DS, Peng Y-M, Leigh S, Davis TP, Woodward DL: Disposition of mitoxantrone in cancer patients. *Cancer Res* 45: 1879–1884, 1985.
217. Stewart JA, McCormack JJ, Krakoff IH: Clinical and clinical pharmacologic studies of mitoxantrone. *Cancer Treat Rep* 66: 1327–1331, 1982.
218. Savaraj N, Lu K, Manuel V, Loo TL: Pharmacology of mitoxantrone in cancer patients. *Cancer Chemother Pharmacol* 8: 113–117, 1982.
219. Chlebowski RT, Bulcavage L, Henderson IC, et al: Mitoxantrone use in breast cancer patients with elevated bilirubin. *Breast Cancer Res Treat* 14: 267–274, 1989.
220. Breast Cancer Trials Group: Adjuvant Tamoxifen in the management of operable breast cancer: the Scottish trial. Report from the Breast Cancer Trials Committee. *Lancet* 2: 171–175, 1987.
221. Love R, Mazess DC, Tormey P, et al: Bone mineral density (BMD) in women with breast cancer treated with tamoxifen for two years. *Breast Cancer Res Treat* 10: 12–16, 1987.
222. Allan SG, Rodger A, Smyth JF, et al: Tamoxifen as primary treatment of breast cancer in elderly or frail patients: A practical management. *Br Med J* 290: 358, 1985.
223. Taylor SG, Gelman RS, Falkson G, Cummings FJ: Combination chemotherapy compared to tamoxifen as initial therapy for Stage IV breast cancer in elderly women. *Ann Intern Med* 104: 455–461, 1986.
224. Fabian C, Sternson L, El-Serafi M, et al: Clinical pharmacology of tamoxifen in patients with breast cancer: Correlation with clinical data. *Cancer* 48: 876–882, 1981.
225. Fromson JH, Pearson S, Bramah S: The metabolism of tamoxifen (ICI 46.474) Part II: in female patients. *Xenobiotica* 3: 711–714, 1973.
226. Sutherland CM, Sternson LA, Muchmore JH, et al: Effect of impaired renal function on tamoxifen. *J Surg Oncol* 27: 222–223, 1984.
227. DeGregorio MW, Wiebe VJ, Venook AP, Holleran WM: Elevated plasma tamoxifen levels in a patient with liver obstruction. *Cancer Chemother Pharmacol* 23: 194–195, 1989.
228. Yap H, Blumenschein GR, Hortobagyi GN, et al: Continuous 5-day infusion vinblastine (VLB) in treatment of refractory advanced breast cancer. *Proc Am Assoc Cancer Res ASCO* 20: 334, 1979.
229. Hammond CB, Borcet LG, Tyrey L, et al: Treatment of metastatic trophoblastic disease: good and poor prognosis. *Am J Obstet Gynecol* 115: 451–457.
230. Nobel RL, Beer CJ: Experimental observations concerning the mode of action of vinca alkaloids, in Shedden WIH (ed): *The Vinca Alkaloids in the Chemotherapy of Malignant Disease*. Alburcham, England, John Sherratt and Sons, 1968, pp. 4–11.
231. Owellen RJ, Donigian DW, Hartke CA, et al: The binding of vinblastine to tubulin and to particulate fractions of mammalian brain. *Cancer Res* 34: 3180–3186, 1974.
232. Nelson RL: The comparative clinical pharmacology and pharmacokinetics of vindesine, vincristine, and vinblastine in human patients with cancer. *Med Pediat Oncol* 10: 115–127, 1982.

233. Holland JF, Scharlau C, Gailani S, et al: Vincristine treatment of advanced cancer: A cooperative study of 393 cases. *Cancer Res* 33: 1258–1264, 1973.
234. Jackson DV, Case LD, Pope EK, et al: Single agent vincristine by infusion in refractory multiple myeloma. *J Clin Oncol* 3(11): 1508–1512, 1985.
235. Anderson RJ, Gambertoglio JG, Schrier RW: *Clinical Use of Drugs in Renal Failure*, Chas. Thomas Publishing, Springfield, Illinois, 1976, pp. 15–17.
236. Mouridsen HT, Faber O, Skovsted L, et al: The biotransformation of cyclophosphamide in man: Analysis of the variation in normal subjects. *Acta Pharmacol Toxicol* 35: 98–106, 1974.
237. Cornwell GG, III, Pajak TF, McIntyre OR, et al: Influence of renal failure on myelosuppressive effects of melphalan: Cancer and Leukemia Group B experience. *Cancer Treat Rep* 66: 475–481, 1983.
238. Powis G: Effects of disease states on pharmacokinetics of anticancer drugs, in Ames M, Powis G, Kovach J (eds): *Pharmacokinetics of Anticancer Agents in Humans*. Elsevier, Amsterdam, 1983, pp. 363–397.
239. Gisselbrecht C, Likiec F, Marty M, et al: Adriamycin pharmacokinetics and abnormal liver function. *Cancer Chemother Pharmacol* 5(Suppl): 20, 1980.
240. Bern MM, McDermott W, Cady B, et al: Intraarterial hepatic infusion and intravenous Adriamycin for treatment of hepatocellular carcinoma. *Cancer* 42: 399–405.
241. Goldsmith MA, Ohnuma T, Roboz J, et al: Phase I clinical and pharmacological evaluation of mitoxantrone. *Proc Am Assoc Cancer Res* 22: 389, 1981.
242. Bender RA, Castle MC, Margileth DA, Oliverio VT: The pharmacokinetics of [^{3} H]-vincristine in man. *Clin Pharmacol Ther* 22: 430–438, 1977.
243. Jackson DV, Castle MC, Bender RA: Biliary excretion of vincristine. *Clin Pharmacol Ther* 24(1): 101–107, 1978.
244. Van den Berg HW, Desae ZR, Wilson R, et al: The pharmacokinetics of vincristine in man: reduced drug clearance associated with raised serum alkaline phosphatase and dose-limited elimination. *Cancer Chemother Pharmacol* 8: 215–219, 1982.
245. Mueller JM, Flaherty MJ: Vincristine-induced quadriparesis. *South Med J* 71: 1310–1311, 1978.
246. Ratain MJ, Vogelzang NJ, Sinkule JA: Interpatient and intrapatient variability in vinblastine pharmacokinetics. *Clin Pharmacol Ther* 41(1): 61–67, 1987.
247. Chalmers AH, Burgoyne LA, Murray AW: Autoneoplastic and immunosuppressive drugs I: Biochemical and clinical pharmacological considerations. *Drugs* 3: 227–253, 1972.
248. Ohnuma RJ, Greenspan E, Holland JF: Initial clinical study with vindesine: tolerance to weekly IV bolus and 24 hour infusion. *Cancer Treat Rep* 64: 25–30, 1980.

CHAPTER

23

DRUG THERAPY OF GASTROINTESTINAL DISEASE

M. Brian Fennerty
Martin Higbee

PEPTIC ULCER DISEASE

Although the pathogenesis of peptic ulcer disease (PUD) is now known to be complex, Schwartz's dictum, which is now nearly a century old, is still true: "no acid, no ulcer." Recent studies investigating the role of *Helicobacter pylori* and alterations in mucosal defensive factors have added much knowledge to the complex pathogenesis and understanding of ulcer disease. However, the sine qua non of treatment still remains focused on neutralization or diminishing secretion of gastric acid as an essential component of ulcer disease pathogenesis.

Overall, duodenal ulcer (DU) is more common than gastric ulcer (GU). However, in elderly patients, GU predominates. The reason(s) for this is unclear, but some have implicated diminishing acid production with age, increasing use of nonsteroidal anti-inflammatory drugs (NSAIDs) with age, and/or altered gastric mucosal defense (e.g., mucus) with age. In addition, the elderly more frequently present with complications of ulcer disease, i.e., bleeding or perforation, without preexisting dyspeptic symptoms. Whether noncomplicated PUD in the aged is also associated with less frequent symptoms is unknown.

Antacids

Magnesium-based, aluminum-based, or a combination of magnesium and aluminum antacids are the only antacids with data regarding efficacy in treatment of either GU or DU. Antacids have been used for the treatment of dyspepsia for many centuries.[1] Their ulcer-healing properties are primarily attributed to their ability to reduce gastric acidity by neutralizing secreted gastric acid. The resulting increase in pH (>3.5) also prevents activation of pepsinogen to pepsin, therefore inhibiting the formation of the acid-pepsin complex. In addition to these actions, antacids may have a direct cytoprotective effect on gastrointestinal mucosa due in part to endogenous prostaglandin release.[2,3]

Therapeutic response to antacids is dependent upon dose and timing of administration in relationship to meals. Since antacids provide adequate buffering for only 30 min in a fasting state, it is recommended to administer doses of 144 meq of neutralizing capacity 1 and 3 h after meals and at bedtime. Administering shortly after meals extends buffering capacity several hours.[2,4] Alternating different preparations of antacids may help alleviate "taste fatigue" and may improve compliance.

The effectiveness of antacids in healing duodenal ulcers was first documented by Peterson in 1977.[5] He noted that 30 mL (144 meq of neutralizing capacity) of antacid taken seven times a day (1008 meq/day of acid-neutralizing capacity) resulted in a healing rate of 78 percent in the treatment group versus 45 percent healing in the placebo group. A similar study performed by Lam in 1979 showed that 175 mmoL/day of acid-neutralizing capacity healed most duodenal ulcers.[6] However, trials showing therapeutic efficacy utilized antacids six to seven times a day, which is inconvenient for most patients. More recent data suggest less frequent antacid use (four times a day) may also be successful in healing ulcer disease; however, even this regimen is inconvenient for many elderly patients, and confirmatory data regarding efficacy remains lacking.[1] Antacids have also been shown by some investigators to be effective in healing GUs when used at high dose (144 meq buffer capacity), while others have failed to confirm efficacy.[4]

It appears that the newer, more potent tablet preparations of antacids are equivalent in efficacy to the above studied liquid preparations, and tablet preparation may result in greater compliance even if frequent use remains necessary.[1] However, tablets need to be chewed or dissolved to sufficient particle size to offer optimal buffer capacity, and this may negate their therapeutic efficacy in elderly patients who chew poorly.

Unfortunately, the use of antacids in sufficient quantity to heal either duodenal or gastric ulceration can result in a number of side effects. Antacids containing aluminum can exacerbate or result in constipation, a frequent preexisting chronic complaint among elderly patients. Antacids containing magnesium may result in diarrhea, which may be poorly tolerated by the aged. Many antacids are prepared as an aluminum and magnesium combination to counterbalance the side effects of either component administered alone. In addition, antacids can result in diminished drug absorption (captopril, cimetidine, digoxin, iron, phenothiazines, salicylates, phenytoin, and tetracyclines). This interaction with other drug's absorption can be minimized by taking medication 1 h prior to the use of antacids. Increased serum levels of aluminum or magnesium (approximately 5 to 10 percent of aluminum and magnesium may be absorbed) can occur, which may be harmful in certain situations frequently found in elderly patients such as chronic renal insufficiency and dementia. Since the elderly frequently have low (below 30 mL/min) creatinine clearances, the possibility for magnesium toxicity must be considered.

Although antacids have been shown to be efficacious in treating ulcerative disease of the upper gastrointestinal tract, their inconvenience and difficulties with compliance as well as frequent annoying side effects make them a less preferred means of therapy in elderly patients.

Histamine H_2-Receptor Antagonists (H_2 Blockers)

Currently the H_2 blockers as a class are the preferred means of treating PUD in elderly patients. Their effects on acid secretion relate to their ability to occupy and block the histamine H_2 receptors of the parietal cell, thus reducing production of intracellular cyclic adenosine monophosphate (AMP), resulting in diminished hydrogen ion secretion. Although not well proven, some investigators have proposed a direct cytoprotective effect from H_2 blockers.[2]

The H_2 blockers share similar pharmacokinetic properties with no demonstrable clinically significant differences among them (Table 23-1). Histamine H_2 antagonists are well absorbed, and while antacids may decrease absorption of cimetidine and ranitidine, administration with food does not alter absorption of these agents. Due to their significant renal excretion, creatinine clearance should be estimated for the elderly in order to adjust their dose appropriately to avoid potential adverse effects (Table 23-2).

All four of the presently available H_2 blockers (cimetidine, ranitidine, famotidine, and nizatidine) have equivalent healing properties for both DU and GU when dosed appropriately; cimetidine 300 mg four times daily, 400 mg twice daily, or 800 mg at bedtime; ranitidine 150 mg twice daily or 300 mg at bedtime; famotidine 20 mg twice daily or 40 mg at bedtime; and nizatidine 150 mg twice daily or 300 mg at bedtime.[7] It is also expected that H_2 blockers that are soon to be released (roxatidine) will have equivalent healing rates. DU healing rates at 6 weeks

Table 23-1 Pharmacokinetic data

H_2 blocking agent	Oral absorption, %	Half-life, h	Protein binding, %	Elimination, %	
				Urine	Hepatic
Cimetidine	60–70	1–2	13–25	48	30–40
Ranitidine	50–60	2–3	15	30–35	<10
Famotidine	40–45	2.5–3.5	15–20	25–30	30–35
Nizatidine	>90	1–2	35	60	<18

Table 23-2 Oral dose adjustments for renal function

	Creatinine clearance, mL/min	Dose
Cimetidine	0–20	300 mg every 12 h
	20–40	300 mg every 8 h
	>40	300 mg every 6 h or 400 mg every 12 h or 800 mg at bedtime
Ranitidine	>50	150 mg every 12 h or 300 mg/h
	<50	150 mg every 24 h
Famotidine	>10	20 mg every 12 h or 40 mg/h
	<10	20 mg every 24–48 h
Nizatidine	>50	300 mg daily
	20–50	150 mg daily
	<20	150 mg every other day

approach 90 percent, and for GU rates approach 80 percent at 8 weeks. Therefore, it is recommended to treat DU for 8 weeks and GU for 12 weeks to maximize healing rates. Should ulcers fail to heal at these times, reevaluation is recommended. Maintenance of H_2 blocker is effective in preventing recurrence of disease in 80 percent of patients. Dosages of H_2 blocker for maintenance are shown in Table 23-3. Maintenance therapy for GU is not currently approved in the United States. However, studies indicate that maintenance doses are the same as therapeutic doses.[7]

Differences between the H_2 blockers reside in their chemical structure. Cimetidine has an imidazole ring structure while ranitidine has a furan and famotidine a thiazole ring structure. These differences in structure account for differences in potency and may account for many of the differences in side effect profiles but do not alter the pharmacologic and clinical therapeutic effect on acid secretion when given at equivalent doses.[8] Therefore, treatment failure with one agent will not be overcome by substituting with another H_2 blocking agent. Ranitidine and nizatidine are 5 to 12 times more potent than cimetidine on a milligram-to-milligram basis. Ranitidine's and nizatidine's half-lives tend to be more prolonged in geriatric patients secondary to diminished glomerular filtration rate. Famotidine is 30 to 60 times more potent than cimetidine on a milligram-to-

Table 23-3 Recommended maintenance doses of H_2 blockers for duodenal ulcer

Cimetidine	400 mg at bedtime
Ranitidine	150 mg at bedtime
Famotidine	20 mg at bedtime
Nizatidine	150 mg at bedtime

milligram basis and has a longer half-life than either cimetidine or ranitidine. These differences only provide advantages in dosing intervals and compliance.

Side effects of H_2 blocking agents are unusual.[7] Das and colleagues evaluated side effects rates of cimetidine and ranitidine in 34,252 patients and found the incidence was less than 3 percent with no significant difference found between the two H_2 blockers. The side effect profile of cimetidine has been the best studied and reported because cimetidine has been available longer and therefore has had a better chance of having side effects reported. Of greatest concern with cimetidine use in the geriatric patient population is the potential for central nervous system (CNS) disturbances including delirium and confusion.[10] Animal studies had shown that little cimetidine crosses the blood-brain barrier. Therefore, the frequency of CNS disturbances was surprising to many. However, cimetidine does cross the blood-brain barrier in humans, especially in the elderly and the very young and with increasing blood levels of drug.[10] Although these CNS disturbances remain infrequent occurrences, occurring in less than 1 in 1000, it is most commonly seen in the elderly and is directly related to serum levels of drug.[11] These side effects can best be avoided by adjusting dose based upon creatinine clearance since the elderly often have reduced renal function.[12]

Gynecomastia has been noted with cimetidine use. It is hypothesized that this occurs secondary to cimetidine's weak antiandrogenic effect. Cholestasis and hepatotoxicity as well as interstitial nephritis have been reported but are rare. However, increases in creatinine are not infrequently seen with cimetidine use. However, these changes are usually minor and occur secondary to cimetidine's competition with creatinine for renal excretion. Bradycardia and hypotension have been observed with rapid IV administration of large IV doses.

Hematologic effects secondary to H_2 blockers are unusual.[7] Famotidine and cimetidine have been associated with thrombocytopenia. There have been cases of neutropenia or agranulocytosis associated with cimetidine and ranitidine. Finally cimetidine has also been associated with pancytopenia.

Perhaps most importantly, cimetidine inhibits the hepatic microsomal enzyme system (cytochrome P-450); therefore, drugs commonly prescribed in the elderly such as warfarin, diazepam, phenytoin, theophylline, propranolol and lidocaine will have serum levels affected by concomitant cimetidine use (Table 23-4). Because of these observed drug interactions, drugs with narrow therapeutic indices need to be avoided or their serum concentration closely monitored during cimetidine therapy.

The efficacy of ranitidine is equal to cimetidine in both duodenal and gastric ulceration. However, ranitidine has only one-tenth of the binding to cytochrome P-450 as cimetidine. This probably results in fewer drug interactions than cimetidine.[13] Side effects with ranitidine are infrequent, with headache occurring most frequently in approximately 2 percent of patients. Increased liver function tests and bradycardia have been reported. Ranitidine is devoid of any antiandrogen activity and gynecomastia has not been reported.[13] Few drug interactions have been reported with ranitidine; antacids may decrease absorption of ranitidine; diazepam

Table 23-4 H_2-blocker drug interactions[a]

Decreased hepatic clearance	
Long-acting benzodiazepines	Carbamazepine
Theophylline	Calcium channel blockers
Warfarin	Chloraquin
Phenytoin	Quinine
Propranolol	Quinidine
Labetalol	Pentoxifylline
Metoprolol	Triamterene
Lidocaine	Tricyclic antidepressants
Sulfonylureas	
Metronidazole	
Decreased absorption	
Iron preparations	Ketoconazole
Indomethacin	Tetracyclines
Digoxin	
Decreased renal clearance	
Procainamide	*N*-acetylprocainamide
Drugs that decrease cimetidine absorption	
Antacids	Metoclopramide
Anticholinergics	

[a]These interactions are more commonly reported with cimetidine.

may have decreased absorption; procainamide's renal clearance is decreased; glipizide may have enhanced hypoglycemic effect; and warfarin clearance may be decreased.

The newer agents such as famotidine show no antiandrogenic effect and no effect on the cytochrome P-450 system and yet are as effective in healing DUs and GUs. Few significant drug interactions have been reported with these newer agents. Nizatidine has been reported to increase serum salicylate concentrations when high-dose aspirin (>3 g/day) is used.

Therefore, in elderly patients, the preferred H_2 blocker would appear to be ranitidine, famotidine, or nizatidine. However, cimetidine could be safely used in the majority of elderly patients as long as other drug use and side effects are carefully monitored.

Sucralfate

Agents that enhance mucosal defense offer efficacy with minimal adverse effects. Agents such as sucralfate, colloidal bismuth, and carbenoxalone do not suppress acid secretion but provide ulcer healing through binding with the ulcer and forming a protective barrier and/or by enhancing the mucosal cytoprotective properties.[4,14]

Presently only sucralfate is available in the United States. Sucralfate is a salt of sucrose octosulfate and aluminum hydroxide, which in an acid environment ($pH < 4.0$) binds with positively charged protein exudates in the ulcer base forming a viscous, adhesive substance which provides protection from acid, pepsin, and bile salts.[15] Binding to the ulcer lasts 6 h, thus requiring multiple administrations per day. This medication should be administered 30 to 60 min before meals and at bedtime to avoid drug binding to food proteins.

In many clinical trials, sucralfate has been shown to be equivalent to cimetidine and more effective than placebo in healing duodenal ulcers. Twice daily dosing with 2 g before breakfast and bedtime has been shown to be as effective as 1 g four times daily.[16] Combination therapy with an H_2 antagonist is often considered. Van Deventer et al[17] compared cimetidine and sucralfate in combination and singularly in the treatment of duodenal ulcers. The healing rates at 4 and 8 weeks did not differ from those obtained by either agent alone.[17] Further studies will be necessary to demonstrate better healing with combination therapy. Although sucralfate is not approved for GU therapy, a limited number of studies have demonstrated effectiveness in treatment. Sucralfate is therefore a reasonable alternative to the H_2 blockers in treating elderly patients with ulcer disease and may have the advantage of less severe side effects.

Less than 5 percent of sucralfate is absorbed. Potential exists for increased aluminum levels in people with uremia or elderly patients with diminished glomerular filtration rate especially if patients are receiving aluminum-containing antacids. Hypophosphatemia may also occur. In addition, sucralfate can cause constipation in 1 to 2 percent of patients; this constipation may occasionally be severe. Sucralfate may alter the absorption of other drugs such as phenytoin, tetracycline, digoxin, ciprofloxacin, norfloxacin, ranitidine, cimetidine, and theophylline and should be administered separately from these drugs by 1 to 2 h.

Colloidal bismuth has been used in other countries as a treatment for peptic ulcer disease. Its mechanism of action is thought to be similar to sucralfate; however, it is also effective in eradicating or suppressing *Helicobacter pylori*, which has recently been implicated in the pathogenesis of DUs. Side effects are minimal: darkening of the stools, teeth, and tongue and an unpleasant taste.[4]

Prostaglandins

In many elderly people with ulcers in the stomach or duodenum, the etiologic factor is not acid, pepsin, or bacteria, but NSAIDs which are most commonly prescribed to patients in this age group.[18] NSAIDs have a profound impact on local prostaglandin production in gastric and duodenal mucosa. As prostaglandins are important, if not essential, for preservation of mucosal integrity, it is not surprising that this class of drugs is associated with a marked increase in both GU and DU occurrence.[19] The elderly are particularly a concern for several reasons: (1) 50 percent of all NSAIDs prescribed are for people at least 60 years old, (2) the incidence of perforated peptic ulcer is increasing in the elderly, and (3) as many as

90 percent of elderly patients present with complications related to NSAID therapy without preceding warning symptoms.[18] Attempts to prevent NSAID GU complications by prophylaxis with H_2 antagonists and sucralfate administration have been studied. These agents have been disappointing and have shown no significant difference between placebo and active drug.[20,21]

A novel approach to treating these patient's mucosal injury is in "replacing" the lost mucosal prostaglandins with oral prostaglandin analogues. Misoprostil is a methyl ester analogue of prostaglandin G_1. Large doses (800 μg/day) of misoprostil result in a dose-dependent suppression in both basal and stimulated gastric acid secretion.[22] Misoprostil also increases mucous production as well as increases mucosal bicarbonate secretion.[22] Misoprostil's effect on increasing or maintaining gastric mucosal blood flow may be its most potent mechanism of cytoprotection. Doses of 800 μg/day result in DU healing at 4 weeks of 70 percent and appear to be as effective as H_2 antagonists in patients with GUs.[23] Misoprostil appears to be much more efficacious than H_2 antagonists in preventing and healing NSAID-induced gastric ulceration and is probably equivalent to H_2 blockers in healing DUs related to nonsteroidals.

Recommended doses of misoprostil are 200 μg orally four times daily with food. If this cannot be tolerated, 100 μg orally four times daily can be tried.

Side effects of misoprostil include 5 to 34 percent incidence of diarrhea with the higher doses used in treating ulcer disease.[23] At lower doses, the incidence of diarrhea is probably less than 5 percent. The diarrhea is usually mild and transient and responds to a temporary reduction in dose. The diarrhea is thought to be secondary to increased intestinal secretion of fluid as well as diminished motility of the bowel. Other side effects reported are nausea (3 percent), abdominal pain (3 percent), vomiting (2 percent), headache (1 percent), and rash (1 percent).

In summary, elderly patients with either GUs or DUs are probably best treated with the H_2 antagonists.[24] Ranitidine, famotidine, or nizatidine may be preferred as cimetidine is also effective but may result in more side effects and drug interactions in this patient population. An acceptable alternative is to use sucralfate, which is both effective and infrequently associated with severe side effects. Misoprostil is approved as prophylaxis against NSAID-induced gastric ulceration. Antacids should only be used for symptomatic relief of ulcer pain. Omeprazole (discussed in the following section) has recently been approved for short-term therapy of duodenal ulcer. It is an alternative treatment in patients with GU or DU, especially in patients refractory to other therapy. Healing rates exceed that of H_2 blockers for both DU and GU.

GASTROESOPHAGEAL REFLUX DISEASE

Gastroesophageal reflux disease (GERD) is a common disorder encountered in adults at any age. The incidence in the elderly is unknown. GERD occurs secondary to the reflux of gastric contents (acid, pepsin, bile, etc.) into the esophagus. In normal people, this occurs physiologically postprandially in an upright position and is rapidly cleared by normal esophageal peristalsis, acid-neutralizing effect of swallowing saliva, and an intact mucosal barrier. In GERD patients, reflux occurs pathologically during fasting and recumbency. Most GERD patients reflux because of diminished lower esophageal sphincter pressure or inappropriate relaxation of the lower esophageal sphincter. Other factors contributing to GERD include delayed gastric emptying, diminished esophageal clearance, decreased saliva bicarbonate, and altered mucosal defensive factors. These pathogenic factors are not infrequently found in elderly patients. Characteristically symptoms include complaints of heartburn and regurgitation.

The cornerstone of medical therapy involves diminishing gastric hydrogen ion secretion and/or neutralizing of gastric acid. However, novel therapies aimed at improving gastric and esophageal emptying, improving lower esophageal sphincter tone, and bolstering mucosal defensive factors are emerging.

Antacids

Antacids are used for the symptomatic relief of heartburn associated with GERD. Antacids have not been shown to be effective either in the long-term relief of symptoms related to reflux disease or in healing of reflux-induced esophageal damage. Antacids containing alginic acid have been reported to diminish gastroesophageal reflux. However, there are no data that indicate that this improvement in reflux results in better symptom control or improved healing of esophagitis. As mentioned under peptic ulcer, antacid use is associated with frequent side effects in the elderly as well as inconvenience, and these drugs should be used only as adjunctive therapy in the setting of reflux disease.

H_2 Antagonists

H_2 antagonists are effective in the symptomatic relief of reflux disease. H_2 antagonists probably heal erosive esophagitis in the majority of patients if treated long enough and with high enough doses. In a trial specifically targeted at elderly patients with reflux disease, a 6-week double-blind study showed decreased symptoms and improved healing with ranitidine 150 mg twice a day versus placebo.[25] However, most studies of H_2 antagonists as treatment of reflux disease demonstrate that many patients with erosive esophagitis fail to heal completely with standard "ulcer-type" doses of H_2 antagonists. It appears that some of these patients will heal and have improved symptom control with increased doses of an H_2 antagonist (i.e., ranitidine 300 mg bid to tid). In spite of this, H_2 antagonists remain the initial drug of choice in treating symptomatic GERD. The pharmacokinetics and side effect profiles of H_2 antagonists have been discussed in the previous section on ulcer disease.

Omeprazole

Omeprazole, which is a substituted benzimidazole, acts by selective, noncompetitive inhibition of the hydrogen/potassium adenosinetriphosphatase (ATPase) enzyme (proton pump) in the parietal cell.[26] The proton pump is the final common pathway of gastric acid secretion, and inhibition will abolish parietal cell response to all types of stimulation. Within the parietal cell, the drug is trapped in the acidic secretory canaliculus, resulting in the formation of the sulfoxide metabolite which is the active form of the drug. This active form of the drug binds to the hydrogen potassium ATPase irreversibly inactivating the enzyme. Antisecretory action is seen within 1 h after oral administration and reaches maximum activity within 2 h. Although the serum half-life is less than 1 h, the antisecretory effect lasts up to 72 h. When omeprazole therapy is discontinued, gastric secretory activity returns to normal in 3 to 5 days. Continued use of this drug in doses of 20 to 40 mg daily results in greater than 90 percent inhibition of both basal and stimulated acid secretion. Since omeprazole is acid labile, the drug is delivered orally in a sustained-release formulation. Absorption is rapid. Elimination is primarily hepatic with excretion of metabolites in the urine. In the elderly, the elimination is slightly decreased and bioavailability slightly increased. Despite these slight pharmacokinetic differences, no recommendations for dosage alteration in the elderly are necessary. Therefore, for treatment of GERD, 20 mg daily should be instituted. Patients should be instructed to take the medication before or with meals.

Omeprazole has proven efficacy in the treatment of GERD. In all reflux studies to date, omeprazole was significantly better than full-dose H_2 blockers used bid in both symptom response and endoscopic healing of esophagitis both at 4 and 8 weeks.[27] Omeprazole is a well tolerated drug with a side effect profile similar to the H_2 antagonists. Headache is most frequent (7 percent). Other side effects are diarrhea, abdominal pain, nausea, vomiting, dizziness, constipation, rash, back pain, and cough occurring in less than 2 to 3 percent.

Omeprazole results in reversible modest elevation in serum gastrin. The clinical importance in humans is probably negligible but remains uncertain. In rats prolonged elevation of gastrin results in carcinoid tumors. This effect has not been observed in humans, and gastrin levels are not elevated to the level seen either after surgical vagotomy or in patients with pernicious anemia. Omeprazole inhibits the hepatic microsomal P-450 enzyme system and will alter certain drugs' metabolism. Caution should be used when administering with diazepam, warfarin, and phenytoin due to increased half-lives of these drugs due to this inhibition.

Prokinetic Agents

The medical treatment of GERD has been traditionally targeted toward neutralizing acid activity or decreasing acid production. However, as mentioned earlier, different pathogenic components contribute to reflux disease. These include an absent or insufficient reflux barrier, the nature of the refluxate (i.e., acid, bile, pepsin), decreased esophageal clearance, decreased gastric emptying, and decreased mucosal tissue resistance.

Delayed gastric emptying may predispose to reflux disease. There is a discrepancy in the literature whether decreased gastric emptying is more common in gastroesophageal reflux disease, but there is a suggestion that this may be a major component in the pathophysiology of selected patients.[28] Compounds capable of increasing upper gastrointestinal motility and therefore increasing gastric emptying include bethanechol, metoclopramide, domperidone, and cisapride.

Metoclopramide is a benzamide derivative that increases resting lower esophageal sphincter pressure as well as improves gastric emptying. Metoclopramide's mechanism of action may be dependent on intramural cholinergic neurons where it augments the release of acetylcholine and sensitizes the muscarinic receptors.[29] Metoclopramide also may act by antagonizing the inhibitory neurotransmitter dopamine's effect on gastrointestinal smooth muscle. Metoclopramide's effect in the stomach is to coordinate the gastric and duodenal motor function to produce an aboral movement. In some adult patients with GERD, symptoms improve with metoclopramide and when used adjunctively with H_2 blockers improves esophagitis in some patients. The dose used in treating reflux disease is 10 mg 15 to 30 min before meals. In older patients, this initial dose should probably be decreased to 5 mg tid or qid. In addition, as metoclopramide is primarily excreted through the kidney, patients with creatinine clearance less than 40 mL/min should have the dose halved.

The side effects of metoclopramide are frequent, especially among the elderly. Neuropsychiatric effects can occur in up to one-third of patients. These neuropsychiatric side effects include agitation, fatigue, drowsiness, extrapyramidal reactions, anxiety, insomnia, confusion, and disorientation.

Newer agents such as domperidone (a benzimidazole derivative) are not available at the present time in the United States. Domperidone acts as a dopamine antagonist. No lower esophageal sphincter effect has been seen with domperidone. Domperidone's clinical efficacy seems to be equal to metoclopramide. This compound acts peripherally and does not enter the CNS and, therefore, seems to be devoid of many of the neuropsychiatric side effects with metoclopramide. Domperidone exhibits a marked prolactin effect seen in 10 to 15 percent of patients.[29] The mechanism of this prolactin effect is unclear.

The newest agent being studied is cisapride, a benzamide derivative which has no antidopaminergic actions. Cisapride facilitates release of acetylcholine at the myenteric plexus and increases lower esophageal sphincter pressure.[29] Cisapride's efficacy has been remarkable in improving both symptoms and endoscopy scores in the small studies done to date. Side effects of cisapride include cramps and diarrhea that can be seen in up to 5 percent of patients.

In summary, elderly patients with infrequent reflux symptoms can be managed with prn use of antacids. Those with frequent or continuous reflux symptoms are best treated with a potent H_2 blocker such as ranitidine, famotidine, or nizatidine in full dose twice daily. Patients with incomplete relief of symptoms with H_2 blocker therapy or those with erosive esophagitis should be treated with omeprazole. Now that potent proton pump inhibitors are available, poorly tolerated adjunctive drugs such as metoclopramide will be rarely needed in the therapy of GERD.

INFLAMMATORY BOWEL DISEASE

As the pathogenesis of inflammatory bowel disease remains an enigma but presumably involves some alteration of immunologic surveillance or function, most of the agents used in treating inflammatory bowel disease have an effect on the immune system. Use and efficacy of sulfasalazine dates back to the 1930s and the use of corticosteroids dates to 1948 in the treatment of inflammatory bowel disease.

Corticosteroids

The hypothesized therapeutic mechanisms for steroids include both anti-inflammatory and immunosuppressive actions.[30] Corticosteroids work by passive entry into the cytosol of the cell where they bind to a steroid receptor. This steroid receptor-drug complex then translocates to the nucleus, inducing messenger ribonucleic acid (RNA) transcription and the subsequent cellular production of proteins. These proteins act at specific target tissues and affect the disease process. In addition to the effect on specific protein production, corticosteroids also cause a redistribution of lymphocytes, inhibit release of interleukin 1 and interleukin 2, and inhibit monocyte-macrophage function, prostaglandin production, and leukotriene production. This last mechanism, inhibition of leukotriene production, is receiving new attention and may be the primary effect of corticosteroids on inflammatory bowel disease.[30] Corticosteroids have been shown to be effective both orally and topically in distal colitis and orally in patients with mild to moderately active ulcerative colitis and Crohn's disease.[31] Corticosteroids are not useful as maintenance therapy of inflammatory bowel disease.

Corticosteroid toxicity is related to inhibition of the hypothalamic-pituitary axis. Newer agents (none of which are presently available) have diminished toxicity secondary to extensive first-pass metabolism by both erythrocytes and the liver, resulting in metabolites with little or no biologic activity.[31] Agents such as beclomethasone dipropionate enemas are equivalent to prednisolone in efficacy but have no effect on serum cortisol. Budesomide is more effective than prednisolone enema but, once again, has no effect on serum cortisol. Tixocortal pivolate is a nonglucocorticoid, nonmineralocorticoid derivative of cortisol devoid of systemic toxicity. These newer agents may become widely used if clinically effective.

Side effects of steroids include cataract formation, diabetes, metabolic bone disease, and skin disorders, making long-term use difficult in patients with inflammatory bowel disease, especially in elderly patients where preexisting cataracts, osteoporosis, and diabetes are frequently found.

Sulfasalazine and Associated Analogs

In the late 1930s, Dr. Anna Svartz, a Scandinavian rheumatologist, popularized sulfasalazine as a treatment of ulcerative colitis.[31] Sulfasalazine resulted in an improvement of symptoms and was widely applied in the treatment of inflammatory bowel disease. Sulfasalazine is a conjugate of 5-aminosalicylic acid (5-ASA, a salicylate) and sulfapyridine (a sulfonamide) linked by an azo bond.[32] The mechanism of sulfasalazine may be an antibacterial effect, immunomodulator function, effect on prostaglandin production, inhibition of polymorphonuclear cell migration, and most importantly, inhibition of lipoxygenase (leukotrienes). Sulfasalazine is partially absorbed intact in the proximal jejunum, but the majority of the drug is delivered unchanged to the large bowel. Here the endogenous microbiologic flora cleaves the azo bond, resulting in both free sulfapyridine and 5-ASA. The sulfapyridine is absorbed across the colonic mucosa, but the 5-ASA is largely unabsorbed by the colon. If ingested orally, each individual drug would have been absorbed by the small bowel. The 5-ASA moiety was shown to be the active ingredient of sulfasalazine by Azad Khan, indicating sulfapyridine as no more effective than placebo in treating patients with inflammatory bowel disease. However, intolerance and toxicity of sulfasalazine is usually related to sulfapyridine.

In both the National Crohn's Cooperative Disease Study and the European Cooperative Study sulfasalazine was shown to be effective in Crohn's colitis or ileocolitis but had no remission-maintaining effect.[33] In ulcerative colitis not only is sulfasalazine capable of inducing remission but it is also effective in maintenance of remission. Sulfasalazine in a dose of 2 to 4 g/day is more efficacious than placebo in both symptom control and endoscopic appearance in mild-to-moderate ulcerative colitis. Sulfasalazine is also effective in maintaining remission in doses of 2 to 4 g.

As many patients are intolerant to the sulfapyridine that is absorbed once the azo bond is split, newer agents containing 5-ASA alone such as mesalamine, olsalazine, and balsalazide have been developed in an effort to improve the side effect profiles.[32] Mesalamine is formulated as a delayed release acrylic resin or a slow-release 5-ASA microsphere. The resin dissolves at a pH greater than 6, which is found in the ileum and colon, whereas the microspheres of ethylcellulose gradually dissolve in the small bowel. Olsalazine is a 5-ASA molecule bonded by an azo bond to another 5-ASA molecule. Balsalazide is a 5-ASA azo bonded to an inert carrier. All these cogeners are effective in inducing remission in patients with inflammatory bowel disease. Four-gram 5-ASA enemas are more effective than hydrocortisone enemas in inducing remission in patients with distal inflammatory bowel disease. 5-ASA suppositories are also effective in ulcerative proctitis in doses between 200 mg and 1 g used two to three times daily. 4-ASA, which is more stable in enema form than 5-ASA, is equivalent to 5-ASA and superior to placebo in inducing remission. Both 5-ASA enemas and suppositories are able to maintain remission of inflammatory bowel disease. Oral 5-ASA is useful in disease proximal to the splenic flexure where the topical formulations may not reach.

Sulfasalazine diminishes folic acid levels by diminishing absorption via competitive inhibition of the jejunal brush border enzyme folate conjugase which hydrolyzes polyglutamate folate to the monoglutamate form for transportation. Iron therapy, a frequent mineral supplement in the elderly, should be avoided with sulfasalazine as iron binds to sulfasalazine, preventing bacterial reduction. Side effects of sulfasalazine occur in 21 percent of patients and include nausea, vomiting, and anorexia, which are probably related to high sulfapyridine levels found in slow acetylaters. Headache, urticaria, maculopapular lesions, blue discoloration of the skin, and toxic epidermal necrolysis have also been described. Reversible male infertility, exacerbation of ulcerative colitis, pancreatitis, liver dysfunction, neutropenia, granulotosis, and hemolytic anemia all have been associated with sulfasalazine use. Some patients demonstrating intolerance to sulfasalazine can effectively be treated by slowly reintroducing the drug. Olsalazine is associated with watery diarrhea in up to a third of patients.[33]

Azathioprine

In Crohn's disease, azathioprine has been shown to be effective over a 2-year period if used adjunctively.[31] Azathioprine has a marked steroid-sparing effect, but its therapeutic onset is delayed by a mean of 3.1 months. Azathioprine is also effective in maintaining remission in Crohn's disease. This remission-maintaining effect in Crohn's disease is not seen with steroids or sulfasalazine. Azathioprine is most effective in treating patients that are steroid-dependent, are relapsing frequently, or have fistulas related to their Crohn's disease. Azathioprine also seems to be effective in patients with ulcerative colitis that are steroid-dependent or steroid unresponsive.

Azathioprine is well absorbed with peak concentrations reached within 2 h of oral administration. The half-life is 1 to 1 half-case h and the drug is 30 percent bound to albumin. The drug is eliminated hepatically by xanthine oxidase, and its metabolites are excreted in the urine. Patients receiving allopurinol should have their azathioprine dose reduced by two-thirds to avoid toxicity due to inhibition of azathioprine metabolism.

Side effects of azathioprine include dose-dependent bone marrow suppression in 2 percent of patients. Pancreatitis has been observed in up to 3 percent and allergic reactions are seen in 2 percent. Infections were noted in 7 percent of patients in a long-term trial. The elderly patient poorly tolerates such adverse effects, and therapy should be instituted only after more conventional therapy has failed.

Metronidazole

Metronidazole has been shown to be effective in Crohn's ileocolitis or colitis but not ulcerative colitis. It seems most effective for refractory perianal manifestations, i.e., fistulas, at a dose of 10 to 20 mg/kg/day.[31] Metronidazole's side effects include gastrointestinal symptoms as well as a peripheral neuropathy and a disulfiram reaction. The neuropathy is usually reversible upon cessation of therapy but in some patients is permanent.

In elderly patients with inflammatory bowel disease, the initial therapy of mild-to-moderate ulcerative colitis or Crohn's ileocolitis is oral sulfasalazine. Those intolerant of sulfasalazine will usually be tolerant to osalazine or mesalamine (when available). Those with more distal disease may be best served by initial treatment with 5-ASA enemas or suppositories, which appear to be more effective than rectal steroids. Those with severe colitis or small-bowel Crohn's disease should be treated with oral corticosteroids, but these should be discontinued as soon as feasible. Newer steroid agents may allow for less morbid steroid therapy in the future.

Maintenance of remission in ulcerative colitis can be accomplished in the majority of patients with oral sulfasalazine or oral or topical 5-ASA.

GALLSTONE DISSOLUTION THERAPY

Twenty million Americans (10 percent) have gallstones. Eighty percent of gallstones are cholesterol stones which are formed secondary to lithogenic bile supersaturated with cholesterol. Most of these patients will remain asymptomatic and, therefore, go undetected. The clinical presentation of cholelithiasis is that of biliary colic. However, the elderly may often present with mild or nonfocal symptoms.[34]

Treatment has traditionally been surgery. However, cholecystectomy mortality rates increase with age; for those over 65 years of age undergoing elective cholecystectomy, the mortality is 2 percent; if bile duct exploration is required, the mortality rate is doubled.[35] For these reasons and recognizing the benign natural history of gallstones, oral dissolution therapy is both desirable and safe in selected elderly patients.

Chenodeoxycholic and Ursodeoxycholic Acid

At the present time, two bile acids are available for oral dissolution therapy: Chenodeoxycholic acid (chenodiol) and ursodeoxycholic acid (ursodiol).[34] Chenodiol causes gallstone dissolution by decreasing hepatic cholesterol synthesis, thus desaturating bile. For all patients with gallstones, chenodiol at 750 mg/day results in stone dissolution in 15 percent. However, this rate of stone dissolution approaches 80 percent in selected patients.[34] Features that increase stone dissolution rates include small stones, floating stones, radiolucent stones, and a functioning gallbladder by oral cholecystography. Ursodiol at a dose of 600 mg/day results in dissolution rates equal to that for chenodiol.

The side effects of chenodiol are diarrhea in 20 to 40 percent, and liver test abnormalities in 25 percent, with 5 to 10 percent of patients demonstrating significant elevations in enzymes.[34] In addition, chenodiol increases low-density lipoprotein (LDL) cholesterol by 10 percent. Ursodiol seems devoid of the side effects mentioned above. However, with either dissolution agent gallstone recurrence occurs in 10 percent of patients per year up to a maximum of 40 to 50 percent. Therefore, patients whose stones have dissolved will require prospective monitoring for the recurrence of gallstones.

In summary, oral dissolution therapy in selected elderly patients with cholelithiasis is an effective and well-tolerated alternative to surgery. Treatment should be initiated with ursodiol or a combination of cheno and urso to prevent the frequent side effects seen with cheno alone.[34]

DIARRHEA

Diarrhea can be a concerning symptom in elderly patients as they are less tolerant to volume depletion. The elderly may be at increased risk from diarrhea, regardless of etiology, due to their increased incidence of comorbid diseases, their inability to tolerate the fluid and electrolyte shifts, and their blunted thirst reflex. Acute diarrhea is most frequently secondary to infection with viral agents or related to inflammatory gut conditions such as diverticulitis. However, chronic diarrhea may be secondary to gut pathogens, inflammatory bowel disease, medications, or idiopathic. Since most diarrhea is self-limited and spontaneously subsides, the goals of therapy are to (1) stop the diarrhea, (2) replace fluid and electrolyte loss, and (3) treat or correct the underlying cause if known or possible. Rehydration is the treatment of choice; therefore, drug therapy is used as adjunctive therapy for symptom control and specific disease treatment. Should adjunctive therapy be desired, a variety of agents are available which have both advantages and disadvantages in use. Selection should be based upon a desired pharmacologic response.

Adsorbents

Adsorbents have been used for centuries to treat diarrhea. The mechanism of action is increased stool mass; however, this may only promote a false sense of security. Their disadvantages lie in their nonspecific adsorption (fluid, electrolyte) and the possibility of causing obstruction.

Kaolin, which is hydrated aluminum silicate clay and pectin, is a carbohydrate gel derived from fruit that has been used for over a century in the treatment of diarrhea. Doses of 30 to 120 mL are recommended after each loose stool. Kaolin and pectin are not absorbed and function as nonspecific absorbents. Kaolin-pectin's efficacy is doubtful, and most concerning, diarrhea has been shown to worsen in some cases by increasing fluid and electrolyte loss.[36] Kaolin-pectin is only mentioned here to recommend against its use in the treatment of diarrheal diseases.

Antimotility Agents

Opiate derivatives and anticholinergics are often used to control diarrhea. Opiate derivatives decrease passage of stool by increasing gastrointestinal and ileocecal tone and decreasing bowel motility. The end result of these pharmacologic actions is to relieve tenesmus, cramping, and decreasing diarrhea. However, disadvantages inherent in these mechanisms are the loss of a protective mechanism and decreased transit time, resulting in prolonged contact of the bowel with toxins and infective agents.

Anticholinergic agents (atropine) inhibit diarrhea by decreasing gastrointestinal tone and decreasing motility. Since the therapeutic range is narrow and side effects are almost certain at therapeutic doses, these agents should be used cautiously if at all in elderly. The elderly are particularly at risk with these agents since the systemic anticholinergic effects often result in urinary retention, dry eyes, blurred vision, and dry mouth (xerostomia), conditions that are frequently seen in patients of this age group. Additionally, since elderly patients frequently take medications which exhibit anticholinergic action (antihistamines, antidepressants, antipsychotics), the possibility exists for increased CNS side effects, especially confusion, due to additive anticholinergic action.

Loperamide and Diphenoxylate with Atropine

Loperamide is a phenylpiperidine derivative related to meperidine that decreases intestinal transit via agonist activity at the gastrointestinal opiate receptors. Loperamide also decreases intestinal secretion. In a comparative trial with diphenoxylate, loperamide was shown to be more effective in controlling diarrhea.[37] Loperamide is for the most part without side effects with the exception of constipation and abdominal distention seen with overly vigorous dosing. Dry mouth, nausea, vomiting, dizziness, and drowsiness can also be observed. Diphenoxylate, also a meperidine derivative, with atropine is also effective in controlling diarrhea but is more commonly associated with side effects such as anorexia, nausea, vomiting, abdominal pain, dizziness, depression, headache, lethargy, confusion, sedation, and dry mouth.

Antisecretory

Bismuth subsalicylate, with its affinity for forming a protective complex with mucosal glycoproteins, acts as a barrier and as a demulcent. Although most often used to treat traveler's diarrhea, bismuth subsalicylate is also used to treat diarrhea associated endemic gastroenteritis with nausea and vomiting. Caution should be used, particularly with frequent administration, in order to prevent salicylate toxicity or salicylate interaction with oral anticoagulants.

Bacterial Replacement

Lactobacillus acidophilus and *L. bulgaricus* preparations have been promoted to replenish colonic microflora in diarrheal states, particularly if diarrhea is related to antibiotic use. Introduction of these bacteria supposedly restores the intestinal microflora and improves function. However, there are no validated studies which confirm this therapy, and the authors do not recommend the use of these bacterial preparations. The ingestion of milk or yogurt would promote recolonization similarly and at much less cost.

Antibiotics and Bismuth for Traveler's Diarrhea

Traveler's diarrhea is caused by noninvasive enterotoxigenic *Escherichia coli* in 20 to 75 percent of cases.[38] *Salmonella* sp., *Shigella* sp., and *Campylobacter jejuni* cause the majority of other cases of traveler's diarrhea.

Therapy of traveler's diarrhea can be accomplished either by treating the patients prophylactically or by active treatment once symptoms begin. Prophylactic treatment with trimethoprim-sulfamethoxazole (TMP-SMX) will diminish attack rates 85 percent, doxycycline 75 percent, and the fluroquinolones 85 percent, whereas bismuth subsalicylate will only decrease attack rates 55 percent.[38] Active treatment with 3 days or less of TMP-SMX diminishes the duration of illness from 60 to 90 to 20 to 30 h, ciprofloxacin from 81 to 29 h, and norfloxacin from 106 to 77 h. Bismuth and loperamide have also been studied but are not as efficacious as antibiotics in treating patients with active disease.

The fluroquinolone ciprofloxacin (500 mg twice a day) has been approved by the Federal Drug Administration (FDA) to treat *E. coli, C. jejuni, Shigella sonnei,* and *Shigella flexneri.* It also is effective for other gram negative rods causing diarrhea very well. Ciprofloxacin's coverage includes *C. jejuni*, which is not seen with TMP-SMX. Side effects of ciprofloxacin include CNS stimulation resulting in insomnia, restlessness, dizziness, and headache for long-term use. Ciprofloxacin can increase theophylline and phenytoin serum concentrations.

Elderly patients with mild-to-moderate diarrhea not associated with systemic symptoms are best managed by initial therapy with loperamide. Caution needs to be used with this agent to prevent constipation/impaction in older patients. Older patients traveling to third world countries are best treated prophylactically as they tolerate infectious diarrhea poorly. Once infection has occurred, treatment with ciprofloxacin is the agent of choice.

CONSTIPATION

One of the major misconceptions among elderly Americans is that daily bowel movements are a prerequisite for good health and that laxatives are harmless. Constipation is a symptom, not a disease. Normal stooling frequency in adults varies from three stools per day to three per week.[39] Constipation has different meaning to individual patients, i.e., infrequent stools, too hard, too small, painful, or straining with stool. Despite the belief that constipation increases with age, there is no direct evidence to support this idea.[39] However, constipation remains one of the most common gastrointestinal symptoms among elderly patients and requires careful diagnostic evaluation and a well-thought-out therapeutic plan.[40] When an elderly patient presents with constipation as a complaint, the physician should exclude diseases such as obstruction, fecal impaction, metabolic disorders, and malignancy. The need to discontinue or change medications associated with constipation or known to induce constipation is not infrequent (the effect of narcotics on bowel function is discussed in Chap. 9). Consideration should also be given to prolonged laxative abuse as this will often lead to difficulties in defecation.

The treatment of constipation in the elderly should be approached non-pharmacologically if possible.[41] Immobile or institutionalized patients often require more aggressive pharmacologic intervention. This pharmacologic approach should be stepped. First an etiology should be sought. Once impaction, obstruction, malignancy, or other medical causes (irritable bowel syndrome, diverticulitis, and fissures, proctitis, hemorrhoids, infections, CNS disease, metabolic disorders) have been ruled out, consider dietary modification and increased physical activity, if possible. Although increased fluid intake as therapy is controversial, the increase in fiber will require increased fluids to be effective and safe. A 1-month trial should be completed to determine effectiveness. Should these simple approaches fail, acute treatment with a stimulant cathartic may be necessary followed by prophylaxis. Prophylaxis can be accomplished with psyllium, stool softeners, and hyperosmotic agents. Stool softeners are unnecessary if stools are well hydrated (wet, soft).

Laxatives

Laxatives can be classified into stimulant, saline, emollient, hyperosmolar, and bulk-forming agents.[42] The stimulant laxatives include castor oil, diphenylmethanes, and anthraquinones. Castor oil is metabolized to ricinoleic acid which, through its action on cellular cyclic AMP, impairs water absorption in the ileum, decreases glucose absorption, and increases contractility of the small bowel. Onset of action is within 1 to 3 h. Side effects of castor oil include cramping, nausea, fluid and electrolyte loss, violent expulsion of fecal material, malabsorption, and with chronic use, cathartic colon. The diphenylmethanes include phenolphthalein and bisacodyl. These drugs stimulate the mucosal nerve plexus and increase intestinal chloride secretion. Onset of action results in a soft or semifluid stool in 6 to 8 h. If bisacodyl is given rectally, the onset of action is within 15 to 60 min. Side effects of these compounds include gastric irritation if the drug comes in contact with gastric mucosa, i.e., if bisacodyl is chewed and swallowed, as well as drug eruptions, Stevens-Johnson syndrome, or a purple polychromatic rash which may leave residual pigmentation. More commonly abdominal cramping, fluid/electrolyte loss, nausea, and changes in urine color (pink-orange) occur with phenolphthalein. The anthraquinones include senna, cascara, and aloe. The mechanism of action of these compounds is not well understood. These drugs cause net increased fluid secretion possibly by stimulating Auerbach's plexus. Side effects include melanosis coli and degeneration of Auerbach's and Meisner's nerve plexus in the gut wall seen with chronic long-term use. For this reason, patients, particularly those in long-term care facilities, should not be given these agents on a daily basis as a prophylaxis for constipation. Stimulant agents should only be used after other less aggressive therapy has failed. Stimulant laxatives should never be used more frequently than once a week.

The saline laxatives include oral magnesium salts and sodium phosphate enemas. These agents osmotically retain water since they are poorly absorbed ions. Magnesium also stimulates secretion of cholecystokinin, which stimulates bowel motility and fluid secretion. The onset of action is 1 to 3 h after oral ingestion and 5 to 15 min if given rectally. Side effects are infrequent and include fluid and electrolyte loss, magnesium and sodium accumulation with renal failure, and congestive heart failure, respectively.

The emollient laxatives include docusate salts and mineral oil. Docusate salts are anionic surfactants that lower fecal surface tension and allow increased mixing of water to soften stool. These agents also cause increased intestinal secretion. Mineral oil penetrates feces, making the fecal mass easier to pass. The side effects of chronic mineral oil use include decreased fat-soluble vitamin absorption, anal leakage of oil, as well as potential for lipoid pneumonitis if aspirated. Generally, the use of mineral oil should be avoided due to the potential for serious pneumonitis, particularly in the bedridden elderly.

Hyperosmolar agents include polyethylene glycol, lactulose, sorbitol, and glycerin. Polyethylene glycol is the active ingredient in most preparations used for bowel cleansing for endoscopy and/or radiographic studies. Polyethylene glycol is an osmotic agent whose only side effect is nausea and bloating if consumed in large quantities. Lactulose is hydrolyzed by bacteria to fatty acids, which not only increases osmolality of the stool but also acidity in the bowel lumen. Glycerine and sorbitol are osmotically active substances. The onset of action for lactulose, sorbitol, and glycerin is 1 to 3 days. In elderly patients, sorbitol is as effective as lactulose but causes less nausea and is less expensive.[43] Side effects of lactulose and sorbitol are generally mild but include flatulence, abdominal cramps, diarrhea, and fluid and electrolyte loss. Glycerin can cause rectal irritation.

The bulk-forming agents include agar, bran, psyllium, alginates, methylcellulose, and carboxyl methylcellulose, which all absorb water and expand, causing increased stool bulk. This results in a decreased stool transit time. Onset of action for bulk agents is 1 to 3 days. Common side effects are bloating, flatus, abdominal cramping, distention, and possibly obstruction.

Other methods used in the treatment of constipation have included soapsuds enemas or tap water enemas. Soapsuds enemas are no longer recommended due to occasional colitis and proctitis. Tap water enemas will result in evacuation within 30 min. However, no more than 200 mL of water should be used. Frequent use may also lead to excess water absorption and could aggravate the renal or congestive heart failure commonly encountered in elderly patients.

The treatment of chronic constipation in the elderly should initially consist of bulk agents as they are the safest to use and devoid of most side effects. Sorbitol, which is well tolerated and cheaper than lactulose, is an alternative. In an acute situation, stimulant, glycerine, or hyperosmolar laxatives are safe to use. Chronic use of stimulant laxatives is inappropriate. Newer investigational agents such as cisapride increase the number of bowel movements and decrease laxative use.[44] This agent may prove useful in the future treatment of chronic constipation.

IRRITABLE BOWEL

Irritable bowel syndrome (IBS) is a syndrome of altered bowel habits and abdominal pain. Its initial onset in the elderly is rare, and these symptoms should prompt a thorough search to exclude malignancy or inflammatory processes.[45] However, many elderly patients have a long history of symptoms dating frequently to young adult life. The etiology of IBS is enigmatic but is felt by many to represent a yet uncharacterized gut motility disorder. Abnormal personality traits and neuropsychiatric disorders are frequently seen in patients with IBS. The association of these personality disorders and IBS is unclear.

The pharmacologic treatment of IBS has consisted of anticholinergics, antidepressants, tranquilizers, and bulking agents. None of these modalities has convincing data for efficacy.

Anticholinergics

The mechanism by which anticholinergics are presumed to work in IBS is their effect on gut smooth muscle preventing "spasm." Among the anticholinergics, dicyclomine hydrochloride has equivocal data on its efficacy.[46] Anticholinergic side effects are very frequent and often intolerable. Interestingly enough, if enough drug is used to effect gastrointestinal motility, which is the presumed mechanism of efficacy, then there will be intolerable anticholinergic side effects.[46] Therefore, this class of drug is not recommended in the elderly, due to potential difficulty with urinary retention, blurred vision, dry mouth, and mental confusion related to anticholinergic effects.

Antidepressants

The antidepressants, including amitriptyline and doxepin, work through an unknown mechanism. There is no data showing unequivocal benefit in treating IBS, and the side effects of tricyclic antidepressants, including anticholinergic and cardiovascular, can be very serious in elderly patients. Antidepressants should only be used when there is associated depression requiring treatment. In this instance, the least sedating, hypotensive, and anticholinergic antidepressant should be utilized. For these reasons, amitriptyline should be avoided. Desipramine, nortriptyline or trazadone may be better, more tolerable alternatives.

Tranquilizers

The tranquilizers, such as diazepam, have no efficacy data in IBS but are frequently used as treatment. They should only be used if associated anxiety disorders are present, as they have no role in the primary treatment of IBS.

Combination Agents and Bulking Agents

There are many combination products available, including Librax, which consists of clidinium and chlordiazepoxide, and Donnatal, which contains hyoscyamine, atropine, scopolamine, and phenobarbital. There are no data showing convincing evidence that these agents are effective. The most commonly used therapy for IBS are bulking agents such as psyllium. Longstreth[47] has shown psyllium to be no more effective that placebo in improving bowel symptoms. Bran has also been evaluated as therapy for IBS in a double-blind, placebo-controlled crossover trial and was shown to be equal to placebo.[48] Most importantly, all studies of therapy for IBS show an enormous placebo effect, and any therapy studied without a placebo arm is therefore likely to show a significant benefit.[49] Therefore, there is no firm support for bran or other bulking agents as therapy for IBS, and the placebo response to any form of therapy is likely to be 30 to 65 percent.

REFERENCES

1. Berstad A, Weberg R: Antacids in the treatment of gastroduodenal ulcer. *Scand J Gastroenterol* 21: 385-391, 1986.
2. Garnett WR, Dukes GE: *Upper gastrointestinal disorders*, in Young Ly, Loda-Kimble MA (eds.): *Applied Therapeutics*, 4th ed, Vancouver, WA, Applied Therapeutics Inc., 1988, pp 447-465.
3. Domschke W: Antacids and gastric mucosal protection. *Scand J Gastroenterol* 21(suppl 125): 144-149, 1986.
4. Barardi RR: *Peptic ulcer disease and zollinger-ellison syndrome*, in DiPiro JT, Talbert RL, Hayes PE, et al (eds.): *Pharmacotherapy: A Pathophysiologic Approach*. New York, Elsevier, 1989, pp 418-436.
5. Peterson WL, Sturdevant RL, Frankl HD, et al: Healing of duodenal ulcer with an antacid regimen. *N Engl J Med* 297: 341-345, 1977.
6. Lam SK, Lam KC, Lai CL, et al: Treatment of duodenal ulcer with antacid and sulpirine. A double-blind controlled study. *Gastroenterology* 76: 315-322, 1979.
7. Lipsy RJ, Fennerty B, Fagan TC: Clinical review of histamine$_2$-receptor antagonists. *Arch Intern Med* 150: 745-751, 1990.
8. Lacey Smith J, Gamal MA, Chremos AN, Graham DY: Famotidine, a new H_2-receptor antagonist: effect on parietal, nonparietal, and pepsin secretion in man. *Dig Dis Sci* 30:308-312, 1985.
9. Das AF, Freston JW, Jacobs J, et al: An evaluation of safety in 34,252 patients treated with cimetidine or ranitidine. *IM-Inter Med Special* 11(1): 3-14, 1990.
10. Freston JW: Cimetidine II: Adverse reactions and patterns of use. *Ann Intern Med* 97: 728-734, 1982.
11. Canth TG, Korek JS: Central nervous system reactions to histamine-2 receptor blockers. *Ann Intern Med* 114: 1027-1034, 1991.
12. McCarthy DM: Acid peptic disease in the elderly. *Clin Geriatr Med* 7(2): 231-254, 1991.

13. Zeidis JB, Friedman LS, Isselbacher KJ: Ranitidine: A new H_2-receptor antagonist. *N Engl J Med* 309: 1368–1373, 1983.
14. Ligumsky M, Karmski F, Rochmilewitz D: Sucralfate stimulation of gastric PGE's synthesis: possible mechanism to explain its effective cytoprotective mechanism. *Gastroenterology* 86: 1164, 1984 (abstr).
15. Richardson CT: Sucralfate. *Ann Intern Med* 97: 269–272, 1982 (editorial).
16. Brandstaetter G, Kratochvil P: Comparison of two sucralfate dosages (2g twice a day versus 1g four times a day) in duodenal ulcer healing. *Am J Med* 7a(suppl 2C): 36–38, 1985.
17. Van Deventer GM, Schneiderman D, Walsh JH: Sucralfate and cimetidine as single agents and in combination for treatment of active duodenal ulcers. *Am J Med* 79(suppl 2c): 39–44, 1985.
18. Griffin MR, Piper JM, Daugherty JR, et al: Nonsteroidal anti-inflammatory drug use and increased risk for peptic ulcer disease in elderly persons. *Ann Intern Med* 114: 257-263, 1991.
19. Armstrong CP, Blower AL: Nonsteroidal anti-inflammatory drugs and life threatening complications of peptic ulceration. *Gut* 28: 527-532, 1987.
20. Roth SH, Bennett RE, Mitchell CS, et al: Cimetidine therapy in nonsteroidal anti-inflammatory drug gastropathy: double-blind long-term evaluation. *Arch Intern Med* 147: 1798–1801, 1987.
21. Caldwell JR, Roth SH, Wu WC, et al: Sucralfate treatment of nonsteroidal anti-inflammatory drug-induced gastrointestinal symptoms and mucosal damage. *Am J Med* 83(suppl 3B): 74–82, 1987.
22. Herting RL, Nissen CH: Overview of misoprostil clinical experience. *Dig Dis Sci* 31: 47S–54S, 1986.
23. Monk CP, Clissold SP: Misoprostil: A preliminary review of its pharmacodynamic and pharmacokinetic properties and therapeutic efficacy in the treatment of peptic ulcer disease. *Drugs* 33: 1–30, 1987.
24. Chiverton SG, Hunt RH: Pharmacokinetics and pharmacodynamics of treatments for peptic ulcer disease in the elderly. *Am J Gastroenterol* 83: 211–215, 1988.
25. Zimmerman TW, Vlahceric S, Behar J, Nardi R: Ranitidine treatment of gastroesophageal reflux disease (GERD) in the elderly. *Gastroenterology* 88: 1644(a); 1985.
26. Friedman G: GI drug column: omeprazole. *Am J Gastroenterol* 82: 188–191, 1987.
27. Harelund T, Laursencs, et al: Omeprazole and ranitidine in treatment of reflux esophagitis: double blind comparative trial. *BMJ* 296: 89–92, 1988.
28. Verlinder M: Review article: A role for gastrointestinal prokinetic agents in the treatment of reflux oesophagitis? *Aliment Pharm Ther* 3113–3131, 1989.
29. McCallum RW: Review of the current status of prokinetic agents in gastroenterology. *Am J Gastroenterol* 80: 1008–1016, 1985.
30. Routes J, Claman HN: Corticosteroids in inflammatory bowel disease: A review. *J Clin Gastroenterol* 9: 529–535, 1987.
31. Peppercorn MA: Advances in drug therapy for inflammatory bowel disease. *Ann Intern Med* 112: 50–60, 1990.
32. Friedman G: Sulfasalazine and new analogues. *Am J Gastroenterol* 81: 141–144, 1986.
33. Peppercorn MA: Sulfasalazine. Pharmacology, clinical use, toxicity, and related drug development. *Ann Intern Med* 3: 377–386, 1989.
34. Salen G, Tint GS, Shefer S: Oral dissolution treatment of gallstones with bile acids. *Semin Liver Dis* 10: 181–186, 1990.
35. Krasman ML, Gracie WA, Strasius SR: Biliary tract disease in the aged. *Clin Geriatr Med* 7(2): 347–370, 1991.
36. Portnoy BL: Antidiarrheal agents in the treatment of acute diarrhea in children. *JAMA* 236: 844, 1976.
37. Bergman L, Djarv L: A comparative study of loperamide and diphenoxylate in the treatment of chronic diarrhea caused by intestinal resection. *Ann Clin Reg* 13: 402–405, 1981.
38. Farthing MJG: Review article: prevention and treatment of traveller's diarrhea. *Aliment Pharm Ther* 5: 15–30, 1991.

39. Read NW, Timms JM: Defecation and the pathophysiology of constipation. *Clin Gastroenterol* 15: 937-965, 1986.
40. Rousseau P: Treatment of constipation in the elderly. *Postgrad Med* 83: 341-345, 1988.
41. Tedesco FJ: Laxative use in constipation. *Am J Gastroenterol* 80: 303-309, 1985.
42. Sekas G: The use and abuse of laxatives. *Practical Gastroenterol* 11: 33-37, 1987.
43. Lederly FA, Busch DL, Mattox KM, et al: Cost-effective treatment of constipation in the elderly: A randomized double-blind comparison of sorbitol and lactulose. *Am J Med* 89: 597-601, 1990.
44. Müller-Lissuer S: Treatment of chronic constipation with cisapride and placebo. *Gut* 28: 1033-1038, 1987.
45. Geboes K, Bossaert H: Gastrointestinal disorders in old age. *Age Aging* 6: 197-200, 1977.
46. Klein KB: Drug treatment of the irritable bowel syndrome. *Practical Gastroenterol* 10: 8-14, 1986.
47. Longstreth GF, Fox DD, Yonkeles L, et al: Psyllium therapy in the irritable bowel syndrome. *Ann Intern Med* 95: 53-56, 1981.
48. Lucey MR, Clark MC, Lown JO, Dawson AM: Is bran efficacious in irritable bowel syndrome: A double-blind placebo controlled crossover study. *Gut* 28: 221-225, 1987.
49. Thompson WG: A strategy for management of the irritable bowel. *Am J Gastroenterol* 81: 95-100, 1986.

CHAPTER

24

BACTERIAL AND VIRAL INFECTIONS

Angela Y. Hirai
Neil M. Ampel

The principles of antimicrobial therapy for the elderly are similar to those in other patients. However, the aged represent a unique group within our population with regard to infectious diseases. In particular, the elderly appear to be at increased risk for complications occurring as a result of infection when compared to younger individuals. The reasons for this are complex and relate, at least in part, to the general increase in the incidence of degenerative and chronic diseases and to the increased rate of hospitalization and institutionalization among those in this population group. While senescence of the specific elements of the immune system is probably not a major factor in this increased incidence,[1,2] breakdown in the nonspecific barriers against microbial invasion is undoubtedly important. Moreover, diseases like chronic pulmonary disease, stroke, and diabetes all affect host resistance to infection and either are more common among the elderly or are at a more severe and advanced stage. The increased use of immunosuppressive drugs, such as corticosteroids and cancer chemotherapy agents, also reduces host resistance and increases the risk of infection. Other drugs more commonly used in the elderly may alter mental status or reduce the cough reflex and result in increased pulmonary infections. Finally, the normal physiologic process of aging may act to decrease normal host defenses by reducing gastric acidity, cough reflex, and skin integrity.[2]

It may be more difficult to diagnose infections among the elderly. While the signs and symptoms are similar to those seen in younger patients, the elderly tend to present with fewer focal findings and demonstrate a more generalized response to infection. For example, pneumonia in the aged patient may present as decreased mental status and fever with cough and pleuritic chest pain being absent or minimal. The meningismus of bacterial meningitis may be masked in the elderly because of cervical osteoarthritis, which also causes neck stiffness.[2,3]

Certain infections are more common among the elderly. The incidence of urinary tract infection increases dramatically in both males and females over the age of 60. Increasing debility and the use of indwelling urinary catheters further increase the incidence of urinary tract infection. While *Escherichia coli* is the most common infecting organism in the elderly, as it is among younger patients, other gram-negative bacilli are more prevalent in the older population. Bacterial meningitis caused by gram-negative bacilli and by *Listeria monocytogenes* also appears to be more frequent in the elderly. Finally, bacterial pneumonia is a common problem in the aged. While *Streptococcus pneumoniae* is a frequent pathogen, other organisms such as *Legionella* and aerobic gram-negative bacilli play an important role, particularly among those who are hospitalized. Mixed pulmonary infection due to aspiration is also a more common problem among the elderly. Epidemic influenza is also more likely to strike the elderly who reside in chronic care institutions. Finally, tuberculosis, either due to reactivation of a previously acquired infection or due to acute infection associated with an active case in an institutionalized setting, is also more frequently encountered.[2,3]

The treatment of infections among the elderly is complicated by the occurrence of more frequent adverse reactions and drug interactions. The age-related decline in renal function makes the use of drugs that are nephrotoxic, such as aminoglycosides and amphotericin B, more difficult. Ototoxicity, which may occur with vancomycin and aminoglycosides, may also reduce already impaired hearing in the elderly patient. Bleeding diatheses seen with certain cephalosporin antibiotics which contain the *N*-methylthiotetrazole side chain are more frequent in the elderly as are seizures due to imipenem-cilastatin. Hepatitis due to the antituberculous drug isoniazid increases with increasing age.[4]

In addition, the elderly are more likely to be on multiple drugs with an increased likelihood of adverse drug interactions. For example, erythromycin and ciprofloxacin may inhibit metabolism of theophylline and result in theophylline toxicity. On the other hand, rifampin may increase the metabolism of warfarin and result in suboptimal anticoagulation.[4]

This chapter is not intended to be encyclopedic. Rather, the authors have tried to focus on the most commonly used antimicrobial agents in the elderly. Specifically, comments have been limited to those agents used in the treatment of bacterial infections, including those due to *Mycobacterium tuberculosis* and to the two most common viral infections, influenza and herpes zoster. For more detailed discussions of particular issues, the reader is recommended to the references.

SPECIFIC ANTIMICROBIAL AGENTS

Beta-lactams

The beta-lactam antibiotics consist of two major groups of agents, the penicillins and the cephalosporins. Because their mechanism of action is the same and their structure is very similar, the section dealing with these issues is combined.

Structure and mechanism of action The discovery of penicillin is now a well-known story in the annals of science. In 1928, Alexander Fleming observed in agar plates which he had previously discarded that areas around a contaminating mold appeared to inhibit the growth of bacteria. Nearly 10 years later, H. W. Florey exploited this discovery when he and his coworkers purified penicillin and used it clinically.[5] Since then, the beta-lactam antibiotics have become the mainstay of the physician's armamentarium against a wide variety of bacterial pathogens.

The basic penicillin nucleus possesses three important structural components: the beta-lactam ring, which must be intact for antimicrobial activity; the five-member thiazolidine ring; and a side chain off of the beta-lactam ring, which defines the antimicrobial spectrum as well as the pharmacologic and pharmacokinetic properties of the specific agent. The cephalosporins differ in that they possess a six-membered ring rather than the thiazolidine ring and have two areas to which side chains can be attached (Fig. 24-1).

Antimicrobial activity of the beta-lactam antibiotics is dependent upon their ability to penetrate the bacterial cell wall, resist inactivation by beta-lactamases, and bind to and inactivate so-called penicillin binding proteins (PBPs). Bacterial resistance may develop when there is interference with any of these steps.

PBPs are enzymes that are important for the biosynthesis of the peptidoglycan component of the bacterial cell wall. Beta-lactam antibiotics bind to and inactivate PBPs located on the inner aspect of the bacterial cell membrane. Each beta-lactam agent has an affinity for certain PBPs; this affinity partially determines the effects of a particular antibiotic on a bacterium. Some PBPs are essential for cell survival, and inactivation results in bacterial death, while others are not essential, and inactivation does not result in death.

The most important mechanism of resistance of microorganisms to the beta-lactams is the production of beta-lactamases, enzymes which are capable of hydrolyzing the beta-lactam ring. There are many different types of beta-lactamases. Some are encoded on plasmids while others are encoded on bacterial chromosomes. Some are constitutively produced while others are induced only in the presence of beta-lactams. Some, like the penicillinases of *Staphylococcus aureus*, are relatively specific for certain antibiotics, while others, like the TEM-1 found in many gram-negative bacilli, can hydrolyze a variety of beta-lactams.[5,6] Much of the effort to produce new beta-lactams has been placed on developing agents which are resistant to the action of beta-lactamases. Methicillin-resistant staphylococci are often resistant to multiple antibiotic agents. The mechanism

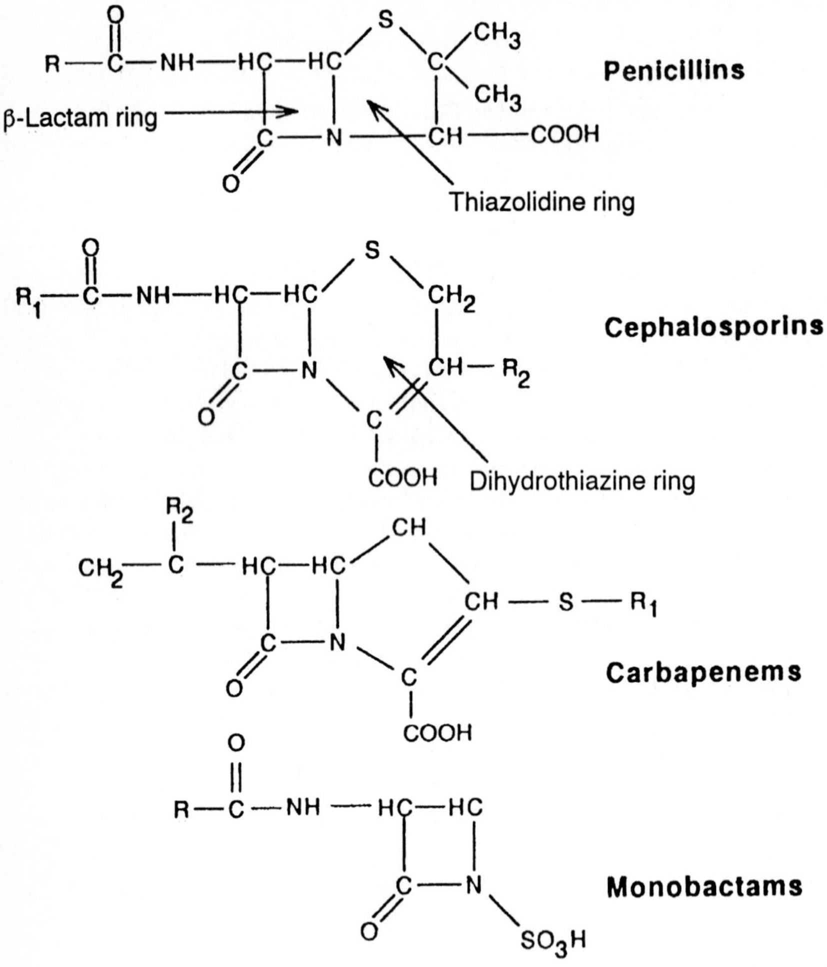

Figure 24-1 Basic structure of the beta-lactams.

of resistance is not fully understood but is not due to production of a beta-lactamase.[7]

Penicillins

Pharmacokinetics Penicillin G, the prototypic penicillin agent, is acid-labile, and much of it is inactivated in the stomach when taken orally. Penicillins that are stable in acid, such as penicillin V, amoxicillin, and dicloxacillin, are absorbed in the proximal duodenum and reach peak serum levels approximately 1 h after ingestion. Penicillins are well distributed throughout the body. Although different compounds have varying amounts of serum protein binding, the significance of this is questionable. The serum half-life of most penicillins is short, around 30 min or less.

Most penicillins are excreted unchanged in the urine by proximal tubule secretion. Hence, very high concentrations of active drug accumulate in the urine and account for the usefulness of these agents in the treatment of urinary tract infections. Tubular secretion can be blocked by probenecid, resulting in a longer serum half-life. Renal dysfunction can also result in a prolonged serum half-life with accumulation of toxic concentrations of drug. Nafcillin is an exception in that it is principally excreted by the liver.[5,8] Peritoneal dialysis removes penicillins in variable amounts, thereby necessitating dosage adjustments for certain agents, such as carbenicillin and ticarcillin. Hemodialysis removes penicillin G, ampicillin, amoxicillin, carbenicillin, ticarcillin, azlocillin, mezlocillin and pipericillin.

Adverse Reactions The major adverse drug reactions encountered with the penicillins are due to hypersensitivity. This occurs least often when the drug is given orally, is higher in frequency after intravenous infusion, and is most common with intramuscular injection of procaine penicillin or when applied topically. The incidence of allergic reactions in the general population is 3 to 5 percent and may be as high as 10 percent in patients who have been previously treated with a penicillin.[8] Common manifestation of penicillin allergy are rash, fever, and serum sickness. Most patients with infectious mononucleosis treated with ampicillin will develop a macular or maculopapular rash indistinguishable from a drug hypersensitivity reaction. This is not, in fact, an allergic reaction.

Hematologic toxicity due to the penicillins is rare. Neutropenia may be caused by any of the penicillins, but nafcillin is probably the most common agent associated with this. Disruption of normal platelet aggregation, particularly with carbenicillin and ticarcillin, has been reported, but the clinical implications of this are not clear. Gastrointestinal side effects are frequently encountered with oral dosage forms, particularly with ampicillin. Although the development of pseudomembranous colitis has been associated with virtually all antimicrobial agents, ampicillin is the most common cause of this potentially serious side effect. Cases of abnormal liver function tests have been reported, particularly with oxacillin, but major hepatic injury is rare. Renal toxicity is also rare. Interstitial nephritis, which may be associated with fever, eosinophilia, eosinophiluria, hematuria, proteinuria, and pyuria, may be associated with all the penicillins, but the majority of conclusive cases have occurred with methicillin, a drug which is rarely used today.

Electrolyte imbalances are not an uncommon side effect with parenteral penicillin therapy. Hypokalemia may occur, particularly with the disodium preparations of ticarcillin and carbenicillin. Most of the commercially available forms of injectable penicillins are manufactured as sodium salts. Attention to the amount of sodium being administered is important in patients with congestive heart failure, hypertension, and renal dysfunction. Central nervous system (CNS) toxicity, manifested as hallucinations, agitation, myoclonus, seizures, and coma, are most commonly associated with the combination of massive penicillin doses given parenterally and diminished renal function, resulting in drug accumulation within the CNS.

Indications and Use The penicillins can be divided into six distinct classes based on structure and function (Table 24-1). Within each class are numerous agents with slightly different pharmacokinetics, toxicities, and spectra of actions. The following discussion has been adopted from Wright and Wilkowske.[8]

Natural penicillins Aqueous penicillin G is the prototypic natural penicillin. Because it is degraded by gastric acid, its use as an oral agent is limited. As a parenteral agent, it is still the drug of choice for severe pneumococcal disease, including pneumonia, meningitis, and endocarditis. It remains a useful drug for the treatment of other streptococcal infections, including those due to enterococci, and is useful for the treatment of meningitis due to *Neisseria meningitidis* and *L. monocytogenes*. Penicillin G remains the agent of choice for infections due to various other organisms including those causing anaerobic infections of the head

Table 24-1 Classification of commonly used penicillins

Class	Commonly used agents	Major antibacterial spectrum of class
Natural	Penicillin G Penicillin V Benzathine penicillin G Procaine penicillin G	Streptococci, enterococci, β-lactamase negative staphylococci, *N. meningitidis*
Penicillinase resistant	Nafcillin Oxacillin Dicloxacillin	β-Lactamase-producing staphylococci
Aminopenicillins	Ampicillin Amoxicillin	Same as for natural penicillins plus some strains of *Haemophilus influenzae*, *E. coli*, and *Proteus*
Carboxypenicillins	Carbenicillin Ticarcillin	Same as for aminopenicillins plus *Pseudomonas aeruginosa*
Ureidopenicillins and piperazine penicillins	Piperacillin Mezlocillin Azlocillin	Same as carboxypenicillins plus *Klebsiella pneumoniae* and more strains of *P. aeruginosa*
Beta-lactamase inhibitor combinations	Amoxicillin and clavulanate Ampicillin and sulbactam Ticarcillin and clavulanate	β-Lactamase-producing strains of staphylococci, gram-negative bacilli, and *Bacteroides fragilis*

Source: Adapted from Ref. 8.

and neck, *Clostridium perfringens* and *C. tetani, Borrelia bergdorferi*, the agent of Lyme disease, and non-penicillinase-producing staphylococci. Penicillin V is similar to penicillin G but is acid stable and can be given orally. Other natural penicillins include benzathine penicillin and procaine penicillin, both of which are given by intramuscular injection. The former agent may persist in the body for up to 4 weeks. Its use now is principally for the treatment of syphilis. Procaine penicillin has been used for the treatment of gonorrhea. Because of the emergence of penicillinase-producing strains of *Neisseria gonorrheae*, this can no longer be recommended. Procaine penicillin is the most likely penicillin to cause allergic reactions.

Penicillinase-resistant penicillins These semisynthetic penicillins resist the breakdown of the beta-lactam ring by penicillinases. Their main use is in the treatment of infections due to penicillinase-producing staphylococci. While methicillin was the original agent in this group, it is almost never used today because of its association with renal toxicity. Oxacillin and nafcillin are currently the parenteral agents of choice. Dicloxacillin is the agent of choice for oral therapy. None of these agents have activity against methicillin-resistant staphylococci and should not be used to treat infections due to these organisms.

Aminopenicillins Ampicillin has a similar spectrum of activity against gram-positive organisms as penicillin but also has activity against a variety of aerobic gram-negative bacilli, including many strains of *E. coli, Proteus mirabilis, Salmonella, Shigella*, and *H. influenzae*. Unfortunately, many strains of the latter three organisms have developed resistance to ampicillin, and activity cannot be ensured without antimicrobial susceptibility testing. Further, ampicillin has no activity against *Klebsiella* species and *P. aeruginosa*. While ampicillin is stable in gastric acid and can be administered orally, the closely related compound amoxicillin is much more completely absorbed and should be used instead of oral ampicillin except for the treatment of shigellosis, where high fecal concentrations of antibiotic are required.

Carboxypenicillins Carbenicillin shares the antibacterial activity of ampicillin but has extended action against *P. aeruginosa* as well as some species of *Proteus* and *Enterobacter*. Like ampicillin, it has no activity against penicillinase-producing staphylococci or *Klebsiella* species. The dosages required to treat *P. aeruginosa* are higher than for other organisms, on the order of 24 g/day for the adult with normal renal function. These high doses in conjunction with a relatively high sodium content (4.7 meq/g) make carbenicillin a less desirable agent for patients with congestive heart failure or other conditions where sodium excess is a problem. Carbenicillin alone is acid labile, but indanyl carbenicillin is a form of the drug that is orally absorbable. However, it does not achieve serum levels capable of inhibiting many bacteria and is only recommended for the treatment of urinary tract infections.

Ticarcillin has an antimicrobial spectrum similar to carbenicillin but is more active against *P. aeruginosa.* Although it has a slightly higher sodium content than carbenicillin, sodium loading is less of a problem because lower doses can be given. Treatment of a serious pseudomonal infection in an adult with normal renal function usually requires 18 g/day. An aminoglycoside is usually combined with either carbenicillin or ticarcillin for the treatment of serious infections due to *P. aeruginosa* since this combination is synergistic in its antibacterial activity against this organism.

Ureidopenicillins and piperazine penicillins Three semisynthetic penicillins, mezlocillin, azlocillin, and piperacillin, belong to this category. These agents have an extended antimicrobial spectrum over carbenicillin and ticarcillin. In particular, they demonstrate increased activity against *P. aeruginosa* and *Klebsiella*. They also have reasonable activity against the anaerobe *B. fragilis*. The roles of these three agents in the treatment of infection is not yet fully established, but in addition to their increased antimicrobial activity when compared to carbenicillin and ticarcillin, they also contain less sodium and require less dosage adjustment in renal failure. Hence, they may offer an advantage over the carboxypenicillins.

Penicillin–beta-lactamase inhibitor combinations Two different beta-lactamase inhibitors, sodium sulbactam and potassium clavulanate, have been combined with penicillins in order to extend the antimicrobial activity of the latter agents by inactivating beta-lactamases produced by a variety of bacteria. One combination, Augmentin, consists of amoxicillin with clavulanate and has activity against beta-lactamase-producing *H. influenzae, Branhamella catarrhalis, Klebsiella, E. coli, B. fragilis*, staphylococci, and many other organisms. Similar antibacterial activity is achieved with Unasyn, a combination of ampicillin and sulbactam. Timentin, the combination of ticarcillin with clavulanate, extends the spectrum of ticarcillin in the same manner. No additional activity against *P. aeruginosa* is achieved by any of these agents since antibiotic resistance by this organism is not due to beta-lactamase production.

Cephalosporins

Cephalosporin antibiotics are all semisynthetic beta-lactam antibiotics. Since the introduction of cephalothin in 1962, numerous cephalosporins have been approved for use in this country. The "generational" concept of classification is widely used. While the term *generation* initially indicated the time the drug was introduced for use, it now conveys the approximate antibacterial spectrum of the agent. In general, first-generation cephalosporins were introduced from the 1960s through the 1970s and have excellent activity against methicillin-sensitive staphylococci, streptococci, and some gram-negative bacilli such as *E. coli, Proteus*, and *Klebsiella*. Second-generation cephalosporins were introduced in the late 1970s and early 1980s and have extended coverage against gram-negative bacilli but slightly less against gram-positive organisms. Finally, third-generation cephalosporins were introduced in the 1980s and have even more activity against gram-negative organisms, some even possessing activity against *P. aeruginosa* but having proportionally less activity against gram-positive bacteria. No cephalosporin of any generation has documented in vivo activity against enterococci, methicillin-resistant staphylococci, *Listeria*, or fungi. Finally, there are both overlaps and gaps in the generational classification system, and its use without a grasp of the specific activity and pharmacokinetics of any particular agent can lead to confusion and misuse.

In general, the cephalosporins differ from one another based on the side chains at R_1 and R_2. However, two agents traditionally classified as cephalosporins are, in fact, structurally distinct moieties. Cefoxitin is a cephamycin with an α-methoxy group at position 7 of the beta-lactam ring, while moxalactam has an oxygen molecule rather than a sulfur in the dihydrothiazine ring.

Pharmacokinetics and adverse reactions Most cephalosporins are excreted by the kidney, and decreases in renal function necessitate reduction in dosage. Exceptions to this are ceftriaxone and cefoperazone, which are hepatically excreted. Both agents are associated with an increased incidence of diarrhea.[9] Drugs with the methylthiotetrazole (MTT) ring at the R_2 position, such as moxalactam, cefamandole, cefoperazone, cefotetan, and cefmetazole, may be more likely to cause bleeding and disulfiram-like reactions. Moxalactam is the drug most frequently implicated in bleeding diatheses associated with the MTT side chain.[9,10]

All cephalosporins are associated with superinfection due to resistant organisms. Enterococcal and yeast infections have been most frequently reported.[6] This is more likely to occur with agents with the most antibacterial activity. In addition, the emergence of resistant organisms has been noted, principally due to the emergence of inducible, chromasomally mediated beta-lactamases.[10]

Although hypersensitivity reactions similar to those seen with the penicillins can be seen with the administration of cephalosporins, they are relatively uncommon. In patients with a history of a rash after the use of a penicillin agent, a cephalosporin can be safely given. However, if the penicillin reaction was anaphylaxis or otherwise severe, the use of cephalosporins should be avoided.[9]

Classification, antibacterial spectrum, and use

First-generation agents There are three first-generation parenteral cephalosporins available: Cephalothin, cephapirin, and cefazolin (Table 24-2). The latter has a significantly longer half-life than the others, allowing it to be given on an 8-h schedule. Moreover, it achieves higher and more sustained blood concentrations. Because of these facts, cefazolin is the preferred first-generation cephalosporin.[10] Cephalexin, cefadroxil, and cephradine are three orally available first-generation cephalosporins. Their activity is roughly equivalent to the parenteral agents, but they appear to have less activity against gram-negative bacilli. None of these agents should be used for the treatment of meningitis.

Table 24-2 Classification of commonly used parenteral cephalosporins, carbapenems, and monobactams

Generation or class	Commonly used agents	Major antibacterial spectrum of class
First	Cephalothin Cephapirin Cefazolin	Methicillin-sensitive staphylococci, nonenterococcal streptococci, *E. coli, Klebsiella* sp., some *Proteus* sp.
Second	Cefamandole	Similar to first generation, some activity against *H. influenzae* and gram-negative bacilli
	Cefuroxime	Same as first generation with increased activity *against H. influenzae* and gram-negative bacilli
	Cefoxitin Cefotetan	Similar to first generation, with activity against *B. fragilis* and some gram-negative bacilli
Third	Cefotaxime Ceftriaxone	Slightly less active against staphylococci but very active against nonenterococcal streptococci and aerobic gram-negative bacilli; not active against *P. aeruginosa*
	Ceftazidime	Poor activity against staphylococci but active against nonenterococcal streptococci and aerobic gram-negative streptococci and bacilli; very active against *P. aeruginosa*
Carbapenem	Imipenem-cilastatin	Active against most staphylococci, streptococci, and aerobic gram-negative bacilli
Monobactam	Aztreonam	Only active against aerobic gram-negative bacilli

Source: Adapted from Ref 9.

Second-generation agents Cefamandole was the first cephalosporin to be introduced in this category. It has increased activity over *H. influenzae* and some gram-negative bacilli when compared to first-generation agents. However, some strains of *H. influenzae* are relatively resistant. Cefonicid has a spectrum of activity similar to cefamandole but has a longer half-life. Intravenous cefuroxime has increased activity against *H. influenzae* and is effective in the treatment of meningitis, although other agents may be superior.[11] The oral form, cefuroxime axetil, is not well absorbed and should not be used for serious infections, particularly those due to *H. influenzae.*[12] All three of the second-generation agents are somewhat less active against susceptible staphylococci and streptococci compared to first-generation drugs.[9,10]

As mentioned, cefoxitin is not a cephalosporin but a cephamycin. It has a distinct antimicrobial spectrum in that it has activity against the majority of strains of *B. fragilis* as well as a variety of gram-negative bacilli. It is not useful for the treatment of infections due to *H. influenzae.* Cefotetan has a similar antimicrobial spectrum but has a considerably longer half-life. Neither are useful in the treatment of meningitis.[5,10] Cefmetazole is another cephamycin agent with pharmacokinetics and antimicrobial spectrum similar to cefoxitin.

Third-generation agents Agents in this category can be divided into those without and those with activity against *P. aeruginosa.* Cefotaxime, ceftriaxone, and moxalactam are representative of the first group. All are useful in the treatment of meningitis due to susceptible organisms. Cefotaxime and ceftriaxone are roughly equivalent in antimicrobial spectrum, but ceftriaxone has a considerably longer half-life. Both have activity against susceptible staphylococci and streptococci equal to the second-generation agents but are much more potent against a variety of nonpseudomonal gram-negative bacilli. Moxalactam has additional activity against *B. fragilis.* Because of numerous reports of bleeding complications, moxalactam is rarely used today.[5,9,10]

Ceftazidime is the major agent in the group of third-generation cephalosporins with antipseudomonal activity. It also provides coverage against a wide variety of gram-negative bacilli. It has limited activity against staphylococci but provides reasonable activity against nonenterococcal streptococci. It is useful for the treatment of meningitis against susceptible organisms. Recent evidence suggests that it may also be useful as a single agent for the empiric therapy of febrile, neutropenic patients.[13] Cefoperazone and cefsulodin are two other agents which possess antipseudomonal activity.[9]

Carbapenems and Monobactams

Imipenen-cilastatin Imipenem is the *N*-formimidoyl derivative of the naturally occurring compound thienamycin and possesses the broadest antimicrobial spectrum of any beta-lactam. It is also has a high degree of resistance to breakdown by beta-lactamases. Because imipenem is rapidly metabolized by the kidney, the commercially available form consists of a combination of imipenem and cilastatin sodium, the latter being a renal dipeptidase inhibitor.[14] Imipenem-cilastatin is strikingly active against gram-positive organisms, including most streptococci, penicillinase-producing staphylococci, and *Listeria.* However, methicillin-resistant staphylococci and one species of enterococci, *Streptococcus faecium,* are relatively resistant. Imipenem-cilastatin is also very active against a large variety of gram-negative aerobic bacilli, including *P. aeruginosa,* and also has significant activity against many anaerobes.[15]

Imipenem-cilastatin is not absorbed orally. It is well distributed in most tissues, including the cerebrospinal fluid (CSF), after intravenous administration. The serum half-life in persons with normal renal function is about 1 h, but this increases to 4 h in those with complete renal failure.[15] It is removed by hemodialysis.

The adverse effects reported for imipenem-cilastatin are similar to those seen with other beta-lactam antibiotics. These include gastrointestinal complaints, such as diarrhea, rashes, and other hypersensitivity reactions, and superinfections secondary to resistant organisms. A disturbing complication has been seizures and other CNS toxicity. Seizures appear to occur more frequently in the elderly and the severely ill. No tendency toward increased bleeding or renal abnormalities has been reported.[14,15]

The role of imipenem-cilastatin, particularly in the elderly, remains unclear. It clearly has a broad range of antimicrobial activity, making it potentially useful for the treatment of a great many infections. However, the employment of this agent should be tempered with its expense, the risks of superinfection and CNS toxicity, the emergence of resistant organisms, and the availability of more established, safe, and inexpensive alternatives.[6]

Aztreonam Aztreonam is the only available agent in a new class of beta-lactams, the monobactams. Aztreonam has a comparatively narrow spectrum of activity which is limited to the aerobic gram-negative bacilli, including *P. aeruginosa*. It has no activity against gram-positive bacteria or against anaerobes.[16]

Aztreonam is not orally absorbed but is widely distributed in the body after intravenous administration. Excretion is principally renal with a half-life of about 2 h in those with normal renal function. This increases to 8 h in complete renal failure. Hemodialysis and, to a lesser extent, peritoneal dialysis remove the drug.[16]

Aztreonam has relatively few adverse effects. A potentially important advantage is that is has minimal cross-reactivity with other beta-lactams in the beta-lactam allergic patient. Therefore, it may be used in those patients who have had significant beta-lactam hypersensitivity reactions who require antibiotic therapy for aerobic gram-negative bacilli. Aztreonam may also have a role in replacing aminoglycosides in the treatment of aerobic gram-negative bacillary infection in select patient populations.[16]

Vancomycin

Vancomycin, introduced in 1956, was initially used extensively because of its activity against penicillinase-producing staphylococci. However, it fell out of favor for the next two decades because of the availability of the penicillinase-resistant penicillins and because of reports of severe nephrotoxicity associated with the drug. With the emergence of methicillin-resistant staphylococci in the 1970s, vancomycin reemerged as a useful antimicrobial agent. Nephrotoxicity was rarely reported with a new highly purified formulation of the drug. Vancomycin is now an important weapon in the antimicrobial armamentarium against gram-positive bacteria.[17]

Vancomycin inhibits the formation of the peptidoglycan polymer of the bacterial cell wall at a different site than the beta-lactams. It has a narrow spectrum of action directed against gram-positive organisms including methicillin-sensitive and methicillin-resistant staphylococci, streptococci including enterococci, corynebacteria, and clostridia species. It has no activity against gram-negative bacteria.[5,18]

Vancomycin is poorly absorbed orally. The high concentrations reached in the gastrointestinal tract have made orally administered vancomycin a useful agent in the treatment of *Clostridium difficile*-associated diarrhea. After intravenous administration, it distributes widely into tissues. It enters the CSF in relatively low concentrations, and its efficacy in treating meningitis due to susceptible organisms is unproven. Vancomycin is cleared almost exclusively by the kidneys. Its half-life in those with normal renal function is 6 h, and the usual dosage is 500 mg to 1 g every 12 h. In renal failure the half-life increases to 7 days. Since it is not removed by hemodialysis or peritoneal dialysis, it may given once per week to patients with renal failure whether or not they are undergoing dialysis.[5,18] A nomogram has been developed for dosing in patients with lesser degrees of renal insufficiency.[19]

A peculiar adverse effect of vancomycin is the development of diffuse erythema and pruritus during intravenous infusion. This reaction is not a true hypersensitivity reaction to vancomycin and is thought to be due to the release of histamine through nonimmunologic mechanisms.[18] Slowing the infusion to over 60 min, giving the drug on a 6-h rather than a 12-h frequency, and pretreatment with antihistamines may ameliorate this side effect in those who develop it. Nephrotoxicity due to vancomycin appears to be uncommon and usually mild. Ototoxicity occurs, particularly when serum levels are greater than 30 μg/mL. Both of these adverse effects may be increased when vancomycin is combined with aminoglycosides.[5,18] Vancomycin should be used cautiously in the elderly, who may be more susceptible to both these adverse effects.

Aminoglycosides

Streptomycin, the first aminoglycoside, was introduced into clinical use more than 40 years ago. Since then, these agents have been a mainstay in the treatment of a variety of infections, particularly those due to aerobic gram-negative bacilli. However, their use has been challenged recently because of the availability of less toxic agents.

Structure and mechanism of action All aminoglycosides are aminocyclitols and consist of two or more cyclical amino sugars bound to a central hexose nucleus by a glycoside linkage.[20,21] The agents available for use in the United States can be divided into two groups. One group, all derived from the fungus *Streptomyces*, consists of streptomycin, kanamycin, neomycin, tobramycin, and amikacin. The latter is synthesized from kanamycin. The second group, derived from *Micromonospora*, is made up of gentamicin and netilmicin. In this section, only gentamicin, tobramycin, netilmicin, and amikacin are discussed.

All aminoglycosides act by binding to the 30S portion of the bacterial ribosome and halting protein synthesis. Since this binding is irreversible, aminoglycosides are capable of killing, rather than just inhibiting, bacteria. Because of their distinct mechanism of action, aminoglycosides can often be used in combination with antibiotics that act at other sites, such as the beta-lactams, to result in enhanced or synergistic bacterial killing. Penetration of aminoglycosides into bacteria requires oxygen-dependent transport. Because of this, aminoglycosides are only active against aerobic bacteria under aerobic conditions.[20,21]

Pharmacokinetics The pharmacokinetic properties of the aminoglycosides are shared by the different agents.[21] None are absorbed after oral administration. Parenteral administration can be performed either intravenously or intramuscularly. However, the preferred route is intravenous since intramuscular absorption may be erratic. The volume of distribution is equivalent to the extracellular fluid compartment, and penetration into the joints, pleural, pericardial, and peritoneal spaces is good. However, aminoglycosides do not enter the CNS or the eye appreciably after parenteral administration.[20]

The aminoglycosides are all excreted unchanged by the kidney. This leads to extremely high concentrations of active drug in the urine. The half-life of gentamicin, tobramycin, and netilmicin in persons with normal renal function is 2 h. For amikacin, it is closer to 3 h. The half-lives are increased proportionally with renal dysfunction. Hemodialysis and, to a lesser extent, peritoneal dialysis are capable of removing aminoglycosides. Because of predictable decreases in renal function with aging,[22] the aminoglycosides should be used with caution in the elderly.

Spectrum of activity The general antimicrobial range of activity is similar for gentamicin, tobramycin, amikacin, and netilmicin. All are broadly active against aerobic, gram-negative bacilli, including *Klebsiella, Salmonella,Shigella, Proteus, Enterobacter, Serratia,* and *P. aeruginosa.* They possess limited activity against gram-positive organisms, including *S. aureus* and many streptococci. A major use of aminoglycosides is in combination with other classes of antibiotics to achieve synergism, or increased activity, against certain organisms. Penicillin G or ampicillin plus gentamicin has been used to treat severe infections due to enterococcus and *Listeria.* Nafcillin or vancomycin plus an aminoglycoside may be useful in treating staphylococcal infections. Antipseudomonal beta-lactams plus aminoglycosides offer synergistic activity against *P. aeruginosa.*

The major mechanism by which bacteria develop resistance to the aminoglycosides is the production of a variety of enzymes, including a phosphotransferase, a nucleotidyltransferase and several acetyltransferases, which break down the aminocyclitol linkages. Amikacin and netilmicin are least likely to be affected by this.[20,21] Much less common mechanisms of drug resistance include defective membrane binding sites and nonpermeable cell walls.[20]

Adverse reactions Unfortunately, the aminoglycosides are inherently toxic agents. Currently, any modification of the aminoglycoside molecule to reduce toxicity would also reduce antibacterial activity.[20] By far the major and important toxic effects involve the kidney and the hearing and vestibular system. Less common adverse effects include neuromuscular blockade, encephalopathy, rashes, and nausea and vomiting.

Aminoglycoside-related nephrotoxicity is secondary to damage to proximal tubule cells, resulting in loss of microvillae, organelle disruption, and cellular necrosis.[23] Early toxicity may be manifested by urinary tubular casts or an increase in urinary β_2 microglobulin. However, these findings are too nonspecific to be of use in predicting the development of clinical renal dysfunction. As toxicity progresses, nonoliguric and eventually oliguric renal failure may occur. The precise incidence of renal dysfunction secondary to aminoglycosides is not known but has been reported as between 10 and 25 percent.[24] One factor associated with nephrotoxicity secondary to aminoglycosides is increasing age, possibly because of already reduced renal function.[22] Others include preexisting renal disease, volume depletion, debilitated state,[20] and the concomitant use of other nephrotoxic agents. Renal failure resulting from aminoglycosides is usually but not always reversible. Nephrotoxicity appears to be most likely when trough serum levels are elevated above 2 μg/mL for gentamicin, tobramycin, and netilmicin and above 10 μg/mL for amikacin for prolonged periods.[20]

Ototoxicity due to aminoglycosides is manifested as either auditory or vestibular dysfunction or both. Symptoms may begin as tinnitus or a feeling of ear fullness. Vestibular toxicity is usually manifested as dizziness, vertigo, or nausea. Toxicity appears to be secondary to irreversible damage to the otic hair cells.[23] The incidence appears to be far less than the incidence of nephrotoxicity but is probably underappreciated. Ototoxicity is most related to sustained peak serum levels greater than 12 μg/mL for gentamicin, tobramycin, and netilmicin and above 35 μg/mL for amikacin.[20] Concomitant use of other ototoxic agents, such as vancomycin, may increase the risk. The elderly, because of underlying loss of auditory function, are at particular risk for this complication. Patients with end-stage renal disease are also at risk because of the increased use of aminoglycosides and less compulsive serum level monitoring in this group.

Clinical indications The indications for aminoglycosides, particularly in the elderly, is changing. Because of their predictable activity against a broad range of aerobic gram-negative bacilli, they still remain useful agents for the empiric treatment of certain infections. However, for other infections, aminoglycosides have been supplanted by the newer, broad-spectrum beta-lactams.

Aminoglycosides remain appropriate agents for the treatment of presumed gram-negative bacillary sepsis, particularly when acquired in the hospital, as combination therapy for peritonitis due to bowel perforation and other intra-abdominal catastrophes, and for the therapy of severe urinary tract infections. Because of their diminished activity under anaerobic and acidic conditions, they are less useful for the treatment of pneumonia, abscesses, and other closed-space infections, even when due to susceptible organisms. Finally, systemic aminoglycosides should never be used as the sole therapy for meningitis or intraocular infections.

There are differences between the available aminoglycosides with regard to antimicrobial spectrum of activity and toxicity, but these are not great. In general, amikacin is the least susceptible to breakdown by bacterial enzymes. However, gentamicin and tobramycin are reasonable choices for empiric therapy if the susceptibility pattern of the hospital or clinic does not indicate a high level of bacterial resistance to these agents. In general, tobramycin has slightly greater activity against *P. aeruginosa* while gentamicin is more active against *Serratia* and offers increased synergism against enterococci.

Dosing and serum level monitoring Regardless of renal function, a loading dose of drug should be given for all aminoglycosides. For gentamicin, tobramycin, and netilmicin, this is 2 to 2.5 mg/kg of lean body weight. For amikacin it is 7.5 mg/kg. For those with normal renal function, dosing of gentamicin, tobramycin, and netilmicin is 1 to 1.7 mg/kg every 8 h. However, there is recent enthusiasm for administering these agents every 12 to 24 h in an attempt to reduce toxicity.[25] For amikacin, dosing is 7.5 mg/kg every 12 h. For patients with various degrees of renal insufficiency, lower doses of all the aminoglycosides should be given. This is based on estimating the creatinine clearance using the Cockcroft-Gault equation[4,20]:

$$\text{Calculated creatinine clearance (mg/100 mL)} = \frac{(140 - \text{age in years}) \times \text{weight in kg}}{72 \times \text{serum creatinine (mg/100 mL)}}$$

For females, the value obtained should be further multiplied by 0.85 to obtain the creatinine clearance. If the serum creatinine is below 1.0 mg/100 mL, it should be assumed to be equal to 1.0. The estimated creatinine clearance is then used as a percentage and multiplied by the interval dose.[20] An alternative approach is to use a nomogram which relates the creatinine clearance to an elimination constant for the drug.[26]

Since serum levels are correlated with otoxicity and nephrotoxicity of the aminoglycosides as well as with therapeutic outcome, levels should be monitored early in the course of therapy, usually after the first three to five doses. It is wise to obtain subsequent levels at weekly intervals. Based on the results, adjustment in the dosing should be made to keep levels in the nontoxic, therapeutic range and follow-up levels obtained. Peak levels should be drawn within 30 min of the end of an intravenous infusion or 1 h after an intramuscular dose. Trough levels should be obtained just prior to the next dose.

Dosing during dialysis requires further adjustment. For hemodialysis, a 1-mg/kg dose of gentamicin, tobramycin, or netilmicin and a 3.75-mg/kg dose of amikacin should be given after dialysis. Dosing in-between dialysis should be as for complete renal failure. For peritoneal dialysis, the drug can be added to the dialysate fluid to reach desired serum levels. For gentamicin, tobramycin, and netilmicin, this would be 8 to 10 mg for every 2-L bag of dialysate, while for amikacin, 40 to 60 mg for each 2 L.[20] Serum levels should be carefully monitored.

Quinolones

Mechanism of action and pharmacology Nalidixic acid, introduced in 1963, is the forerunner of all quinolones. It has never been a widely used antimicrobial because bacteria rapidly develop resistance to it. However, the addition of a 7-piperazine and a 6-fluorine to the nalidixic acid molecule results in the fluorinated piperazinyl quinolones, which are potent, broad-spectrum antibiotics.[27] All quinolones inhibit DNA gyrase, an essential bacterial enzyme which is required for DNA replication, transcription, and repair.[28] It is assumed that the bactericidal activity of the fluorinated quinolones is related to gyrase inhibition.[29] Bacterial resistance to the fluorinated quinolones occurs but at a relatively low rate.[28-30] Moreover, quinolones do not appear susceptible to plasmid-mediated resistance factors as are the beta-lactams.[28,29]

The fluorinated quinolones have several pharmacologic properties that make them attractive as antimicrobial agents. They are generally well absorbed from the gastrointestinal tract and have a wide volume of distribution and a relatively long serum half-life allowing twice-a-day dosing in patients with normal renal function.[31] As well, they achieve high concentrations within monocytes and polymorphonuclear leukocytes, making them useful for the therapy of infections involving intracellular organisms. The major route of excretion is the kidneys, and the serum half-lives of all the agents are increased significantly in renal failure. Because there is some liver metabolism, increased serum levels may also occur in patients with severe hepatic dysfunction.[32]

Adverse effects and drug interactions The quinolones are well tolerated. Less than 5 percent of patients complain of gastrointestinal discomfort, including nausea, vomiting, and abdominal pain. Antibiotic-associated diarrhea associated with *C. difficile* has been reported.[30,31] Quinolones are not recommended for children or pregnant women because of the potential for cartilage damage in the young.[31,32] This is not an issue in the elderly. However, rare instances of seizures and CNS toxicity have been reported, particularly in the elderly.[32]

Absorption of the quinolones may be decreased by antacids containing magnesium, aluminum, or calcium.[31] The metabolism of theophylline and warfarin may be decreased by the quinolones, potentially leading to toxic levels of these drugs. This effect may be greater with ciprofloxacin than with other currently available quinolones.

With the recent reports of servere toxicity associated with temafloxacin therapy in the elderly, quinolones should be used cautiously in these patients, with close monitoring of renal and hepatic function.

Spectrum of activity Currently three fluoroquinolones, norfloxacin, ciprofloxacin, and ofloxacin, are approved for use in the United States.[31] All these agents have antibacterial activity against a wide range of gram-negative bacilli, including *P. aeruginosa*. In addition, they have good activity against both methicillin-sensitive and methicillin-resistant staphylococci but have less activity against streptococci, including enterococci. They have little or no activity against anaerobes, including *B. fragilis* and *C. difficile.*[31,32] Of the available agents, ciprofloxacin is the most potent.

Clinical indications All three available fluoroquinolone antibiotics are useful in the treatment of urinary tract infections, bacterial gastroenteritis not due to *C. difficile,* and gonococcal urethritis.[32] They may also have efficacy in the therapy of bacterial prostatitis. Norfloxacin and ciprofloxacin have also been used to prevent bacterial infection in neutropenic patients.[33,34] Ciprofloxacin has been useful in the treatment of osteomyelitis, malignant external otitis, pneumonia due to susceptible organisms, and skin and soft-tissue infections. Although bacterial meningitis has been successfully treated with ciprofloxacin, too little experience exists to advocate the use of the available fluoroquinolones for this indication. In contrast to norfloxacin and ciprofloxacin, ofloxacin may be useful for the treatment of chlamydial infections.[31]

The quinolones have already enjoyed extensive utilization since their introduction. However, the precise indications for these agents are still not fully defined, and caution should be exercised in their use until more clinical experience is gained. It is clear that norfloxacin should be limited to the treatment of urinary tract infections and bacterial gastroenteritis. Ciprofloxacin has broader applications. However, there are little data comparing the efficacy of ciprofloxacin to other agents. One application where it may be superior to conventional therapy is for the oral therapy of bacterial osteomyelitis, particularly that due to *P. aeruginosa.* The role of ofloxacin remains to be established.

Erythromycin

Erythromycin was introduced for clinical use in 1952. It is a macrolide antibiotic which consists of a 14-membered macrocyclic lactone ring attached to two sugar moieties. There are currently four oral preparations and two formulations for intravenous administration. The drug should not be given intramuscularly.[35]

Mechanism of action and antimicrobial spectrum Erythromycin binds to the 50S subunit of the 70S ribosome of susceptible microorganisms, resulting in inhibition of protein synthesis.[36] Erythromycin is active against many gram-positive and gram-negative bacteria, with notable activity against *S. pneumoniae,* group A beta-hemolytic streptococci, *Legionella, Mycoplasma pneumoniae, Campylobacter jejuni, Bordetella pertussis*, chlamydia, rickettsia, and many strains of nontuberculous mycobacteria. Isolates of *S. aureus* are generally susceptible, but resistant strains are not uncommon. While some anaerobic organisms are susceptible to erythromycin, *B. fragilis* is usually resistant.[35-37]

Antimicrobial resistance to erythromycin is being increasingly reported and is particularly problematic with staphylococci and streptococci.[35,36] It appears to be due to demethylation of specific adenine residues of ribosomal ribonucleic acid.[36] Initially susceptible staphylococci may develop resistance to erythromycin during therapy and cross-resistance to other related compounds, such as clindamycin, may occur.[35,36]

Clinical pharmacology The four oral preparations, erythromycin base, erythromycin stearate, erythromycin estolate, and erythromycin ethylsuccinate, are all relatively well absorbed from the gastrointestinal tract. The base, stearate, and ethyl succinate formulations are better and more completely absorbed in the fasting state, while absorption of the estolate form is not as affected by food. However, no one form of oral erythromycin appears superior to another with regard to blood levels of erythromycin.[35] Higher blood levels than those achieved with oral preparations can be obtained with the intravenous administration of either erythromycin lactobionate or erythromycin gluceptate.

Erythromycin penetrates into most tissues, including the prostate. However, it does not enter the CSF or brain in any appreciable amount.[35,37] Erythromycin is concentrated and excreted by the liver, which results in high bile and stool concentrations. Less than 5 to 15 percent of the total amount of drug is excreted by the kidneys. Although the serum half-life is prolonged from about 2 h in normal renal function to approximately 5 h in anuria, no dosage adjustment is necessary for renal failure. Erythromycin is not removed by hemodialysis or peritoneal dialysis.[35]

Adverse effects and drug interactions Erythromycin is generally considered to be a very safe agent. By far, the most common side effect is gastrointestinal distress, usually nausea, vomiting, and diarrhea, which can occur with either intravenous or oral doses. This may be related to its ability to increase the propulsive motor activity in the stomach and small bowel, acting as a motilin agonist.[38] Thrombophlebitis is common with intravenous infusion but can be reduced by diluting the drug and avoiding rapid infusion. Less common adverse reactions include cholestatic hepatitis, which occurs most frequently with erythromycin estolate, and sensorineural hearing loss. The latter may occur with both oral and intravenous erythromycin[35,39] but usually occurs when high doses are given, particularly in patients with reduced hepatic or renal function. As with many other antibiotics, *C. difficile*-associated diarrhea has been reported to occur after erythromycin use.

Erythromycin has numerous drug interactions through its ability to inhibit the hepatic cytochrome P-450 system. Theophylline, warfarin, methylprednisolone, carbamazepine, and cyclosporine levels[40] may all be increased in those concurrently taking erythromycin because of inhibition of metabolism of these agents by the liver.

Clinical indications Because of its activity against *S. pneumoniae* and other streptococci, *Mycoplasma,* and *Legionella*, the major indication for the use of erythromycin is in the treatment of community-acquired pneumonia. While oral formulations are adequate in most cases, intravenous erythromycin in doses up to 1 g every 6 h is often required for the treatment of serious infections due to *Legionella.*

Erythromycin is still useful for the therapy of minor infections due to staphylococci and streptococci, particularly in the penicillin-allergic patient. However, because of the development of resistance during therapy, other agents should be considered for the treatment of serious infections due to these organisms. Erythromycin is also valuable for the treatment of a variety of other conditions, including gastroenteritis due to *C. jejuni*, chlamydial infections, and erythrasma, a superficial cutaneous infection due to *Corynebacterium minutissimum.*[35]

Trimethoprim-Sulfamethoxazole

Introduced in 1968, trimethoprim-sulfamethoxazole consists of a fixed combination of the diaminopyrimidine trimethoprim and the sulfonamide sulfamethoxazole. Trimethoprim-sulfamethoxazole represents one of the few examples of an effective combination antimicrobial available for clinical use.[41]

Mechanism of action Trimethoprim-sulfamethoxazole was specifically developed to provide sequential and synergistic inhibition of folate metabolism by susceptible microorganisms.[42] Sulfonamides, including sulfamethoxazole, block the synthesis of dihydrofolic acid from *para*-aminobenzoic acid and pteridine by the enzyme tetrahydropteroic acid synthetase. Trimethoprim acts at a subsequent step to inhibit the reduction of dihydrofolic acid to tetrahydrofolic acid by the enzyme dihydrofolate reductase. The result is a marked decrease in microbial DNA

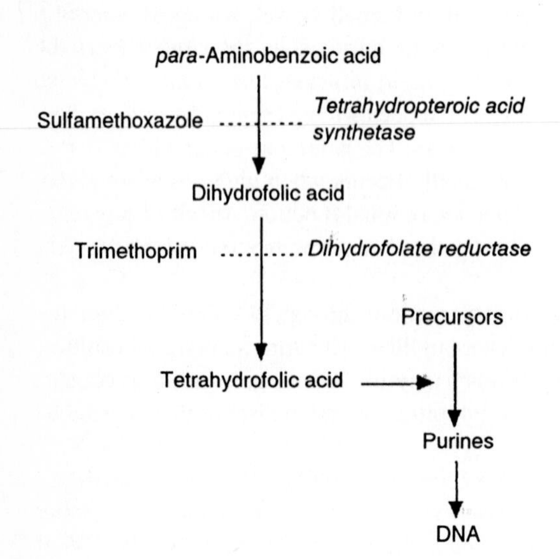

Figure 24-2 Mechanism of action of trimethoprim-sulfamethoxazole.

synthesis (Fig. 24-2). Because mammals are not able to synthesize folic acid and because trimethoprim is 50,000 times more active against bacterial than mammalian dihydrofolate reductase, a high therapeutic-to-toxic ratio is achieved.[42]

Spectrum of activity Trimethoprim-sulfamethoxazole has a broad range of activity for a wide variety of organisms. It possesses high activity against *H. influenzae*, including beta-lactamase-producing strains, and many strains of *E. coli, Klebsiella, Shigella,* and *Salmonella*. It is less predictably active against strains of *Serratia, Proteus,* and *Providencia*. It has no activity against *P. aeruginosa* and very little activity against anaerobic organisms. Many gram-positive organisms are susceptible, including *S. pneumoniae* and *Streptococcus pyogenes, S. aureus*, and *L. monocytogenes*. Enterococci are not routinely susceptible. Trimethoprim-sulfamethoxazole also is active against *Nocardia*, some strains of nontuberculous mycobacteria, and *Pneumocystis carinii*.[41-43]

The critical determinant for the antimicrobial activity of trimethoprim-sulfamethoxazole appears to reside in trimethoprim.[42,43] There are several mechanisms by which organisms express trimethoprim resistance. Some are intrinsically resistant, while others are able to acquire resistance through transferable factors. Emergence of high-level trimethoprim resistance has already been observed in *E. coli* isolated from the stools of individuals treated with trimethoprim-sulfamethoxazole.[44]

Pharmacokinetics Trimethoprim-sulfamethoxazole is supplied as a fixed combination of one part trimethoprim to five parts sulfamethoxazole. This results in a steady-state serum concentration ratio of 1 : 20, which is optimal for antimicrobial activity. Both trimethoprim and sulfamethoxazole are well absorbed from the gastrointestinal tract with peak serum levels of trimethoprim occurring about 1 h after ingestion and about 4 h after ingestion for sulfamethoxazole.[41] Trimethoprim-sulfamethoxazole is supplied for oral use as either single strength, containing 80 mg of trimethoprim and 400 mg of sulfamethoxazole, or double strength, containing 160 mg of trimethoprim and 800 mg of sulfamethoxazole. It is also supplied in an intravenous formulation.

Trimethoprim-sulfamethoxazole reaches therapeutic concentrations in a wide range of tissues. In general, trimethoprim is more widely distributed throughout the body than sulfamethoxazole. Because of this unequal distribution, there is variation in the concentration ratios of the two drugs in various tissues. However, the synergistic activity of the combination is probably still preserved.[42,43]

In patients with normal renal function, the serum half-life of trimethoprim is approximately 11 h, and that of sulfamethoxazole is 9 h. A typical dose of oral trimethoprim-sulfamethoxazole is one single-strength or double-strength tablet every 12 h. Intravenous trimethoprim-sulfamethoxazole dosing is usually based on the dosage of trimethoprim. For most bacterial infections, this is 6 mg/kg/day in two divided doses.[45] The half-life of both agents is increased in renal failure. When the creatinine clearance is less than 30 mL/min, a reasonable approach is to reduce the dose by one-half to one-third of normal after loading with a single, full dose.[42] Because the half-life of sulfamethoxazole is so greatly increased in complete renal failure, it is advised that trimethoprim-sulfamethoxazole either not be used when the creatinine clearance is less than 15 mL/min or that serum sulfamethoxazole levels be obtained to guide dosing in this circumstance.[45] For patients on hemodialysis, normal loading doses may be given after each dialysis with intervening doses administered based on serum sulfamethoxazole drug levels,[41] aiming for levels below 120 μg/mL. The use of trimethoprim-sulfamethoxazole in patients on peritoneal dialysis is not established.[46]

Adverse effects and drug interactions Serious adverse reactions to trimethoprim-sulfamethoxazole are relatively uncommon.[41,42] The most common involve gastrointestinal symptoms, including nausea, vomiting, abdominal cramps and diarrhea, cutaneous reactions, and hematologic toxicity. These appear to occur in 3 percent or less of patients treated.[41-43]

The most concerning adverse reactions are hematologic, including megaloblastic anemia, hemolytic anemia, neutropenia, and thrombocytopenia. These are more likely to occur in those with diminished folate stores and in those with conditions leading to depressed bone marrow function, such as renal transplant recipients receiving azathioprine.[47] Acute megaloblastic anemia has been reported after administration of high doses of trimethoprim-sulfamethoxazole intravenously.[48] In addition, there have been several reports of liver toxicity, principally occurring as intrahepatic cholestasis,[49,50] and at least one report of fatal hepatic failure due to trimethoprim-sulfamethoxazole.[51] Trimethoprim-sulfamethoxazole should be used with care in patients with severe renal dysfunction, as it may induce crystalluria.[41] The incidence of adverse reactions to trimethoprim-sulfamethoxazole is markedly increased in patients infected with the human immunodeficiency virus (HIV). The reasons for this are unclear, but the drug should be used cautiously in these patients.

Trimethoprim-sulfamethoxazole may interact with several medications. O'Reilly has shown that it enhances the effect of warfarin[52] through a stereoselective mechanism which results in an increase in the plasma levels of S-warfarin.[53] It may also potentiate the activity of phenytoin, tolbutamide, and chlorpropamide.[41]

Clinical indications Trimethoprim-sulfamethoxazole has a variety of clinical uses. It has been used successfully in the treatment of genitourinary tract infections, including cystitis, pyelonephritis, and acute bacterial epididymitis and prostatitis. It is also useful in the treatment of gastrointestinal infections due to susceptible strains of *Shigella* and for the therapy of traveler's diarrhea. However, the increasing prevalence of trimethoprim resistance may limit its usefulness for these infections in the future. It also possesses efficacy for the treatment of acute bronchitis and pneumonia due to susceptible organisms.

Trimethoprim-sulfamethoxazole is useful in the therapy of several miscellaneous infections. It is one of the preferred agents to treat *P. carinii* pneumonia in immunocompromised patients, including those infected with HIV. However, the dosage given is much higher than for bacterial infection, 20 mg/kg of trimethoprim per day given in four divided doses. Trimethoprim-sulfamethoxazole has been used for the therapy of infections due to *Nocardia* species and for meningitis due to *L. monocytogenes* in penicillin-allergic patients. It may have efficacy in the treatment of some infections due to *Legionella.*[54] Like norfloxacin and ciprofloxacin, trimethoprim-sulfamethoxazole has been reported to reduce the incidence of infection in patients with profound granulocytopenia. However, because it may prolong bone marrow recovery due to its antifolate effect, it should be used cautiously in such patients.

Agents Active against Mycobacteria

Tuberculosis remains a significant problem among the elderly. Fortunately, current therapy is effective and relatively nontoxic. However, treatment modalities have evolved rapidly during the last decade, both because of the introduction of new agents and because of new regimens employing shorter courses of therapy. The discussion below will be limited to the treatment of tuberculosis and will focus on four agents: isoniazid, rifampin, ethambutol, and pyrazinamide (Table 24-3).

Isoniazid Isoniazid or isonicotinic acid hydrazide (INH) was discovered and introduced as an antituberculous agent in the early 1950s. Its precise mechanism of action is not known, but it is highly active against most strains of *M. tuberculosis.*

Table 24-3 Recommendations for the most commonly used agents for the treatment of tuberculosis

Drug	Daily dose/body weight	Maximum daily dose	Twice weekly dose	Major adverse reactions
Isoniazid	5 mg/kg orally or intramuscularly	300 mg	15 mg/kg (900 mg maximum)	Hepatitis, peripheral neuropathy, hypersensitivity reactions
Rifampin	10 mg/kg orally	600 mg	10 mg/kg (600 mg maximum)	Orange discoloration of secretions, nausea, hepatitis, flulike syndrome, thrombocytopenia
Pyrazinamide	15–30 mg/kg orally	2 g	—	Hepatitis
Ethambutol	15–25 mg/kg orally	2.5 g	—	Optic neuritis

Source: Adapted from Ref. 55.

Resistance to isoniazid has been increasing over the last two decades and is particularly prevalent in southeast Asia, Africa, and Latin America. Fortunately, this is not yet a major problem in the United States.[55]

Isoniazid is well absorbed from the gastrointestinal tract and reaches peak serum levels within 2 h after ingestion. It is widely distributed through the body, including the CSF.[56] Hepatic acetylation followed by renal excretion is the major route of elimination. Individuals can be phenotyped into slow and rapid acetylators, the latter being more common among Eskimo and Oriental populations.[56]

The major toxicity of isoniazid is hepatotoxicity. Elevation of serum transaminases to less than two or three times normal occurs in 10 percent or more of all individuals taking isoniazid. Frank hepatitis with markedly elevated serum transaminases is much less common, occurring in less than 1 percent of all those treated and usually within the first 12 weeks of therapy.[57] Because mildly elevated liver function tests are common with isoniazid therapy and clinical hepatitis is rare, patients should be monitored for evidence of clinical hepatitis monthly for the first few months and then less frequently. Liver function tests can also be obtained at these times, but most clinicians would not discontinue therapy unless serum transaminases were greater than three to five times normal.[56]

Several factors have been associated with an increased risk of hepatitis due to isoniazid. One study by the U.S. Department of Public Health indicated that hepatotoxicity increases markedly at ages above 50 years, suggesting that isoniazid should be used with extreme caution in the elderly.[56] However, recent experiences by Stead[58] indicate that isoniazid may be given safely in the aged. Individuals who are rapid acetylators of isoniazid may also be at increased risk of developing hepatitis, possibly due to the production of a toxic metabolite, acetylhydrazine.[59] Daily doses compared to intermittent doses may also be associated with increased hepatic injury.[56] Finally, the use of alcohol may also increase hepatotoxicity due to isoniazid. Patients should be instructed to avoid consumption of large amounts of alcohol while on therapy.

Peripheral neuropathy due to increased metabolism of pyridoxine or vitamin B_6 may occur in some patients, particularly those with diabetes, uremia, alcoholism, and malnutrition, who are also taking isoniazid. These patients should be given daily pyridoxine supplementation. Rarely, isoniazid is associated with hypersensitivity reactions, including rash, urticaria, and fever.[56]

Isoniazid may interact with other medications. It decreases the metabolism of phenytoin and carbamazepine, resulting in higher and potentially toxic levels of both agents. In addition, carbamazepine may potentiate isoniazid-associated hepatotoxicity by inducing the production of acetylhydrazine. In addition, serum levels of ketoconazole may be reduced by the concomitant use of isoniazid,[45] and the therapeutic effect of isoniazid and rifampin may be decreased by ketoconazole.[60]

Rifampin Rifampin acts by inhibiting mycobacterial DNA-dependent RNA polymerase and is very active against *M. tuberculosis* as well as a variety of other microorganisms. However, it should never be used alone for the treatment of tuberculosis. It is well absorbed after oral ingestion and has a wide volume of distribution, including the CSF. It is excreted in both the urine and the bile. In general, rifampin is well tolerated, and adverse effects occur in less than 2 percent of individuals.[56] Rifampin predictably causes an orange discoloration of saliva, urine, and other body secretions, and patients should be warned about this. Intermittent therapy has been associated with a variety of adverse effects, including thrombocytopenia, neutropenia, and an influenzalike syndrome. Clinical hepatitis occurs in about 1 percent of all those treated with rifampin, and this is slightly increased in those also taking isoniazid.[45] Rifampin may increase the metabolism of several medications and reduce their effectiveness. These include corticosteroids, warfarin, digoxin, oral hypoglycemic agents, ketoconazole, and cyclosporine.[55,56]

Pyrazinamide Pyrazinamide was once abandoned as a first-line agent for the treatment of tuberculosis because of unacceptable hepatic toxicity. However, it has had a resurgence in use since the employment of lower, less toxic doses. It is well absorbed orally, and its major route of excretion is by glomerular filtration.[56] Its major toxicity remains liver injury, occurring in 1 to 5 percent of patients treated with the currently recommended doses of 15 to 30 mg/kg/day.[55,56]

Ethambutol Ethambutol has enjoyed less use for the treatment of tuberculosis since the introduction of rifampin. Its precise mechanism of action against *M. tuberculosis* is unknown. Because it inhibits but does not kill *M. tuberculosis,* its main function is as a companion drug to other agents to retard the development of drug resistance. Ethambutol is well absorbed after oral ingestion, and approximately half is excreted unchanged in the urine. Its major adverse effect is ocular toxicity, presenting as blurry vision, red-green color blindness, or central scotomata. This occurs in less than 1 percent of patients treated with 15 mg/kg/day.[55] However, all patients receiving ethambutol should be instructed to report a change in vision during therapy. The major current indication for the use of ethambutol is as an additional agent when isoniazid resistance is suspected.[55]

Indications for antituberculous therapy There are two major indications for the use of chemotherapy for tuberculosis. The first is for preventive therapy. Preventive therapy should be considered for household contacts or any others in close association with an individual with active tuberculosis. Preventive therapy should also be considered for anyone with evidence of prior infection with *M. tuberculosis.* Groups at particular risk for reactivation of previously acquired infection include those with recent skin test conversions, those with positive skin tests and chest radiographs indicative of previous tuberculosis without evidence of active disease, and those with underlying conditions which increase the chance of reactivation. These conditions include diabetes mellitus, underlying immunosuppressive conditions, including infection with HIV, prolonged treatment with corticosteroids, lymphoreticular malignancies, and end-stage renal disease. Preventive therapy consists of isoniazid 300 mg/day for at least 6 and no more than 12 months.[55]

The second indication for the therapy of tuberculosis is to treat active disease, usually defined as the identification or isolation of *M. tuberculosis* from a clinical specimen. Two major regimens currently exist for the treatment of active tuberculosis. The first is a combination of isoniazid and rifampin for a total of 9 months. Drugs may be given daily for this period or, after daily administration for the first 2 months, they may be administered twice weekly. A second regimen consists of a total of 6 months of therapy. For the first 2 months, isoniazid, rifampin, and pyrazinamide are given daily. For the remaining 4 months, daily or twice weekly isoniazid and rifampin is given as in the 9-month regimen. A recent trial of this regimen in the United States indicated that it was successful and relatively nontoxic.[61] More detailed discussions of the treatment of tuberculosis can be found elsewhere.[55,56]

Treatment of Viral Infections (Table 24-4)

Influenza and herpesvirus infections are the two most common viral infections which affect the elderly. Although these infections have been difficult to treat in the past and remain problematic even now, there have been recent advances in therapy which make intervention more successful than in the past.

Influenza There are more than 10,000 excess deaths each year in the United States due to influenza, and nearly 90 percent of these deaths are in patients over 65 years of age.[62] Hence, influenza is a major health risk among the aged. Currently, there are two methods available for the prevention of influenza, immunization and prophylaxis with amantadine.

Immunization While not a pharmacologic agent, immunization is of major importance in the prevention of influenza. The influenza vaccine is made from highly purified, egg-grown viruses that have been inactivated and are therefore not infectious. Each year's vaccine usually contains three viral strains felt to be most likely to cause disease in the United States in the upcoming winter. Generally, two strains of influenza A and one strain of influenza B are included. The vaccine can be prepared as "split," or chemically treated to reduce pyrogenicity, or "whole." Either preparation may be used in the adult.[63]

The only major contraindication to giving the influenza vaccine is anaphylactic hypersensitivity to eggs. The most common adverse effect of influenza immunization is local redness or soreness, which may occur in up to one-third of recipients. Occasionally, fever, malaise, and myalgias occur, suggesting to the patient the onset of influenza. These symptoms usually dissipate after 1 or 2 days. It is recommended that patients with febrile illnesses have their immunization postponed until the symptoms abate. The Guillain-Barré syndrome, occurring in

Table 24-4 Use and dosage recommendations for amantadine and acyclovir

Infection	Indication	Drug	Dosage	Route
Influenza A	Prevention	Amantadine	100 mg once daily[a,b]	Oral
	Treatment	Amantadine	100 mg once daily[a,b,c]	Oral
Herpes zoster	Localized	Acyclovir	800 mg five times daily[a,c]	Oral
	Disseminated	Acyclovir	10–15 mg/kg every 8 h[a]	Intravenous
Herpes simplex	Prevention	Acyclovir	200 mg two to three times daily[a]	Oral
	Treatment, mild cutaneous disease	Acyclovir	200 mg five times daily[a]	Oral
	Treatment, severe cutaneous disease	Acyclovir	5 mg/kg every 8 h[a]	Intravenous
	Treatment, encephalitis	Acyclovir	10 mg/kg every 8 h[a]	Intravenous

[a]Dosage reduction necessary for renal dysfunction.
[b]Dosage for those 65 years and older.
[c]Should be started within 72 h of signs and symptoms.
Source: Adapted from Refs. 65, 66, 72.

association with the swine flu vaccine of 1976, has not been associated with subsequent influenza immunization products.

All persons over 65 years of age and those living in nursing homes or other chronic care facilities should be vaccinated. Although the elderly may not develop postimmunization serum antibody titers as high as those in younger age groups, the vaccine has been shown to be effective in preventing complications of illness associated with influenza in this group of patients. Health care workers in these facilities should also be vaccinated to prevent spread of the infection. Immunization should be done in the late fall to allow time for neutralizing antibodies to develop before the peak epidemic period, usually beginning in December.[62]

Amantadine and rimantadine Amantadine has efficacy approximately equal to influenza immunization in preventing influenza A-related disease. However, it has no efficacy against influenza B, which accounts for 20 percent of all cases of influenza. A related compound, rimantadine, has antiviral activity similar to amantadine but is yet not approved for use in the United States.[62,63]

Both amantadine and rimantadine appear to act by blocking the uncoating of viral RNA within host cells. Amantadine is well absorbed after oral ingestion. In healthy young adults, 100 mg of amantadine twice daily results in therapeutic peak plasma concentrations of 0.5 to 0.8 μg/mL. In persons over 65 years of age this same level is reached with just half of this dosage. Amantadine is excreted unchanged in the urine, and plasma half-life is increased in those with renal dysfunction. Only a small amount is removed by dialysis. Rimantadine differs from amantadine in that it has a larger volume of distribution and a longer plasma half-life and its pharmacokinetics are not significantly altered by liver or renal disease.[62]

The most common adverse effects of amantadine are gastrointestinal upset and CNS toxicity, manifesting as increased nervousness, lightheadedness, difficulty concentrating, insomnia, and impaired psychomotor performance. The CNS effects are related to elevated serum levels and are more likely to occur in the elderly and in those taking antihistamines and anticholinergic drugs. Rimantadine has the same incidence of gastrointestinal side effects as amantadine but rarely causes CNS toxicity.[62]

Amantadine is recommended for use during influenza A epidemics under several circumstances. When there is a documented outbreak of influenza A in institutions or among high-risk persons, amantadine should be started in those who are unvaccinated and in any patient who may be expected to have had a poor response to vaccination, such as those with HIV infection. All individuals without contraindications who have not been vaccinated should be vaccinated at the time amantadine is started, and amantadine should be continued for 2 weeks, the time it takes for a protective antibody response to develop. For those in whom influenza vaccination is contraindicated, amantadine should be continued during the entire course of the epidemic, usually 5 to 7 weeks. Amantadine may also be prescribed for unvaccinated persons who have frequent contact with high-risk persons, such as health care workers in institutional settings. The recommended prophylactic dosage of amantadine is 100 mg a day for those over 65 years. Further dosage reductions may be required for those with renal impairment.[62,63]

Amantadine may also be used in high-risk patients with suspected or established influenza A infection. In such cases, it should be started within 48 h of the onset of symptoms and continued for 7 days.[62,63] The dosage is not established, but 100 mg/day in those over 65 years of age is a reasonable dosage. If and when rimantadine is approved for use in the United States, it will be the preferred agent for the prevention and treatment of influenza A infection over amantadine because of its equal efficacy and lower incidence of CNS toxicity.[64]

Acyclovir and herpesvirus infections Acyclovir is an acyclic analog of guanosine. Its specific antiviral activity is dependent upon the production of two viral enzymes. When taken up by virus-infected cells, acyclovir is selectively phosphorylated by herpes-specific thymidine kinase to acyclovir monophosphate. Host cellular enzymes then further phosphorylate it to acyclovir triphosphate. This form of acyclovir is capable of inhibiting herpes-specific DNA polymerase by acting as a DNA chain terminator.[65,66]

In vitro, acyclovir is most active against herpes simplex types 1 and 2. It has less activity against herpes varicella zoster and Epstein-Barr virus. Acyclovir is not active in vitro against cytomegalovirus, possibly because this virus lacks thymidine kinase. However, a recent report suggests that acyclovir may still have some efficacy against cytomegalovirus in vivo.[67] The development of resistance to acyclovir among initially sensitive herpesvirus strains has been described both in vitro and in vivo. The most common mechanism is the replication of thymidine kinase-deficient mutants.[68]

Acyclovir is slowly and incompletely absorbed after oral administration with a bioavailability of only 15 to 30 percent.[65,66] With intravenous administration in those with normal renal function, the serum half-life is approximately 3 h, and dosing at 5 mg/kg three times daily achieves serum levels above those needed to inhibit herpes simplex virus in vitro. However, higher doses are needed to achieve the same level of inhibition for herpes zoster. Acyclovir is distributed to all tissues, with highest levels occurring in the kidney and lowest levels in the CNS.[66] Elimination of acyclovir is principally through renal filtration and excretion with a renal clearance of three times that of the creatinine clearance. Probenecid reduces renal clearance and increases serum levels. As expected, renal dysfunction increases the serum half-life, up to 20 h in the anuric patient. Acyclovir is readily hemodialyzable.[65,66]

Acyclovir is a safe and relatively nontoxic drug. Its major adverse effect is nephrotoxicity, possibly due to crystallization of the drug within the renal tubules. Nephrotoxicity has been associated chiefly with high-dose (>5 mg/kg every 8 h) intravenous therapy and is not usually seen with oral therapy. Dehydration, bolus rather than infusion therapy, and underlying renal dysfunction appear to be associated risk factors. In addition, there have been some reports of CNS toxicity due to acyclovir. Acyclovir does not appear to suppress bone marrow production of blood cells.[65,66]

In the elderly, the major clinical indications for acyclovir are for the treatment of herpes zoster and, to a lesser extent, for the treatment and prevention of herpes simplex infections. Herpes zoster is a common disease in the elderly and is often associated with acute severe pain followed by protracted postherpetic neuralgia. In immunocompromised patients, the infection can become disseminated and result in encephalitis, hepatitis, and severe cutaneous involvement. In general, treatment of the elderly noncompromised patient with localized herpes zoster is aimed at speeding recovery and preventing the development of postherpetic neuralgia. A recent study has shown that oral acyclovir started within 72 h of rash at 800 mg five times daily for 7 days resulted in decreased new lesion development, faster loss of vesicles, and fuller crusting of lesions than seen patients on placebo.[69] Despite these results, acyclovir has not been shown to prevent postherpetic neuralgia.[70,71] Because of this, the use of acyclovir in the noncompromised elderly patient with localized herpes zoster is limited.

For patients with localized herpes zoster and an underlying immunodeficiency disease which makes them susceptible to dissemination, such as lymphoma, corticosteroid therapy, or HIV infection, or in patients who already have evidence of dissemination, acyclovir plays a more defined role. In such cases, high-dose oral therapy as described above may be started initially. However, intravenous therapy using doses of 10 to 15 mg/kg every 8 h for 10 days is indicated in those patients with evidence of encephalitis or other severe manifestations of infection. Dosage adjustments are recommended in patients with decreased renal function. The goal of such therapy is to arrest the spread of the virus.

Acyclovir has been shown to be useful for acute therapy and prevention of herpes simplex infections of the genitals and lips in both immunocompromised and noncompromised patients. For acute infection in patients with normal renal function, oral acyclovir 200 mg five times per day is efficacious. Intravenous therapy in these situations is usually not required. However, in those patients with herpes simplex encephalitis and normal renal function, treatment with intravenous acyclovir 10 mg/kg every 8 h for 10 days is indicated. Preventive therapy with oral acyclovir is also indicated in patients with certain conditions predisposing them to immunodepression and reactivation of herpes simplex infection, such as allogeneic bone marrow and solid organ transplantation recipients.

CONCLUSION

While most of this chapter discusses specific issues regarding particular antimicrobial agents, we would like to reemphasize some of the major principles of treating infections in the elderly. The process of aging, while not associated with a specific immunologic defect, leads to an overall lowering of host defenses. Because of this, the elderly are more likely than the nonaged adult population to develop a variety of infections. They are particularly susceptible to pneumonia, urinary tract infections, and skin infections. Chronic diseases and institutionalization compound this risk. In addition, physiologic changes associated with aging, particularly the loss of renal function, make the elderly more likely to develop toxicity from a number of antimicrobial drugs. Combining these principles with a knowledge of specific antimicrobial agents should enhance the clinician's ability to manage infections in the elderly.

REFERENCES

1. Saltzman RL, Peterson PK: Immunodeficiency of the elderly. *Rev Infect Dis* 9: 1127–1139, 1987.
2. Garibaldi RA, Nurse BA: Infections in the elderly. *Am J Med* 81(suppl 1A): 53–58, 1986.
3. Berk SL, Smith JK: Infectious diseases in the elderly. *Infect Dis Clin North Am* 67: 273–293, 1983.
4. Gleckman RA, Czachor JS: Reviewing the safe use of antibiotics in the elderly. *Geriatrics* 44(7): 33–39, 1989.
5. Pratt WB, Fekety R: *The Antimicrobial Drugs*. New York, Oxford University Press, 1986.
6. Gleckman RA, Bergman MM: Newer antibiotics: their place in geriatric care. Part II. *Geriatrics* 42(2): 61–70, 1986.
7. Brumfitt W, Hamilton-Miller J: Methicillin-resistant *Staphylococcus aureus*. *N Engl J Med* 320: 1188–1196, 1989.
8. Wright AJ, Wilkowske CJ: The penicillins. *Mayo Clin Proc* 62: 806–820, 1987.
9. Thompson RL: Cephalosporin, carbapenem, and monobactam antibiotics. *Mayo Clin Proc* 62: 821–834, 1987.

10. Gleckman RA, Bergman MM: Newer antibiotics: their place in geriatric care. Part I. *Geriatrics* 41(12): 51–55, 1986.
11. Schaad UB, Suter S, Gianella BA, et al: A comparison of ceftriaxone and cefuroxime for the treatment of bacterial meningitis in children. *N Engl J Med* 322: 141–147, 1990.
12. Carson JW, Watters K, Taylor MR, Keane CT: Clinical trial of cefuroxime axetil in children. *J Antimicrob Chemother* 19: 109–112, 1987.
13. Hathorn JW, Rubin M, Pizzo PA: Empirical antibiotic therapy in the febrile neutropenic cancer patient: Clinical efficacy and impact of monotherapy. *Antimicrob Agents Chemother* 31: 971–977, 1987.
14. Pastel DA: Imipenem-cilastatin sodium, a broad-spectrum carbapenem antibiotic combination. *Clin Pharm* 5: 719–736, 1986.
15. Barza M: Imipenem: first of a new class of beta-lactam antibiotics. *Ann Intern Med* 103: 552–560, 1985.
16. Brogden RN, Heel RC: Aztreonam. A review of its antibacterial activity, pharmacokinetic properties and therapeutic use. *Drugs* 31: 96–130, 1986.
17. Cook FV, Farrar WE Jr: Vancomycin revisited. *Ann Intern Med* 88: 813–818, 1978.
18. Hermans PE, Wilhelm MP: Vancomycin. *Mayo Clin Proc* 62: 901–905, 1987.
19. Moellering RC Jr: Vancomycin therapy in patients with impaired renal function: A nomogram for dosage. *Ann Intern Med* 94: 343–346, 1981.
20. Pancoast SJ: Aminoglycoside antibiotics in clinical use. *Med Clin North Am* 72: 581–612, 1988.
21. Edson RS, Terrell CL: The aminoglycosides: streptomycin, kanamycin, gentamicin, tobramycin, amikacin, netilmicin, and sisomicin. *Mayo Clin Proc* 62: 916–920, 1987.
22. Robertson D: Pharmacology and aging—pharmacokinetics and pharmacodynamics, in Brocklehurst JC (ed): *Textbook of Geriatric Medicine and Gerontology*, 3d ed. New York, Churchill Livingstone, 1985, pp 145–156.
23. Garrison MW, Zaske DE, Rotschafer JC: Aminoglycosides: Another perspective. *DICP Ann Pharmacother* 24: 267–272, 1990.
24. Eisenberg JM, Koffer H, Glick HA, et al: What is the cost of nephrotoxicity associated with aminoglycosides? *Ann Intern Med* 107: 900–909, 1987.
25. Chan GLC: Alternative dosing strategy for aminoglycosides: impact on efficacy, nephrotoxicity, and ototoxcity. *DICP* 23: 788–794, 1989.
26. Chan RA, Benner EJ, Hoeprich PD: Gentamicin therapy in renal failure: A nomogram for dosage. *Ann Intern Med* 76: 773–778, 1972.
27. Fass RJ: The quinolones. *Ann Intern Med* 102: 400–401, 1985.
28. Wolfson JS: Norfloxacin: A new targeted fluoroquinolone antimicrobial agent. *Ann Intern Med* 108: 238–251, 1988.
29. Nix DE, DeVito JM: Ciprofloxacin and norfloxacin, two fluoroquinolone antimicrobials. *Clin Pharm* 6: 105–117, 1987.
30. Neu HC: Quinolones: A new class of antimicrobial agents with wide potential uses. *Med Clin North Am* 72: 623–636, 1988.
31. Hooper DC, Wolfson JS: Fluoroquinolone antimicrobial agents. *N Engl J Med* 324: 384–394, 1991.
32. Walker RC, Wright AJ: The quinolones. *Mayo Clin Proc* 62: 1007–1012, 1987.
33. Karp JE, Merz WG, Hendricksen C, et al: Oral norfloxacin for prevention of gram-negative bacterial infections in patients with acute leukemia and granulocytopenia. A randomized, double-blind, placebo-controlled trial. *Ann Intern Med* 106: 1–7, 1987.
34. Dekker AW, Rozenberg AM, Verhoef J: Infection prophylaxis in acute leukemia: A comparison of ciprofloxacin with trimethoprim-sulfamethoxazole and colistin. *Ann Intern Med* 106: 7–11, 1987.
35. Gribble MJ, Chow AW: Erythromycin. *Med Clin North Am* 66: 79–89, 1982.
36. Washington JA II, Wilson WR: Erythromycin: A microbial and clinical perspective after 30 years of clinical use. *Mayo Clin Proc* 60: 189–203, 271–278, 1985.
37. Wilson WR, Cockerill FR III: Tetracyclines, chloramphenicol, erythromycin, and clindamycin. *Mayo Clin Proc* 62: 906–915, 1987.

38. Hastening gut transit [editorial]. *Lancet* 2: 974-95, 1990.
39. Schweitzer VG, Olson NR: Ototoxic effect of erythromycin therapy. *Arch Otolaryngol* 110: 258-260, 1984.
40. Martell R, Heinrichs D, Stiller CR, et al: The effects of erythromycin in patients treated with cyclosporine. *Ann Intern Med* 104: 660-662, 1986.
41. Cockerill FR, Edson RS: Trimethoprim-sulfamethoxazole. *Mayo Clin Proc* 62: 921-929, 1987.
42. Rubin RH, Swartz MN: Trimethoprim-sulfamethoxazole. *N Engl J Med* 303: 426-432, 1980.
43. Wormser GP, Keusch GT: Trimethoprim-sulfamethoxazole in the United States. *Ann Intern Med* 91: 420-429, 1979.
44. Murray BE, Rensimer ER, DuPont HL: Emergence of high-level trimethoprim resistance in fecal *Escherichia coli* during oral administration of trimethoprim or trimethoprim-sulfamethoxazole. *N Engl J Med* 306: 130-135, 1982.
45. Kucers A, Bennett NM: *The Use of Antibiotics*. Philadelphia, J. B. Lippincott, 1987.
46. Bennett WM: Guide to drug dosage in renal failure. *Clin Pharmacokinet* 15: 326-354, 1988.
47. Bradley PP, Warden GD, Maxwell JG, Rothstein G: Neutropenia and thrombocytopenia in renal allograft recipients treated with trimethoprim-sulfamethoxazole. *Ann Intern Med* 93: 560-562, 1980.
48. Kobrinsky NL, Ramsay NKC: Acute megaloblastic anemia induced by high-dose trimethoprim-sulfamethoxazole. *Ann Intern Med* 94: 780-781, 1981.
49. Coto H, McGowan WR, Pierce EH, Thomas E: Intrahepatic cholestasis due to trimethoprim-sulfamethoxazole. *South Med J* 74: 897-898, 1981.
50. Nair SS, Kaplan JM, Levine LH, Geraci K: Trimethoprim-sulfamethoxazole-induced intrahepatic cholestasis. *Ann Intern Med* 92: 511-512, 1980.
51. Ransohoff DF, Jacobs G: Terminal hepatic failure following a small dose of sulfamethoxazole-trimethoprim. *Gastroenterology* 80: 816-819, 1981.
52. O'Reilly RA, Motley CH: Racemic warfarin and trimethoprim-sulfamethoxazole interaction. *Ann Intern Med* 91: 34-36, 1979.
53. O'Reilly RA: Stereoselective interaction of trimethoprim-sulfamethoxazole with the separated enantiomorphs of racemic warfarin in man. *N Engl J Med* 302: 33-35, 1980.
54. Rudin JE, Evans TL, Wing EJ: Failure of erythromycin in the treatment of *Legionella micdadei* pneumonia. *Am J Med* 76: 318-320, 1984.
55. Bass JB Jr, Farer LS, Hopewell PC, Jacobs RF: Treatment of tuberculosis and tuberculosis infection in adults and children. *Am Rev Respir Dis* 134: 355-363, 1986.
56. Van Scoy RE,Wilkowske CJ: Antituberculous agents. *Mayo Clin Proc* 62: 1129-1136, 1987.
57. Comstock GW: New data on preventive treatment with isoniazid. *Ann Intern Med* 98: 663-665, 1983.
58. Stead WW: Tuberculosis among elderly persons: An outbreak in a nursing home. *Ann Intern Med* 94: 606-610, 1981.
59. Mitchell JR, Zimmerman HJ, Ishak KG, et al: Isoniazid liver injury: Clinical spectrum, pathology, and probable pathogenesis. *Ann Intern Med* 84: 181-192, 1976.
60. Engelhard D, Stutman HR, Marks MI: Interaction of ketoconazole with rifampin and isoniazid. *N Engl J Med* 311: 1681-1683, 1984.
61. Cohn DL, Catlin BJ, Peterson KL, et al: A 62-dose, 6-month therapy for pulmonary and extrapulmonary tuberculosis. A twice-weekly, directly observed, and cost-effective regimen. *Ann Intern Med* 112: 407-415, 1990.
62. Douglas RGJ: Prophylaxis and treatment of influenza. *N Engl J Med* 322: 443-450, 1990.
63. CDC: Prevention and control of influenza. Recommendations of the Immunization Practices Advisory Committee (ACIP). *MMWR* 39(RR-7): 1-15, 1990.
64. Dolin R, Reichman RC, Madore HP, et al: A controlled trial of amantadine and rimantadine in the prophylaxis of influenza A infection. *N Engl J Med* 307: 580-584, 1982.
65. Dorsky DI, Crumpacker CS: Drugs five years later: Acyclovir. *Ann Intern Med* 107: 859-874, 1987.
66. Laskin OL: Acyclovir. Pharmacology and clinical experience. *Arch Intern Med* 144: 1241-1246, 1984.

67. Balfour HH Jr, Chace BA, Stapleton JT, et al: A randomized, placebo-controlled trial of oral acyclovir for the prevention of cytomegalovirus disease in recipients of renal allografts. *N Engl J Med* 320: 1381–1387, 1989.
68. Hirsh MS, Schooley RT: Resistance to antiviral drugs: the end of innocence. *N Engl J Med* 320: 313–314, 1989.
69. McKendrick MW, McGill JI, White JE, Wood MJ: Oral acyclovir in acute herpes zoster. *Br Med J* 293: 1529–1532, 1986.
70. Surman OS, Flynn T, Schooley RT, et al: A double-blind, placebo-controlled study of oral acyclovir in postherpetic neuralgia. *Psychosomatics* 31: 287–292, 1990.
71. McKendrick MW, McGill JI, Wood MJ: Lack of effect of acyclovir on postherpetic neuralgia. *Br Med J* 298: 431, 1989.
72. Hermans PE, Cockerill FRI: Antiviral agents. *Mayo Clin Proc* 62: 1108–1115, 1987.

Index

Page numbers ending in italic *t* or *f* refer to tables or illustrations, respectively.